Cancer:
Improving Your Odds

1st Edition

A Science-Based Approach to Naturally Preventing and Treating Cancer

John G. Herron

Eagle Stock Publishing

12162019

ISBN 13: 9781709219931

First edition: 12/16/2019

Updates at - https://improvingyourodds.com

Support at - https://www.facebook.com/groups/cancer.improving.your.odds

Table of Contents

Updates at - https://improvingyourodds.com

Support at - https://www.faccbook.com/groups/cancer.improving.your.odds

Updates at - https://improvingyourodds.com

Support at - https://www.facebook.com/groups/cancer.improving.your.odds

Updates at - https://improvingyourodds.com

Support at - https://www.facebook.com/groups/cancer.improving.your.odds

◆ ❖ ◆

Introduction

Let's start by analyzing the title of this book.

"***Cancer.***" You or a loved one probably have it, or you most likely wouldn't be reading this. I love to tell myself that most people reading this book are trying to prevent their first cancer, but that probably isn't true. The "C" word is often spoken of in whispers, as it can be synonymous with death. However, survival rates from conventional medicine truly have improved. Today, many cancers that used to be death sentences are survivable, especially if caught early.

"***Improving Your Odds***" means that there are many natural treatments that have been scientifically shown to improve one's odds of successfully fighting or preventing cancer. Most of these natural treatments are complementary to conventional therapies, including immunotherapy, chemotherapy and radiation. The preponderance of the scientific evidence shows that you can *Improve Your Odds* of preventing, delaying, beating and surviving cancer by adding some simple natural treatments. "*Improving Your Odds*" means exactly that: Your odds of beating cancer will improve. It does not mean everyone who follows this advice will beat cancer, but the evidence indicates that significantly more will.

"***A Science-Based Approach to Naturally Preventing and Treating Cancer***" – Everything recommended in this book is backed by scientific research, and often lots of it. I've tried to avoid studies where the research hasn't been peer reviewed, has obvious financial conflicts of interest, cannot be duplicated, or didn't follow good scientific methods (e.g., tests done on two mice with no controls would not be very scientific, nor would "Patient 'A' had their cancer go into remission from taking X." The sample size is very important). The studies included in this book are of a quality level such that you can show them to your doctor and not get laughed at (but if they do laugh, that might be a sign to look for another doctor). There are plenty of "alternative" and "natural treatments" out there, and I've researched most of them. But if there is no scientific evidence of their safety and efficacy, they are not discussed in this book (except perhaps to tell you to avoid them).

This book isn't about giving you hope (though it should); it is truly about giving you science-based ways to *Improve Your Odds* of beating cancer naturally. Strategies with clear scientific evidence of efficacy, strategies that you can undertake without a medical degree or a six-figure income, strategies that you won't be embarrassed to discuss with your oncologist (be sure to bring the book with you and highlight the research studies that apply to you ahead of time).

With this book I hope to begin a cancer treatment revolution, so that people can help themselves (and their medical treatments) without having to trust some guy simply making stuff up and posting it on the internet from his parents' basement.

Now, let me tell you what this book is not about.

There are many books out there preaching the virtues of alternative treatments (and there are probably thousands of websites). Some of these "treatments" are not only worthless, but also dangerous; these methods can make your cancer worse, cause other significant health issues or convince people to avoid medical treatments that do work. Most of these alternative treatments have no scientific research to support them whatsoever, or worse, there is high-quality science showing they do not work. There are hundreds of such worthless treatments, everything from coffee enemas to frequency generators (such as the Rife machine). Even one book where the author gets their advice from spirits (non-denominational, of course) who talk only to the author (the rest of us aren't worthy, I guess). If a treatment has no scientific evidence of efficacy I would avoid it. There are literally tens of thousands of research studies on natural treatments, some with strong evidence of efficacy, those are what are discussed in this book.

> *I'll be glad to show any spirit my sources, if the spirit will show me theirs.*

So, what makes this book different? Unless a treatment has valid scientific literature showing strong evidence of at least in vitro (in the test tube) efficacy, it will not be recommended in this book, which puts a greater emphasis on treatments that have been proven effective through in vivo (in the body) research. The evidence I include comes from major universities, scientific journals, government funded projects, etc. Some of the evidence presented is as strong as that for FDA-approved treatment options (e.g., more studies, larger number of research subjects, etc.) They simply do not have the backing of drug companies. All of this is brought to you in an easy-to-understand format, but the book also includes abstracts from research studies so you can verify my sources of information (without undertaking a séance).

You also will not read anything here suggesting that you delay (or forgo) conventional medical treatment. I believe in the "kitchen sink" approach: Throw everything at the cancer that won't make the cancer worse or harm your health, and that has been scientifically shown to "*Improve Your Odds.*" Thus, this book presents a complementary approach, something that "*Improves Your Odds*" when combined with your medical treatment. If you decide to avoid certain medical treatments, it should not be because of what you've read here. However, I know some people may choose not to go through chemotherapy or radiation, and I understand that. Medical options don't always have a clear and convincing track record for all forms and stages of cancer (though they can also save lives in many situations where oncologists recommend them). That decision should be between you and your oncologist. I cannot help you make it. The treatments in this book can be used with or without other medical treatments; you'll see why as you read on.

Updates at - https://improvingyourodds.com

Support at - https://www.facebook.com/groups/cancer.improving.your.odds

You will find that I let the research studies do some of the talking. Anyone can write an opinion book (as we all have opinions); it takes scientific research, and peer review of that research, to verify potential cancer treatments, even natural ones. I don't include all the methodology from the studies, and I try to get to what is most important—the study conclusions. I cannot and do not take credit for discovering any of the cancer treatments found here. I give credit where it belongs, to the thousands of research scientists who have spent their careers looking for cancer preventatives, treatments and cures (in some cases with no hope of making a profit). Most researchers must fight tooth and nail for even the smallest grants in order to research anything natural (as these rarely lead to anything patentable that can make a company rich). These researchers do not work for large drug companies. I call myself a "meta-researcher." I research the research. You don't want me, or anyone else (other than your oncologist), telling you how to treat your cancer based just on theory, their opinion or some philosophy (theirs or their spirits').

How I Got Involved

This book is not about me and my cancer. It truly is about "*Improving Your Odds*," but I thought I would mention my cancer here in the introduction so you know why I started researching this topic. I was diagnosed in September 2017 with "nodular melanoma" (on the side of my left leg above my knee), a very aggressive form of melanoma. Standard melanoma is already a very dangerous form of skin cancer, and nodular is much worse. I was staged at IIc, basically meaning that it was very deep and had ulcerated, but it had not yet spread to any of the organs. I had a second melanoma tumor removed from my right arm in January 2018 (it was already there in September). It was a standard melanoma and considered a "second primary" (not caused by the first one); it was wide, but not deep. At the time, I chose not to undergo the therapy I was offered (for a stage IIc) as it had very poor evidence of success and came with a lot of side effects. I didn't make that decision because I thought I could beat it through natural means (there are much better forms of immunotherapy, but they're very expensive, and thus reserved for stage III/IV). I did undergo a mass excision, surgery where they removed a very large chunk of flesh from around the two tumors. This was not fun, but I'm glad I did it.

Just as I was starting to research natural treatments for the first two cancers, the one in my leg came back with a vengeance. At first, I thought the bump under my skin was a large horsefly bite, as I had been around them just a couple days before I discovered it. It didn't look anything like my other cancers. Over the next two months it continued to grow, so I decided I should get it checked out (you think?!?). Turns out it was a recurrence of the original nodular melanoma cancer, but under the skin. On the ultrasound they found that it was huge (10cm or 4") and had smaller satellite tumors. Pretty nasty, and now my cancer showed a propensity to metastasize.

That is when I got really serious about researching ways that I could Improve My Odds! My last book, *The Gut Health Protocol*, required a lot of research (it has over 1,200 research study abstracts), so I'm used to interpreting the science and I dug into it. I was already doing some things for my immune system, and it turned out that was very fortuitous (see Chapter 2).

Because I had local metastasis, my oncologist was now able to put me on a much newer immunotherapy, a PD-1 inhibitor (Keytruda). This is a great class of drugs, certainly better than chemo and radiation, especially for my type of cancer. But still the "complete remission" rate is not very good. Turns out that many of the things I had started doing had evidence of improving outcomes with PD-1 inhibitor treatment (see Chapter 2). In a bold (and rarely tried) move, my oncologist and I decided not to surgically remove the tumor, as leaving it might help train the immune system on what to attack (PD-1 inhibitors basically unhide cancers so that the immune system can see them). I really upped what I was doing naturally, and probably found some natural adjuvant treatments just in time. It all paid off: Within 3 treatments of Keytruda, my tumor was gone! The research on Keytruda shows that only about 6% of people have a complete response like this, and my oncologist had never had a patient see a large tumor like this disappear so quickly. All without surgery, chemo or radiation. I still have a melanoma "tattoo" on the surface of the skin; it had grown there 2 to 3 weeks before I sought treatment. It is black pigmented skin, which is a hallmark of melanoma, but mine is now benign. Doctors who don't know my story freak out when they see it as it looks like I have melanoma, but I don't (this is almost always removed during surgery, so it is very rare to see one that is benign).

Even though I currently have no signs of cancer (I was told that I am in "complete remission"), that may not mean that I've "improved <u>my</u> odds" enough to prevent a recurrence. Or enough to prevent some unrelated cancer from coming along. Only time will tell. I continue to do many of the things outlined in this book and will do so until I die of something else! When flipping a coin, you can *Improve Your Odds* of coming up with heads if you flip it 5 times rather than once, but there is no guarantee that heads will come up. So, I do everything I can to *Improve My Odds*, and so should you.

Thus, the title of this book: *Cancer: Improving Your Odds*.

You can find updates and articles at - https://improvingyourodds.com/

Support at - https://www.facebook.com/groups/cancer.improving.your.odds

◆ ❖ ◆

Goals of This Book

- Introduce you to the term "complementary medicine."

- Help you understand how something as simple as natural foods and supplements can help you "*Improve Your Odds*" at fighting cancer, improve your immune system, and perhaps help save your life.

- Provide you with solid scientific evidence to back up all such claims.

- Show you that diet, sleep and mild exercise are also valuable tools in your fight against cancer.

- Explain "detoxifying," why it is important and why this term is often misused and misunderstood.

- Discuss EMF and the practical things you can do to avoid it.

- Present convincing evidence that the health of the gut is vital to beating and preventing cancer. It is perhaps one of the most important parts of the immune response against cancer (even skin cancers!).

- Present these complementary concepts in clear language. My goal is to provide scientific evidence for everything presented here, but in a manner that makes it easy to understand (with links to the full research studies for you and your doctor). I try to narrate most research abstracts so that you can read them with a better understanding of what is being discussed.

- Help you improve your general and immune health in ways that *Improve Your Odds* against getting future cancers. These are actionable strategies that you can start doing today, most at little to no cost.

- Leave you with a genuine reason for hope. Cancer is no longer a death sentence!

◆❖◆

How to Use This Book

I've tried to make this book readable as well as valuable as a reference tool. I would advise you to make full use of the Table of Contents, Index, and glossary to help you locate the natural treatment you're interested in, or what might work especially well with your type of cancer. Using these resources, you'll be able to put together a list of everything that research shows is beneficial in treating (or preventing) your form of cancer. When combined with the base protocol in Chapter 9 this can help you develop your treatment plan. I highly recommend people read the paperback version of this book—read the whole thing—and highlight as they go. There is nothing sacred about this book: Write in the margins, dogear the pages, whatever it takes for you to customize it to your treatment. A well highlighted book also helps you discuss your treatment plan with your oncologist should you wish to do so. If you have one of the eBook versions, many of those also have a highlighting feature and some give you the ability to bookmark and take notes.

When looking to put together a natural treatment plan, you need to understand that most natural supplements are not nearly as narrowly targeted as pharmaceuticals (and this can be a good thing). Instead of impeding a very specific aspect of a cancer cell's biology, they empower your immune system to fight cancer. It is thought that we actually develop many cancers over our lifetime, but our immune system gets rid of them before they can grow out of control. Do not limit yourself to only looking for natural treatments that have been shown to treat your particular form of cancer. Instead, also include those that have shown immune system benefits in fighting several kinds of cancer. Research money to investigate natural cancer treatments is very hard to come by, so no natural treatment option has been tested against all types of cancer. You will most likely not win your battle against cancer with a poorly functioning immune system, and there always seems to be room for improvement, so be sure to include natural treatments that have been shown to improve it.

I've included excerpts from a large number of scientific research studies. Don't feel you have to understand every word in these studies; they're here to show you that there is good scientific evidence (sometimes very strong evidence) of efficacy. The parts I've included are usually from the study's abstract or conclusion, so the information is often presented in a more concise and understandable manner. If you see words you don't understand, you can look them up in the glossary or simply read past them. I sometimes define them in the text if I think it is important to the narrative. Just don't let the complexity scare you; there won't be a test afterwards. There are no drug companies involved in natural treatments/adjuvants (things that improve the main therapy or the therapy response), so there are no multimillion-dollar ad campaigns. No one holds a monopoly over any of these treatment options. So, you won't find any slick advertising with the same people who were selling timeshare properties a few months ago, making promises that barely adhere to FDA regulations. There simply is not much money behind natural supplements. This means you'll need to trust the research;

personally, I would much rather trust the scientific research community than a pharmaceutical advertising agency.

You also should not simply believe what you read on the internet, in a book or even what I have to say (especially if you meet me at some airport bar after a long layover!). I've come across a great deal of misinformation and misinterpretations of science while searching the internet; some of these websites (and a few book authors) are downright dangerous. However, when a large amount of reproducible scientific evidence is presented, you can rest assured that you are doing your due diligence to verify that the information is accurate. Every research study included in this book has enough information accompanying it that you will be able to verify its authenticity and efficacy. If you click through to the studies, you'll often find links to dozens more studies—I just could not include abstracts from every research study I came across (this book is already able to press out wrinkles from clothes). You'll also probably find more great information in some of those studies; I'm often limited in how much I can include here due to copyright restrictions and space limitations. BTW: The study abstracts are included *as is* with no corrections to spelling, grammar, variations in language structure, etc. Some were originally written in other languages and translated to English before they were posted to PubMed.

You will notice that most of the research studies reference "PubMed." PubMed is run by the US National Institutes of Health (part of the US government). PubMed "comprises more than 28 million citations for biomedical literature from MEDLINE, life science journals, and online books." Think of it as an index (with abstracts) to scientific research, regardless of where that research may reside or who published it. Being able to reference PubMed ID numbers makes it much easier for you to find a study's full abstract; the easiest way is to simply search for "PubMed 23668749" (replacing the number here with the PubMed ID number you are looking for—or simply click on the link if reading this as an eBook). The search results will show the PubMed abstract first (or in some cases, the whole study) as .gov sites are considered authoritative; these links will then be followed by other studies and websites where the study is mentioned. Just make sure the search result shows "https://www.ncbi.nlm.nih.gov/" in the link.

Some excerpts in this book are from the full study, and some are from the publicly available abstracts. Most excerpts are quite short unless the study is available under a more liberal use license (due to copyright law). You paperback readers will find the complete link in the endnotes at the end of the book (reference the superscript number following the study abstract). If the link was very long, I used a short-link service to make it easier to type in. (for you paperback readers).

Lastly, I highly recommend joining the book's Facebook group; you will find a lot of support there. You'll also find me there from time to time; though I can't answer everyone's questions, I answer enough that you may be able to find an answer to your question by using the Facebook search function. From my experience with my previous book, I've found a support group like this to be a very valuable resource for people.
https://www.facebook.com/groups/cancer.improving.your.odds

The book's website will have updated information and articles of interest. This will help keep the book up to date between releases.
https://improvingyourodds.com

The website also contains links to the recommended supplements on Amazon. These are the ones that I use or have at least researched myself. Though I make a very small amount of money on each sale (through Amazon), the website serves more as a reference tool for you (and you can always purchase the listed supplements elsewhere if you find them cheaper).

Chapter 3 is about the relationship between gut health and cancer. If you would like to learn more, I am also the author of *The Gut Health Protocol*, available on Amazon at:
http://amzn.to/2f5RRec

There are also plenty of articles on gut health at the book's website:
https://www.theguthealthprotocol.com

Important Note

If you have any other health conditions or are taking medications, you should check the Memorial Sloan Kettering database "About Herbs, Botanicals & Other Products" for interactions with any supplements you plan to start taking. Here you can look up most natural supplements to see if they interfere with your medications (disclaimers apply). [1]

Updates at - https://improvingyourodds.com/

Support at - https://www.facebook.com/groups/cancer.improving.your.odds

❖

Chapter 1
A Complementary Approach

> *"He who takes medicine and neglects to diet wastes the skill of his doctors."* ~ *Chinese Proverb*

As was explained in the Introduction, this book outlines a complementary approach to treating and preventing cancer. In other words, you should usually do what your oncologist is telling you to do and make medical treatment decisions irrespective of what is found in this book. Regardless of what you may have read on the internet, everything your oncologist is recommending does have evidence of efficacy, or they wouldn't be allowed to prescribe it and insurance wouldn't pay for it.

For some types of cancer, what your doctor is offering may only *Improve Your Odds* a little, but the same treatment may significantly improve your odds if you have another type of cancer, or even if you have slightly different genetics than another person. Yes, there can be some serious side effects to some of these medical treatments, but they have also helped a lot of people. Remember, the goal here is to *"Improve Your Odds,"* not "thumb your nose at modern medicine" or simply trust the latest conspiracy theory.

It is also OK to quiz your doctor about how much their recommended treatment is likely to *Improve Your Odds,* and then weigh this information against the possible side effects. I've found most oncologists to be honest about the information they provide you. I've even had one tell me that they didn't think a certain treatment was worth the side effects; it simply was not effective enough. Do not ignore modern treatments: They have saved thousands of lives. But don't ignore alternative treatments either. There is a lot of evidence that they can help you as well, especially in conjunction with your medical treatment.

Most people have their minds sent reeling when they hear they have cancer. We start trying to grasp the fact that death might be just around the corner, and everything that means. A million things begin running through our minds, and time is of the essence. We start planning for death, not life.

> *I created a list of things for my wife to take care of in the first month after my death. I also created a list of all bank accounts, retirement accounts, etc., including phone numbers. I started throwing out things she wouldn't need. I created a spreadsheet and budget that she could use after I was gone. It was a very emotional time.*

We may also start looking for someone, or something, to blame for the situation we're in. Was it preservatives in food? Was it all those family vacations to the beach as a kid? Is it that coal-fired power plant a couple miles down the road? Was it growing up in a home where parents smoked? Is it those contrails (or "chemtrails") from planes overhead? Someone must be to blame for this.

I would encourage you not to fall into that trap. Even if one or more of these things are true, most people around you who had similar exposures didn't get this cancer; you did. You can also blame it on bad luck or genetics. But chances are the cancer can be blamed on a combination of things. We know that genetics do play a strong role in determining who is more *susceptible* to cancer (or perhaps just a specific type of cancer). However, this does <u>not</u> mean all these people will get cancer in their lifetime. It means that along with other factors, they have less ability to prevent getting that cancer. People with very good genetics can still get cancer; they are just less likely to. Combined with the large number of environmental and inherited risks, there is an element of luck (or possibly just vulnerabilities we don't understand yet).

This book does not adhere to any specific alternative approach—and there are hundreds of them, such as: orthomolecular medicine, traditional Chinese medicine (TCM), Ayurvedic medicine, homeopathy, reiki, shiatsu, cupping, colon cleansing, coffee enemas, the Alkaline Diet, Budwig Protocol, Gerson therapy, faith healing, spirits, religion, etc. There may be some benefits with a few of these, either physiologically or psychologically, but the approach taken in this book is to include only those natural substances/therapies that have scientific evidence of "*Improving Your Odds*" of surviving cancer. If I couldn't find creditable evidence of efficacy, then that natural treatment wasn't mentioned here. If all I could find was evidence that an approach doesn't work or is dangerous, then I may call it out as ineffective or a hoax. Some of these alternative approaches have huge followings, and I'm sure to get a lot of negative feedback for calling them out. But I'm OK with that; this book is about evidence, not wishful thinking or some misplaced philosophy.

When faced with a life-changing, dramatic (or traumatic) event, we must try to use objective reasoning (such as from scientifically based research) in making decisions. At a time like this, we tend to want to think emotionally and our judgement becomes clouded; we must not give in to the false hope of a miracle cure (nor uneducated naysayers telling you to avoid medical treatments). There are currently no miracle natural cures. Right now, there are only ways that we can help the body, and mostly our immune system, fight cancer (and some work quite well at this!). Nature has been dealing with cancer for millions of years. It has a huge head start; we

Updates at - https://improvingyourodds.com

Support at - https://www.facebook.com/groups/cancer.improving.your.odds

just need to follow its lead and give it a helping hand. We need to *improve the odds* that our immune systems will be successful!

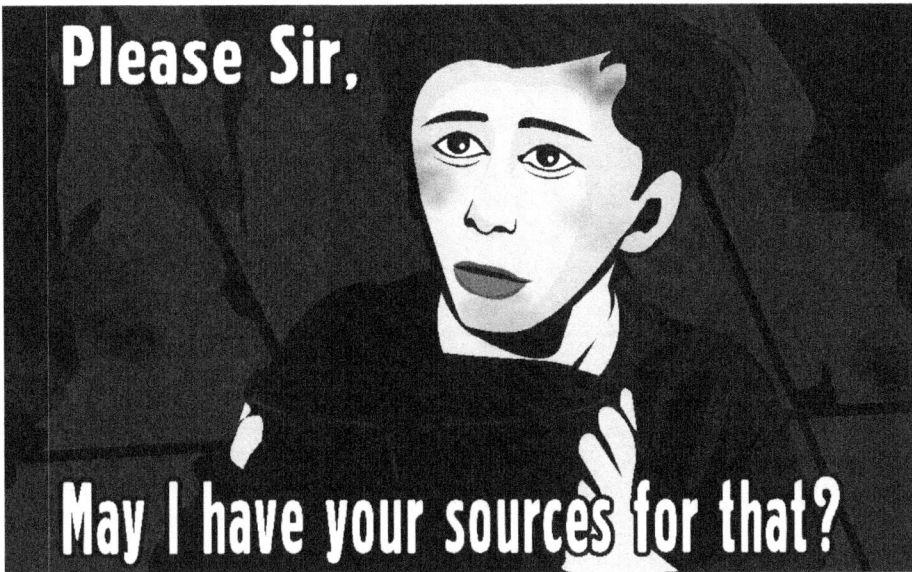

While researching this book I came across a LOT of misinformation, hoaxes and simply dangerous advice. One thing they all had in common was that there was no peer-reviewed scientific research to back up their claims. Most of them had "theories" that, on the surface, may sound good. But in most cases those theories don't hold up to scientific scrutiny. If you don't get anything else from this book, there are two things I would like you to remember: 1) Don't trust anything, or anyone, that isn't backed up with high-quality, peer-reviewed research; 2) There is no vast conspiracy by drug companies to prevent research into natural treatments. If there is such a conspiracy, it isn't working very well, as there are thousands upon thousands of research studies on natural cancer treatments. Granted, some of those are not from the US or Europe, but that doesn't make the studies any less valid. Western countries have hitched their wagon to pharmaceuticals and expensive treatments. This is where the money is at, and some of that money gets poured into research, but generally, only research into more patentable drugs. No conspiracy is necessary; as the age-old adage says, just follow the money. Lucky for us, there are still universities all over the globe (including in Western countries) doing research on natural treatments, often with the help of government grants. Of course, we still need a lot more research. There are a lot of natural substances and many different types of cancers and genetic confounders, and proper research is very expensive.

When doing your own research, I would be very careful about the quality of the research papers and studies. If a paper has not appeared in a peer-reviewed journal, that is a bad sign. If it appears in a non-medical or poorly known journal, that can be a bad sign. If the study was not randomized, that is another bad sign. If it was written by a clinic that specializes in the treatment discussed in the paper, then the quality of evidence needs to be even stronger (they have a financial interest in showing good results). I tried hard to include mostly higher-quality studies in this book.

I will focus mostly on immunomodulators (things that help our immune system fight cancer) rather than cytotoxins (such as chemotherapy that outright kills cancer cells, usually while killing many non-cancerous ones as well). Immunomodulators usually have broader applications with benefits applying to several, or sometimes all, cancers. Where cytotoxins are often more specific (benefiting only one, or a few, cancers), they usually have far more side effects as well. There are some natural cytotoxins, but they too have side effects and dangers. While a cytotoxin may only work on one specific type of cancer, immunomodulators help the immune system fight nearly all cancers it is capable of recognizing (and new checkpoint inhibitor drugs can help the immune system see much better! See Chapter 2). Cytotoxins, even natural ones, are not discussed in this book unless research shows a high level of safety.

> The word "adjuvant" comes from the Latin word "adiuvare," meaning to aid or help.

Chemotherapy and radiation may save lives, but they also take some lives; nobody denies that. However, research shows they generally add more time on this planet than they subtract. Natural supplements with similarly dangerous properties will not be discussed here, as they would require human trials and more research before I would feel comfortable recommending them. Even with surgery, chemotherapy and radiation, it is our immune system that prevents metastasis by cleaning up any stray or loose cancer cells. Chemotherapy and radiation both damage the immune system; surgery is rarely done without antibiotics, and that has now been shown to severely impact the immune system as well. Metastatic cancer causes 90% of cancer deaths, and while primary tumors can usually be removed through surgery, metastasizing cells cannot. Radiation can't be used for metastasizing cells. Though chemotherapy is somewhat effective against metastatic cells, these cells are not easily killed by chemotherapy. For the most part, this only leaves the immune system and immunotherapies to fight metastasizing cancer cells. So, improving the immune system is nearly always an excellent idea! Therefore, it is a good idea to work on the immune system before, during and after these other treatments (OK, maybe not during surgery). Thus, the primary focus of this book: improving the immune response to cancer.

Cancer cells are characterized by several hallmarks, including excessive cell growth, reprogramming of energy metabolism that supports their uncontrolled proliferation, resistance to cell death by suppression of apoptosis (programmed cell death when cells age or malfunction), induction of angiogenesis, the ability to invade and metastasize to distant sites, and suppression of an immune response against tumor cells. These are the functions that natural supplements can often return to normal functioning, thus leading to the death of cancer cells without harming healthy ones.

I think you'll find what follows to be a fascinating overview of just how complex nature can be (again, there won't be any pop quizzes, so just enjoy the ride). With over 60% of current cancer drugs being derived from nature, it shouldn't surprise us that nature can help us fight cancer. This leads us to our first abstract.

> "Most (> 60%) anticancer drugs that are in clinical use and have demonstrated significant efficacy for combatting cancer originate from natural products derived from plants, marine organisms, and microorganisms. The anticancer activity of most natural products often act via regulating immune function, inducing apoptosis or autophagy, or inhibiting cell proliferation." – PubMed ID#PMC5679595 (2017) [2]

The supplements and foods discussed in this book are natural products that simply must be consumed or extracted, and thus cannot receive a patent (though a synthetic version might be patentable). Without the ability to receive a patent, drug companies are not the least bit interested in them. I wouldn't blame them too much; receiving FDA approval to market a drug for fighting cancer now costs over $3 billion (*Washington Post* [3])! That is a lot of money in anyone's book; without the ability to recoup those costs, why should anyone want to make an investment in research? Thus, the reliance on university research, foreign research and government grants to study these substances. Countries with socialized medicine are more likely to subsidize non-patentable research; this is because any discoveries would be very inexpensive to implement and would help lower the costs of their medical program.

What you'll find here are the orphan treatments: those that no one wants to finance and no one wants to promote, but that may have just as much benefit as many of the medical treatments on the market—and the science to prove it! They can also have very powerful adjuvant benefits (adjuvant treatments are those that can increase the effectiveness, and/or reduce the side effects, of a primary treatment. You'll see that word used a lot in this book and in the research).

EVOLUTION

A hat tip to those who do not believe in "evolution." I use this word quite a bit throughout the book. However, nothing here precludes a higher power's involvement. The more I read about how our immune system works, how it works with nature, and the sheer complexity of it, the more I can see the hand of God in it. I see the word "evolution" as a way of trying to describe the overwhelming complexity of the biological world and how we've adapted to it over time. Science has only scratched the surface of this complexity. I think most people who believe in God realize that while we are on this planet, we can never truly understand the full complexity of human biology and the universe around us. However, I think it is possible that all this complexity was put here to keep us busy and entertained, so science should never be ignored. We should keep digging for answers. So, when you see the word "evolved," just know that this helps to explain how things are connected and how they change; you can just as easily substitute words like "God created."

WHY DOESN'T MY DOCTOR RECOMMEND THESE THINGS?

Some do, but not enough. Doctors are trained to prescribe FDA-approved prescription drugs for ailments. The FDA process very rarely approves natural botanicals as drugs; this is because the process of approval is very, very expensive and no one will pony up the money for it. Because natural botanicals cannot receive a patent, there is no way for a drug company to recoup those costs; once something non-patentable receives FDA approval, competitors can then sell the product without having paid any of the FDA approval costs (no patent means no protection from competition). Natural treatments simply are not taught in medical school, as doctors will not be prescribing them. Ongoing training is often paid for by drug companies, so natural treatments are rarely mentioned then, either. No one is paying for TV advertising showing that certain nutrients can help cure cancer (the FDA has made this illegal, even if it is factual, as these nutrients are not FDA approved to treat disease). So, unless doctors read books like this one, or are curious enough to scour through research studies on the topic (in their off time), they are really never exposed to this information.

Doctors are trained in "rescue medicine," not preventative medicine. When is the last time you heard of someone receiving a prescription medicine (other than an immunization) to help prevent disease? However, doctors have hundreds of drugs that can be prescribed to treat disease once a person gets sick; thus, "rescue medicine."

Another problem with natural supplements is liability. If a doctor tells you to take natural supplements and your cancer doesn't improve, or you have an allergic reaction to them, you may sue the doctor. If the doctor had only provided prescription drugs, that liability would shift to the drug manufacturer. Since the drugs were the "standard of care," the doctor would have done no wrong. Non-FDA approved supplements are not the standard of care, so there is no way to defer the liability and the doctor can be held liable for malpractice. Even though the natural supplement may be more effective, and most likely far safer, what little residual risk there may be is more than the doctor wants to deal with.

You can help your doctor by bringing natural treatments to their attention. Offer to loan them your copy of this book! Ask them questions about the topic, or even copy a few pages for them. Your doctor will want to see the studies behind your assertions. Maybe this will be enough to whet their appetite for more. Doctors are busy people, but many of them have a passion for medicine. Perhaps you can light the spark that will cause them to take the time to learn more. They don't have to prescribe natural options to their patients; they can simply recommend a book or discuss it with them informally.

> *"The art of medicine consists of amusing the patient while nature cures the disease."* ~ *Voltaire*

How Can Nutritional Supplements Possibly Help If Modern Drugs Can't?

As mentioned earlier, over 60% of the current drugs used to fight cancer come from the natural world. Most of these substances have been modified to make them patentable, but that doesn't always mean that the patentable drug is better than the natural source that it came from. Plants have spent literally billions of years devising new molecular structures, or compounds, for their own purposes. These compounds are used by plants to fight off disease, infections, parasites, insects, tumors, etc. Over time plants might find multiple uses, some very diverse, for the same compounds. Animals consume these plants and have evolved with them; their bodies also discovered ways of utilizing these compounds. Often the uses are similar to what plants used them for, fighting off diseases and infections.

Plants can also get cancerous tumors, such as burls, or burs, on trees. In plants, tumors are often caused by bacteria, viruses and fungi, though most anything that can cause structural damage to the plant cells can cause it. The cancer manifests itself a little differently; that is due to the biology of plants, but the excessive multiplication of cells is basically the same as in humans. Plant cells are held in place; they don't move around like they do in animals. This prevents metastasizing, so cancers, once they form, stay where they formed and simply grow from there. If this were the case with humans, doctors would simply cut out the tumor, and that would the end of it. But humans are not plants, and metastasis is the primary concern with human cancer; metastasis to organs is what usually kills a person. Many theories over the years (some of which persist today) have tried to link human cancers to bacteria, viruses and fungus (such as molds and yeasts). Though there are a few human cancers linked to these infections (human papilloma virus (HPV), *Helicobacter pylori* (gastric cancers) and hepatitis B and C viruses), this is not the primary cause of cancer in humans.

Plants have had to create chemical compounds to deal with these problems. Many of these compounds have been shown to be active against cancer (in plants and animals as well as humans).

> "Promise of bitter melon (Momordica charantia) bioactives in cancer prevention and therapy… These results are significant as inhibition of EBV-EA induction is recognized to be correlated with anti-tumor promoting activities in cancer chemoprevention studies… showed significant cyto-toxic effects (in MTT assay) against MCF-7 (breast cancer), HepG2 (hepatocellular cancer), HEp-2 (laryngeal cancer), and WiDr (colon cancer) cells" – PubMed ID#PMC5067200 [4]

> "An estimated 15 percent of all human cancers worldwide may be attributed to viruses… Epstein-Barr virus, human papilloma virus, hepatitis B virus, and human herpes virus-8 are the four DNA viruses that are capable of causing the development of human cancers. Human T lymphotrophic virus type 1 and hepatitis C viruses are the two RNA viruses that contribute to human cancers."
> – PubMed ID#PMC1994798 (2006) [5]

All of this means that the plant and fungus worlds are ripe for researching new cancer treatments. Such compounds can be found in nearly every plant; it's just a matter of whether they are suitable for treating human cancers (and many are).

> The link between healthy diet and cancer has been revealed in numerous studies. An inverse association between the consumption of fruits and vegetables and cancer risk was evident by an epidemiological study in Netherlands. It has been found that the consumption of 21 vegetables and 9 fruits decreased the tumor growth in urothelial cancer patients. It has also been reported that Asians have lower incidence of cancer than the residents of Western countries, and the rate increases substantially among Asians who have migrated to the West. Consumption of diet rich in plant products may be one of the important reasons for the low incidence of cancer in Asia. A wide variety of natural products containing anticancer properties have been reported in the literature. – PubMed ID#PMC4369959 (2015) (Open Access Attribution available at the link) [6]

I try to avoid conspiracy theories in this book, and there are plenty of cancer books and websites already indulging in this paranoid reasoning. However, conspiracy theories are not needed to understand that if most cancer research is done (or paid for) by drug companies, then any research results that do not lead to large profits are going to be ignored. This, of course, not only means that research failures (that is, research that didn't show anticancer results) will be ignored, but also that any successful research that doesn't lead to a patentable drug will also be ignored (in the pharmaceutical world, this is still thought of as a failure as the research didn't lead to profit). I would say that it is possible that cures for some cancers may have already been discovered, and the research buried. However, this research may be repeated in other countries and by universities, so it may not be lost forever.

The plant and fungus worlds are full of cancer-fighting compounds. Are they cures? That depends on how you define *cure*. Immunomodulating drugs (and natural compounds in that class) do not actually kill cancer; they give your immune system what it needs to fight cancer better. So, it isn't the immunologic substance that cures the cancer—it is the person's own immune system. The immunologic is simply ***improving your odds*** (sometimes dramatically).

The countries that consume the greatest variety, and quantity, of natural plants and spices also have the least amount of cancer (even when adjusted for age, as an aging population would have more cancers). This data has been backed up by several studies that have shown when populations move from a low-cancer-risk area to a high-cancer-risk area, their risk of cancer increases considerably. Cancer doesn't usually "just happen" to people. It is their lifetime of accumulated environmental choices and exposures that matters the most—not just what they <u>are</u> exposed to, but what they <u>are not</u> exposed to (e.g., a wide variety of plant compounds, exercise, a different diet, diverse probiotic bacteria, etc.). A person's DNA does influence many cancers, but infrequently does it actually "cause" these cancers. The added risk of having certain genes can be offset by making better environmental choices, such as: better diet, less stress, more exercise, no smoking, less alcohol, avoiding pollutants, etc. You should be *improving your odds* at every turn and with every decision.

Share of population with cancer, 2016
Share of total population with any form of cancer, measured as the age-standardized percentage. This share has been age-standardized assuming a constant age structure to compare prevalence between countries and through time

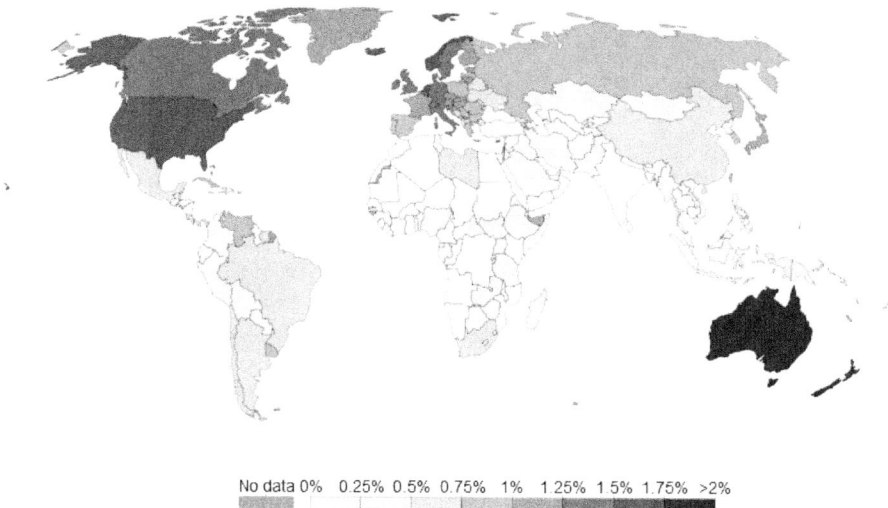

No data 0% 0.25% 0.5% 0.75% 1% 1.25% 1.5% 1.75% >2%

Source: IHME, Global Burden of Disease   OurWorldInData.org • CC BY-SA 7

The above map shows the share of the population in each country with any form of cancer. Westernized countries with diets high in processed foods and low in vegetables, herbs and spices have, by far, the highest rates of cancer. **These statistics are adjusted for age**, meaning that the data isn't skewed simply because people may live longer in countries with better medical care, lower crime, good sanitation, etc. See https://ourworldindata.org/cancer for more information. In countries with European backgrounds, people are at much higher risk of contracting cancer, and immigrants to these countries see their risk of cancer increase. It isn't genetics and it isn't the land mass, so it must be environmental choices (such as diet).

I highly recommend that you discuss the information in this book with your oncologist, for two reasons. The first: A few things in this book can be contraindicated—in other words, they may interfere with your treatment (by supplementing certain antioxidants, for example). The second reason is that most oncologists love to learn new things, but they are very particular, and they want scientific evidence of efficacy. They are busy people and don't want to waste their time or clutter their brains with something that is useless (or worse yet, may harm people). I think this book should include enough science to at least whet their appetite to learn more. If you can afford it, I would encourage you to purchase a copy of this book for your oncologist. This will not only help them understand natural treatment options, but it will also likely help you as they will be able to advise you better (and it costs less than most copayments).

> *"Today we fight. Tomorrow we fight. The day after, we fight. And if this disease plans on whipping us, it better bring a lunch, 'cause it's gonna have a long day doing it."* ~ *Jim Beaver,* Life's That Way

CONTRAINDICATIONS

Herbs, foods and other natural treatments are very biologically active. Nearly everything listed in this book has been a part of the human diet for many generations. Concentrated extracts can still sometimes be problematic, and those should be discussed with your oncologist or general practitioner if you are on other medications. Some of these substances can interfere with certain medications. Often it is because the natural substance here does the same job as your medication (and dosing might be affected); in other cases, it may interfere with your medication. In general, everything mentioned in this book is safe when used as directed; most are probably no more dangerous than a recommendation to drink coffee, which is very biologically active (and it sometimes needs to be restricted as well). However, everyone is different. Just don't think that simply because something is "natural," it is harmless in every situation—that simply isn't true.

Again, when in doubt you should consult your doctor. You can also use online tools to do a quick check for contraindications. Here is one of the better tools, one that I use frequently (I'm afraid I can only shove so much data into my head):
Memorial Sloan Cancer Center – Search About Herbs [8]

Also, be sure to read the disclaimer in Appendix Z. It contains very important information about any risks you may be taking if you choose to treat yourself.

Allergies

There is also a chance that you may be allergic to something mentioned in this book. It is thought that for every botanical on this planet, there is someone allergic to it. I would advise adding one new food or supplement at a time and watching for new symptoms. New symptoms may indicate an allergy, but other conditions are also possible (e.g., a food intolerance, exacerbating an existing intestinal bacteria overgrowth, histamine intolerance, etc.) But if you suffer the classic signs of an allergy, such as shortness of breath, difficulty breathing, nausea, vomiting or diarrhea, you should stop taking the botanical. If the symptoms are severe or long-lasting, you should see a doctor or call a medical help line.

Very few people will have adverse symptoms or contraindications with their medications. These botanicals, vitamins and minerals are based on foods and herbs that have been consumed for centuries. But we should always be cautious.

◆ ❖ ◆

Chapter 2
The Immune System

> *Once a disease has entered the body, all parts which are healthy must fight it: not one alone, but all. Because a disease might mean their common death. Nature knows this; Nature attacks the disease with whatever help she can muster. ~ Paracelsus (1493-1541)*

Our immune system is what prevents and cures cancer. If we have cancer, we like to think that it is the surgery, chemotherapy, radiation or the natural protocol we're on that are going to cure us. But that simply isn't true; those can only help. It is our own immune system that cures our cancer, prevents its return or prevents cancer in the first place.

Let's look at surgery; for an example, I'll use melanoma as it is often visible. When a person is diagnosed with melanoma, the first thing doctors do is schedule them for surgery and do what is called a "wide local excision" (WLE).

> *"WLE" is the removal of the tumor and surrounding tissue; it is a rather crude procedure that reminds me of using a melon baller on watermelon. Of course, they must be careful when doing this, but the results still look like they used a melon baller until things grow back. Don't worry—the tissue generally fills back in.*

The object of this procedure is to remove as much of the cancer as possible. However, doctors know they can never remove everything; metastasizing cancer cells are already circulating in the body, some nearby, some far and wide. It is the immune system that will clean up what is left (or try to). The surgery was done to reduce the load on the immune system as much as possible. Very few surgical procedures for cancer are declared 100% effective, as there is always a chance some cancer cells were missed or that metastasizing cells are in the blood or lymphatic system.

The stronger your immune system is, the better your *odds* are of preventing or beating cancer; there is no disagreement about that. Though doctors have some targeted immune system therapies, they have little in the way of drugs to improve the overall immune system (which is why they do not discuss it very much). This is where complementary approaches can be very useful. Most of this book is not about killing cancer cells with cytotoxic substances; it is about improving the immune system so that your body can better fight cancer naturally.

Though most of this book is about natural adjuvant treatments, I decided to include some information on immunotherapies. Not only are these treatments very promising (I might have died without them), but this allows me to better cover the workings of the immune system while also covering these drugs. Therefore, this chapter is applicable to everyone, whether you are going to be treated with immunotherapy or not, and whether you are treating cancer or trying to prevent it. The immune system is important regardless, and you need to know how it works. Nearly anything that improves immunotherapy treatment will improve other treatments as well (exceptions are possible, but none are included here as they would be uncommon).

Immunotherapies can greatly "*Improve Your Odds*" by allowing your own immune system to do its job. In this context, that means allowing your immune system to see and destroy cancer cells! There are several types of immunotherapy. There are also several natural adjuvant treatments that have been shown to greatly improve immunotherapy outcomes. Most (but not all) immunotherapies work by allowing your body to "see" cancer cells; most do not actually otherwise improve the ability to kill cancer cells. The adjuvant treatments mentioned in this book can improve the immune system, and therefore, they can help you whether you are on immunotherapy or not! Even better, if your doctors decide to put you on immunotherapy later, you'll most likely have a better response if you start the natural therapies ahead of time.

One of the newer classes of immunotherapy drugs is called checkpoint inhibitors (though they go by several names). They block signals given off by cancer cells that trick the immune system into ignoring them; this allows them to hide from the immune system. This includes PD-1/PD-L1 inhibitors. PD-L1 tells T cells (a major part of our immune system) that the cells are normal (not foreign invaders and not cancerous), and it is important in regulating the immune system. Some cancer cells create large amounts of PD-L1. T cells contain a matching protein called PD-1, and when PD-L1 attaches to the PD-1, it tells the T cells not to attack that cell. PD-1 inhibitors prevent T cells from being "turned off" by cancer cells trying to hide from them. PD-1/L1 inhibitors stop this from happening. Immunotherapy drugs are far more selective than chemotherapy drugs, which means they generally don't cause damage to healthy cells, though they are not without other side effects. Because they can be far more effective and less harmful to patients, expect to hear much more about them in the next few years.

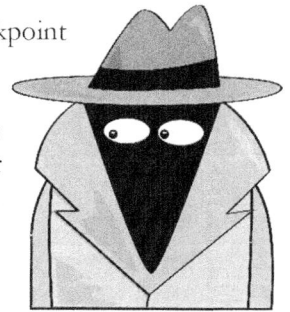

PD-1 inhibitors include:

- Pembrolizumab (Keytruda)
- Nivolumab (Opdivo)
- Cemiplimab (Libtayo)

PD-L1 inhibitors include:

- Durvalumab (Imfinzi)
- Atezolizumab (Tecentriq)
- Avelumab (Bavencio)

Another type of checkpoint inhibitor is called CTLA-4 inhibitors. These include:

- Ipilimumab (Yervoy)

You can find information about other types of immunotherapy in this WebMD article. [9] The one thing they all have in common is that they rely on your own immune system to do the heavy lifting. Immunotherapy drugs do not kill cancer; your body does. The drugs simply allow your immune system to do its job.

New drugs are becoming available all the time, so this should not be considered a complete list. Your oncologist will know which checkpoint inhibitor or combination of them is best for your cancer, what your insurance will pay for and whether there may be any clinical trials open for new drugs. Sometimes they will use more than one of these drugs for maximum effectiveness.

Cancer cells can hide from the immune system. They lie and tell the immune system that they are normal cells, when clearly, they are not. Checkpoint inhibitors basically allow your immune system to see cancer cells for what they are: defective cells that need to be removed. Until this occurs, your immune system is at a severe disadvantage in detecting cancer cells.

First, the bad news: Not everyone responds to these drugs. For example, Keytruda (the drug I was on) has one of the better overall response rates; for melanoma it has a 33% overall response rate (27% partial response and 6% complete remission). This is still far better than chemotherapy, for which the partial response rate was 4% (for melanoma) and there were no complete responses in that study group. These drugs do have possible side effects, though generally less than chemotherapy or radiation, and the side effects are often treatable. Again, your oncologist will talk you through this.

> *I started improving my immune system a year before I went on immunotherapy. I'm convinced this is why I was in that 6% complete remission group. I had a 4" tumor that disappeared in fewer than 8 weeks after starting immunotherapy, which is an exceptional response. My immune system was certainly up to the challenge once it could see the tumor for what it was.*

Now, some good news: What researchers are finding is that there are things within our control that can *Improve Your Odds* of being one of those for whom these drugs work! The rest of this chapter will be about what you can do to *Improve Your Odds* with immunotherapy. Throughout the book I'll be sure to tell you what I was doing to improve my immune response (but don't ignore the research). Remember, what improves the immune system for immunotherapy can most likely help any other therapy as well; it's just that the results can often be dramatic with immunotherapy.

Once your immune system is better able to detect cancer cells, it still must have the ability to do something about them. What researchers are finding is that many people do not have an immune system capable of mounting an effective attack against established tumors. One could just chalk this up to bad genetics (and for years, doctors and researchers did exactly that). However, when they found the same patterns in mice and found that they could significantly improve survival in mice, with nothing more than probiotics and dietary changes, that got them thinking. Would this also be possible in humans? New in vivo (in the body) research on humans has shown that without a doubt, there are things that you can do to *Improve Your Odds* to help beat cancer, especially with (but not limited to) immunotherapy.

❖ MICROBIOME/PROBIOTICS

Several recent in vivo studies have shown connections between the health of the gut, its microbial population and better outcomes with checkpoint inhibitors (and probably all immunotherapy medications). The results have been dramatically better when test groups with already healthy guts were given certain probiotics. Note that if you are having gut issues or eat a poor diet, you'll need to work on that as well.

In this **human in vivo** study out of the University of Texas MD Anderson Cancer Center, they found a significant difference in the gut microbiome between people who responded to PD-1 immunotherapy and those who did not. Those who responded to PD-1 therapy had significantly higher diversity and a relative abundance of beneficial bacteria in the gut.

> "Metagenomic studies revealed functional differences in gut bacteria in responders, including enrichment of anabolic pathways. Immune profiling suggested enhanced systemic and antitumor immunity in responding patients with a favorable gut microbiome as well as in germ-free mice receiving fecal transplants from responding patients. Together, these data have important implications for the treatment of melanoma patients with immune checkpoint inhibitors." – PubMed ID#29097493 (2018) [10]

Recent research has shown that having a strong, healthy microbiome is very important to the success of immunotherapy (and generally for a strong immune system). The following study (out of the University of New South Wales, Sydney, NSW, Australia) looked at PD-1 and PD-L1 inhibitors and found a very strong association with Bifidobacterium. The species identified here were *Bifidobacterium longum*, *Bifidobacterium adolescentis* and *Bifidobacterium breve*. It is thought that the probiotic bacteria activate dendritic cells in the intestines; these dendritic cells are key modulators that shape the immune system through their beneficial effects on CD8+ T cells. It is the T cells that attack and destroy cancer cells. But again, this can only occur after the immune system can spot cancer cells, which is the job of the immunotherapy.

"In recent years, the blockade of immune checkpoint proteins and molecules that deliver inhibitory signals to activated T cells, have shown great promise in cancer treatment. However, the beneficial effects of these treatment strategies were seen only in a subgroup of patients. In this review, we summarize the emerging evidence of improving immune checkpoint protein blockade therapy efficacy by modulating gut microbiota… A very interesting study by Sivan et al. provided strong evidence that the efficacy of PD-L1 blockage therapy can be improved by the modulation of gut microbiota… to identify the responsible bacterial species, they used 16S ribosomal RNA (16S rRNA) sequencing and identified Bifidobacterium species, particularly Bifidobacterium breve, Bifidobacterium longum, and Bifidobacterium adolescentis as the candidate species… This experiment resulted in Bifidobacterium-treated mice having significantly improved tumor control as compared to mice that did not receive Bifidobacterium. Sivan et al. also showed that the possible mechanisms by which Bifidobacterium species inhibited tumor growth were through activating DCs (dendritic cells), which in turn, improves the effector function of tumor-specific CD8+ T cells. **Given that the enhanced anti-melanoma effect from Bifidobacterium species had occurred at the innate immunity level, the authors anticipated that Bifidobacterium species also provide anti-tumor beneficial effects to other types of tumors**… The findings by Sivan et al. using mice models suggest that it is possible to enhance the anti-tumor efficacy of PD-L1 blockade therapy in treating cancer patients by modulating their gut microbiota… A recent study by Frankel et al. using metagenomic shotgun sequencing method showed that melanoma patients who responded to immune checkpoint inhibitors were enriched with Bacteroides caccae. Furthermore, they showed that the bacteria that are enriched within responders are most likely to be antibody dependent. Patients who responded to nivolumab (PD-1 antibody) were enriched with Fecalibacterium prausnitzii, Bacteroides thetaiotamicron, and Holdemania filiformis" – PubMed ID#PMC5845387 (2018) [11]

Several studies have made it clear that a strong and diverse microbiome is very important to achieve a good response from immunotherapy, and especially checkpoint inhibitors. If you have recently undergone systemic antibiotic therapy (most oral antibiotics), your gut is most likely compromised (see the following research study), and your microbiome is not as strong or as diverse as it should be. You may have no symptoms from this, but it could significantly hinder your immune response to cancer cells. At this point I would recommend taking immediate measures to rebuild the microbiome. If you have recently taken broad-spectrum antibiotics, you may want to start a program to strengthen your microbiome, such as the one discussed in Chapter 2 of *The Gut Health Protocol* or Chapter 3 in this book. Then, boost that even more with Bifidobacterium probiotics and a significant increase in soluble fiber in your diet.

> "In mice subcutaneously injected with melanoma and bladder cancer, response to anti-PD-L1 therapy was significantly correlated with Bifidobacterium-treated mice (oral gavage) compared to non-Bifidobacterium-treated mice… Of note, Bifidobacterium was not detected in mesenteric lymph nodes, spleen, or tumor suggesting that systemic antitumor immune responses occurred independently of bacterial translocation… In a separate melanoma-bearing mouse model, response to anti-PD-L1 therapy significantly correlated with fecal transplantations from patients abundant in Ruminococcaceae family and Faecalibacterium spp… In mice established with sarcoma and melanoma, 2 weeks of broad-spectrum antibiotics and rearing in specific pathogen-free conditions adversely affected survival with PD-1 $\pm$ CTLA-4 blockade." – PubMed ID#PMC6423251 (2019) [12]

The following is a **human in vivo** study that looked at 221 metastatic melanoma (MM) patients (Pts). As with the mouse study, they found that a healthy microbiome made a significant difference in response rates to anti-PD-1 therapy. This is very important research on human cancer patients that anyone on immunotherapy should pay attention to (though it most likely applies to any cancer patient, or to anyone wanting to prevent cancer, as a strong immune system is required to fight cancer). This research was done at the MD Anderson Cancer Center and appeared in the *Journal of Clinical Oncology*.

> "we evaluated the microbiome in a large cohort of pts with MM, focusing on responses to anti-PD-1… Pts on anti-PD1 were classified as either responders (R) or non-responders (NR)… Significant differences in diversity and composition of the gut microbiome were noted in R vs NR to anti-PD-1, with a higher diversity of bacteria in R vs NR (p = 0.03). Differences were also noted in the composition of gut bacteria, with a higher abundance of Clostridiales in R and of Bacteroidales in NR… Immune profiling demonstrated increased tumor immune infiltrates in R pts , with a higher

density of CD8+T cells; this correlated with abundance of specific bacteria enriched in the gut microbiome."

Journal of Clinical Oncology, DOI: 10.1200/JCO.2017.35.15_suppl.3008 35, no. 15_suppl (May 20 2017) 3008-3008. [13]

It's been shown that supplementation of Bifidobacterium (again, available in some common off-the-shelf probiotics) has the same benefit as PD-1 inhibitor immunotherapy. Combining the two shows even greater benefits! Do not underestimate the importance of a strong microbiome and Bifidobacterium probiotics.

"Bifidobacterium as associated with the antitumor effects. **Oral administration of Bifidobacterium alone improved tumor control to the same degree as programmed cell death protein 1 ligand 1 (PD-L1)– specific antibody therapy (checkpoint blockade), and combination treatment nearly abolished tumor outgrowth.** Augmented dendritic cell function leading to enhanced CD8+ T cell priming and accumulation in the tumor microenvironment mediated the effect. Our data suggest that manipulating the microbiota may modulate cancer immunotherapy." – PubMed ID#PMC4873287 (2015) [14]

With 80% of plasma cells—mainly immunoglobulin A (IgA)-bearing cells (a huge part of our immune system)—residing in the gut, it should come as no surprise that the gut plays a very large role in immune health. I think anyone on any type of immunotherapy should discuss taking these very specific probiotics, as well as taking prebiotic fibers, with their oncologist. The benefits are large and the risks are very low, so I feel this is usually a no-brainer.

Recent research also shows that taking antibiotics in the months before immunotherapy can significantly reduce patients' life expectancy. This was found regardless of the type of antibiotic or the type of cancer! This is simply because the antibiotics killed the beneficial bacteria that support the immune system in fighting cancer.

"Antibiotics reduce survival rates in cancer patients taking immunotherapy… prior antibiotic use had a median overall survival of just two months, compared to 26 months for those with no antibiotic use prior to treatment. A similar effect was seen across all cancer types." – Imperial College London (2019) [15], PubMed ID#31513236 (2019) [16]

❖ MUSHROOMS

When you read the section on mushrooms in Chapter 6, you'll see why medicinal mushrooms can work very well with immunotherapy drugs. They increase the number and effectiveness of NK (natural killer) cells (a type of lymphocyte, which is a white blood cell) and feed the beneficial bacteria mentioned above.

> "Defect of dendritic cell maturation in tumor microenvironments is an important immunological problem limiting the success of cancer immunotherapy. Cordyceps militaris extracts significantly induced level of IL-18 transcription via enhancing of P1 promoter region in mouse brain and liver and activated the IFN-γ production in mouse leukemic monocyte macrophage cell line (RAW 264.7). The result indicates its potential as an immune activator or anti-cancer drug" – PubMed ID#PMC3339609 (2012) [17]

The following research looks at the evidence from over 80 studies on mushrooms and their effect on immunomodulation and immunotherapy in cancer. It is clear from the overwhelming amount of evidence that mushrooms exhibit strong immune system benefits, especially in the context of treatment and prevention of cancers.

> "Following an oral uptake of mushrooms/mushroom compounds, intestinal immune factors are activated, that is, dendritic cells and macrophages that secrete cytokines that initiate local or systemic immunity. Intestinal epithelial cells are also stimulated to secrete IL-7, an important cytokine in cancer immunotherapy… extracts confer antitumor effects by promoting maturation of lymphocytes and NK cells and increasing macrophages proliferation, T helper cells, and CD4/CD8 ratio and population, which is accompanied by increase in weight and size of spleen, and this increase is attributed to the higher numbers of monocytes and granulocytes among other immune cells… consumption of mushroom compounds initiates innate and adaptive immunity by enhancing immune-surveillance against cancer by involving monocytes, macrophages, NK cells, and B cells, CTLs secretion antitumor related cytokines and activation of immune organs, getting rid of cancers, and strengthening the weakened immune system. These actions by mushroom compounds lead to cancer cell apoptosis, cell cycle arrest, and prevention of angiogenesis and metastasis." – PubMed ID#PMC5937616 (2018) [18]

Open Access Creative Commons Attribution
Evidence Based Complement Alternative Medicine 2018 Published online 2018 Apr 22. doi: 10.1155/2018/7271509

This study looked at the effect of polysaccharopeptides (PSP) from *Coriolus versicolor* (turkey tail, or "CV") mushrooms on the immune system. The authors found a large increase in NK cells, lymphocyte counts and CD8+ T cells (which are so important for immunotherapy) with CV use. Turkey tail mushrooms are discussed at greater length in Chapter 6.

> "CV extract was administered after the completion of radiotherapy and was shown to increase NK cytotoxic function and lymphocyte counts, with CD8+ T cells and CD19+ B cells increasing dose dependently… more than 80 previously treated breast cancer patients were given PSP/Danshen capsules for 6 months, leading to increased T-helper and B cell counts and proportions… Increases in leukocyte and neutrophil counts, as well as serum IgG and IgM levels, were observed in non-small cell lung cancer patients randomized to PSP treatment… In lung, gastric and esophageal carcinoma, PSP was also associated (to varying degrees) with alleviated symptoms, improved NK activity, increased IL-2 production and CD4 T cell levels, protective effects against radiation-induced lymphopenia, and improved survival rates when combined with radiotherapy… Preclinical in vitro and in vivo data suggest that PSP has immunomodulatory (largely immunostimulatory) effects that may be beneficial, particularly when combined with anticancer treatment." – PubMed ID#PMC5592279 (2017) [19]

Open Access Attribution - Journal Frontiers in Immunology, 2017, vol 8, DOI:10.3389/fimmu.2017.01087 – Saleh Mohammad H., Rashedi Iran, Keating Armand

> "it has been extensively demonstrated both preclinically and clinically that aqueous extracts obtained from CV display a wide array of biological activities" – PubMed ID#12211223 (2002) [20]

Several different medicinal mushrooms have been found to increase T cell proliferation and infiltration, as well as NK cells and other markers of a strong immune system. This is vitally important in order to destroy the cancer tumor and the free-floating metastatic cells once the immune system is able to see the cancer cells (e.g., while on checkpoint inhibitors such as anti-PD-1 inhibitors). Remember, it isn't good enough to expose the cancer cells to the immune system (un-cloak them)—our immune systems must be able to destroy the cells once it sees them.

> "concerning the exploration of the immunomodulatory potential of H. erinaceus (Lion's Mane), it can be stated that polysaccharide fractions of the mushroom ethanol extract and derivatives thereof are able to promote dendritic cell maturation and dendritic cell-mediated cytokine production and T-cell proliferation, as well as to activate macrophages and increase TNFα production. Stimulatory effects on intestinal immune system, manifested

mainly through increase of surface IgA expression and natural killer cell activation, have also been reported in mouse in vivo experiments, when the polysaccharide fraction of H. erinaceus was given as a food supplement… a Hericium-derived protein HEP3, which demonstrated a complex immunomodulatory impact in mice, has also been able to strongly reduce growth of CC531 cell xenograft tumors after intraperitoneal injection. The immunomodulatory effect was induced through stimulation of the gut microbiota with the protein and involved activation of the proliferation and differentiation of T-cells and stimulation of the intestinal antigen-presenting cells" – PubMed ID#PMC6044372 (2018) [21]

❖ BETA-GLUCANS

Beta-glucans make up part of the cell wall of certain plants, fungi and bacteria. They make up part of the mushroom's structure, which is one of the reasons why mushrooms are so beneficial. Different sources of beta-glucans provide different benefits, and the structure varies by what are referred to as "side chains." Therefore, it is best to consume a variety of foods that contain beta-glucans, such as oats, barley, seaweed, mushrooms and nutritional yeast. There is even an over-the-counter phage complex that kills unwanted bacteria throughout the intestines; the dead cells of that bacteria provide beta-glucans to the systemic environment and a prebiotic food to beneficial bacteria. Phages are very specific in the bacteria they kill. This can be an excellent way to both feed good bacteria, eliminate some unwanted bacteria and provide beta-glucans to the systemic environment. Even though mushrooms contain beta-glucans, it is best to get a variety of beta-glucans in your diet. Beta-glucans are discussed in more detail in Chapter 6.

The following paper does a very good job of presenting the benefits of using beta-glucans as an adjuvant supplement along with immunotherapy (such as anti-PD-1 and anti-PD-L1 therapies).

"Recent clinical success with immune checkpoint inhibitors, chimeric antigen receptor T-cell therapy, and adoptive immune cellular therapies has generated excitement and new hopes for patients and investigators. However, clinically efficacious responses to cancer immunotherapy occur only in a minority of patients. One reason is the tumor microenvironment (TME), which potently inhibits the generation and delivery of optimal antitumor immune responses… Polysaccharides, also known as β-glucans, can be extracted from the cell walls of natural resources such as plant, fungi, and bacteria. They are biomolecules that can adopt pathogen-associated molecular patterns and can modulate host immune responses via priming and/or stimulating innate immune cells such as macrophages, neutrophils, and granulocytes… β-glucan molecules are potential immune modulator that can manipulate innate and adaptive immune responses within the TME and improve clinical responses of current cancer immune-therapies… In vivo studies have shown that β-(1–3) glycosidic backbone of yeast glucan could not be digested in stomach so that most glucans enter the proximal small intestine, where the yeast glucans were captured by macrophages and digested into small fragments within macrophages. Glucan fragments could be transported by macrophages to bone marrow and the endothelial reticular system… there are multiple β-glucan-based clinical trials in cancer immunotherapy… Recently, a combination therapy using β-glucan and mAbs targeting immune checkpoint molecules such as PD-1 and PD-L1 has been investigated in preclinical models with promising antitumor efficacy, and is anticipated to be translated into a phase I clinical trial… β-glucans with different structures appear to stimulate antitumor responses in completely different manners" – PubMed ID#PMC5834761 (2018) [22]

Creative Commons attribution - Zhang M, Kim JA, Huang AY. Optimizing Tumor Microenvironment for Cancer Immunotherapy: β-Glucan-Based Nanoparticles. Front Immunol. 2018;9:341. Published 2018 Feb 26. doi:10.3389/fimmu.2018.00341

The first sentence of the following article from a major oncology journal says a lot; the health of the immune system is critical in both preventing and fighting cancer. Without a very well-functioning immune system, most oncology treatments are not going to be successful. Immunotherapy checkpoint inhibitors certainly have an important role—allowing the immune system to detect cancer cells—but without a strong immune system to fight cancer cells, these therapies will not be very successful. Mushrooms and other beta-glucans can help with this, along with many other adjuvant therapies found in this book.

"The functioning of the immune system is critically engaged in the progression of tumors, and immunotherapy is the foremost strategy for cancer treatment. Cancer therapy highlights the role of B and T lymphocytes, DCs, NK cells, and mononuclear phagocyte cells. Mushrooms exhibit interesting immune-regulating properties that may be useful in cancer management. Successful immunotherapy requires both the increase in tumor-specific immunity and the reversal of tumor-associated immune suppression… **Ingestion of oral β-glucans in medicinal mushrooms has been found to activate various immune system components, including macrophages, NK cells, DCs, and T helper lymphocytes, which affects tumor cell viability** and potentiates the release of various mediators including lymphokines and interleukins (ILs)… Several studies have demonstrated that DCs are functionally defective in tumor-bearing hosts. MD-fraction can directly activate macrophages and DCs and can induce both helper T cells (Th) and tumor-specific cytotoxic T cells to inhibit tumor cell growth." – PubMed ID#PMC5973856 (2018) [23]

Creative Commons License Attribution - Rossi P, Difrancia R, Quagliariello V, et al. B-glucans from Grifola frondosa and Ganoderma lucidum in breast cancer: an example of complementary and integrative medicine. Oncotarget. 2018;9(37):24837–24856. Published 2018 May 15. doi:10.18632/oncotarget.24984

"Orally administered beta-glucans are absorbed through the gastrointestinal tract and taken up by tissue-resident macrophages. Here, they are fragmented, transported to the bone marrow and reticuloendothelial system and eventually released and taken up by other immune cells, leading to various immunological effects" – PubMed ID#PMC5069311 (2016) [24]

❖ OTHER

This section discusses a few more things that might help make immunotherapy more responsive.

Aspirin – There is some evidence that a COX2 inhibitor, such as aspirin (even low-dose aspirin), may enhance the effectiveness of checkpoint inhibitors. Be sure to work with your oncologist on this; even though aspirin is available over the counter, that doesn't mean it is without risks. Also see PubMed ID#27057439. [25]

"COX Inhibitors Enhance the Efficacy of Immunotherapy with an Anti-PD-1 Blocking Antibody… Aspirin blocks both COX-1 and COX-2… even a modest degree of COX inhibition might help enhance the efficacy of immunotherapies, including those based on immune checkpoint blockade… Mice that fully eradicated COX-sufficient tumors upon treatment with aspirin + anti-PD-1 were immune to a subsequent challenge in the absence of further treatment" – PubMed ID#PMC4597191 [26]

I started a low-dose aspirin about halfway through my immunotherapy. After about 6 weeks I found that it was thinning my blood too much (needle pokes took longer to stop bleeding), so I started taking it every other day. Again, my goal was to Improve My Odds, not bleed half the day.

Metformin – This is a widely prescribed oral anti-diabetic (prescription) drug. CD 8+ TIL exhaustion (where the immune system can no longer infiltrate tumor cells) is one of the main reasons for a poor response (or poor ongoing response) to immunotherapy. Though trials have yet to get underway, adding metformin may help prevent TIL exhaustion and extend the benefits of immunotherapy (especially checkpoint inhibitors) to more people. Metformin is a prescription drug, and you would have to work with your oncologist if this is something you want to try.

> "In-vitro and in-vivo analysis of metformin has exhibited anti-proliferative activity… It has also been observed that metformin activates the T cell mediated immune response against cancer cells… Meta-analysis of data obtained from cohort and observational studies has revealed that metformin use was associated with a decrease in both cancer related and all-cause mortality… Evidence from preclinical trials has described that metformin, at least in part, exerts an anti-cancer effect by inhibiting immune exhaustion of CD 8+ TILs [26], thus amplifying the existing immune action against cancer cells." – PubMed ID#PMC5130043 (2016) [27]

> Open Access Attribution - Chae YK, Arya A, Malecek MK, et al. Repurposing metformin for cancer treatment: current clinical studies. Oncotarget. 2016;7(26):40767–40780. doi:10.18632/oncotarget.8194

Modified Citrus Pectin (MCP) – This is discussed more in Chapter 6; it is included here in relation to the immunotherapy drug Keytruda. MCP is a galectin-3 inhibitor and may show some benefits as an adjuvant combination with Keytruda (pembrolizumab) and perhaps other PD-1 inhibitors.

> "Excitingly, one of these trials showed that the combination of pembrolizumab with the galectin-3 inhibitor GR-MD-02 gave promising early results in the treatment of patients with advanced melanomas in a phase Ib clinical trial… Immunotherapy using monoclonal antibodies blocking immune checkpoint molecules has shown promising progress. However, to increase overall responsiveness, several investigators started to combine these with galectin inhibitors to enhance the therapeutic effect." – PubMed ID#PMC5855652

❖ STRATEGY

This is an area that may really fascinate your oncologist. Many already know about some of this (but can't really prescribe it, for reasons covered earlier in the book), but most love talking about it. How our bodies work is truly fascinating, and very complex. I mean, who would have thought that a simple forest mushroom could help us kill cancer? It usually can't do much on its own because cancer is cagey; it hides from the immune system in ways that almost seem like it is an intelligent life form. But combine these natural immune-enhancing botanicals with modern science (e.g., immunotherapy), and you have a very strong combination!

Everything listed below is either a food, derived from food or lives on organic food (the probiotics). Doses are not extreme; in fact, our ancestors probably consumed far more mushrooms and plant fibers than people do today. Nevertheless, feel free to discuss your plans with your oncologist.

1. A strong, healthy and diverse microbiome is extremely important for a good response to immunotherapy. I would pay close attention to the recommendations in Chapter 3. In addition, take a good probiotic that contains Bifidobacterium and perhaps a phage complex to boost its benefits even more (see the book's website for recommendations).

2. Consume a good mix of prebiotic supplements to feed the microbiome; be sure to include larch tree fiber and modified citrus pectin, as these are identified in Chapter 6 as having anticancer properties.

3. Consume a diet high in plants and vegetables that contain soluble fiber. Soluble fiber feeds Bifidobacteria; insoluble fiber and cellulose do not. I recommend that most of the vegetables you consume are well cooked, as this frees the nutrients and soluble fiber from the bonds of insoluble fiber. Pressure cooking is an excellent way to cook vegetables for this purpose. Moist cooking as in a casserole, soup or stew is also a very good way to consume vegetables. Boiling is not a good idea as it leaches nutrients. If frying, I recommend al dente as to not denature the plant fibers. Some raw vegetables are OK, but the hyped benefits of raw foods are more fad than fact (humans have been cooking foods for over a million years!).

4. Consume a variety of medicinal mushrooms. I think it is especially important to take a high-quality powdered medicinal mushroom mix—one that is made from the fruiting bodies of the mushroom and hot-water extracted. If you are on immunotherapy, I would consider supplementing with a mushroom powder to be of vital importance, second only to a Bifidobacteria supplement and feeding the microbiome. See Chapter 6 for much more information on using medicinal mushrooms.

5. Consume foods high in beta-glucans, as well as taking a beta-glucan supplement. These show similar benefits to mushrooms (which are high in beta-glucans). See the Beta-glucans section in Chapter 6 for more information.

6. With your doctor's OK, take a low-dose aspirin. Work with your doctor to take a dose that does not thin your blood too much.

◆ ❖ ◆

Chapter 3
Gut Health, The Key to Immune Health

"The doctor of the future will give no medicine, but will interest his patients in the care of human frame, and in the cause and prevention of disease." ~ *Thomas Edison*

As the author of the book *The Gut Health Protocol*, [28] I have a lot of material for this section, but I'm going to keep this chapter to the essentials of how gut health relates to cancer (all cancers, not just those of the gastrointestinal tract). If I didn't, this book would be twice the size. If you feel your gut has issues (gas, bloating, frequent constipation, diarrhea—that is, loose stools—more than once per week, chronic heartburn, etc.), then you should also read *The Gut Health Protocol*. It has truly helped thousands of people restore the health of their gut, and thus improve their immune system. If you *think* your gut is in pretty good shape, this chapter might be enough for you.

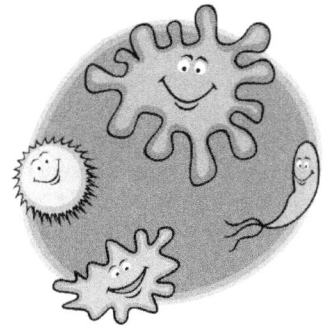

Very recent research has shown that gut health, microbiome diversity and some specific beneficial bacterial strains are essential for our immune system's ability to fight cancer. Current immunotherapy basically unhides cancer cells so that the immune system can identify those cells as cancerous (sometimes you'll see it described as "taking the brakes off the immune system"). These drugs do not kill cancer cells; your immune system must do that. If your immune system isn't up to the task (and that is often the case with people on immunotherapy), then the drugs will do little or even no good. This is thought to be why the complete remission rate for these drugs is as low as 6%, though partial remission (which might mean stopping the disease's progression completely, but not getting rid of it) is as high as 40%. Certainly worth trying, especially with the help of the advice in this book! In this article, the authors show how healthy gut microbiota can assist immunotherapy's fight against melanoma (yes, gut microbes can help fight skin cancer! Who knew!?):

> "The second and third studies found that melanoma patients with plenty of healthy gut bacteria responded well to immunotherapy. In contrast, the patients who didn't have success with immunotherapy had imbalanced gut flora, which also was correlated with lower immune cell activity. The researchers in both studies concluded that cancer patients who maintain healthy gut flora are more likely to have positive results from immunotherapy." – Ubiome (2018 – Includes links to several research studies) [29]

When you consider that the gut is responsible for "70% of the entire immune system," you can start to get a picture of just how important it is to general health, as well as to preventing and fighting cancer.

> "The gastrointestinal system plays a central role in immune system homeostasis… The crucial position of the gastrointestinal system is testified by the huge amount of immune cells that reside within it. Indeed, gut-associated lymphoid tissue (GALT) is the prominent part of mucosal-associated lymphoid tissue (MALT) and represents almost 70% of the entire immune system; moreover, about 80% of plasma cells [mainly immunoglobulin A (IgA)-bearing cells] reside in GALT." – PubMed ID#PMC2515351 (2008) [30]

This chapter is vitally important to anyone fighting or trying to prevent cancer, not just to those on immunotherapy.

New research shows that immune system T cells and dendritic cells (which help identify threats and activate an immune response against tumors) are modified by gut bacteria in ways very beneficial to fighting cancer. The topic of Immunotherapy is discussed more in Chapter 2, though this information applies to everyone. Without healthy gut bacteria, our immune system does not fight cancer cells (and probably many other diseases) nearly as well as it would otherwise. Infiltration of T cells (again, a major component of the immune system) into the tumor is one of the strongest signs of a successful outcome. If T cells cannot penetrate the tumor, they cannot kill it (it would be like shooting a BB gun at a fortress). One of the best prognosticators, and one that you might see on test results from a tumor biopsy, are tumor-infiltrating lymphocytes (TIL). Lymphocytes that attack and kill tumor cells are T lymphocytes (or "T cells"). On test results, TILs are usually graded as "absent," "non-brisk," or "brisk." Brisk is what you want, in contrast to "absent." The risk of dying from melanoma (for example) was 30% less for "non-brisk," and 50% less for "brisk." Obviously, this is an important number and one that is very much affected by gut health, as I'll describe below.

> "Subgroups of patients who have tumor-infiltrating lymphocytes in the stroma may have better response to chemotherapy and favorable long-term prognosis.

Updates at - https://improvingyourodds.com

Support at - https://www.facebook.com/groups/cancer.improving.your.odds

Accumulating evidence shows that the immune system plays a crucial role in the outcomes of some BC (Breast Cancer) subgroups, especially more aggressive, proliferative ones such as triple-negative and HER2-positive BC. This review article will present data on the role of lymphocyte infiltration in BC prognosis and response to therapy." – PubMed ID#29061314 (2017) [31]

"Therefore, in TNBC (triple-negative breast cancer), **the more stromal TILs a patient has at diagnosis, the better their outcome** after adjuvant anthracycline-based chemotherapy... core biopsies from more than 3000 patients have been assessed for correlation between immune markers...stromal TILs are associated with higher rates of pathological complete remission (pCR), independent of other clinico-pathological prognostic factors or the chemotherapy regimen" – PubMed ID#PMC6267863 (2015) [32]

Recently, researchers have been able to extract TILs from patients and essentially grow them to much larger numbers in the lab. These TILs are then injected back into the patient as another form of immunotherapy. These approaches have shown promise in clinical trials, with some studies showing overall response rates of 40% in metastatic melanoma, 90% in acute lymphoblastic leukemia and 40% in chronic lymphoblastic leukemia. However, this method relies on TILs that are capable of easily infiltrating the tumor, and not everyone has these. Therefore, improving the immune system first is still beneficial.

One of the main reasons why TILs aren't more potent against tumors (in many people) is that cancer cells adapt and deploy mechanisms to evade detection by TILs, and they also take measures to suppress the anti-tumor immune response by releasing various factors to change the tumor microenvironment (TME) that blocks T cells. Tumors can also learn to hide from TILs. So, TILs that worked before may be rendered useless by tumors adapting.

Important: To successfully beat cancer we need to improve the immune system (especially TIL T cells' quantity and quality), prevent cancer cells from hiding from the TILs (e.g., immunotherapy drugs), and prevent the tumor from successfully changing its own microenvironment (e.g., by buffering the acidity with sodium bicarbonate, see Chapter 6, pH Buffering). The first two measures are the most important. This is the more natural approach and one that will probably replace chemotherapy and radiation therapy for many types of cancer.

> *This combination of immunotherapy and natural adjuvant therapy is already being used to replace chemotherapy and radiation for some cancers. In treating my melanoma, I've had neither chemo nor radiation, and I don't expect to. I didn't even have surgery for my last, and largest, tumor—all thanks to immunotherapy (to unhide the cancer) and adjuvant natural therapy to boost the immune system as described in this book.*

So, what does this have to do with gut health? (Get to the point, John!)

"T cell infiltration of solid tumors is associated with favorable patient outcomes... **Oral administration of Bifidobacterium alone improved tumor control to the same degree as programmed cell death protein 1 ligand 1 (PD-L1)-specific antibody therapy (checkpoint blockade), and combination treatment nearly abolished tumor outgrowth.** Augmented dendritic cell function leading to enhanced CD8(+) T cell priming and accumulation in the tumor micro-environment mediated the effect... Bifidobacterium-treated mice displayed significantly improved tumor control in comparison with their non-Bifidobacterium treated counterparts, which was accompanied by robust induction of tumor-specific T cells in the periphery and increased accumulation of antigen-specific CD8+ T cells within the tumor. These effects lasted several weeks." – PubMed ID#PMC4873287 (2015) [33]

Department of Pathology, University of Chicago. Sivan, A., Corrales, L., Hubert, N., Williams, J. B., Aquino-Michaels, K., Earley, Z. M., ... Gajewski, T. F. (2015). Commensal Bifidobacterium promotes antitumor immunity and facilitates anti-PD-L1 efficacy. Science (New York, N.Y.), 350(6264), 1084–1089. doi:10.1126/science.aac4255

As you can tell from this research study abstract (the full study appeared in the major medical journal *Science*), taking a simple probiotic supplement may be just as important as any of the game-changing (and ultra-expensive) PD-1/PD-L1 immunotherapy drugs! This is huge! Even better, the two can work together synergistically. **This appears to be a highly effective way of "***Improving Your Odds***," one I would not overlook.** In fact, I didn't overlook it; I'm convinced that my efforts to rebuild my gut, which included taking a highly effective Bifidobacterium probiotic and consuming prebiotics, are why I did so well on my immunotherapy.

By coincidence I had started taking an excellent probiotic/prebiotic (which I still take) shortly before my original cancer diagnosis. It contains Bifidobacterium strains as well as a phage complex that amplifies these strains throughout the colon. (The beneficial bacteria in most probiotic supplements normally die long before reaching the end of the colon. The phage complex helps prevent this.) My TIL levels were measured as "Brisk," the best score and one that isn't overly common, and my treatment outcome put me in the 6% of people who have complete remission. I feel lucky and blessed that I found out about this just in time.

The probiotic bacteria improve your immune system (in part through "T cell priming"). They are not improving the effectiveness of the immunotherapy drug, and they are not poisoning you or the cancer cells. Therefore, taking specific probiotics will likely benefit most cancer treatments, not just immunotherapy. Though there is no research on this yet, it should also be highly effective in helping to prevent cancer! Or at least killing it off in the fetal stage (before you even know it is there).

I am limited in how much of the above study I can include here, but the full paper is available online (at the link specified in the endnote). This is one study you certainly should bring to your oncologist's attention.

Several other probiotic strains have also shown anticancer benefits against certain cancers (especially colon cancer). These include *Lb. plantarum*, *B. infantis*, *Lb. rhamnosus* and *S. thermophilus*. However, the research is not as strong, and the effect may not be as broad as what is shown above. The immune-modulating benefits of Bifidobacterium are especially important. Another bacterium species found to benefit the immune system, and to *Improve Your Odds* with cancer, is *Akkermansia muciniphila*. However, this species is not available as an over-the-counter supplement or by prescription. *A. muciniphila* often shows up low on stool tests, and the best way to increase its numbers is through the use of PREbiotics. This will also increase the levels of Bifidobacterium; this important topic will be discussed below.

> "stool samples at diagnosis revealed correlations between clinical responses to ICIs and the relative abundance of Akkermansia muciniphila Oral supplementation with A. muciniphila… restored the efficacy of PD-1 blockade in an interleukin-12-dependent manner by increasing the recruitment of CCR9+CXCR3+CD4+ T lymphocytes into mouse tumor beds." – PubMed ID#29097494 (2018) [34]

> "Here, we show that Akkermansia muciniphila, an intestinal bacterium associated with systemic effects on host metabolism and PD-1 checkpoint immunotherapy, induces immunoglobulin G1 (IgG1) antibodies and antigen-specific T cell responses… A. muciniphila-specific T cell responses in individuals due to differences in microbiota composition or other environmental signals may have profound systemic effects." – AAAS journal Science DOI: 10.1126/science.aaw7479 (2019) [35]

The immune system was discussed at length in Chapter 2, but a discussion of it here is necessary to see how gut microbiota fit into this picture (your immune system is very important to cancer treatment, with or without immunotherapy). Several research studies have found that these T cells become more abundant and far more effective when exposed to certain bacteria in the gut (especially Bifidobacterium, as well as a rich diversity of beneficial strains from *Bacteroidetes* and *Firmicutes*). We don't need to get too caught up in learning all the strains we need in our gut (we can't supplement some of them, anyway, but I have covered the most important ones that we can supplement). What is important is that we promote a healthy gut. If we have too much dysbiotic bacteria (unwanted bacteria) in the gut, it will prevent the beneficial bacteria from thriving. If there is no gut dysbiosis, then mostly what we need to do is provide the proper *bacteria food* to the gut: "Feed them, and they will come."

I highly recommend that everyone read Chapter 2 (The Immune System), even if you are not on any type of immunotherapy. You'll quickly see just how important gut health and a healthy microbiome are to our immune system's ability to fight cancer.

❖ PREBIOTICS - BENEFICIAL BACTERIA FOOD

What is beneficial bacteria food? We've covered some of this already, without even calling it that. Most of these are covered in Chapter 6 in more detail.

- Fucoidan/Seaweed
- Aloe Vera
- Sweet Potatoes
- Flaxseed
- Cruciferous Vegetables
- Mushrooms
- Beta-Glucans

Soluble Fiber Supplements

- Larch Tree Arabinogalactan
- Acacia Senegal (gum arabic)
- Partially Hydrolyzed Guar Gum (PHGG).
- Glucomannan (konjac plant, konjac noodles)

These prebiotics all <u>preferentially</u> feed beneficial bacteria! All are highly beneficial in their own right (e.g., containing fractions that have anticancer properties), but their ability to improve the makeup and diversity of our gut bacteria is a very special bonus! In addition to these very special foods, anything containing "soluble fiber" will also feed good bacteria, though some do this better than others. Consuming a diverse diet of vegetables and low-sugar fruit (as discussed in Chapter 4) will provide a variety of these fibers, as well as nutrients, needed by our gut's microbiota.

Possibly avoid (especially as supplements):

- Galacto-oligosaccharide (GOS) – Some people may get gas, bloating or diarrhea from this one. If so, you should avoid it.
- Pectins – Some people are allergic to these. Symptoms, especially at first, may only include bloating or mild diarrhea. But some people may have a more severe reaction.
- Psyllium seed husk – This can be harsh for some people and difficult to adjust to for others. If it works for you, it's fine to take.
- Inulin – This can be very hard to adjust to for some people. Symptoms include gas, bloating and diarrhea.

The key here is that these foods "selectively" stimulate beneficial bacteria, such as Bifidobacteria. This means they can feed good bacteria while not feeding the bad. As shown here, you need to consume a variety of non-digestible carbohydrates.

> "Bifidobacteria can utilize a diverse range of dietary carbohydrates that escape degradation in the upper parts of the intestine, many of which are plant-derived oligo- and polysaccharides… Different bifidobacterial strains may possess different carbohydrate utilizing abilities… the growth and metabolic activity of beneficial gut bacteria, such as bifidobacteria, can be selectively stimulated by non-digestible carbohydrates, termed "prebiotics"… Bifidobacteria are Gram-positive, heterofermentative, non-motile, non-spore forming microorganisms"
> – PubMed ID#PMC3145055 (2011) [36]

Pokusaeva, Karina et al. "Carbohydrate metabolism in Bifidobacteria." Genes & nutrition vol. 6,3 (2011): 285-306. doi:10.1007/s12263-010-0206-6

Bifidobacteria manufacture over 40 different enzymes to break down various carbohydrates (that we could not break down otherwise). These include some enzymes that specifically break down tough polysaccharides such as chitinase, which breaks down the chitin in mushrooms, and alpha- and beta-mannosidase, to break down mannose from the mushroom. It is obvious that mushrooms provide a rich source of beneficial prebiotics to Bifidobacteria (or they wouldn't have the enzymes to break them down). Vegetables and green leafy plants are also a rich source of soluble fibers and other prebiotics to feed Bifidobacteria (see the partial list above), not to mention lots of vitamins, minerals and other cancer-fighting bioactive phytochemicals.

Although beating and preventing cancer are a little more complex than simply eating these foods, they certainly (and conclusively) help. Though there are no numbers out on this, my guess is if everyone simply ate more of these foods, and less of the foods that feed bad bacteria, our overall cancer rates could be cut considerably, perhaps by 50% or more (my bet is on more). Survival rates for cancer would also go way up. This isn't based on my opinion or personal beliefs, but on the considerable amount of scientific research on the subject (some of which has already been presented).

So, what do the foods above have in common? All of them contain prebiotics. Prebiotics are essentially carbohydrates that we humans cannot digest or assimilate, but beneficial bacteria can. Much like humans, our beneficial bacteria need a diverse diet of their prebiotic foods; you can't simply buy a bottle of fiber powder and call it good.

You can find out much more on this topic by reading about each of the above foods in Chapter 6, Chapter 2 on Immunotherapy and Chapter 4 about Diet. Gut health is also discussed in detail in my book *The Gut Health Protocol*.

❖ OPPORTUNISTIC BACTERIA FOOD

Why do I use the term "preferentially feed" to describe how these foods support beneficial bacteria? The prebiotics in these foods are what our guts expect to see. Humans cannot digest them; therefore, the undigested prebiotics get moved on as "waste" (one person's waste is a microbe's gourmet meal!). Our beneficial bacteria have been expecting to be fed like this since humans first inhabited this planet (and before, as the same thing happens in primates and most other mammals). Our beneficial microbes not only tolerate this waste, they require it.

On the other hand, opportunistic bacteria are waiting for something else. They're called "opportunistic" because they are waiting for their opportunity to thrive, and what many of them thrive on are more simple sugars (mostly monosaccharides and disaccharides) that have been "malabsorbed" in our gut. Sugars that don't assimilate (digest and absorb) in our gut get mixed with the waste and go on to feed the unwanted bacteria, the opportunistic bacteria, in our gut. Our gut does not expect these sugars. Historically, they rarely made it to the colon, and by and large our ancestors didn't have this problem. Our ancestors consumed very little sugar, drank no alcohol and took no antibiotics, and thus, their guts usually worked much better than ours. Unwanted and opportunistic bacteria push out good bacteria, which we need for a healthy immune system.

One of the main malabsorbed sugars is lactose. Lactose is the sugar found in milk; it is designed to feed baby mammals (such as calves and human babies). Nature provides babies with an enzyme that helps them break down lactose (into the simple sugars glucose and galactose) for easy absorption. When the baby absorbs lactose, it doesn't malabsorb, and therefore it doesn't feed bad bacteria below. In our biological history adults didn't consume dairy; it was given to babies by their mothers. Nature is very efficient, and it discovered early on that adults didn't drink milk; therefore, after we were about 5 to 8 years old, our bodies didn't need to keep making the enzyme (lactulose) that breaks down lactose. About 7,500 years ago, there was a genetic change in some Europeans that allowed them to continue to make some lactase enzyme into their adult years. This is believed to have occurred after Europeans started dairy farming and commonly consuming milk as adults. However, even among people of European descent, many are still at least partially lactose intolerant. You can be lactose intolerant and not know it, as you might be lucky enough to have certain gut bacteria that consume lactose without causing symptoms (thus compensating for the lack of the lactase enzyme). However, this is still not the natural state, and these bacteria generally are not what you want in large numbers in your gut. It is also likely that opportunistic bacteria will eventually move in to consume that lactose. So, it is best to just avoid lactose.

Another commonly malabsorbed sugar is fructose, sometimes called fruit sugar. Fructose takes a rather different route to absorption and conversion than glucose and other sugars. It must travel to the liver to get converted to glucose (no other sugar does this). This route is prone to problems, especially as we age (it is also a major cause of non-alcoholic fatty liver disease, or NAFLD). Everyone has a different capacity for how much fructose they can absorb, and how quickly. Things that affect this are age, small intestinal bacterial overgrowth (SIBO), IBS, IBD,

---

intestinal yeast, medications, past cases of food poisoning, reactions to antibiotics, certain medications, etc. To some degree these causations are cumulative. After you've consumed more fructose than you can absorb, the rest goes on to feed bad bacteria in the large intestine. Drinking fruit juices is even more problematic because the gut often cannot absorb fructose in liquid form fast enough, and again it will malabsorb.

Simply overeating, especially carbohydrates, can lead to a dysbiosis of unwanted, opportunistic and sometimes pathogenic bacteria. Our gut can only process so much food at a time; it then basically runs out of stomach acid and digestive enzymes (until the next meal). This undigested/unassimilated food will then continue to the colon where, again, it will feed unwanted bacteria. Always strive to eat in moderation; 3 moderate meals are better for you than one very large meal, even if it means more calories.

Poor nutrition will lead to adrenal fatigue, thyroid issues, anxiety, depression, hair loss, depressed immune system (so more disease) and even, eventually, more cancers. Poor nutrition in most countries today is not due to too little food (with exceptions of course), but rather from a poor diet (many of us make poor food choices) and poor digestion/absorption. Medications such as antacids and over-the-counter pain medications (mostly NSAIDS) can cause gut issues that can lead to the malabsorption of certain nutrients. We're often our own worst enemies. If we lived like our recent ancestors of just 150 years ago, we wouldn't have many of these issues. We would, of course, have other issues that would probably be even worse (such as dysentery). **So, the trick is to keep one foot in the past and one foot in the now, with a vision of the future!**

Most people probably understand the importance of good nutrition in being able to fight cancer and improving the immune system. What a lot of people may not understand is that without a well-functioning digestive system and good intestinal health, you are not getting proper nutrition, regardless of what you eat or the supplements you take. In fact, if you are malabsorbing nutrients, you are feeding opportunistic bacteria. As the author of *The Gut Health Protocol*, I often hear people tell me about all the nutritional supplements they take, and yet they have many of the symptoms of nutritional deficiencies. Some of these people even have test results showing nutritional deficiencies. You can take the most expensive nutritional supplements you want, but if your gut isn't functioning properly, you are not going to absorb and assimilate that nutrition. The common adage is true: You'll simply be making expensive urine. Good nutrition is very important for a well-functioning immune system (various nutrients will be discussed much more in Chapter 6).

The gastrointestinal tract is a well-choreographed machine. Hundreds of processes must take place in the correct order, and if one of those processes fails, it impacts the functionality of the gut below it. This process starts in the mouth. Food needs to be well chewed, mixing it with saliva and the amylase enzyme it contains. About 30% of starch digestion takes place in the mouth. This chyme is then transported down the esophagus to the stomach. In the stomach the food is mixed (churned) with strong gastric juices, consisting of hydrochloric acid (HCl), potassium chloride (KCl) and sodium chloride (NaCl). Many people, especially as they grow older or if they have a *Helicobacter pylori* infection, do not make enough stomach acid (this normally gets made in the parietal cells of the stomach lining). People often make the problem worse by taking antacids, as the symptoms of too little stomach acid mimic those of too much. Without proper acidity, plant and meat fibers are not broken down properly, do not get transported in a timely manner, and food can ferment in the stomach (causing acid reflux and other abnormalities).

Up to this point, nutrients still haven't been absorbed. The chyme then makes its way to the small intestine. If everything has gone right up to this point (and that isn't always the case), then the small intestine takes over. At this point the very acidic chyme is mixed with sodium bicarbonate to raise the pH of the chyme from about 3 to 4 pH up to about 6 pH. As the food enters the small intestine, it is then dosed with digestive enzymes (to further break down protein, fats and carbohydrates) and bile (to further break down fat). Even if all of this is working fine—and there is a lot that can go wrong—, the microvilli in the small intestine still need to be working properly in order to absorb all of this goodness. Malabsorption here is often brought on by inflammation from small intestinal bacterial overgrowth (SIBO), excessive alcohol consumption, medications, etc.

As you can see, even in this simplified explanation there is a lot that can go wrong. Chronic imbalances of the gut microbiota can cause a lot of gut issues, but so can aging and medications.

> "This is where a lot of the important stuff occurs, and where the nutrients in food are assimilated. Because of all the nooks and crannies, folds, and micro 3D surfaces (such as villi and microvilli) the functional surface area of the small intestine is the size of a football field! If things aren't working correctly in the small intestine you can die from malnutrition, even if eating a good diet! Very small amounts of food chyme, mixed with stomach acid, is squirted from the stomach into the duodenum (the first part of the small intestine) about every 20 seconds. Where it is bathed in bicarbonate (basically baking soda) to raise the pH (make it less acidic). It is also bathed in enzymes and bile salts from the gall bladder and pancreas to further break down the food in to more assimilable components (e.g.,breaking proteins down in to amino acids and starches in to sugars). The villi and microvilli absorb the vitamins, minerals, sugars, etc., into the bloodstream. It takes food about 3-5 hours to move through the small intestine into the colon. If the food travels through faster, you are not properly assimilating nutrients from your food." – _The Gut Health Protocol_ [37]

There are many things that can go wrong with the small intestine, and all of them will affect nutritional absorption. One of the more common problems is small intestinal bacteria overgrowth (SIBO). SIBO generally occurs when colonic bacteria, often unwanted coliform bacteria, make their way to the small intestine. Here they cause fermentation of food, releasing damaging toxins and in short, preventing us from obtaining much of the nutritional benefit from our food.

> *Did you know that there are as many bacteria cells in your body as there are human cells?*

People tend to think of the colon as just waste piping. Though this, of course, is true, there is a lot more going on here. One of the colon's primary jobs is to remove excess fluids from the stool. In addition to this, the trillions of bacteria (our microbiome) in our gut go about producing many nutritional components.

> "Here is a partial list of nutrients manufactured in the colon and made available to us: vitamins K, K2, B1, B2, B6, B12, biotin, folate, fatty acids (such as butyrate, propionate, acetate). All of these nutrients, and more, are manufactured in our gut by bacteria and then used by us. Recent studies also show that bioactive chemicals that reduce inflammation are also manufactured by healthy gut bacteria." – _The Gut Health Protocol_ [38]

Vitamin K2 is covered in Chapter 6, and unless you consume homemade sauerkraut, homemade kimchi or meat labeled as "grass-fed," you are unlikely to get enough of this important vitamin. Our guts can produce some of these vitamins (due to the miracle of our microbiome), but only if gut health is optimal. Another important product of microbiome fermentation is butyrate. Butyrate is also discussed in Chapter 6, but in short, it is responsible for many cancer-preventing and immune-boosting benefits. Though we can obtain a small amount of butyrate from butter (which is where butter gets its name), it is not enough and not in the right place (we need most of our butyrate to be produced in the colon; what we consume gets absorbed and most never makes it to the colon). Even though vitamin B12 is manufactured in the colon, it cannot be absorbed from there; this is one vitamin that we must obtain from eating meat (or if you're a vegan, you must take a supplement. Vegan-friendly B12 is made from a bacterial process). Many of the "B" vitamins can be made by our microbiome.

Proper stomach and intestinal health are vital to mineral absorption. Gastric juices in the stomach work to make minerals more bioavailable, which makes it easier for the small intestinal microvilli (microscopic projections of absorptive cells that line the small intestine) to absorb them into the bloodstream. Intestinal issues, such as leaky gut and SIBO, can prevent the microvilli from properly absorbing minerals and some vitamins. Over time this can have a devastating effect on the immune system.

Often, we may think that our gut is in good shape, but in reality, it may not be. Simply because we don't have diarrhea, constipation, pain or acid reflux doesn't mean our gut is at its optimal condition. Most Westerners do not have a strong microbiome (again, the trillions of bacteria that produce vitamins, enzymes, short-chain fatty acids and other beneficial chemicals for us). Poor diet, sterile food, chlorinated water, stress, antibiotics, antacids, alcohol and other medications have all combined to greatly weaken our microbiome. Not only do we not have enough beneficial bacteria, but the diversity has been severely impacted. Because we inherit some of our microbiome from our mothers (during vaginal childbirth or close contact just after birth), we are increasingly getting off to a bad microbial start. If our mothers had a weak microbiome, or even dysbiosis (a poor mixture of unwanted and commensal bacteria), then this poor beginning can compound over generations. Unless you consume a lot of prebiotic-containing foods, avoid sugar, drink in moderation (and no more than twice per week), haven't had antibiotics in a few years, etc., your microbiome is probably not optimal.

Studies have shown that between 16% and 23% of all cancers are microbial-driven—that is, driven by bacteria, viruses, yeast and parasites. These are just the known, direct causes. Most often the original cause of a cancer is unknown. Bacteria may translocate from the gut into the bloodstream, causing cancers that cannot later be traced to bacteria as the causative factor. Researchers in the future will surely find more cancers are due to infectious agents than is currently believed. Even more cancers are due to a lack of beneficial bacteria, as opposed to bad bacteria causing the cancer.

> "Helicobacter pylori, hepatitis B and C viruses, and human papillomaviruses were responsible for 1·9 million cases, mainly gastric, liver, and cervix uteri cancers. In women, cervix uteri cancer accounted for about half of the infection-related burden of cancer; in men, liver and gastric cancers accounted for more than 80%." – PubMed ID#22575588 (2012) [39]

> "The symbiotic relationship between microbiota and the host is mutually beneficial. The host provides an important habitat and nutrients for the microbiome, and the gut microbiota support the development of the metabolic system and the maturation of the intestinal immune system by providing beneficial nutrients, e.g., by the synthesis of vitamins and short chain fatty acids (SCFAs). Therefore, the interaction between the microbiome and intestinal immune system is critical to maintain mucosal homeostasis… The intestinal mucosal immune system constitutes the largest immune component in vertebrates, functioning closely with the intestinal microbiome. The balance of the intestinal mucosa immune system plays a key role in host homeostasis and defense." – PubMed ID#PMC5408367 (2017) [40]

❖ MICROBIOME AND CANCER

You can probably tell by now that gut health is a big deal. The right beneficial bacteria can help improve your immune system and fight cancer; the wrong bacteria can weaken the immune system and cause or worsen cancer (and further push out beneficial bacteria). The right kind of bacteria can also greatly improve the effectiveness of immunotherapy (see Chapter 2). The microbial environment in the gut is called the "microbiome," and it is a very complex system of over a thousand bacteria species, yeasts and viruses (beneficial, harmful and freeloaders/commensal, known as "microbiota"). Maintaining the microbiome is of the utmost importance and you should not take anything that is going to screw it up (unless your doctors tell you that it might save your life or a limb, etc.) You can certainly "*Improve Your Odds*" against cancer by improving your gut microbiome and gut health.

I'm afraid there are many over-the-counter supplements that can damage the microbiome. Some are labeled to make you think they will help kill bad bacteria in the gut; however, most of these have been found to have antiseptic properties, that is, they are substances that can kill all microbes, good and bad. I cover all of this in much more detail in *The Gut Health Protocol* (and the Facebook group of the same name). Wiping out the good bacteria in your gut is not what you want!

Humans frequently have an altered immune response (where the immune system may ignore the bad cells or microbes while attacking the good ones) when exposed to certain components of unwanted and pathogenic bacteria, and this can result in autoimmune diseases. One of these compounds is lipopolysaccharide (LPS), found in the shell of certain gram-negative bacteria such as *E. coli* and *Klebsiella*; LPS is also known as an endotoxin. The other component mentioned in the study below is flagellins, which are found in the lash-like appendage, or whip-like tail, of certain bacteria such as *E. coli* and *H. pylori*. What the authors found was that when these bacteria were present in the gut, they could translocate to the pancreas and "shift macrophages, the key immune cells in the pancreas, into immune suppression." This will block the immune system's ability to attack cancer cells (and in this study, severely limit the effectiveness of PD-1 immunotherapy. But the same would also apply to other therapies; the immune system would not attack the cancer cells). The use of antibiotics has been shown to increase the number of T cells that can infiltrate and kill tumor cells; this is simply because it killed unwanted bacteria in the gut (but at the same time, antibiotics will weaken the microbiome, so there are often better ways of balancing the microbes in the gut). The key takeaway point here is that a healthy microbiome can benefit immune health (in several ways) and thus "*Improve Your Odds*" of beating cancer! You should strive to reduce unwanted bacteria and increase beneficial bacteria (which reduce and prevent unwanted bacteria, as well as directly benefit the immune system, as explained in Chapter 2).

> "bacteria that are more abundant in pancreatic cancers – including groups of species called proteobacteria, actinobacteria, and fusobacteria – release cell membrane components (e.g.,lipopolysaccharides) and proteins (e.g.,flagellins) that shift macrophages, the key immune cells in the pancreas, into immune suppression… Adding antibiotics improved the performance of a checkpoint inhibitor in a mouse model of PDA, as shown by an increase in T cells that could attack the tumors" – NYU.EDU (2018) [41]

The following research paper appeared in the prestigious journal *Science*. It found that gut microbiota could have a huge impact on many types of cancer—and not just of those of the gut, but also cancers including skin, breast and liver cancer. This is strong evidence that gut health exerts systemic influences over cancer (not just intestinal cancers), most likely through its powerful influence over the immune system.

> "alterations of the gut microbiota also influence the incidence and progression of extraintestinal cancers, including breast and hepatocellular carcinoma… the gut microbiota influences oncogenesis and tumor progression both locally and systemically… Accumulating evidence demonstrates that intestinal bacteria influence oncogenesis, tumor progression, and response to therapy." – PubMed ID#PMC4690201 (2015) [42]

Certain unwanted bacteria can promote cancer and release toxins. Developing a strong microbiome of beneficial bacteria will help get rid of unwanted bacteria in the gut (such as *E. coli*, mentioned below. Most strains of *E. coli* are strong endotoxin producers).

> "Bacteria are carcinogens and tumor promoters. Bacteria produce toxins that disrupt the cellular signal thus perturbing the regulation of cell growth. Also, they are potential tumor promoters through inducing inflammation" – PubMed ID#PMC5856380 (2018) [43]

> "bacteria that cause persistent infections produce toxins that specifically disrupt cellular signalling to perturb the regulation of cell growth or to induce inflammation. Other bacterial toxins directly damage DNA. Such toxins mimic carcinogens and tumour promoters and might represent a paradigm for bacterially induced carcinogenesis" – PubMed ID#15806096 (2005) [44]

> "Bacteria are the primary cause of UTIs, with the vast majority (70–80%) attributed specifically to infection with E. coli… A recurring theme in the link between bacterial infection and carcinogenesis is that of chronic inflammation, which is often a common feature of persistent infection. Conclusion: These findings suggested that urinary bladder infection by E. coli may play a major additive and synergistic role during bladder carcinogenesis." – PubMed ID#PMC3511874 (2012) [45]

Though the following research was focused on immunotherapy, it is becoming clear that a healthy microbiome can allow the immune system to fight and prevent cancers—not just gut cancer, but even malignant melanoma skin cancers! Our bodies create little cancers all the time (often just a few cells); it is our immune system that usually destroys them before they grow into harmful tumors and spread.

> "Evaluating the Role of the Gut Microbiome to Bolster Immunotherapy Response in Melanoma - Based on data seen in several mouse studies in

> Chicago and France, it is suggested that altering the microbiome may be necessary to promote responses to checkpoint inhibition. While this approach is being evaluated in non-small cell lung cancer and renal cancers, a group at the University of Pittsburgh, led by Hassane M. Zarour, MD, has designed a trial involving a subset of patients with melanoma." – Targeted Oncology [46]

Once again, we see where certain microbiota in the gut (and even some over-the-counter probiotics) can benefit the immune system in ways that treat and prevent cancers.

> "host immune responses to environmental microbes significantly impact and inhibit cancer progression in distal tissues such as mammary glands… This leads us to conclude that consuming fermentative microbes such as L. reuteri may offer a tractable public health approach to help counteract the accumulated dietary and genetic carcinogenic events integral in the Westernized diet and lifestyle." – PubMed ID#24382758 (2014) [47]

Lipopolysaccharide (LPS) molecules are endotoxins created by gram-negative bacteria; it is part of their cell wall. It can be found in bacteria such as *Shigella*, *E. coli*, *Klebsiella*, and *Salmonella*. Some strains of these bacteria are opportunistic and can live in the human gut without causing symptoms for long periods of time. However, given the right conditions, they can bloom forth and lead to disease or chronic conditions (such as diarrhea and abdominal bloating or pain). LPS are strongly proinflammatory and have been linked to at least a worsening of many forms of cancer. LPS are often produced by bacteria in our gut (especially *E. coli*), where they translocate into the systemic environment (the blood, organs and even our brain), or they can be produced by bacteria growing in the systemic environment (where an infection can be much more dangerous).

LPS can produce a strong immune response in humans. Besides eliciting a strong proinflammatory reaction (which can lead to cancer progression), LPS can basically keep the immune system preoccupied. We want the immune system focused on fighting cancer cells, not on fighting a gram-negative bacterial overgrowth. Worse yet, LPS can cause an overstimulation of the immune system, which then releases histamine (and other proinflammatories) that can end up harming healthy cells and making us feel cruddy. This histamine response leads to even more inflammation.

By rebalancing the microbiome and strengthening our gut's beneficial bacteria, we can help push out these unwanted opportunistic strains. In fact, beneficial bacteria can actually produce bactericides that help kill or hinder these unwanted competing bacteria (all the while providing health benefits to us).

> "bacterial lipopolysaccharide (LPS), and histamine in breast cancer cell adhesion to vascular endothelial cells… Histamine augmented the TNF-α effect… LPS is an important risk factor for cancer metastasis and that the elevated serum level of histamine further increases the risk of LPS-induced

cancer metastasis. Preventing bacterial infections is essential in cancer treatment" – PubMed ID#24333719 (2014) [48]

"Lipopolysaccharide induces inflammation and facilitates lung metastasis in a breast cancer model … Inflammation is a potent promoter of tumor metastasis… the number and size of metastatic lesions… were significantly greater in the lungs of LPS☐treated mice, as compared with those in control mice" – PubMed ID#25625500 (2015) [49]

"Lipopolysaccharide (LPS) increases the invasive ability of pancreatic cancer cells through the TLR4/MyD88 signaling pathway… Inflammation plays a multifaceted role in cancer progression, and NF-kappaB is one of the key factors connecting inflammation with cancer progression. We have shown that lipopolysaccharide (LPS) promotes NF-kappaB activation in colon cancer cells and pancreatic cancer cells… LPS increased the invasive ability of pancreatic cancer cells… TLR/MyD88/NF-kappaB signaling pathway plays a significant role in connecting inflammation and cancer invasion and progression." – PubMed ID#19722233 (2009) [50]

"Lipopolysaccharide-induced metastatic growth is associated with increased angiogenesis, vascular permeability and tumor cell invasion… Endotoxin/lipopolysaccharide (LPS), a cell wall component of Gram-negative bacteria, is a potent inflammatory stimulus… LPS-induced growth and metastasis of 4T1 experimental lung metastases is associated with increased angiogenesis, vascular permeability and tumor cell invasion/migration with iNOS expression implicated in LPS-induced metastasis." – PubMed ID#12216068 (2002) [51]

Since most of us now have some level of LPS-producing bacteria in our gut, we can all benefit from taking measures to reduce their levels.

❖ STRATEGY

Gut health is a huge topic, so I would like to again recommend that you read *The Gut Health Protocol* (available on Amazon), especially if you think you have any gut issues, but also even if you don't. As you can tell from this chapter and Chapter 2, proper gut health is vital to

---

preventing and fighting cancer. It is especially important to encourage the growth of beneficial bacteria in the gut, especially (but not limited to) Bifidobacterium strains.

Here are some of the major takeaway points from this chapter.

- If you have any diarrhea, or loose stools, once per week or more, you need to figure out why and deal with it. Diarrhea is not a natural condition, and it is harmful to the microbiome, general health and the immune system.

- Take a probiotic with Bifidobacterium strains. One that contains a phage complex to boost these strains throughout the intestine is preferred. See the book's website for recommendations.

- Consume a healthy diet that is low in sugar and refined foods and high in a variety of vegetables. Consume a small amount of low-sugar fruit daily, and engage in moderate consumption of organic grass-fed meats (organ meat is even better), which are high in nutrition. Also see Chapter 4 - Diet.

- Consume vegetables high in soluble fiber, as they are very important to a healthy microbiome. I would also try to consume more mushrooms (and powdered mushroom supplements) and brown seaweed if possible; both contain great sources of prebiotics. Mushrooms have excellent immunomodulating properties (see Chapter 6). You can take all the probiotics you want, but if you don't feed these bacteria, they won't do you nearly as much good.

- Many of the other supplements found in Chapter 6 are also beneficial to the microbiome. Be sure to include as many of these in your diet as you can.

- Consume more fermented foods, especially kefir, real sauerkraut, kimchi, miso and other wild fermented vegetables. These foods contain a diversity of beneficial bacteria strains (in amounts high enough to do a lot of good). They also contain a wide variety of other beneficial bacteria, bioavailable vitamins and minerals, and unique peptides with possible anticancer properties. Just make sure the brands you purchase contain live cultures.

Many Westerners tend to eat like children (and even children shouldn't be eating the way they do). Because we were brought up this way, changing our eating habits as adults is very difficult. However, if you have cancer, this is one of those things where your life may depend on trying.

We must decrease our intake of processed foods, refined carbohydrates, artificial sweeteners (stevia and monk fruit are fine), sugary sweets, milk/cream, etc. None of these foods were consumed by our ancient (and even not so ancient) ancestors. Our bodies simply aren't capable of living on these *unnatural* foods; day after day, year after year, they take their toll. Just as importantly, we lose out on some of the extraordinary benefits from healthier foods that we may not be accustomed to, such as seaweed, mushrooms, dark green leafy vegetables, and even vegetables we may never have heard of. I would recommend that you start by consuming something outside your comfort zone every day (and variety truly is important), working your way up to eating something new 2-3 times per day. Add mushrooms to an omelet, put some seaweed flakes in a casserole, drink a cup of kefir, eat a handful of walnuts, add some diced jicama to a salad, mix some mushroom powder in with your morning coffee (really, you'll hardly notice, and it doesn't hurt the flavor), etc., etc. The options are endless.

I would like to reiterate one last time: If you have gut issues, work on them. A healthy gut is key to immune system health, and the immune system is the most important part of preventing and fighting cancer.

If you would like more information on gut health, I would like to highly recommend my book, The Gut Health Protocol, available on Amazon. [52] I also have a specially formulated probiotic/prebiotic called "Phage Complete" that has helped thousands of people with their gut health. I formulated this myself and both my wife and I take it twice daily! [53] In accordance with FDA regulations, I make no cancer claims for this product. This product is not intended to diagnose, treat, cure or prevent any disease.

Updates at - https://improvingyourodds.com/

Support at - https://www.facebook.com/groups/cancer.improving.your.odds

◆ ❖ ◆

Chapter 4
Diets, A Scientific Approach

The good physician treats the disease; the great physician treats the patient who has the disease." ~ William Osler

We tend to think of a "diet" as something low-calorie, designed to make us lose weight, when in truth it simply means "a way of eating." We all consume our own "diet." There are many different diet plans out there depending on the outcome we need to achieve: lose weight, gain weight, control diabetes, consume no animal products (vegan diet), improve blood pressure, improve general health, etc. Changing our diet is something that most of us dread; it not only involves willpower, but also a change to our daily routine. Often it affects those around us as well; for example, will two different meals need to be prepared? Do we need to change what restaurant we eat at? What about telling Aunt Clara you can't eat her cake?

There have been many diets proposed to help treat or prevent cancer. Anyone can throw out theories, and (sorry) "dead people tell no tales," so without high-quality research, these theories are useless (otherwise, there may be 10 dead people out there for every 1 glowing testimonial, as the diet actually made the cancer worse for those 10). You'll find very few cancer diets that have a lot of good scientific evidence to support them. Keeping with the theme of this book, I'm only going to recommend those diets that have scientific research that shows efficacy (and I will steer you away from some that have evidence that the diet can make your cancer worse).

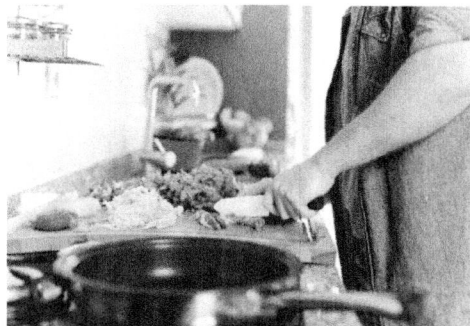

You cannot separate diet and nutrition; our diet is what normally provides us with nutrition. Chapter 6 will cover individual nutrients, and nutritional supplements, in much greater detail. This chapter is going to discuss the food we eat and reference the nutrients they contain, the latter of which are discussed in Chapter 6. I've looked at the science behind nearly every diet you can think of, and what is included here is what has been shown to work. When I say a diet "works," that means it has numerous scientific studies showing that it benefits cancer treatment and prevention. I will then cover a couple of the most popular diets that people use to fight cancer, but they may not work nearly as well as people think.

There are almost as many theories on a diet for cancer as there are people with cancer. Everyone has an opinion on this. Here are just a few of the things I've heard: fruit diet, no fruit diet, high carb, low carb, watermelon diet, vegan, vegetarian, Seventh-day Adventist, Breuss cancer treatment, Brandt Grape Cure, cabbage juice diet, celery juice diet, whole food diet, liquid diet, raw food diet, juice diet, paleo diet, alkaline diet, Budwig diet, Gerson Diet, metabolic diet, etc., etc. All are claimed to cure and/or prevent cancer. That cannot be possible as some of these diets are the complete opposites of each other.

Another thing I've noticed about diet is that many people take it very, very personally. Diets can become a religion to some people. We sometimes see this with vegans; after all, consuming meat means first killing an animal. All these diets have some number of devotees who are willing to say almost anything to support their diet and gain followers.

> *I get this image in my head of diet proselytizers at the farmer's market, with me playing the part of Captain Clarence Oveur (Peter Graves) in the 1980 spoof* Airplane! *I'm fighting my way past the vegetable stands through the throngs of zealots all trying to convince me that only their path is the right one.*

Yet, there is an increasing emphasis in the research community on the importance of diet in the prevention and treatment of various cancers. Judging from the hundreds of research studies on this topic, it is obvious that our diet can affect cancer outcomes. It can also increase or decrease our chances of contracting cancer in the first place. The right diet can certainly "*Improve Your Odds*" in the battle against cancer.

There is a lot of hype out there that someone with cancer—or trying to prevent cancer—should avoid red meat, or any meat. This will be covered later in this chapter when discussing vegan and no-meat diets. However, let me whet your appetite a little (or not). Red meat is not the problem; our ancestors have always consumed red meat—every generation and almost every tribe ever studied. Today, the problem is the quality of meat and the way it is prepared. You cannot consume an animal that was raised its entire life confined in a concrete bunker, constantly exposed to waste products (literally breathing in germs from waste all day), eating grains rather than green grass, getting no fresh air or sunlight, constantly under stress and fear, getting very little exercise and being pumped with hormones and antibiotics, and expect their meat to equal that which our ancestors consumed. Then we take this meat and process it with nitrates and other preservatives. We finish that by cooking it until the outside is charred (which creates carcinogens). All the while, we usually ignore the healthiest parts of the animal, the organs. Then we get sick and blame all meat? Buzzards eat better meat than we do! We need to eat more like our ancestors.

Evidence shows a much stronger cancer correlation with high-glycemic index foods, such as sugar, bread, wheat, pasta and potatoes, than it does with red meat. People eating more of these types of foods had a 49% increase in lung cancer and a whopping 92% increase in squamous cell carcinoma! To think, some people may see a reduction of 50% or more in cancer risk simply by changes to their diet! There are 268,600 new cases of invasive breast cancer each year, and researchers expect over 1,900,000 new cases of cancer (all types) in 2020! That is up 23% since 2010. Think about how many lives can be saved simply by changes in diet!

> Postprandial glucose (PPG) and insulin responses play a role in carcinogenesis… We observed a significant association between GI (glycemic index) and lung cancer risk and GIac (total available carbohydrate) and lung cancer risk. We observed a more pronounced association between GI and lung cancer risk among never smokers, (5th vs 1st Q OR=2.25, 95% CI: 1.42–3.57), squamous cell carcinomas (SCCs) (5th vs 1st Q OR=1.92, 95% CI: 1.30–2.83) – PubMed ID#PMC4780226 (2016) [54]

> "Participants with high free fructose and glucose intake were at a greater risk of developing pancreatic cancer (highest compared with lowest quintile, RR, 1.29; 95% CI" – PubMed ID#PMC2687095 (2009) [55]

> "A prospective cohort analysis of dietary carbohydrate and fiber intakes was conducted among 62,739 postmenopausal women… Rapidly absorbed carbohydrates are associated with postmenopausal breast cancer risk among overweight women and women with large waist circumference. Carbohydrate intake may also be associated with estrogen receptor-negative breast cancer." – PubMed ID#18469262 (2008) [56]

In part, this correlation with sugar (and carbs) is because cancer cells have a 10- to 17-fold higher consumption of glucose than nonmalignant cells. All that excess sugar in the blood literally feeds cancer. This is a well-known phenomenon called the Warburg effect, wherein cancer cells rely on glucose to support their high growth rate and cellular processes. Most cancer cells cannot utilize ketos (discussed in the next section), whereas normal cells can thrive on them (see PubMed ID#PMC2849637 [57]). This is the basis of the PET scan for detecting cancer, in which clinicians inject the patient with radioactive glucose prior to the scan. Cancer cells will absorb this at a much higher rate than normal cells.

> *Do you know what the most commonly consumed "vegetable" is? The potato, and yet it has a glycemic index (GI) of 83-89 (where pure glucose is 100). Compare this to sugar-sweetened ice cream, which has a GI of 61! The glycemic index is how well a food converts to glucose and how quickly. So, when I say you need to consume more vegetables, I am not talking about French fries!*

❖ STRATEGY

As the evidence will show, a ketogenic diet is the best diet for fighting and preventing cancer. However, not everyone does it correctly. A ketogenic diet for treating and preventing cancer should be diverse, high in nutritious foods, and vitamin- and mineral-dense, with plenty of low-carbohydrate vegetables, low-sugar fruit, soluble fiber and other prebiotic carbohydrates to feed our beneficial bacteria. If you cannot go low-carbohydrate enough to stay in ketosis (this will be discussed in the next section), then follow the rest of these guidelines while staying as close to ketosis as you can. Judging by the research, there is little doubt that sugar (all digestible carbohydrates convert to sugar in the body) feeds cancer. Sugar is one of the few foods for which there is evidence that it feeds cancer. Just remember that a ketogenic diet is not an all-meat diet; it doesn't even have to be a high-meat diet. Ketogenic book recommendations will be discussed later (with ketogenic vegan/vegetarian advice later in this chapter).

The object of this book is to improve people's odds at preventing and curing cancer, and thus saving their lives. It aims to do this by scouring as much research on the topic as I can find. In so doing, religion and philosophy will take a backseat. It is up to you to fit this information into your world and spiritual view; because of this, there is no one-size-fits-all diet. However, if you simply don't want to try a diet because you don't like it, or that it isn't what you grew up eating, don't expect to get very far in your efforts to *Improve Your Odds* of beating cancer. Cancer is serious, deadly serious. Do what you need to do to beat it. That doesn't mean simply switching to another diet that tells you pasta and honey will beat your cancer (with zero evidence to back up those claims). Follow the science, not your cravings, and not the person trying to placate you to sell more books or con you into taking them on as your health coach. I'm afraid there are a lot people out there doing this.

Best Diets for Beating Cancer (ranked in order)

1. Ketogenic diet combined with intermittent fasting – This must be done correctly with plenty of vegetables. See the next section for details.
2. Pure ketogenic diet – Stay barely in ketosis all the time. This means no sugar, very low carbs, high fat and moderate protein.
3. Low-carb diet – This diet is similar to the above, but usually with lower amounts of fat, ketogenic for only a few weeks, and again, plenty of vegetables. Try to combine with intermittent fasting.
4. Intermittent fasting – See that diet later in this chapter. Again, no sugar.
5. Vegan diet plus meat – WHAT?! OK, blasphemous, I know. But basically, eat like a vegan, with a small amount of meat or fish once or twice per day (along with vegetarian options). Fish and eggs are fine. Try to keep it as low in sugar and starches as you can. Intermittent fasting while on this diet helps even more.
6. Vegetarian/Seventh-Day Adventist – See vegan diet plus meat above.
7. No-sugar diet – Explained later, but pretty much what it says.

KETOGENIC DIET

Ötzi is the 5,300-year-old man found frozen in a glacier high up in the Ötztal Alps on the Austrian-Italian border. Shortly before I wrote this book, new research came out regarding the contents of Ötzi's stomach when he died. Ötzi, better known as "The Iceman," is discussed more in Chapter 6 regarding mushrooms, but it turns out he also showed evidence of nearly being on a ketogenic diet. Humans throughout history preferred nutrient-dense foods (such as the organs of animals) when they were available, as well as high-caloric foods (which at the time meant animal fat). Plant matter was often consumed (probably daily for most people), but when meat was available, it was usually consumed. Animal fat was a prized food.

Approximately 46% to 50% of Ötzi's full stomach consisted of fats. Most of the rest of the food was protein from ibex (a type of mountain goat) and red deer. Charcoal particles found in the stomach indicate that the food was cooked over fire. There was a small amount of einkorn seed (heritage wheat, but apparently unground so it didn't provide much nutritional value) as well as some inedible, and slightly toxic, fern (probably used to treat a parasite infection).

> "Iceman's last meal: fat and game meat from ibex and red deer supplemented with cereals from einkorn… He seems to have had a remarkably high proportion of fat in his diet, supplemented with fresh or dried wild meat, cereals, and traces of toxic bracken… The most abundant elements found in the stomach content were the nutritional minerals iron, calcium, zinc, magnesium, and sodium, consistent with the consumption of red meat or dairy products… These data suggest that the Iceman's last meal was well balanced in terms of essential minerals required for good health with no evidence of toxic heavy metals such as lead, cadmium, or arsenic. – Current Biology Journal (2018) (Creative Commons attribution available at the link) [58]

The analysis of one meal does not show that ancient people followed a ketogenic diet, but it does tend to indicate that meat was commonly consumed, and that fat was preferred over lean muscle meat. This assertion is one supported by many other research studies and archeological evidence. Since both deer and ibex are low in fat, it tends to indicate that the Iceman's last meal probably consisted mostly of the organ meats, which are much higher in fat and contain far more nutrition. The grain consumed by Ötzi is seasonal and may have been a much smaller part of his diet in the winter months.

The ancient diet was high in animal fat when animal fat was available to people. The organs were highly sought after because they were both high in fat (and thus calories and energy) and highly nutritious. Before agriculture became commonplace (8,000 to 10,000 years ago), grains were consumed sparingly; it was just far too much work to collect grains and mill them by hand to make them edible. The amount of energy used in this effort could often exceed the amount of energy received. Only once agriculture, and more modern milling techniques, became available did the energy-expended-to-energy-received ratio tilt in favor of grain consumption. Humans evolved on a diet high in animal fat and protein, supplemented with what they could gather. They also experienced a lot of lean times, when they would be in ketosis. Ketosis was not by choice, but rather due to a lack of sufficient calories; also, in the winter months the reliance was on meat and fish, rather than plants.

Humans have experienced ketosis since the beginning of their time on this planet (and probably quite often). The first recorded use of a ketogenic diet (rather than just a calorie-restricted diet that produces ketosis) was in the 1920s. The Mayo Clinic discovered that a ketogenic diet worked quite effectively to control seizures in epileptic children. This replaced fasting as a way of controlling epilepsy. They found that children thrived on a ketogenic diet (whereas they did not thrive on a calorie-restricted diet or when fasting) and they were much more likely to stay on the diet. This diet quickly became a worldwide first-line treatment for epilepsy and is still sometimes used for this condition (see "The Charlie Foundation for Ketogenic Therapies" [59] for more information).

By the way, nutritional ketosis is very different from diabetic ketosis. In non-diabetics, blood sugar levels will remain within normal ranges while in ketosis. When a diabetic goes into ketosis, they also have very high glucose levels due to a lack of insulin (or insulin not being effective for them). Nutritional ketosis has been found to be very safe in numerous research studies (and again, is prescribed to children for epilepsy).

No other diet has shown the same level of anticancer activity as the ketogenic diet. There is quite a bit of research on this diet and cancer, and some of it shows dramatic improvements in cancer outcomes. Cancer relies on high levels of blood glucose to survive, as most tumors cannot utilize fatty acids or ketones for energy. In fact, ketones can inhibit tumor growth and damage cancer cells (but not normal ones). These facts have been shown in study after study (abstracts to follow). Normal human cells, including brain cells, can thrive on ketones for energy, whereas cancer cells require glucose, so a ketogenic diet starves them. When you can feed healthy cells and starve cancerous cells, anything else you may do to kill or treat cancer simply works better. A ketogenic diet makes a perfect adjuvant treatment, starving cancer cells to put them at a distinct disadvantage when being treated with chemotherapy, radiation therapy, even immunotherapy. These therapies all benefit from a ketogenic diet.

The basics of a ketogenic diet are simple: Consume few enough carbohydrates and enough fat to cause your body to switch from burning sugars for energy (all carbohydrates are converted to glucose sugar in the body) to burning fat for energy. This diet can be calorie-neutral or one that causes weight loss; that is up to you. It is also possible to remain vegan and do a ketogenic diet, though it is more difficult (I've included a reference at the end of this section). You can consume more fat to make up the difference in calories from reducing carbohydrates; protein intake should remain about the same as normal. As some of the studies below indicate, a person who is underweight should not waste (lose excessive weight) on this diet if the calories are kept at normal levels. For someone underweight, there may be a little weight loss at first, but it should level off quickly. People who need to lose weight will probably lose weight while in ketosis, sometimes significantly, at least until their weight falls to an ideal level. There are

---

over-the-counter tests (and devices) for measuring whether you are in ketosis or not (but if you follow the rules, you'll most likely be in ketosis).

To be in a state of ketosis means to be burning fat for energy (dietary fat, and your body fat if you have excess), and to get there means going on a ketogenic diet. A true ketogenic diet is grounded in the basics of macronutrients, the types of calories you consume.

> "A calorically controlled very high-fat diet that should be at least 70 to 81% FAT, no more than 20% protein (optimally less than 15%) and absolutely no more than 5% total carbs." – KnowTheCause.Com [60]

Most people enter "ketosis" (the state of burning fat for energy, rather than sugar/carbohydrates) once they reduce their carb intake to less than 20 to 50 grams per day (this will vary from person to person). This switch may take 3 to 4 days (depending on your activity level and metabolism). They will stay in ketosis for as long as they keep their carb and protein levels at the levels needed for ketosis. Activity is encouraged, up to your abilities; even a small amount of activity is beneficial.

An important thing to remember about a ketogenic diet is that it is _not_ an all-meat diet. If you know someone on a ketogenic diet and meat is all they eat, they are doing it wrong. In fact, there are vegan versions of the ketogenic diet. Ketogenic simply means burning fat for energy, rather than carbohydrates. You can, and should, consume plenty of healthy, low-carbohydrate vegetables while eating ketogenic. These vegetables should be high in soluble fiber to keep your microbiome (the beneficial bacteria in your gut) alive and well. Many studies are showing a healthy microbiome is essential not only to staying well, but also to a strong immune system and to fighting cancer (new research is showing that people with a strong microbiome do much better on immunotherapy than those with a weakened microbiome). So, in short, a ketogenic diet can be described as: high fat, moderate protein, low carbohydrate, very low sugar, high dietary fiber, nutritionally rich foods, and lots of low-carbohydrate vegetables.

While reading information about ketogenic diets, remember that your main goal is to stay slightly ketogenic, all the time. You'll find many variations of the ketogenic diet. Some of these diets are geared towards bodybuilders, people wanting to lose weight, those coping with anxiety or depression, etc. Some of these ketogenic diets may be more extreme than what you need. You may also need to ignore some of the other information you come across, as it doesn't apply to you. What is important for you is to be ketogenic (in a state of ketosis) while eating very healthy food (again, including a wide variety of low-carbohydrate vegetables).

A ketogenic diet looks a lot like the Atkins Diet; in fact, some of the research mentions using a "modified Atkins Diet." However, there are some important differences. On the ketogenic diet you should try to avoid sugar alcohols; these are allowed on Atkins as they are often used as sugar substitutes. Atkins also uses a "phased" approach to weight loss, meaning that you can consume more carbs as time goes on; phase 4 of the Atkins Diet is no longer ketogenic. The Atkins Diet also does not cap protein intake; protein is capped on the ketogenic diet (you still consume plenty to meet the body's needs). This is because our bodies can convert protein to glucose if carbohydrate intake is too low, and this can cause us to stop burning fat for energy, thus halting ketosis. However, the diets have more similarities than differences, and it is easy to use Atkins Diet recipes to remain ketogenic with a few minor modifications.

You may have heard about the "glycemic index" in regard to food; if you visit a dietitian, they often bring it up. The glycemic index measures how much a food raises glucose levels two hours after consuming. But the glycemic index is not always the best way to measure how much of a food converts to sugar. A lot of food takes longer to convert. Basically, <u>all</u> carbohydrates that humans can digest and assimilate convert to glucose; some just take longer. The glycemic load should also be considered, as it is a better indicator of how much of the carbohydrates can be absorbed by the body (total). I've found it much easier to simply look at the carbohydrate number on packaged foods or look it up online. I then just keep my daily total below about 40 grams. On a ketogenic diet, after considering the total carb count, then consider the glycemic index (as you do not want blood sugar and insulin spikes).

For packaged foods, the amount of carbohydrates should be listed. For fresh foods, use any of the online calculators that show carbohydrates.

- http://nutritiondata.self.com/
- https://ndb.nal.usda.gov/ndb/search/list

Do not fall into the trap of consuming something high in carbohydrates simply because it may (or may not) have other healthy attributes. Honey is a prime example of this; people think that it has some sort of magical healing powers and that "natural" sugars are somehow better for us than processed sugars. When it comes to cancer and ketogenic diets, sugar is sugar, and cancer doesn't care, so you should avoid all forms of it (be sure to read the research abstracts below).

> *In terms of sugar content, honey is actually worse for you than a Snickers candy bar using either the glycemic index (GI) or the glycemic load. A Snickers bar (113 grams) has a GI of 55, but just ONE Tbsp of honey also has a GI of 55!!! That same Snickers bar (again, 113 grams) has a glycemic load (GL) of 35. 113 grams of honey has a glycemic load of over 48!!! Almost 50% higher than the Snickers bar!!! Raisins are even worse. A 113-gram serving of raisins has a GL of 53. So, if you're worried about cancer, diabetes, metabolic syndrome, etc., don't reach for honey, raisins or the Snickers bar!!*

I'm not saying the candy bars are better for you, but many people have a misconception about honey and natural sugars ("fruit good, refined factory sugar bad"), when in reality, cancer doesn't care where the sugar comes from.

In short, all commonly consumed digestible simple sugars are bad, regardless of where they come from. Since carbohydrates convert to sugar, they can be "bad" as well, especially if you consume more than you are burning off. In moderation our body can usually handle some "bad." A healthy person getting plenty of exercise doesn't have much to worry about from consuming moderate amounts of sugar and carbohydrates. But someone with cancer needs to

---

avoid dietary sugar (table sugar, fructose, lactose, dextrose, honey, etc.). Other carbohydrates should be consumed in strict moderation while following a ketogenic diet (perhaps with a little intermittent fasting).

The exception to the above is medicinal polysaccharides (such as those found in mushrooms). These are technically sugars; however, due to their complexity, humans cannot utilize them as a calorie source. Thus, these medicinal polysaccharides do not convert to glucose, and therefore they do not feed cancer; however, most beneficial bacteria in the gut do utilize them. Even when consumed in small amounts, they have anticancer properties; these are discussed in detail in Chapter 6.

Regardless of which ketogenic diet you use, I would encourage you to consume plenty of low-carb healthy vegetables and mushrooms. Vegetables contain a lot of nutrition, far more than just high levels of vitamins and minerals. The beneficial microbes in our gut, our microbiome, are a major component of our immune system (see Chapter 2), and these microbes need to be properly fed. The food they consume consists of soluble fibers, indigestible polysaccharides, resistant starch, beta-glucans and other substances only found in vegetables. The Standard American Diet (SAD) is not cancer preventative, and trying to eat SAD while on a ketogenic diet is not nearly as beneficial as trying to eat healthy and ketogenic.

The Resources section below will point you towards a lot more information to help get you started.

❖ RESEARCH

There is a large body of evidence showing the benefits of a ketogenic diet on cancer treatment. Most of the in vivo research, including xenografts, has been adjuvant alongside traditional therapies (such as chemotherapy). This is due to funding and grant bias (bias towards traditional medical therapies). However, when you see this kind of benefit across multiple types of cancer and multiple types of treatments, you can be pretty sure that a ketogenic diet has benefits of its own (with or without other treatments). Much of the in vitro research clearly shows the benefits of a ketogenic diet across a wide range of cancers, even without other treatments being used.

The following meta-analysis looked at 13 research studies that examined the effects of a ketogenic diet (KD) on tumor growth. 9 of them looked at both tumor growth and survival time. All 13 studies showed the diet to have clear benefits for inhibiting tumor growth, and all 9 studies that looked at survival time found significant improvements to survival time for those in the KD groups.

> "A ketogenic diet consists of high fat, with moderate to low protein content, and very low carbohydrates, which forces the body to burn fat instead of glucose for adenosine triphosphate (ATP) synthesis. Generally, the ratio by weight is 3:1 or 4:1 fat to carbohydrate+protein, yielding a diet that has an energy distribution of about 8% protein, 2% carbohydrate, and 90% fat…

studies have shown that ketogenic diets reduce tumor growth and improve survival in animal models of malignant glioma, colon cancer, gastric cancer, and prostate cancer. Furthermore, ketogenic diets have been hypothesized, with some supporting evidence, to potentiate the effects of radiation in malignant glioma models as well as in non-small cell lung cancer models... Evidence of ketogenic diets increasing cancer cell oxidative stress is present both clinically and in animal models... Combining a ketogenic diet with hyperbaric oxygen therapy decreased tumor growth rate, increased mean survival time, and increased β-hydroxybutyrate compared to controls in a metastatic mouse cancer model. Thus combining a ketogenic diet with hyperbaric oxygen may further increase the oxidative stress inside of tumor cells." – PubMed ID#PMC4215003472 (2014) [61]

Open Access attribution - Allen BG, Bhatia SK, Anderson CM, et al. Ketogenic diets as an adjuvant cancer therapy: History and potential mechanism. Redox Biol. 2014;2:963–970. doi:10.1016/j.redox.2014.08.002

Increasing survival time is very important. Besides the fact that it means you're walking the planet longer, it also slows down the progression of cancer, giving other therapies more time work, and thus *Improving Your Odds*. The following meta-study reviewed 268 research articles, and of those, 13 were eligible for inclusion in the study. This once again shows that a ketogenic diet clearly benefits cancer treatment; the diet also works very well with other treatments, increasing their effectiveness. (KD = Ketogenic Diet, SD = Standard Diet)

"mice with systematic metastatic cancer that used KD represented a significant increase in survival time compare to control group. Also, bioluminescent signal showed a clear trend of reduced tumor growth." In another study "Mice were injected with gastric tumor cells and then, randomly were divided into two feeding groups; either a KD or a standard diet (SD). The tumor growth and mean survival time in the KD group were significantly reduced and induced respectively, compared to the SD group... In this study, all included articles indicate that KD had a inhibitory effect on tumor growth and 9 researches expressed that KD could enhance survival time. Among these researches, the greatest effect was seen for the KD with omega 3 fatty acids 21.8%, MCT 36.2%, lard 11%, carbohydrate 3% and protein 20%" – PubMed ID#PMC5450454 (2017) (Open Access attribution available at the link) [62]

Most cancers require large amounts of glucose; without this glucose supply, their growth and proliferation are greatly reduced. When combining a ketogenic diet with hyperbaric oxygen therapy, there was a significant decrease in the tumor growth rate and a 77.9% increase in mean survival time compared to controls. This again shows that decreasing sugar/carbs in the diet and increasing oxygen to the cells can have a dramatic impact on cancer survival.

> "Abnormal cancer metabolism creates a glycolytic-dependency which can be exploited by lowering glucose availability to the tumor. The ketogenic diet (KD) is a low carbohydrate, high fat diet which decreases blood glucose and elevates blood ketones and has been shown to slow cancer progression in animals and humans… KD alone significantly decreased blood glucose, slowed tumor growth, and increased mean survival time by 56.7% in mice with systemic metastatic cancer." – PubMed ID#23755243 (2013) [63]

Combining different treatments often provides better results than simply the sum of the two. The following research looked at lung cancer tumors (using a xenograft model of human lung cancers grafted into mice). Treatment consisted of radiation therapy combined with a ketogenic diet. The study found that adding a ketogenic diet slowed tumor growth compared to the controls. Other studies have shown that a ketogenic diet helps people better tolerate radiation therapy.

> "The ketogenic diets combined with radiation resulted in slower tumor growth in both NCI-H292 and A549 xenografts (P < 0.05), relative to radiation alone. The ketogenic diet also slowed tumor growth when combined with carboplatin and radiation, relative to control… These results show that a ketogenic diet enhances radio-chemo-therapy responses in lung cancer xenografts" – PubMed ID#23743570 (2013) [64]

This research, appearing in the journal *Frontiers in Molecular Neuroscience*, shows clear benefits of a ketogenic diet in glioma (an aggressive type of brain cancer) treatment. The diet was especially beneficial in conjunction with radiation treatments (adjuvant therapy). In a study where mice were implanted with human glioma cells, those receiving just radiation therapy (and standard mouse chow) survived about 70 days, and all were dead after about 150 days. **In the mouse group that both received radiation therapy and were on a ketogenic diet, 80% of the mice were still alive after 250 days.** The paper goes on to evaluate human clinical trials where a ketogenic (KD) or a caloric restriction (CR) diet were used (the CR diets also caused a state of ketosis).

> "a reduction in tumor growth could be achieved by decreasing glucose availability, which can be accomplished through pharmacological means or through the use of a high-fat, low-carbohydrate ketogenic diet (KD). The KD, as the name implies, also provides increased blood ketones to support the energy needs of normal tissues… The variety of effects seen when glucose in lowered and/or ketones are increased suggests that this may also potentiate other therapies, including newer immune- and targeted therapies… This

suggests that the ketone bodies themselves possess antitumor effects… Taken together, the preclinical data provides strong support for the clinical use of the KD or CR as an adjuvant therapy for the treatment of gliomas and other cancers." In regards to human studies "The case reports described above along with numerous anecdotal reports suggest that the KD may be a promising anti-cancer therapy" – PubMed ID#PMC5110522 (2016) (Open Access attribution at the link) [65]

A strict calorie-restricted diet will induce ketosis. However, studies have shown that calorie restriction is neither necessary nor desirable. As outlined earlier, one can enter ketosis simply by restricting carbohydrates and increasing fat intake (to maintain calories). This provides the desired benefits and allows for a diet that is much easier to follow. Here a ketogenic diet was shown to "significantly decrease" neuroblastoma growth.

"Ketogenic diet and/or calorie restriction significantly reduced tumor growth and prolonged survival in the xenograft model. Neuroblastoma growth reduction correlated with decreased blood glucose concentrations and was characterized by a significant decrease in Ki-67 and phospho-histone H3 levels in the diet groups with low tumor growth… targeting the metabolic characteristics of neuroblastoma could open a new front in supporting standard therapy regimens… we propose that a ketogenic diet and/or calorie restriction should be further evaluated as a possible adjuvant therapy for patients undergoing treatment for neuroblastoma." – PubMed ID#26053068 (2015) [66]

In this study, tumor growth was significantly delayed with a ketogenic diet, compared to that in the standard diet group. The ketogenic diet was unrestricted, meaning the mice could consume as much food as they wished.

"Tumors are largely unable to metabolize ketone bodies for energy due to various deficiencies in one or both of the key mitochondrial enzymes, which may provide a rationale for therapeutic strategies that inhibit tumor growth by administration of a ketogenic diet with average protein but low in carbohydrates and high in fat… The tumor growth in the MKD and LKD groups was significantly delayed compared to that in the SD [Standard Diet] group… Application of an unrestricted ketogenic diet delayed tumor growth in a mouse xenograft model." – PubMed ID#25773851 (2015) [67]

This study out of the University of Nebraska Medical Center shows how a ketogenic diet can be beneficial against pancreatic cancer. This study was a xenograft in vivo model using mice; a xenograft is where human cancer cells are grafted onto the organs of mice. Here the cancer cells grow, or are inhibited, as if they were in humans. The ketogenic diet significantly inhibited the growth of pancreatic cancer cells and induced apoptosis (causing the death of just cancer cells).

"We observed reduced glycolytic flux in tumor cells upon treatment with ketone bodies. Ketone bodies also diminished glutamine uptake, overall ATP content, and survival in multiple pancreatic cancer cell lines, while inducing apoptosis… Ketone body-induced intracellular metabolomic reprogramming in pancreatic cancer cells also leads to a significantly diminished cachexia in cell line models. Our mouse orthotopic xenograft models further confirmed the effect of a ketogenic diet in diminishing tumor growth and cachexia… our studies demonstrate that the cachectic phenotype is in part due to metabolic alterations in tumor cells, which can be reverted by a ketogenic diet, causing reduced tumor growth and inhibition of muscle and body weight loss." – PubMed ID#25228990 (2014) [68]

Cancer cells rely on large amounts of glucose to survive; the studies are overwhelming in this regard. Without glucose, cancer cells cannot proliferate. In fact, when you get a PET scan to detect cancer, they use a radioactive form of glucose. This glucose gets rapidly taken up by the cancer cells and is easily differentiated from normal cells on the PET scan. A ketogenic diet restricts the amount of glucose available to cancer cells and provides "ketones," a form of energy that normal cells can easily utilize, but again, most cancer cells cannot.

"markedly increased uptake and utilization of glucose have been documented in many human tumor types, most readily by noninvasively visualizing glucose uptake using positron emission tomography (PET) with a radiolabeled analog of glucose (18F-fluorodeoxyglucose, FDG) as a reporter." – Cell journal doi: 10.1016/j.cell.2011.02.013 [69]

The following study looked at a ketogenic diet's ability to benefit cachectic cancer patients (those who experience physical wasting caused by advanced cancer, with symptoms including weight loss, wasting of muscle, and loss of appetite). It is important to include good levels of high-quality fats, including omega-3, MCT and saturated fats.

"Overall, application of the unrestricted ketogenic diet was highly significantly associated with survival… Compared to the applied standard diet, the unrestricted ketogenic diet had a retarding effect on tumour growth and resulted in larger necrotic areas within the tumours… cancer cachexia accounts for about 20% of cancer deaths… Ketogenic diets, however, with high fat, adequate protein and low carbohydrates, have been shown to prevent or limit the protein catabolism in skeletal muscle… A non-restricted ketogenic diet may thus indeed be capable of benefiting cachectic cancer patients when supplemented with adequate lipids. The ketogenic diet described in this study induced both a slight increase in body weight and a slower growth rate of human tumour cells… a carbohydrate-restricted diet supplemented by lipids rich in omega-3 fatty acids and MCT delays the growth of glucose fermenting tumours. The effect did not depend on caloric restriction and there was no loss of body weight." --- PubMed ID#PMC2408928 (2008) (Open Access license attribution available at the link) [70]

The following 2017 meta-study looked at 468 clinical trials and human research studies that examined ketogenic dieting for treating cancer, which took place between the years 1985 and 2017. This number was eventually whittled down to 214 that met the study's criteria.

"preclinical studies have shown the effect of ketogenic diet to reduce tumor growth and improve survival in animal models of malignant glioma, prostate cancer, colon cancer, and gastrointestinal cancer… As described above, we could conclude that in order to see any significant progression or improvement by ketogenic diet, at least 3 to 4 weeks of ketogenic diet is required." – PubMed ID#PMC5624453 (2017) [71]

In the following meta-analysis, the authors looked at 29 animal and 24 human studies. The studies varied widely in what cancers were studied, length of study, reasons for excluding patients from the study, and how well compliance was monitored. Still the results showed that a ketogenic diet clearly has anti-tumor benefits, especially when combined with other treatments.

"All available human studies were systematically analyzed and supplemented with results from animal studies. Evidence and confirmation were treated as separate concepts. In total, 29 animal and 24 human studies were included in the analysis. The majority of animal studies (72%) yielded evidence for an anti-tumor effect of KDs… Feasibility of KDs for cancer patients has been shown in various contexts. The probability of achieving an anti-tumor effect seems greater than that of causing serious side effects when offering KDs to cancer patients." – PubMed ID#28653283 (2017) [72]

The following paper summarizes a few of the many research studies on ketogenic diets treating and preventing cancer. As with many of the studies quoted here, each of the statements below point to actual research studies as evidence. It is clear that a ketogenic diet provides several benefits in the fight against cancer tumors and the prevention of cancer formation.

> "**Insulin** has been shown to stimulate mitogenesis (even in cells lacking IGF-1 receptors) and it **may also contribute by stimulating multiple cancer mechanisms, including proliferation, protection from apoptotic stimuli, invasion and metastasis**… Considering the obvious relationship between carbohydrates and insulin (and IGF-1) a connection between carbohydrate and cancer is a possible consequence… **insulin inhibition caused by a ketogenic diet could be a feasible adjunctive treatment for patients with cancer.** In summary, perhaps through glucose 'starvation' of tumour cells and by reducing the effect of direct insulin-related actions on cell growth, ketogenic diets show promise as an aid in at least some kind of cancer therapy… In the 1980s, seminal animal studies by Tisdale and colleagues demonstrated that a ketogenic diet was capable to reduce tumour size in mice, whereas more recent research has provided evidence that ketogenic diets may reduce tumour progression in humans, at least as far as gastric and brain cancers are concerned… ketogenic diets show promise as an aid in at least some kind of cancer therapy and is deserving of further and deeper investigation" – PubMed ID#PMC3826507 (2013) (Creative Commons attribution at the link) [73]

This long-term study looked at over 62,500 men and women and found that a moderately low-carbohydrate, high-protein diet—regardless of the quantity of fat intake—was not related to cancer or other health risk factors. This study did not look at truly ketogenic diets, which are even lower in carbohydrates. However, this indicates that high-protein diets are not a risk factor for cancer.

> "Results - LCHP (low-carbohydrate, high-protein) score was not related to cancer risk, except for a non-dose-dependent, positive association for respiratory tract cancer that was statistically significant in men… These largely null results provide important information concerning the long-term safety of moderate carbohydrate reduction and consequent increases in protein and, in this cohort, especially fat intakes." – PubMed ID#PMC3654894 (2013) [74]

The following is based on an actual human trial (ClinicalTrials.gov#NCT01535911 [75]) involving glioma (brain cancer) patients.

> "We conclude that 1. KD is safe and without major side effects; 2. ketosis can be induced using customary foods; 3. treatment with KD may be effective in controlling the progression of some gliomas; and 4. further studies are needed to determine factors that influence the effectiveness of KD, whether as a

monotherapy, or as adjunctive or supplemental therapy in treating glioma patients." – PubMed ID#PMC4371612 (2015) [76]

In this research they looked at supplementing ketones in a controlled in vivo study with mice with metastatic cancer. This study looked to maintain calories while increasing ketones in the body. This ruled out calorie restriction as the reason for the benefits shown. They found a 50% to 69% increase in survival time in the mice fed the ketone precursors.

"Ketone supplementation prolonged survival and induced a trend of reduced tumor burden in mice with metastatic cancer… dietary administration of ketone precursors, BD (1,3-butanediol) and KE (ketone ester), increased mean survival time by 51 and 69%, respectively, in VM-M3 mice with metastatic cancer. These data support the use of supplemental ketone administration as a feasible and efficacious cancer therapy" – PubMed ID#PMC4235292 (2014) [77]

Here the authors show that brain tumor cells cannot utilize ketone bodies for energy, whereas normal cells can. In the full study it is pointed out that as long as brain tumors are provided proper glucose levels, they will survive; when glucose is restricted (and ketones take its place), their growth will either be severely restricted, or the tumor cells will perish.

"Targeting energy metabolism in brain cancer with calorically restricted ketogenic diets… Information is presented on the calorically restricted ketogenic diet (CRKD) as an alternative therapy for brain cancer. In contrast to normal neurons and glia, which evolved to metabolize ketone bodies as an alternative fuel to glucose under energy-restricted conditions, brain tumor cells are largely glycolytic due to mitochondrial defects and have a reduced ability to metabolize ketone bodies. The CRKD is effective in managing brain tumor growth in animal models and in patients, and appears to act through antiangiogenic, anti-inflammatory, and proapoptotic mechanisms." – PubMed ID#19049606 (2008) [78]

"ketone bodies possess many characteristics that can impair cancer cell survival and proliferation… Clearly, ketone bodies exhibit several unique characteristics that support their use as a metabolic therapy for cancer… dietary administration of ketone precursors, BD and KE, increased mean survival time by 51 and 69%, respectively, in VM-M3 mice with metastatic cancer (Fig. (Fig.3).3). These data support the use of supplemental ketone administration as a feasible and efficacious cancer therapy, which should be further investigated in additional animal models to determine its potential for clinical use." – PubMed ID#PMC4235292 (2014) [79]

Open Access Attribution - Poff AM, Ari C, Arnold P, Seyfried TN, D'Agostino DP. Ketone supplementation decreases tumor cell viability and prolongs survival of mice with metastatic cancer. Int J Cancer. 2014;135(7):1711–1720. doi:10.1002/ijc.28809

"Evidence exists that chronically elevated blood glucose, insulin and IGF1 levels facilitate tumorigenesis and worsen the outcome in cancer patients… Epidemiological and anthropological studies indicate that restricting dietary CHOs (dietary carbohydrates) could be beneficial in decreasing cancer risk… Studies conducted so far have shown that such diets are safe and likely beneficial, in particular for advanced stage cancer patients… CHO restriction mimics the metabolic state of calorie restriction or - in the case of KDs - fasting. The beneficial effects of calorie restriction and fasting on cancer risk and progression are well established. CHO restriction thus opens the possibility to target the same underlying mechanisms without the side-effects of hunger and weight loss… a multitude of mouse studies indeed proved anti-tumor effects of KDs for various tumor types, and a few case reports and pre-clinical studies obtained promising results in cancer patients as well." – PubMed ID#PMC3267662 (2011) [80]

Open Access attribution - Klement RJ, Kämmerer U. Is there a role for carbohydrate restriction in the treatment and prevention of cancer?. Nutr Metab (Lond). 2011;8:75. Published 2011 Oct 26. doi:10.1186/1743-7075-8-75

❖ SAFETY

Ketogenic diets have been used for many years to treat a variety of conditions, most notably seizures in children. The approach has been used to treat epilepsy in China since 400 BCE and has been used at the Mayo Clinic in the US since 1921. The diet continues to be used today for this purpose, especially in young children for whom surgery isn't an option.

The safety of a ketogenic diet has been shown in many different research studies. The following are just a few of them.

"The present study shows the beneficial effects of a long-term ketogenic diet. It significantly reduced the body weight and body mass index of the patients. Furthermore, it decreased the level of triglycerides, LDL cholesterol and blood glucose, and increased the level of HDL cholesterol. Administering a ketogenic diet for a relatively longer period of time did not produce any significant side

> effects in the patients. Therefore, the present study confirms that it is safe to use a ketogenic diet for a longer period of time than previously demonstrated."
> – PubMed ID#PMC2716748 (2004) [81]

All systems go… in this 2017 study a very low-carbohydrate ketogenic diet was shown to be completely safe. They compared a low-carbohydrate ketogenic state to diabetic ketoacidosis. These two states were shown to be very different in nature, with the main difference being that glucose levels are significantly higher in diabetic ketoacidosis (and yet the cells are unable to utilize this glucose). In short, ketogenic dieting is safe and healthy; diabetic ketoacidosis is dangerous.

> "blood pH; plasma bicarbonate; plasma glucose as well as anion gap or osmolarity were not statistically modified at four months after a total weight reduction of 20.7 kg in average and were within the normal range throughout the study. Even at the point of maximum ketosis all variables measured were always far from the cut-off points established to diabetic ketoacidosis… During the course of a VLCK diet there were no clinically or statistically significant changes in glucose, blood pH, anion gap and plasma bicarbonate. Hence the VLCK diet can be considered as a safe nutritional intervention" – PubMed ID#PMC5608861 (2017) [82]

The "temporary constipation and fatigue" below are usually just that, temporary, and relieved by increasing water consumption, increasing soluble fiber intake and maintaining calories by consuming more fat. But again, no other adverse side effects were noted, including to cholesterol levels.

> "Except for temporary constipation and fatigue, we found no severe adverse side effects, especially no changes in cholesterol or blood lipids… a KD is suitable for even advanced cancer patients. It has no severe side effects and might improve aspects of quality of life and blood parameters in some patients with advanced metastatic tumors." – PubMed ID#21794124 (2011) [83]

❖ R ESOURCES

A full "how to" is beyond the scope of this book; however, there are dozens of books, and cookbooks, about ketogenic dieting. If you search Amazon, you'll easily find them; there is also a very large amount of free information on the internet. Ketogenic dieting is all the rage right now, so there is no shortage of books and resources. There are even a few books written specifically for using a ketogenic diet to fight cancer.

- *Keto for Cancer: Ketogenic Metabolic Therapy as a Targeted Nutritional Strategy* by Miriam Kalamian and Thomas N. Seyfried, October 2017 [84] – This book will pick up where this one leaves off on understanding and implementing a ketogenic diet for cancer. Though it can help you figure out how to eat keto, it is not a recipe book.

- *The Easy Keto Meal Prep: 800 Easy and Delicious Recipes* by Aphanie Kalton [85] – As the title mentions, a whole lot of keto recipes. Each recipe lists the carb count, so it will be easy to come up with your own meal plans and snacks.

- *Keto Meal Prep* by Liz Williams, December 2018 [86] – Some of the recipes have too high of a carb count to stay in ketosis (consuming 3 meals per day). You may need to modify some of the recipes a little.

- *KetoFast* by Dr. Joseph Mercola [87] – Spends a lot of time covering the benefits of ketogenic dieting and fasting. The approach is sort of a combination of intermittent fasting, long fasting and ketogenic dieting. I liked the overview and benefits of the approach more than the implementation.

There are also a large number of online resources, including blogs, how-to websites, Facebook support groups, etc. Here are a few online resources to get started:

Websites

- Keto Dash (https://ketodash.com)
- Perfect Keto (https://www.perfectketo.com)
- Ketogenic Forums (https://www.ketogenicforums.com)

Facebook Groups

- Ketogenic Lifestyle (over 900,000 users!)
- Ketogenic Diet Recipes (over 170,000 users)
- Ketogenic Diet Beginners (over 150,000 users)

Ketogenic books usually do not have cancer treatment or prevention in mind, so you'll need to make some minor tweaks. So, whether you read one of these books or you are already familiar with ketogenic dieting, there are a few things to keep in mind.

- Avoid polyunsaturated oils (PUFA for short), such as "vegetable" oil, sunflower seed oil, peanut oil and even canola oil. These oils are highly reactive and go rancid easily. Though it can happen in the bottle, this is even more of a problem at the cellular level. Reactive oils are not good for cancer or the immune system.

- Another thing to consider is our ancestors (and all mammals) consumed a much lower ratio of omega-6 to omega-3 PUFAs. Today most Westerners consume a ratio of about a 20:1 omega-6 to omega-3 fats, whereas our ancestors had a ratio of about 1:1; even about 200 years ago, this was about 3:1. This is a huge (2,000%) difference, and one our body is not built to handle. Try to keep the amount of omega-6 (e.g., vegetable oils) to a minimum.

- There are both plant and animal sources of omega-3, with most animal sources coming from fish. The plant source is alpha-linolenic acid (ALA), and it can be found in hemp seeds, flax seeds, pumpkin seeds, tofu, soy beans and walnuts. The type of omega-3s found in fish are eicosapentanaenoic acid (EPA) and docosahexaenoic acid (DHA). EPA and DHA are much healthier for us than ALA, and although the body can convert AHA to EPA and DHA, this is a very inefficient process. Therefore, 1 gram of AHA does not convert to 1 gram of EPA/DHA. For this reason, it is much better to obtain your omega-3s from fish and fish oils. This topic will be discussed more in Chapter 6 as it is an important one for fighting cancer and improving the immune system.

- Many ketogenic diets do not stress the importance of eating a diet high in vegetables and low-calorie fruit. Though I discuss this earlier in this section, it is worth repeating. Do not eat a caveman/carnivore diet; it is not necessary and is certainly not preferred. Include a low-carbohydrate vegetable of some kind in every meal. Variety is important, so you may want to eat a small amount of several vegetables with your meal. Salads are great for this (avoid iceberg lettuce; it is all but useless nutritionally). So be sure to consume a wide variety of low-starch/low-carbohydrate vegetables. You can always add some diced chicken, bacon, etc., for flavor and protein.

- Try to consume most of your vegetables <u>cooked</u>. Though raw vegetables are in vogue right now, cooked vegetables are more nutritious. Raw vegetables have much of their nutrition bound up in the insoluble fiber (such as cellulose), and they also contain antinutrients that mostly get neutralized by cooking. For these reasons much of the nutrition in raw vegetables never gets absorbed by the small intestine. Cooking releases these bonds and allows us to absorb the vitamins and minerals. Cooking also makes some insoluble fiber better available to our microbial friends. Consuming some raw vegetables is fine, but focus on cooked vegetables. Either way, try to consume organic when you can.

- Avoid sugar alcohols. Some recipes, especially diet dessert recipes, may include ingredients that contain sugar alcohols. These taste sweet, but our bodies cannot utilize them as a carbohydrate. However, they feed the wrong kind of bacteria in our gut and harm the microbiome (a huge part of our immune system). Sugar alcohols are commonly found in commercial diet treats (such as Atkins bars). Here is a partial list of sugar alcohols to avoid: erythritol, hydrogenated starch hydrolysates (HSH), isomalt, lactitol, maltitol, mannitol, sorbitol and xylitol. Any ingredient ending in "itol" should be suspect. Glycerin is also a sugar alcohol and is commonly found in processed foods and some nutritional supplements.

- Purchase a ketogenic cookbook. Though there are thousands of very good recipes online, this will give you the motivation to try something new.

Once you understand the basics of a ketogenic diet and the tweaks for treating cancer, you should be able to easily modify the thousands of online recipes. You can even do things like combining a good vegan vegetable recipe with a pork chop recipe.

❖ MCT OIL

Medium-chain triglycerides (MCT) are a type of fat commonly found in coconut and palm oils. Lesser amounts can also be found in cheese, butter, milk and yogurt. MCTs are rapidly absorbed into the portal venous system and subsequently enter cells without the need for fatty acid transport proteins. This process is much more efficient than the long-chain fatty triglycerides more commonly found in our diet. The word "triglycerides" simply refers to fats or lipids carried in the blood. The triglycerides that show up on your cholesterol test mostly come from sugars and carbohydrates (in your diet) that the body converts to fat for storage. MCTs, on the other hand, can help reduce body fat while increasing lean muscle mass. MCTs can also be used to reduce cholesterol levels and reduce blood levels of triglycerides. MCTs have been used to treat various medical conditions, such as gallbladder disease, AIDS, cystic fibrosis, Alzheimer's disease, and seizures in children. [88]

MCT oil has also been researched for cancer treatment and prevention. MCT oil should be used conjunctively with a ketogenic diet. It is important that your MCT oil only contains C8 and C10 carbon chains (look for it on the bottle).

> "The ketogenic diet used here provides average protein and is low in carbohydrates and high in fat enriched with omega-3 fatty acids and MCT (MKD) or with lard only (LKD). Compared to the applied standard diet, the unrestricted ketogenic diet (both LKD and MKD) had a retarding effect on tumor growth and resulted in larger necrotic areas within the tumors. Although the difference is not significant, there is a tendency that MKD is more efficient than LKD. Blood glucose levels in MKD and LKD group were unaltered, while their ketone body levels were significantly elevated compared to those of the SD group. **In contrast to most conventional cancer chemotherapies, which indiscriminately target both normal cells and tumor cells, ketogenic diets are the only known therapies that can target tumor cells while enhancing the health and vitality of normal cells.** In this regard, the ketogenic diet for cancer management stands apart from all conventional therapeutic approaches." -- journal.waocp.org (2015) [89]

> Open Access citation - DOI:http://dx.doi.org/10.7314/APJCP.2015.16.5.2061Growth of Human Colon Cancer Cells in Nude Mice is Delayed by Ketogenic. Guang-Wei Hao&, Yu-Sheng Chen&, De-Ming He, Hai-Yu Wang, Guo-Hao Wu1, Bo Zhang

The following study looked at supplementing MCT C8 and C10 in neuroblastoma (NB) cancer lines (in a xenograft mouse study. In a xenograft, human cancer cells or tumors are grafted onto mice). This was done in conjunction with a ketogenic diet (KD).

> "Based on our findings in the present study, we hypothesize that enrichment of an ad libitum KD with specific triglycerides can increase the efficacy of NB therapy similar to that achieved with calorie-restricted KDs. Furthermore, such lipid-modified KDs may enable to use reduced doses of chemotherapy, according to the synergy we observed here between the KDs and the metronomic CP treatment." – PubMed ID#PMC5630289 (2017) [90]

Many of the studies looked at supplementing omega-3 fatty acids and MCT while on a ketogenic diet.

> "therapeutic strategies that inhibit tumour growth by administration of a ketogenic diet with average protein but low in carbohydrates and high in fat enriched with omega-3 fatty acids and medium-chain triglycerides (MCT)... Application of an unrestricted ketogenic diet enriched with omega-3 fatty acids and MCT delayed tumour growth in a mouse xenograft model." – PubMed ID#18447912 (2008) [91]

MCT oil increased serum ketone levels, which assists a ketogenic diet.

> "Consumption of 56 g/day of MCTs for 24 weeks increases serum ketone concentrations" – PubMed ID#PMC4669977 (2015) [92]

> "These results suggest that diets containing MCT would provide the best ketogenic regime to reverse the weight loss in cancer cachexia with a concomitant reduction in tumour size." – PubMed ID#3219268 (1988) [93]

❖ LOW-SUGAR DIET

Much of this topic is covered under the ketogenic diet section above, and the details won't be repeated here. I have included a few more facts regarding sugar and why avoiding it can be very helpful when treating cancer.

> *Cancer cells have a 10- to 17-fold higher consumption of glucose than nonmalignant cells.*

Fructose (found in fruit) is sugar, and it is every bit as dangerous to us as refined sugar (in fact, table sugar is 50% fructose). Cancer cells can utilize fructose when glucose is not available to them; they cannot utilize amino acids (e.g., from protein).

> "Rapid proliferation and Warburg effect make cancer cells consume plenty of glucose... Recent studies have revealed a close correlation between excessive fructose consumption and breast cancer genesis and progression... we found that fructose, not amino acids, could functionally replace glucose to support proliferation of breast cancer cells. Fructose endowed breast cancer cells with the colony formation ability and migratory capacity as effective as glucose...

Furthermore, we demonstrated that the fructose diet promoted metastasis of 4T1 cells in the mouse models… fructose can be used by breast cancer cells specifically in glucose-deficiency, and suggest that the high-fructose diet could accelerate the progress of breast cancer in vivo." – PubMed ID#PMC5622605 (2017) (Open Access license attribution at the link) [94]

In addition, fructose "is tightly linked to many metabolic diseases, such as non-alcoholic fatty liver disease, insulin resistance, diabetes, hypertension, hyperlipidemia, cardiovascular and cerebrovascular diseases, obesity and chronic consumption" (quote from above study).

The following study clearly showed that carbohydrate intake (which includes sugar and fructose) is associated with breast cancer risk, with the strongest association found with sucrose (table sugar) and fructose (fruit sugar). No increase in breast cancer risk was found with total fat intake. This study kept the calorie intake equal in all study groups.

"Carbohydrate intake was positively associated with breast cancer risk. Compared with women in the lowest quartile of total carbohydrate intake, the relative risk of breast cancer for women in the highest quartile was 2.22… Among carbohydrate components, the strongest associations were observed for sucrose and fructose. No association was observed with total fat intake." – PubMed ID#15298947 (2004) [95]

❖ RECOMMENDATION

There is a very large body of evidence showing that a ketogenic diet can be used to help treat and prevent a large number of cancers. Cancer cells have a 10- to 17-fold higher consumption of glucose than nonmalignant (normal) cells, and most cannot utilize ketones effectively, whereas normal cells can. This allows the normal cells to function normally on a ketogenic diet while selectively starving cancer cells. A ketogenic diet may not be enough by itself to successfully treat an aggressive cancer, but it sure should be part of an overall strategy.

A ketogenic diet can be difficult at first, as it not only involves a mostly new way of eating, but there is also a metabolic adjustment period. The first couple of weeks on a ketogenic diet can be tough, but after that adjustment period, most people report higher energy levels and better mental focus.

It is beyond the scope of this book to outline exactly "how" to eat a ketogenic diet. There are plenty of books on this topic already. There are also a number of websites and Facebook support groups that do a very good job of helping you through it and providing free recipes.

INTERMITTENT FASTING

There is evidence that various forms of intermittent fasting can be beneficial to cancer treatment. It seems to be especially effective as an adjuvant treatment (combined with other cancer treatments). Though I believe that intermittent fasting probably is beneficial for cancer treatment and prevention, the evidence was not strong enough to include here. What few studies there are did not control for total calorie intake (so was intermittent fasting beneficial on its own, or simply because the test subjects were consuming fewer calories?). In contrast, a ketogenic diet was found to be highly beneficial even if calorie intake remained the same. There is evidence that calorie restriction can be helpful.

Intermittent fasting does seem to have several health benefits, and it may well turn out to be beneficial for treating and preventing cancer. However, I would recommend combining the concept of intermittent fasting with a ketogenic or low-carbohydrate diet.

> "Cycles of starvation were as effective as chemotherapeutic agents in delaying progression of different tumors and increased the effectiveness of these drugs against melanoma, glioma, and breast cancer cells. In mouse models of neuroblastoma, fasting cycles plus chemotherapy drugs--but not either treatment alone--resulted in long-term cancer-free survival. In 4T1 breast cancer cells, short-term starvation resulted in… increased oxidative stress, caspase-3 cleavage, DNA damage, and apoptosis. These studies suggest that multiple cycles of fasting promote differential stress sensitization in a wide range of tumors and could potentially replace or augment the efficacy of certain chemotherapy drugs in the treatment of various cancers." – PubMed ID#22323820 (2012) [96]

For more information I would recommend the following websites:

Wikipedia – Intermittent Fasting [97]

Healthline – Intermittent Fasting 101 [98]

There are also several Facebook support groups on intermittent fasting.

LOW-FAT DIETS

Low-fat diets seem to be prescribed for just about every aliment you can think of. Yet when one digs into the research, especially more recent studies, there just isn't much evidence that a low-fat diet is beneficial. Most of these studies have people eating healthier foods to substitute for the calories lost by lowering fat (e.g., cutting out meat and replacing with it vegetables).

"I've read lots of studies showing that a low-fat diet has several anticancer benefits, including increased apoptosis, lower cell proliferation, anti-metastasis, etc. Are you saying they just made this stuff up?"

No. The studies are accurate: A low-fat diet did improve anticancer markers—but whether they meant to or not, they sort of cheated. These studies looked at reducing specific types of fat, namely omega-6 polyunsaturated fatty acids (PUFA), mostly corn oil and hydrogenated fats. These have been linked to cancer, where other fats (such as omega-3) have not. This was done in a controlled environment with mice. There are no studies that I'm aware of that compared a low-fat diet to a diet containing a healthy balance of fats (e.g., a diet with a 1:1 ratio of omega-6 to omega-3s that also contained healthy saturated fats). Other studies that showed benefits looked at reducing "total fat." Westerners consume a diet far too high in polyunsaturated fats (20 times too high on average), and therefore, reducing total fat will be significantly reducing harmful polyunsaturated fats. You do not need to reduce total fat to achieve this effect; simply reducing polyunsaturated fats is enough.

In numerous studies, corn oil diets both decreased apoptosis (which can lead to cancer growth) and increased cancer cell proliferation, whereas olive oil has just the opposite effect. The study below clearly states that a "corn oil-enriched diet has a clear stimulating effect on mammary carcinogenesis." In other words, corn oil and other high-omega-6 polyunsaturated fatty acids (PUFA) clearly increase one's odds of getting "breast, colorectal and prostate cancers." Because a high-omega-6 diet decreases apoptosis and increases proliferation, one should certainly want to decrease omega-6 fatty acids in their diet if treating an existing cancer. On the other hand, adding omega-3 fatty acids from fish lowers cancer risk.

> "n-6 polyunsaturated fatty acids (PUFA), particularly linoleic acid (18:2n-6), have shown a strong stimulating effect on breast, colorectal and prostate cancers… histological detection of apoptotic cells by TUNEL confirmed a decrease in apoptosis in the epithelial cells in HCO group. These data suggested that changes in the apoptotic capacity of the mammary gland may be one of the molecular mechanisms by which the corn oil-enriched diet has a clear stimulating effect on mammary carcinogenesis… glands from LF-HOO group had down-regulated expression of S100a6 at both adult ages tested. S100 genes have a role in breast cancer progression… the diet rich in n-6 PUFA had a clear stimulating effect on breast carcinogenesis… results from the olive oil fed groups had no significant differences compared to controls… there was also a clear stimulating effect of the diet rich in n-6 PUFA, whereas the groups fed the high EVOO diet were more similar to the low-fat control… while the

stimulating effect of the high-corn-oil diet is clear and strong, the more variable and weaker influence of the high EVOO diet, despite being high fat, suggests that this type of oil has some beneficial effect that may partially counteract the total fat intake. Several active components of olive oil have been suggested to have health benefits" – PubMed ID#PMC4875377 (2016) (Open Access attribution at the link) [99]

> Moral, Raquel et al. "Diets high in corn oil or extra-virgin olive oil differentially modify the gene expression profile of the mammary gland and influence experimental breast cancer susceptibility." European journal of nutrition vol. 55,4 (2016): 1397-409. doi:10.1007/s00394-015-0958-2

When reviewing research studies that examined low-fat diets and cancer risk/recurrence, nearly all of them used corn oil, soy oil or some other omega-6 polyunsaturated fatty acid (PUFA) oil. This type of fat has since been shown to increase cancer risk. When studies used olive oil or saturated fats, the cancer risk of a normal "Western" diet (higher in fat) was not found. This tends to support other studies that show the real cancer culprit is not total fat, or even saturated fat, but rather certain PUFA oils, the omega-6 to omega-3 ratio, and high PUFA consumption. The exception is that a strong correlation was found between saturated "trans fats" and cancer—these artificial fats should always be avoided.

The following research was published in the prestigious *American Association of Cancer Research* journal. It looked at the effects of various fats on the different skin cancers, including total fat intake, cholesterol, saturated fat, monounsaturated, polyunsaturated, omega-6 and omega-3 fats. The study examined over 36,000 cases of cancer and found a higher association of cancer with omega-6 in SCC, BCC and melanoma cancers. Slightly higher risk was associated with high levels of omega-3 for basal cell carcinoma (BCC). This tends to indicate that the other fats studied do not have a systemic cancer risk, as the only fat associated with various skin cancers was polyunsaturated.

> "No other fats were associated with melanoma risk... Conclusions: Polyunsaturated fat intake was modestly associated with skin cancer risk." – PubMed ID#PMC6035072 (2018) [100]

In the following study of prostate cancer, researchers found that a diet high in corn oil enhanced (worsened) prostate cancer. A diet low in omega-6 fats but high in saturated fats had no negative effects.

> "In this xenograft model, we found no difference in tumor growth or survival between low-fat- vs. Western-fed mice, when the fat source was saturated fat. Given these results conflict from those when corn oil is used in which low-fat

diets have been shown to delay PCa growth, these findings suggest type of fat may be as important as amount of fat in the setting of PCa." – PubMed ID#PMC3766524 (2013) [101]

These results were also found in another study funded by a National Institutes of Health (nih.gov) grant. This study found that corn oil stimulated prostate cancer growth, whereas saturated fats did not. It also found that a high-starch or high-glycemic index diet increased prostate cancer risk.

"our prior study used corn oil (a rich source of polyunsaturated fat) as opposed to milk fat and lard (a rich source of saturated fat) in the current study. Though a direct comparison would be necessary, this suggests that at least in the current tumor model, corn oil may stimulate prostate cancer growth to a greater extent than saturated fats. Future studies are needed to assess not simply the amount of dietary fat, but also the composition of the fat (i.e., saturated vs. unsaturated) and how this can be optimized to reduced tumor growth… two recent human studies have suggested that either a high-starch diet or a high glycemic index diet increases prostate cancer risk… a high carbohydrate diet stimulates insulin production and insulin is a known prostate cancer growth factor" – PubMed ID#PMC3959866 (2008) [102]

This meta-analysis of 38 different studies on olive oil clearly pointed to a cancer-protective role for olive oil: "The highest category of olive oil consumption was associated with lower odds of having any type of cancer."

"In total 38 studies were initially allocated; of them 19 case-control studies were finally studied (13800 cancer patients and 23340 controls were included). Random effects meta-analysis was applied in order to evaluate the research hypothesis. It was found that compared with the lowest, the highest category of olive oil consumption was associated with lower odds of having any type of cancer… the latter was irrespective of the country of origin (Mediterranean or non-Mediterranean). Moreover, olive oil consumption was associated with lower odds of developing breast cancer and a cancer of the digestive system, compared with the lowest intake. The strength and consistency of the findings states a hypothesis about the protective role of olive oil intake on cancer risk." – PubMed ID#PMC3199852 (2011) [103]

When studies increased "saturated fat" to show that this is unhealthy, they often used hydrogenated vegetable oil. Hydrogenation converts this normally polyunsaturated fat to one that is saturated. This type of artificial fat has been shown in numerous studies to be unhealthy and is linked to increased cancers. I know of no studies linking coconut oil (a natural saturated fat) with increased cancer risk.

Previous studies of fat and breast cancer were based on mouse studies. In those studies tumors were induced, and then high-fat diets were assigned to half the mice, while standard mouse chow was fed to the other half. The mice were monitored for cancer outcomes. A high-fat diet is very unnatural for mice and would have little bearing on how humans should eat.

The following research followed over 180,000 women from the well-known "Nurses' Health Study" and the "Nurses' Health Study II" and found that there was no relation between dietary fat intake and lethal breast cancer risk; if anything, the authors found that those consuming a higher-fat diet had a slightly lower risk of lethal breast cancer.

> in relation to lethal breast cancer risk in 88,759 women in the Nurses' Health Study (NHS; 1980–2010) and 93,912 women in the Nurses' Health Study II (NHSII; 1991–2010)… Higher total fat intake was associated with a slightly lower lethal breast cancer risk (top vs. bottom quintile hazard ratio [HR] 0.85; 95 % CI 0.72, 1.01; p trend = 0.05). Specific types of fat were generally not associated with lethal breast cancer risk… Conclusions: Higher pre-diagnosis fat intake was not associated with greater risk of lethal breast cancer in these large prospective cohort studies, consistent with the weight of the evidence against a causal role for fat intake and breast cancer incidence" – PubMed ID#PMC4124826 (2014) [104]

Recommendation

Current research suggests that a low-fat diet is unlikely to help treat or prevent cancer. The important thing is the quality of the fat. In animals, fat is where toxins can accumulate, especially in less healthy animals. If you consume animal fat, I recommend organic and grass-fed when possible. The fat from grass-fed animals also contains vitamin K2 (see Chapter 6 for its anticancer benefits).

- Consume a variety of high-quality fats, such as: extra virgin olive oil, coconut oil, organic grass-fed beef, organic grass-fed butter/ghee, fatty fish, and omega-3 fish oils (high in EPA/DHA). When consuming animal fat, focus on high-quality organic fat to avoid fat-soluble toxins.

- Avoid "vegetable" and grain oils (AKA polyunsaturated omega-6 fats). There is far too much recent evidence showing how detrimental they can be. You can't always control this when eating out, so make up for it at home.

- If you are vegan or vegetarian, use olive, coconut and palm oils. Consider making an exception for fish oils (see Chapter 6 for more information).

VEGAN/VEGETARIAN/NO-RED-MEAT DIETS

If you are already a vegan or strict vegetarian, you may take umbrage with this section. Let me start by saying there are legitimate ethical and philosophical reasons for avoiding animal products and I understand that. This section will discuss this topic as it relates to cancer, the immune system, and to a lesser degree, general health. This can be a highly controversial topic, with plenty of biases on both sides, and some of this bias, unfortunately, has crept into research. Bias is often shown in full force in many books and websites.

I'm going to start this section with a clear fact: Eating a diet high in nutritious plant matter is beneficial in the fight against cancer, for improving the immune system, for improving gut health and for general health. I think there is little doubt about that. For meat eaters, consuming more plant matter will probably entail consuming less meat in the diet, as there is only so much room in the gut.

That said, I can find no convincing evidence that consuming organic grass-fed meat in moderation either causes cancer or makes it worse.

It is true that there are a few studies that compared vegan diets to a high-meat diet. The conclusion was usually that the meat diet caused some condition or another, when compared to a diet with no meat. On the surface this may appear to indicate that the meat-free diet was better. But these studies weren't designed to reach that conclusion. To even begin to reach such a conclusion, the study would need to control for the amount of vegetable matter consumed (and quality), total calorie intake, quantity and quality of the meat consumed, and type of vegetable matter. In other words, both the vegan diet and the meat-eating diet would need to include the same amount and type of vegetables and total calories (calorie restriction is known to benefit cancer treatment). This is how any well run research study is done; all things must be equal in the two groups under study except for the variable being studied (meat versus no meat). Only then can you say that meat consumption is what led to a poorer health outcome (rather than simply consuming more vegetable matter or fewer calories). To my knowledge, no such study has been done on humans (and mice do not naturally eat red meat, so they shouldn't be used in such a study).

The following study states that in the absence of fermentable resistant carbohydrates, bacteria will ferment protein. If sufficient resistant carbohydrates (such as soluble fiber and non-digestible polysaccharides) are not available, then the gut bacteria will consume protein as their energy source. When bacteria ferment protein (including plant protein) as an energy source, they produce toxic compounds, such as ammonia, phenols, cresols, hydrogen sulfide and amines. It is believed that these toxic compounds increase cancer risks and genetic instability. The takeaway point here is to always properly feed your gut bacteria by consuming low-carbohydrate vegetables high in soluble fibers, mushrooms high in beta-glucans (and other resistant polysaccharides), and resistant starches ("resistant" means that these carbohydrates are resistant to digestion by humans but are consumed by our gut bacteria as their preferred energy source). An all-meat diet is, admittedly, not a healthy diet.

"Solubilized wheat AX (arabinoxylan) has the potential to counteract the effects of dietary red meat by reducing protein fermentation and its resultant toxic end products such as ammonia, as well as leading to a positive shift in fermentation end products and microbial profiles in the large intestine." – PubMed ID#26740253 (2016) [105]

Long-term consumption of higher-protein diets is likely to predispose individuals to a range of diseases, particularly those related to the presence of toxic metabolites from protein fermentation. This deleterious effect has been shown to be counteracted by carbohydrate fermentation from resistant starch, inulin-type fructans, and secondary metabolites of plant metabolism. -- DOI: 10.1016@j.nut.2015.10.008 (2015) [106]

Phys.org (an online news research service) analyzed a 2016 study appearing in *Nature Biology*. This study found that bacteria that ferment protein are much slower growers. What the study found was that when our gut is fed (resistant) fermentable fibers (e.g., prebiotics) this gives carbohydrate fermenters a strong competitive advantage over protein fermenters (thus reducing their numbers considerably). This prevents the fermentation of protein, and the associated toxins it produces. Phys.org, [107] DOI: 10.1038/ nmicrobiol.2016.88 [108]

As I've mentioned earlier, consuming plants and vegetables has a lot of health benefits. However, eliminating all meat does not. The research I've seen that tries to reach that conclusion is usually seriously flawed. For instance, a study that tries to compare a vegan diet to a carnivorous (nearly all-meat) diet is flawed; cutting out all vegetables and plant matter is not healthy (granted). You cannot use such a study to try and prove that people should give up all meat. That would be like saying that everyone should go on a high-meat diet because people eating a 100% sugar diet aren't healthy; the correlation is flawed. Another problem with some of these studies is that some have shown that a high-fat diet is unhealthy and leads to cancer. Since red meat is often high in fat, they draw the conclusion that red meat causes cancer. This too is a flawed correlation. Nearly all of the high-fat studies used mice that were fed corn or vegetable oil (see the Low-Fat Diets section above), not animal fat. Turns out that corn oil was the problem, not all fat. When other fats were used (olive oil or animal fats), the negative consequences were not seen. It's quite a stretch to go from mice being force-fed corn oil, to stating that meat causes cancer in humans, but that is what is being done.

Regarding prevention of breast cancer, this meta-research study out of Poland reached very similar conclusions: Avoid foods high in polyunsaturated fatty acids (PUFA), increase your omega-3s and get enough vitamin D, soluble fiber and folate. Avoid "grilled" meats and alcohol. In this research, only a very "weak association" was found with saturated fat, and this may be due to trans fats (which are an artificial saturated fat now known to increase the risk of cancer). There are also known cancer risks associated with the quality of animal products consumed (e.g., grilled / charred meats and deli meats, which are high in nitrates, are both known cancer risks). This risk isn't due to saturated fat but was not controlled for in this study. Another very large study referenced below found absolutely no association with saturated fat and cancer. This study's researchers did find a significant difference in the type of PUFA consumed and the risk of contracting breast cancer. Omega-3 is considered a PUFA, but it was found to be protective against breast cancer, whereas omega-6 (e.g., corn /vegetable oils) is also a PUFA and was found to increase the risk of breast cancer.

> "The evidence to date from epidemiologic studies suggests that diet may be associated with both increases and reductions of breast cancer risk, which may be related to the amount and type of foods consumed. Higher intake of foods containing n-3 PUFA, vitamin D, phytoestrogen, fiber, and folate, together with lower intake of saturated fat, n-6 PUFA, grilled meat, and alcohol, may be beneficial… Low intake of marine-derived n-3 PUFA and high intake of n-6 PUFA have been reported to increase risk of breast cancer" – PubMed ID#PMC4829739 (2016) [109]

The following study out of Sweden (involving over 49,000 women) found no association between breast cancer risk and saturated fat, or total fat. They did find benefits associated with monounsaturated fats (e.g., olive oil) for women over 50.

> We investigated whether dietary intakes of total fat, monounsaturated fat (MUFA), polyunsaturated fat (PUFA) and saturated fat (SFA) were associated with breast cancer risk in a prospective cohort of 49,261 Swedish women… Our study did not find evidence for the entire cohort of an association between total fat, MUFA, PUFA or SFA intakes and breast cancer risk… However, possible differential effects of type of fats during premenopausal years were suggested on risk above the age of 50 years… There was a statistically significant trend for a decreased risk across the quintiles of MUFA intake… Our study provides no evidence that total fat, MUFA, PUFA or SFA is associated with overall breast cancer risk" – PubMed ID#PMC2360254 (2007) [110]

The point here is that there does not seem to be a link between total fat or saturated fat and cancer risk. When an increased risk was shown with saturated fat, it was small and most likely due to the quality of the meat in the study participants' diets (this was not controlled for). For example, the people were consuming deli meats high in nitrates and other preservatives or consuming grilled meat (both are known cancer risk factors). Many of those studies also included trans fats as saturated fats; again, this is an artificial saturated fat that should always be avoided.

❖ THE CHINA STUDY

The China Study (the book by T. Colin Campbell) is the vegan's bible when it comes to arguing the health benefits of a vegan diet. I cannot count the number of times I've had a vegan almost slap me in the face with *The China Study* if I dared question their assertion that eating meat is what causes cancer, or that 90% of cardiovascular disease is caused by meat consumption (neither are true). If you're already a vegan and don't own a copy of this book, I recommend that you purchase it right now; this book will serve as great argument material against a meat-eating father-in-law (or some other non-believer). It is a how-to guide to convince others that a vegan lifestyle will prevent almost every disease and that eating meat will kill whoever you are speaking with.

However, I can find <u>no</u> study that shows that eating clean meat or fish causes cancer, and no double-blind human trials have been done on this (as you'll find throughout this book, I never advise anyone to take advice that doesn't have good scientific evidence to support it and the original "China study" does not show what the popular book of the same name asserts). Studies that control for the quality of meat consumed (e.g., grass-fed versus confined feeding operations or preserved meat versus fresh) showed no association between animal fats (or any saturated fat) and cancer risk.

The World Health Organization (WHO) has classified <u>processed meats</u> as being a carcinogen, but not other meats.

> "Processed meat includes hot dogs, ham, bacon, sausage, and some deli meats. It refers to meat that has been treated in some way to preserve or flavor it. Processes include salting, curing, fermenting, and smoking."

I would agree with this to some extent; however, from what I've seen, the research used retrospective studies (questionnaires about people's eating habits). The results of the questionnaires were heavily weighted towards commercially processed meats that use nitrates and other chemicals to preserve the meat. This study did not examine people that consumed organic grass-fed meat and more natural (traditional) preservation methods and whether that would be a problem or not. Even so, the lifetime risk of contracting colon cancer only went from 5% for people that ate no processed meats, to a little less than 6%. Nevertheless, I recommend eating the cleanest, most natural meat possible.

The problem with *The China Study* (the book) is that it is nearly a total work of fiction. The book claims to be based on a large study called the "China–Cornell–Oxford Project" from the 1980s. That study examined the diets of 6,500 rural Chinese and the diseases and conditions they had. The study produced a large amount of statistical information and serves as a valuable research tool. The problem with T. Colin Campbell's book is that it started off with an agenda to make people stop eating meat, and it set out to select data that helps promote that agenda, leaving out anything that contradicts the message. Very little of his book is based off the study;

most of it is simply opinion. Only one chapter of the book even focuses on the China study—that is 39 pages out of 350! Every word of that has been disputed ad nauseam, and in my humble opinion, convincingly. To make matters worse, the evidence is presented very selectively, with the author picking statistics and evidence that support his agenda (especially when taken out of context), while conveniently leaving out a large amount of information that counters the dogma.

> *As Samuel Clemens/Mark Twain would often say: "There are three kinds of lies: lies, damned lies, and statistics."*

As discussed earlier in this chapter, it isn't meat that is the problem for meat eaters. It is the lack of enough plant matter in the diet (and perhaps too many calories). You may need to consume less meat in order to make room for more vegetables and green leafy plants, but consuming clean meat will not cause or worsen cancer—at least no more than consuming too much of any one vegetable (as most contain substances to ward off insects that can also be carcinogens). As with most natural foods that our ancestors would have consumed, "the dose makes the poison" (Paracelsus).

Yet there are plenty of very good reasons to consume meat. Archeologists have found no large ancient population groups (especially prior to 10,000 years ago) that have ever been vegan. They haven't even discovered any smaller tribes that lasted more than about 100 years that ate purely vegan. The closest any society has come was under the Chinese Emperor Liang Wudi (502-549 CE), who basically mandated vegetarianism across China for a few decades; however, this was not a vegan diet, and even this way of eating did not last very long (there was also considerable cheating).

There is good reason for that. Humans require nutrients best obtained (and sometimes only obtainable) from eating animals (whether those be field mice, fish or antelope) or animal products (e.g., eggs). Especially if you believe in science and evolution, I can see no reason for you to believe that a pure vegan diet is best for human health; humans evolved eating meat. No societies <u>ever</u> consumed a pure vegan diet for very long. How do I know this? Perhaps recorded history missed something. That's an easy question to answer; there are <u>no</u> natural, vegan-friendly foods that contain vitamin B12, which can only be obtained from animal sources. Even today, vegans must supplement vitamin B12. Recent vegan converts may survive for several years without supplementing B12 (as our body stores quite a bit of it—that is just how important it is). However, in fewer than 10 years from going vegan, they will have to supplement B12, eat meat, or suffer some awful neurological consequences (and soon after, death). So, it is very safe to say that life-long veganism is a very recent sociological phenomenon (B12 supplements were not available until recent times). We definitely evolved eating animal products.

If you do not believe in evolution and are Christian, just know that the Bible says that Jesus ate both lamb and fish (but does not command, or even really advise, anyone to eat meat). Fish was probably consumed almost daily. There are even references to his disciples consuming locusts.

But again, if you have philosophical reasons not to eat meat, go for it. Just be sure to do a very, very good job of educating yourself on the best ways to do it in a healthy manner.

To do a proper job of debating this topic is a book unto itself. Since I doubt many vegans would be convinced regardless of the evidence, I don't plan to try (and if a person is vegan for philosophical reasons, I don't want to try). Therefore, if you would like more information, I recommend the following links (over time, some of these may become unavailable). They do a good job of refuting the faux science of the *China Study* book. They also contain many additional links to scientific studies or quotes from research scientists. Again, this topic is too large to repeat everything here.

- "Rest in Peace, China Study" by Chris Kresser. This article is routinely updated with new information. [111]
- "The China Study: Fact or Fallacy?" by Denise Minger. A very intelligent young woman who picks apart every aspect of this book with facts and statistics, all in a way that you'll understand and enjoy. I also recommend her book *Death by Food Pyramid*, available on Amazon. [112]

> *The book* The China Study *often uses fat (regardless of the source) to point out how meat causes cancer (especially breast cancer). In Denise Minger's analysis of the evidence presented in the book, she points out that sugar, wine, alcohol and fruit all have a greater association with breast cancer than fat intake! Animal protein has an even lower correlation than fat, lower even than light-colored vegetables, legumes and several other purportedly healthy plant foods! By those standards we should not only give up meat, but many vegan staples as well.*

- "T. Colin Campbell's *The China Study*: Finally, Exhaustively Discredited" by Richard Nikoley. Free the Animal blog post. [113]
- "The China Study: Evidence for the Perfect Health Diet" by Paul Jaminet (author of the book *The Perfect Health Diet*, which I highly recommend reading). [114]

❖ VITAMIN B12

I am only bringing this topic up in case there are any uninformed vegans reading this. There are no vegan-friendly, food-based sources of vitamin B12, and our bodies do not produce it.

> *Vitamin B12 is produced in limited amounts in the large intestine by our gut bacteria, but unfortunately, it can't be absorbed from there. B12 is absorbed by the small intestine (north of the colon; it is a top-to-bottom system), and that B12 is well on its way out of us by the time it's produced.*

As mentioned earlier, vegans must supplement vitamin B12; there are no ways around it. Luckily there are some vegan-friendly supplements on the market that are made from bacteria. Some processed vegan foods are also supplemented with vegan-friendly B12. However, if you eat a vegan diet, you need to make sure you are getting enough vitamin B12. Otherwise you will suffer some very nasty consequences. You also need good B12 levels for a properly functioning immune system to fight cancer. As mentioned in Chapter 2, CD8+ T cells and NK cells are vitally important to fighting cancer, and they require vitamin B12.

> "results indicate that B12 might play an important role in cellular immunity, especially relativing to CD8+ cells and the NK cell system, which suggests effects on cytotoxic cells. We conclude that B12 acts as an immunomodulator for cellular immunity." – PubMed ID#PMC1905232 (1999) [115]

❖ E P A / D H A O M E G A - 3 s

This topic is very important as EPA/DHA omega-3s are an essential piece of fighting and preventing cancer (see Chapter 6). Because these fatty acids can only be obtained from animal fats, that leaves a huge gap in a true vegan's ability to ward off cancer.

Though the body can make both EPA and DHA from plant-based alpha-linolenic acid (ALA), the conversion efficiency is very poor; only 5% to 10% of ALA can be converted to EPA, and less than 1% of ALA can be converted to DHA (and for some people, the conversion rate is even worse). As the study below indicates, "EPA and DHA, must be consumed in the diet." As with many natural supplements mentioned in this book, EPA and DHA are most likely beneficial for many cancers, not only the ones mentioned here (and in Chapter 6); there just aren't a lot of studies with these other cancers.

> "PUFAs, the major structural components of cell membranes, are considered to be pivotal nutrients for preventing non-alcoholic fatty liver disease, autoimmune responses, and other chronic diseases such as cardiovascular disease, cancers, and diabetes… treatments using these fatty acids were shown to prevent colon and breast cancers… humans are able to convert only a small portion of fatty acids to more than 20-carbon PUFAs; the conversion rates of 18-carbon fatty acids to EPA and from ALA to DHA were reported to be 5%–10% and less than 1%, respectively. Therefore, fish and their oils, which contain high levels of more than 20-carbon PUFAs such as EPA and DHA, must be consumed in the diet." – PubMed ID#PMC4728637 (2016) [116]

> "Breast cancer (BC) is the most common cancer among women worldwide. Dietary fatty acids, especially n-3 polyunsaturated fatty acids (PUFA), are believed to play a role in reducing BC risk. Evidence has shown that fish consumption or intake of long-chain n-3 PUFA, such as eicosapentaenoic acid

(EPA) and docosahexaenoic acid (DHA), are beneficial for inhibiting mammary carcinogenesis." – PubMed ID#25412153 (2014) [117]

Though I completely respect a person's decision to eat vegan, this is one area where I think a cancer patient needs to reconsider their choice. Adding fish, and a fish oil supplement, to a vegan diet will go a long way in making a vegan diet into a much healthier vegetarian diet.

"In adult humans, an EPA plus DHA intake greater than 2 g day seems to be required to elicit anti-inflammatory actions" – PubMed ID#22765297 (2013) [118]

For more information, see the Omega-3 Fatty Acids section in Chapter 6; it will have much more information regarding the cancer-protective and cancer-fighting benefits of EPA and DHA.

❖ RECOMMENDATION

Based on the evidence, the best diet for fighting cancer is the low-carb ketogenic diet, including consuming a good amount of low-carbohydrate vegetables. If you want to remain vegan or vegetarian, it is still possible to eat ketogenic; however, it will be difficult, especially if you need to maintain or gain weight. You will need to work hard to maintain your nutritional levels (B12 and iron are especially difficult to obtain on a vegan diet) while avoiding both meat and carbohydrates. There are no vegan-friendly sources of EPA and DHA omega-3s. Though the body can convert ALA, a plant-based omega-3, this process is not efficient and not as healthy as a fish-sourced EPA/DHA supplement. Some people are also genetically predisposed to have very poor ALA conversion.

Here are just a few of the vegan ketogenic diet books I found on Amazon; there are dozens of them (most are cookbooks).

- *Vegan Ketogenic Diet: Top 100 Low Carb Plant-Based Recipes for Keto Vegans* by Anna Solis

- *The Ketogenic Vegan Cookbook: Vegan Cheeses, Instant Pot & Delicious Everyday Recipes for Healthy Plant Based Eating* by Eva Hammond

- *30 Day Ketogenic Vegetarian Meal Plan: Delicious, Easy, and Healthy Vegetarian Recipes To Get You Started On The Keto Lifestyle* by Sharon Kemper

- *30 Day Ketogenic Vegetarian Meal Plan: Top 90 Healthy and Delicious Vegetarian Recipes to Help You Enjoy The Perfect Keto Lifestyle* by Janine Colon

---

ALL-FRUIT DIET

> *Let me start off with an editorial: "This is bananas!"*

An all-fruit diet, by definition, is a very limited vegan diet. So, the previous section should cover most of this topic. It is difficult to remain healthy on a vegan diet (but at least it is possible); it is impossible on an all-fruit diet. The need for B12 alone means you can die on an all-fruit diet, as no fruit contains B12. [119] When you look at everything you'll be missing—all fatty acids, essential amino acids and vitamins (for example, vitamin K2 and B12)—any one of those can cause you to become seriously ill, or die, from a nutritional deficiency. You will certainly be missing out on a lot of cancer-fighting nutrients (again, see Chapter 6)!

When a fruitarian (people who only eat fruit) tells you that our ancestors were fruitarian, they are not talking about humans; they're talking about primates millions of years ago (then ask them why they take a B12 supplement if our ancestors didn't). There have been a LOT of changes to humans since then (science isn't even sure that ancient primates were vegan; there is a very good chance that they ate insects, lizards, etc., as do many current primates). Humans will die on a pure fruitarian diet without supplementation (it might take a few years, but it will happen).

> "The Health Promotion Program at Columbia University reports that a fruitarian diet can cause deficiencies in calcium, protein, iron, zinc, vitamin D, most B vitamins (especially B12), and essential fatty acids." – Columbia.edu [120]

Please, if you care about your health, don't fall for this. You will eventually regret it.

GENERAL DIET STRATEGIES

> *A joyful heart is good medicine, but a broken spirit dries up the bones.*
> ~ Proverbs 17:22

High glucose and fructose consumption feeds cancer; there is little doubt about this. Related to high glucose levels are high insulin levels. People with Type II diabetes have much higher levels of cancer (and insulin) than people without diabetes; people with Type I diabetes do not have higher cancer rates. Type I diabetics do not make insulin, or they do not make enough; Type II diabetics often make too much insulin, but it doesn't get used properly. Thus, the difference in cancer rates. Glucose and insulin levels need to be kept in check through a low-sugar diet (preferably also a low-carbohydrate diet, such as a ketogenic diet), intermittent fasting, exercise and supplements.

> "The cohort included 383,799 subjects without diabetes and 23,358 with diabetes… found an overall 15–30% higher cancer incidence among subjects with diabetes in comparison to those without diabetes." – PubMed ID#PMC5657107 (2017) (Open Access license attribution at the link) [121]

As pointed out in the beginning of this chapter, a diet containing foods high on the glycemic index scale can increase the risk of contracting some types of cancer by up to 92%! This number may be a very low estimate, as the study excluded people with diabetes and other diseases that are also caused by a high-carbohydrate/high-glycemic index diet.

Always try to avoid meats high in hormones, toxins and nitrates, or those that have been char cooked. When possible, only consume grass-fed organic beef, free-range organic chicken/eggs and organic pork.

> "Breast cancer is the most common cancer among women worldwide and the incidence has continued to rise over time. Nutrition influences cancer etiology in about 35% of cancer cases." – PubMed ID#PMC4829739 (2016) [122]

Kotepui, Manas. "Diet and risk of breast cancer." Contemporary oncology (Poznan, Poland) vol. 20,1 (2016): 13-9. doi:10.5114/wo.2014.40560

"Higher intake of foods containing n-3 PUFA, vitamin D, phytoestrogen, fiber, and folate, together with lower intake of saturated fat, n-6 PUFA, grilled meat, and alcohol, may be beneficial." – PubMed ID#PMC4829739 (2016) [123]

The Overall Diet Recommendation

Fighting Cancer – The best way to *Improve Your Odds* is to follow a strict ketogenic diet as described earlier in this chapter. There are many online resources to help you do this. To stay in ketosis, cheat days are not possible (I'm afraid cancer doesn't take a holiday). If you cannot do a ketogenic diet, a low-sugar diet with intermittent fasting is the next best thing. What carbohydrates you do eat should be low on the glycemic index with a low glycemic load.

Prevention and NED – Here there is more flexibility. A low-sugar diet with intermittent fasting should be sufficient. Again, consume foods low on the glycemic index.

Whether you are fighting cancer or preventing cancer, you should eat a clean diet. Eating organic is always best, but it is especially important when eating meat. Make sure the food you eat is high in nutrition.

Consume the following foods as often as possible:

- Mushrooms, mushrooms and more mushrooms – Don't just stick to button mushrooms; get adventurous. Consume the medicinal mushrooms when possible.
- Blueberries and other low-sugar berries
- Cruciferous vegetables, especially the sprouts of these vegetables
- Flaxseed – Purchase sprouted organic when possible. I use about 1 to 2 Tbsp per day.
- Kefir – even if only ¼ cup (dairy, when consumed, should always be organic)
- Wild-caught salmon and other fish high in omega-3 and low in mercury
- Purple sweet potato – Regular sweet potato is also good. Excellent in soups and stews.
- Walnuts and pecans – Moderation is best, as they are high in oxalates.
- Bitter melon – Works well in stir-fries.
- Garlic – Consume it as often as possible. See its section on how to prepare.
- Ginger – Good for Asian stir-fries, tea and baked desserts.
- Green tea – Consume daily (assuming you don't have the COMT genetic issue described in the Green Tea/EGCG section).
- Stevia – Use this to sweeten drinks, such as green tea and vegetable smoothies. There are also recipes out there for stevia-sweetened desserts.
- Turmeric – It really isn't hard to include turmeric in your diet. Just purchase a jar of turmeric powder and sprinkle in soups, stews, casseroles, salad dressings, pot pies, etc. It's easy to if you're cooking your own meals.

❖ Avoid

If you are having chemotherapy or radiation treatments, your oncologist may have a list of foods for you to avoid (such as this one [124]). The following list shows some of the foods that everyone should avoid if treating cancer, and you may also wish to cut back or avoid them if you want to prevent cancer (or improve your immune system).

- Alcohol – See the explanation in Chapter 9 in the Baseline Protocol. Binge drinking is especially problematic. (Don't blame me; I just follow the evidence.)

- Sugar – This is discussed in depth earlier in this chapter; especially avoid high-fructose foods and high-fructose corn syrup. (Again, not my fault.)

- Artificial sweeteners – There is more and more evidence that these mess with insulin, contribute to Type II diabetes/metabolic syndrome and cause a range of health issues. This means avoiding nearly all diet sodas (unless sweetened with stevia). Stevia is by far the preferred sweetener as there is evidence that it helps prevent and possibly even treat some cancers. Monk fruit, another natural low-calorie sweetener, can also be used.

- Highly processed meats – Fresh meat, especially organic, is fine. But processed meats can contain several chemicals that can problematic. Especially avoid added nitrates.

- Omega-6 polyunsaturated fats – Though you shouldn't eliminate these completely, nearly everyone should cut back on them. Especially avoid rancid forms (and these oils go rancid quickly), foods deep-fried in vegetable oils, and never use them for pan frying. See the Omega-3 section earlier in this chapter.

- Trans fats – Hopefully everyone knows this by now. Read the labels.

- Char seared or blackened foods – Yes, this includes beef. Charring creates carcinogens (such as heterocyclic amines and polycyclic aromatic hydrocarbons).

- Fish likely to be high in mercury. See Chapter 6, Omega-3, for more information.

- Foods high in pesticides – In short, eat organic when possible.

- GMO (genetically modified)? – Maybe; evidence is currently lacking, and any risk will vary greatly depending on the food and how it was genetically modified.

❖ DAIRY

There is a growing body of evidence that dairy consumption is linked to cancer and avoiding dairy can benefit cancer treatment. This risk is most likely due to specific aspects of dairy. This may allow for the consumption of some types of dairy (such as organic hard cheeses).

The first problem with dairy is lactose. Most adults malabsorb lactose (milk sugar) at some level. The unabsorbed lactose goes on to feed bad bacteria; gut health was discussed more in Chapter 3. This causes a dysbiosis of bacteria in the colon (it is one of many possible causes), and a dysbiosis can cause cancers throughout the body (not only in the colon). This dysbiosis also pushes out beneficial bacteria (such as Bifidobacterium, discussed in Chapter 2).

> "Dysbiosis can be caused not only by pathogenic organisms and passenger commensals but also by aging and environmental factors such as antibiotics, xenobiotics, smoking, hormones, and dietary cues; these are also well-established risk factors for the development of intestinal or extraintestinal neoplasms… **alterations of the gut microbiota also influence the incidence and progression of extraintestinal cancers, including breast and hepatocellular carcinoma, presumably through inflammatory and metabolic circuitries… Thus, the gut microbiota influences oncogenesis and tumor progression both locally and systemically.**" – PubMed ID#PMC4690201 (2015) [125]

The second problem with dairy is that it substantially raises blood insulin levels. Recent studies have shown that dairy increases blood insulin levels despite having a relatively low glycemic index. Even lactose-free dairy produces higher insulin secretion than white bread (even though white bread has a higher glycemic index (GI) than dairy). Dairy increases blood insulin levels almost 200% more than white bread.

> "the postprandial blood glucose response after the test meal with reconstituted skim milk powder was low, the insulin response after milk was not significantly distinguishable from that after the WWB (white-wheat-bread) reference. Thus, the present results confirm those from a previous study in which the ingestion of pasteurized milk resulted in a discrepancy between blood glucose (GI = 30) and the insulin response (II = 90)… the insulin response to the whey meal was even more pronounced than that to milk… food proteins differ in their capacity to stimulate insulin release" – PubMed ID#15531672 (from the full study 10.1093/ajcn/80.5.1246) (2009) [126]

> *I personally consume unsweetened pea or flax milk. I sweeten with a little bit of stevia. Both are healthy alternatives to milk. The stevia-sweetened pea milk actually tastes quite good.*

The studies below show that higher insulin levels cause increased carcinogenesis.

> "In conclusion, elevated fasting glucose and insulin, and insulin resistance were independently associated with risk of liver cancer" – PubMed ID#PMC5093066 (2016) [127]

> "High fasting concentrations of insulin may be an independent risk factor for poor outcomes in women with breast cancer... Researchers from the University of Toronto Mount Sinai Hospital led by Dr Pamela Goodwin followed 535 women with breast cancer for 10 years and studied the relation between breast cancer grade and stage and insulin concentration" – PubMed ID#PMC1118103 (2000) [128]

In the first study below, insulin resistance (IR) was associated with breast cancer (BCa) in overweight premenopausal women. Higher IR numbers are associated with higher insulin levels (in people who are non-diabetic). The additional studies are a small sampling of those showing that higher insulin levels increase carcinogenesis (cancer formation).

> "findings suggest a bidirectional relationship between dysregulated glucose /insulin metabolism and BCa, as both, tumor- and IR-related markers are correlated with the severity of glucose/insulin metabolism impairment in overweight/obese premenopausal BCa patients." – PubMed ID#PMC5655300 (2017) [129]

> "This evidence suggests that insulin resistance plays a central role in endometrial cancer development." – PubMed ID#22449736 (2012) [130]

> "High serum levels of insulin and IGFs in DM (diabetes mellitus) patients have been shown to increase cellular proliferation and activation of the oncogenic epidermal growth factor receptors, resulting in mitogenic and antiapoptotic effects and inducing malignant cell transformation." – PubMed ID#PMC4937962 (2016) [131]

> "Insulin is known to activate the PI3K/Akt pathway and thus increases carcinogenesis... in many types of cancer cells, insulin induces resistance to chemotherapeutic drugs and may contribute to poor prognosis" – PubMed ID#PMC3933667 (2014) [132]

Updates at - https://improvingyourodds.com

Support at - https://www.facebook.com/groups/cancer.improving.your.odds

In addition to increasing insulin, dairy also contains hormones that increase hormone-responsive cancers, such as breast and prostate cancer. This is especially true for milk from cows given rbST. Always consume organic dairy products.

> "A potent link to dairy seems to exist for three hormone-responsive glands. Acne, breast cancer and prostate cancer have all been linked epidemiologically to dairy intake… dairy-sourced hormones, not being subject to any innate feedback inhibition, may be the source of the androgenic and mitogenic progestins that drive acne, prostate and breast cancer." – PubMed ID#PMC2715202 (2009) [133]

A number of recent studies have shown that dairy products are probably the number-one cause of acne. So, if you or your children have acne, cutting all sources of dairy from the diet should be the first thing to try. Interestingly, a history of acne has been shown to be associated with both breast cancer and prostate cancer (this association hasn't been examined for most other cancers, but it may exist for some other cancers as well). [134]

> "A frequent history of more severe acne appears to be related to a higher prevalence of prostate cancer later in life… Acne appears to be a visible indicator of systemically exaggerated mTORC1 signalling, an unfavourable metabolic deviation on the road to serious mTORC1-driven diseases of civilisation, especially overweight (increased BMI), obesity, arterial hypertension, insulin resistance, type 2 diabetes mellitus, cancer, and Alzheimer's disease" – PubMed ID#23975508 (2013) [135]

Fermenting dairy removes the lactose, denatures the proteins and degrades bovine hormones, thus perhaps eliminating some of the risk associated with dairy. In fact, there is research showing that kefir can help prevent and treat various forms of cancer.

> "some of the bioactive compounds of kefir such as polysaccharides and peptides have great potential for inhibition of proliferation and induction of apoptosis in tumor cells. Many studies revealed that kefir acts on different cancers such as colorectal cancer, malignant T lymphocytes, breast cancer and lung carcinoma." – PubMed ID#28956261 (2017) [136]

Hard cheeses are also fermented (more so than kefir), so hard cheeses may be safer to consume. However, they do not seem to have the cancer-preventative properties of kefir. Unfermented dairy consumption leads to additional cancer formation and a poorer cancer prognosis. The recommendation would be to cut all dairy from your diet, except for hard cheeses, kefir (especially homemade), and possibly homemade yogurt. Any dairy you consume should be organic. Cheese concentrates fat and any hormones and toxins that were in the milk; therefore, always consume organic cheese or other high-fat dairy.

Updates at - https://improvingyourodds.com/

Support at - https://www.facebook.com/groups/cancer.improving.your.odds

◆❖◆

Chapter 5
Sleep, Stress and Exercise

"The only way to keep your health is to eat what you don't want, drink what you don't like, and do what you'd rather not." ~ Mark Twain

Too little sleep and poor sleep quality have been shown to be associated with increased risk of several medical conditions, including obesity, diabetes, cardiovascular disease, hypertension, even total all-cause mortality. An increasing body of evidence shows that a lack of sleep increases the risk of contracting several cancers and their severity. Because the research is limited, it is too early to say if this association is to be found with all cancers, but the evidence is trending in that direction.

There is a direct relationship between sleep disturbances and melatonin (a sleep hormone); therefore, some of the research below studied the relationship between melatonin disturbances and cancer. If you are a night shift worker or your lack of sleep is due to disturbances in circadian rhythms, be sure to read the section on Melatonin in Chapter 6.

Research shows that a single 4- to 5-hour night of sleep can lower your body's "natural killer" (NK) cells by 70%! You need as many of these cells circulating as possible, every day—they've earned their name!

The following colonoscopy-based study looked at 1,240 participants. It was designed to screen for colorectal adenoma, a benign tumor of the colon and rectum that is a precursor lesion to colorectal adenocarcinoma (a form of colon cancer).

"we found a statistically significant association of colorectal adenoma... Cases were more likely to average less than 6 hours of sleep per night... individuals averaging less than 6 hours per night had an almost 50% increase in risk of colorectal adenomas (OR=1.47, CI =1.05-2.06, p for trend=0.02) as compared with individuals sleeping at least 7 hours per night… Shorter duration of sleep significantly increases risk of colorectal adenomas." – PubMed ID#PMC3021092 (2011) [137]

Here, people with the fewest hours of sleep per night had a higher (worse) recurrence score for breast cancer returning.

"OncotypeDX is a widely utilized test to guide treatment in early stage hormone receptor positive breast cancer by predicting likelihood of recurrence… We analyzed data from 101 breast cancer patients with available OncotypeDX recurrence scores to test the hypothesis that shorter sleep is associated with greater likelihood of recurrence… We found that OncotypeDX recurrence scores were strongly correlated with average hours of sleep per night prior to breast cancer diagnosis, with fewer hours of sleep associated with a higher (worse) recurrence score (R=−0.30, p=0.0031)" – PubMed ID#PMC3409927 (2012) [138]

Night workers are known to have a variety of health problems, mostly due to disrupted circadian rhythms. These rhythms guide our hormones, regulate cell regeneration, affect brain wave activity, can negatively impact glucose regulation, etc. They can also, of course, disrupt sleep, including both quality and length of sleep.

"Night workers have lower levels of melatonin, which may predispose them to develop cancer. Endometrial cancer risk is influenced significantly by hormonal and metabolic factors… Of the 121,701 women enrolled in a prospective cohort study, 53,487 women provided data on rotating night shift work in 1988 and were followed through on June 1, 2004… Women who worked 20+ years of rotating night shifts had a significantly increased risk of endometrial cancer… Women working rotating night shifts for a long duration have a significantly increased risk of endometrial cancer, particularly if they are obese." – PubMed ID#17975006 (2007) [139]

In short, either too little or too much sleep is associated with increased risk of death in cancer patients.

"a curvilinear relationship was observed between sleep duration and mortality: short and long sleep duration were associated with increased mortality" – PubMed ID#28366336 (2017) [140]

In this very large study (nearly 300,000 people), they found an association between several cancers and too little or too much sleep. These cancers included: bladder, stomach, head, neck, thyroid, non-Hodgkin's lymphoma, myeloma and ovarian cancers.

> "We assessed the associations between sleep duration and incidences of total and 18 site-specific cancers in the NIH-AARP Health and Diet Study cohort, with 173,327 men and 123,858 women aged 51-72 years at baseline." – PubMed ID#27611440 (2016) [141]

This study included women from the Women's Health Initiative Observational Study. It was pretty clear that women who received less than 7 to 8 hours of sleep per night were more likely to be diagnosed with more aggressive breast cancer.

> "The study included 4171 non-Hispanic whites (NHW) and 235 African Americans (AA) diagnosed with incident, primary, invasive breast cancer in the Women's Health Initiative (WHI) Observational Study… In NHW, women who reported 6 h of sleep/night were more likely to have tumors classified as regional/distant stage at diagnosis compared to women who slept 7-8 h/night (adjusted odds ratio (OR): 1.25, 95% confidence interval (CI): 1.05-1.48). AA women who reported their typical night's sleep as 'average quality' or 'restless or very restless sleep' were more likely to be diagnosed with triple-negative tumors than those who reported 'sound or restful' sleep (adjusted ORs: 2.91 (1.11, 7.63) and 3.74 (1.10, 12.77), respectively)." – PubMed ID#28417334 (2017) [142]

The following meta-study examines many different studies that looked at sleep disturbances and cancer. Though much research remains to be done in this area, the current consensus seems to be that either too little or too much sleep can increase a person's odds of contracting cancer, or of having a worse prognosis after being diagnosed with cancer.

> "There is beginning evidence that some aspects of sleep disturbance may contribute to the development of cancer and substantial evidence that sleep disturbance is associated with many aspects of cancer treatment, cancer symptoms and morbidity, mortality and quality of life… sleep disruption leads to increases in inflammatory mediators, that may contribute to excess morbidity and mortality among people with cancer… review of a large data base revealed that 33–50% of patients undergoing chemotherapy for a variety of cancers reported clinically significant insomnia, with the highest rates in lung cancer patients. These rates were approximately three times as high as those in the general population." – PubMed ID#PMC4346497 (2016) [143]

The following meta-study looked at 10 different studies and found that women who slept longer had decreases of between 38% and 72% in their risk of breast cancer (which is a huge reduction in risk!). They also found those with a higher level of melatonin to have up to a 34% decrease in breast cancer risk.

> "Articles were extracted from the PUBMED database between 2000 and 2012 with the following keywords "sleep duration", "sleep quality", "breast cancer risk" and "melatonin". In total, 10 articles were selected. Most prospective cohort studies found a decrease in the risk of breast cancer varying from 38 to 72% for "long sleepers". Furthermore, a meta-analysis of the studies assessing the link between breast cancer risk and urinary concentration of 6-sulfatoxy-melatonin (6MT), which is melatonin's main metabolite, found a 34% decrease for patients with the highest 6MT concentration." – PubMed ID #23395427 (2013) [144]

In addition to this chapter, be sure to see the section on Melatonin in Chapter 6. Melatonin is known as the "sleep hormone" and has anticancer benefits of its own.

❖ CIRCADIAN RHYTHMS

Sleep and circadian rhythms go hand in hand. One affects the other, and both affect cancer. Circadian rhythms are a roughly 24-hour physiological process that is found in plants, animals, humans, fungi and even some microorganisms. In humans it is strongly linked to sleep; circadian rhythms in humans affect hormones, alertness, body temperature, eating habits, digestion and hundreds of other biological functions. Every cell in the body has its own clock that controls its daily cellular functions; these clocks are all kept pretty much in sync with each other. Some of these functions are important to cancer development and proper function of the immune system.

Our circadian rhythms are endogenous to us, meaning they come from within; they are a part of us. However, they do take cues from our environment in order to keep our internal clock in sync with the environment. These cues include light (including various frequencies of light), temperature, and external chemical changes, such as those produced by bacteria within us and reactive oxygen species (ROS) levels in response to sunlight. Our internal clock is very complex and very important to our health.

> "It is widely accepted that light exerts a powerful influence on the human circadian system, including melatonin synthesis, and it is becoming more widely accepted that the circadian system plays a role in breast cancer. For example,

the efficacy of breast cancer treatment varies with circadian timing" – PubMed ID#PMC1557490 (2006) [145]

With circadian rhythms being so ubiquitous within nature, it should come as no surprise that disruptions to them can have negative consequences to our health—especially to sleep and hormones, but also to our odds of contracting cancer. Cancer prognosis is also worse if circadian rhythms are disrupted.

The following study examined 4,036 women who worked shift work, comparing those who did not work nights to those who did; women who only worked a day shift were used as the control group. Those who did not work nights had a 23% chance of breast cancer over the course of the study, but those who worked shift work that included night work had over 100% greater risk of breast cancer than women in the control group. A pretty startling difference considering the only difference between the two groups was that one group worked shifts that included working at night, and the other group did not. These results have been verified by other studies.

"In total, 94 women developed breast cancer during follow-up. The average follow-up time was 12.4 years. The hazard ratio for breast cancer was 1.23 [95% confidence interval (95% CI) 0.70-2.17] for shifts without night work and 2.02 (95% CI 1.03-3.95) for shifts with night work. When including only women <60 years of age, the risk estimates were 1.18 (95% CI 0.67-2.07) for shifts without night work, and 2.15 (95% CI 1.10-4.21) for shifts with night work… Our results indicate an increased risk for breast cancer among women who work shifts that includes night work." – PubMed ID#23007867 (2013) [146]

In this study published in January 2018 in the journal *Nature,* the researchers showed that two compounds that bind to cells to help regulate cell division, which helps kill several different types of cancer, including glioblastoma cells in mice. These compounds are a part of the circadian rhythm process. Though they killed cancer cells, they caused no harm to normal cells. This is a recent study and has not yet been used in treatment.

"The circadian clock imposes daily rhythms in cell proliferation, metabolism, inflammation and DNA damage response. Perturbations of these processes are hallmarks of cancer and chronic circadian rhythm disruption predisposes individuals to tumour development… the selective anticancer properties of these REV-ERB agonists impair glioblastoma growth in vivo and improve survival without causing any overt toxicity in mice. These results indicate that pharmacological modulation of circadian regulators is an effective novel antitumor strategy" – PubMed ID#PMC5924733 (2018, Nature) [147]

Just more evidence that what we think of as the conveniences of normal, modern life can have a negative effect on human health. The following paper (especially the "full study" link) looks at the accumulated evidence of day-to-day disruptions to our circadian clock. Simple things such as frequent international travel (where multiple time zones are crossed) can have negative consequences for cancer survival and progression.

> "Frequent transmeridian flights or predominant work at night can increase cancer risk. Altered circadian rhythms also predict for poor survival in cancer patients… Tumor grew faster in the jet-lagged animals as compared with controls… Altered environmental conditions can disrupt circadian clock molecular coordination in peripheral organs including tumors and play a significant role in malignant progression." – PubMed ID#15520194 (2004) [148] (Full Study [149])

Blue Light

Blue light seems to get a lot of bad press, and this is unfortunate. Blue light is very important to our circadian rhythms, to the body making melatonin, and thus to good health. However, as with anything having to do with our circadian rhythms, timing is very important. You want your eyes (and skin if possible) exposed to blue light in the morning, and to a lesser extent, early afternoon. You should restrict blue light at dusk and after. This is how nature has worked for millions of years and across nearly every animal species, and humans may be even more sensitive to this process.

Nighttime blue light exposure is a very recent phenomenon—old-fashioned incandescent light bulbs emitted light more in the red spectrum. Old, picture tube-type TVs were balanced in the light they emitted. Today's laptops, TVs and cell phones use LED backlighting that produces far more blue light. As people switch to more energy-efficient LED lightbulbs, these too can emit more blue light. More recent LED bulbs are available with more "white" light, as these bulbs use a phosphor coating to produce this whiter light. You can also get these bulbs in a "warm white" that looks much more like the old incandescent light bulbs (it is slightly reddish in color and is generally thought of as softer). Though LED bulbs are not the equivalent to natural daylight, they are closer than they used to be.

When we are exposed to blue light at night, it disrupts our circadian rhythms and interrupts melatonin release. Too much blue light may also be linked to permanent eye damage (though just how much blue light is needed for this is still being researched). Regarding cancer, the main effect of evening/nighttime blue light is its effect on circadian rhythms and melatonin production. We need blue light for proper circadian rhythms and for melatonin production, both of which are important to fighting and preventing cancer.

> "A major milestone came with the 1998 discovery of melanopsin retinal ganglion cells, a new type of photoreceptor in the eye. These cells provide

> signals to the suprachiasmatic nucleus (SCN), the brain's master clock. They project to many other brain regions as well, influencing myriad aspects of human physiology. Moreover, research would show, they are uniquely sensitive to blue light… blue's benefit, and its detriment, are both a matter of timing. In one experiment, Kunz showed that exposing healthy subjects to 30 minutes of 500 lux polychromatic blue light an hour before bedtime, in their natural home environment, delayed the onset of rapid eye movement sleep by 30 minutes." – PubMed ID #PMC2831986 (2010) [150]

The following study found some correlation between blue light exposure and uveal melanoma (UM, melanoma of the eye). However, there were many other factors involved. Outdoor blue light is also accompanied by some level of UV radiation, and UV radiation is also associated with UM, therefore it might be the UV responsible for uveal melanoma and not visible spectrum blue light. Other factors include iris color (lighter iris color is associated with higher UV risk) and genetics. And yet, other studies have shown that sunlight exposure does not show a strong association with UM.

> "cumulative epidemiological and experimental evidence indicates that blue light is a credible risk factor for the development of UM (Uveal Melanoma)" – PubMed ID#PMC4449937 (2015) [151]

Blue light during the day is associated with higher nighttime melatonin levels (which is what you want). It has also been shown to "significantly" improve prostate cancer.

> "These data show that the amplification of nighttime melatonin levels by exposing nude rats to blue light during the daytime significantly reduces human prostate cancer metabolic, signaling, and proliferative activities… Light profoundly influences circadian, neuroendocrine, and neurobehavioral regulation in all mammals and is essential to life on our planet. The light–dark cycle entrains the master biologic clock, located in the suprachiasmatic nucleus of the brain, in an intensity-, duration-, and wavelength-dependent manner." – PubMed ID#PMC4681241 (2015) [152]

So, when you hear people talking trash about "blue light," just remember that it isn't the blue light that is the problem; it is timing. Blue light exposure during the day (especially sunlight) is a beneficial part of the circadian rhythm cycle and melatonin production. Blue light exposure in the evening and at night has just the opposite effect.

Regarding blue light, here is my advice:

- Try to get outside in the morning and look at the world around you. Look at the sky, but avoid looking at the sun. Try to do this in as natural an environment as possible.

- Limit night exposure to blue light. Use software on your computer and phone that automatically limits blue light after the sun goes down. The one I use on my desktop and laptop is called f.lux (available for Windows, Mac, iPhone/iPad and Android devices). My phone has this function built in, but if yours does not, you can use the f.lux app. Another good one for Android is Twilight: Blue Light Filter.

- When purchasing new light bulbs, make sure you use "warm" bulbs. The white light bulbs aren't that beneficial for the morning cycle. For that, you need to get outside, even if it is cloudy, or purchase a full-spectrum light therapy lamp (and use it as directed; how much time depends on its "Lux" rating).

- Watching television is another source of blue light. This is where some blue light filtering glasses can help when watching TV at night. Some newer TVs have a nighttime setting that will produce far less blue light when activated.

- On rainy days when you can't get outside, take a melatonin tablet before bed. See the section on Melatonin in Chapter 6. This only helps with part of the problem, but it is better than nothing.

Tips for Better Sleep

- Make sure you get outside before noon and get sunlight. Do not look at the sun, but spend at least 30 minutes without sunglasses on bright days, or an hour if cloudy. Just look around at nature. It seems to help to focus on things far away and at parts of the sky that won't cause you to face the sun.

- Afternoon sun is fine, but if you go to bed early and the sun sets late, make sure you restrict strong light at least 2 hours before bed. You can still go outside; just wear sunglasses.

- Avoid all caffeine. Some people are very slow metabolizers of caffeine and it may affect them for over 24 hours! There are other substances in coffee and tea (even decaffeinated varieties) that can interfere with sleep, so it's best to avoid all forms, especially if testing your sensitivity. Any self-testing should last for at least two weeks.

- No more than two alcoholic drinks per day, and nothing within 3 hours of bedtime. I know, that can be rather restrictive. But if you're having problems sleeping, this can help.

- Install software on your phone and computer to remove blue light, such as f.lux [153] (which is free for personal use). This software changes the color temperature of your screen to remove much of the blue light from the screen after sunset. It is this blue light that tells the brain it is time to stay awake and active. The color

---

temperature of the light we see is a very important part of the circadian rhythms. Too much blue light at night can make it harder to get to sleep, stay asleep and sleep well.

- If you spend a lot of time on your computer, you should get a pair of computer glasses, or clip-ons for prescription glasses. These have a mild tint that removes much of the blue light. These should be used after the sun has gone down or for the last 4 hours of your day (before going to bed). These are not needed if you use software to change the color temperature at sunset.

- Set a schedule. Getting up and going to bed at the same time each day helps set the circadian rhythm. Vary too much and it can throw off your body's internal clock.

- "Early to bed, early to rise" (attributed to Benjamin Franklin) is still the best policy. This allows us to synchronize with the forces of nature that push us to be awake during the day and to sleep at night.

- No naps. If you have trouble sleeping at night, a nap can sound really good, but it may also throw off your sleep schedule. However, if you're one of those people who can still go to sleep at your normal time, naps do not seem to have negative consequences. PubMed ID#11560181 (2001) [154]

- Do not eat before bed. There are several reasons for this. Besides being bad for sleep, it can also lead to gut issues such as SIBO and acid reflux, and perhaps worsen *H. pylori*. Avoid any food for at least 3 hours before bed. Trust me on this one; you may have gotten away with it for years, but the older we get, the more likely this can cause problems. Eating late is especially a problem for people who already have the conditions mentioned here.

- Exercise. Several studies have shown the benefits of even light exercise on sleep. Exercise strengthens circadian rhythms and stimulates longer periods of slow-wave sleep, the deepest and most healing period of the sleep cycle. Exercise should be moderate for your health condition (too much or too strenuous exercise can interfere with sleep) and should not cause inflammation that lasts more than an hour. Exercise should also be completed at least 3 hours before bedtime.

"a single bout of exercise can increase the amount of subsequent SWS (slow wave sleep). Secondly, exercise shortly before going to bed could also produce a stress effect that can reduce the amount of subsequent SWS." – PubMed ID#PMC3317043 (2012) [155]

The following study was conducted on healthy, non-obese, elderly women.

"Our data showed that a single moderate-intensity aerobic exercise session improved sleep quality in older women." – PubMed ID#PMC4326238 (2014) [156]

- Noise – Though some people like to sleep with a TV or radio going, this can actually reduce the quality of sleep. Try sleeping with a fan on or use a white noise machine. This type of noise is less stressful to the mind and is similar to the sound of wind or waves that the mind is adapted to hear when sleeping. Try not to have it any louder than necessary, and perhaps try to turn it down a little every week or two. Noise, and especially unnatural noise, is a form of stress for the brain.

- Stress – I know this is easier said than done, but reducing stress in your life will not only help you get to sleep easier, but also can lead to a deeper, more rejuvenating sleep. Stress also negatively affects the immune system, so reducing it can have direct benefits for fighting and preventing cancer. If you cannot reduce the stressors in your life, I recommend that you at least make a strong effort at coping with them better. The following section will touch on stress.

❖ STRESS

Stress is an often overlooked factor in disease, especially cancer. We like to believe that cancer is just something that happens randomly, that it is totally outside of our control. Doctors certainly don't want to blame the patient for their disease, so the myth that cancer is totally random continues. However, research continues to show that environmental factors, many within our control, can significantly contribute to our risk of cancer and can either improve our odds of fighting cancer, or worsen them. Genetics are also one of the risk factors, but cancer is usually not 100% random, and we can do things to help prevent it. Even if cancers were random, our ability to fight them (and kill them in their infancy) depends on a strong, well-tuned immune system, and there is nothing random about that. One of the factors that can worsen our odds of beating cancer is chronic stress, and avoiding or dealing with stress can *Improve Your Odds* of preventing and treating cancer.

It appears that occasional stress is not a cancer risk factor, and it may even be beneficial if handled properly. It is the chronic stress that causes hopelessness, negativity, depression, ruminating and brooding, which lead to poor health and higher cancer risks (and poorer prognosis). Often these are within our control (e.g., a change of attitude, being grateful for what we have, comparing our problems with those of the less fortunate, etc.), though sometimes they may not be (a death of a loved one, disease, loss of a job, etc.). However, there are many ways of dealing with stress: exercise, breathing exercises, yoga, spiritualism, etc.

Ultimately this type of stress is psychological, meaning even if we have good reason to feel hopeless, we must fight it. Adding cancer to our list of problems is not going to help the situation. It is up to us to force ourselves to feel better. This may mean doing what you've always been told not to do. Be selfish; you have to think about yourself and your happiness, and you need to force yourself to do things that may be fun. Watch a movie that makes you laugh (even if you don't want to laugh), associate with more easygoing people when possible, etc. If helping others helps you feel good and relieves stress, then by all means do so. But in doing so, do not forget to help yourself. You cannot help others if you're a stressed-out mess dealing with cancer.

If you find yourself in a relationship with a negative person, it may be difficult to control the external stressors. However, you should know that if you don't find a way to control the stress or escape the relationship, you are greatly worsening your odds of preventing cancer or preventing cancer progression. This isn't just feel-good mumbo jumbo; there is strong scientific evidence behind it. Stress and hopelessness not only negatively affect humans, but also have a strong impact on animals as well (and this can easily be demonstrated in animal research).

Research shows that chronic stress can not only worsen one's odds of contracting cancer, but also lead to a greater risk of metastasis. This risk has been seen in both animal and human studies. Stress hormones, such as cortisol, have a direct impact on the immune system and cancer. Increased hormone levels can be measured under chronic stress conditions, and they are found to be lowered when people and animals receive social support and participate in stress reduction activities.

The following studies do a good job of describing how stress affects cancer and metastasis progression. The first research paper includes references to dozens of additional studies. It is quite clear that various forms of stress can worsen cancer outcomes and increase metastasis.

"Chronicity of negative affect, as manifested by depressed mood or hopelessness, appears to have stronger relationships with outcomes than do stressful events, suggesting that sustained activation of negative affective pathways may provide the strongest links to cancer progression… Several studies have linked high levels of social support to improved clinical outcomes in cancer patients. For example, in breast cancer patients, social support has been related to longer survival in several large-scale studies" – PubMed ID#PMC3037818 (2011) [157]

"Stress promotes development of ovarian cysts in rats: the possible role of sympathetic nerve activation." – PubMed ID#9741836 (1998) [158]

"Animals exposed to acute stress showed a substantial decrease in NK cell cytotoxicity against this tumor in an in vitro assay and, when intravenously injected with this tumor, showed a twofold increase in surface lung metastases. The critical period during which stress increases metastases appears to be the same as that during which this tumor is known to be controlled by NK cells. These findings support the hypothesis that stress can facilitate the metastatic process via suppression of the immune system." – PubMed ID#1654166 (1991) [159]

"In conclusion, breast cancer metastatic cells may be affected by sympathetic cues in various manners, directly or indirectly, depending on their origin (breast, prostate, ovary, skin and so on) and stages of tumor development… it appears from these preclinical studies that interventions aimed at reducing sympathetic nerve activity or downstream signals (including RANKL) may hold promise for limiting tumor cell dissemination to distant organs and thus for improving the prognosis of patients with cancers at risk for metastasis." – PubMed ID#PMC4432778 (2015) [160]

❖ EXERCISE

This section is going to cover why exercise is important; the type of exercise is less important. Even the type of cancer is not a huge factor; exercise helps to prevent and treat nearly every type of cancer studied. To underscore this point I'm going to focus on studies that looked at melanoma (a cancer we might not think exercise would help) and breast cancer (again, a cancer type where the relationship with exercise is not intuitively obvious). Do not lose focus on the fact that exercise has benefits against all types of cancer.

The following study looked at exercise by itself but also discusses the possible benefits as adjuvant treatment when used in conjunction with new immunotherapy drugs (such as checkpoint inhibitors like Keytruda and Opdivo).

"We recently demonstrated that voluntary exercise leads to an influx of immune cells in tumors and a greater than 60% reduction in tumor incidence and growth across several mouse models… tumor incidence was decreased from 70% to 30% by exercise and the tumors that did develop were smaller. Given that fact that the immune infiltrate in the B16 (melanoma) model showed a significant increase not only in NK cells, but also in dendritic cells, B cells, and T cells" – PubMed ID#PMC4972115 (2016) [161]

Here they compared different types of exercise based on their metabolic equivalent task (MET). What they found was that simply walking 3 to 5 hours per week at an average pace could reduce the risk of death after a breast cancer diagnosis.

"Objective: To determine whether physical activity among women with breast cancer decreases their risk of death from breast cancer compared with more sedentary women… Compared with women who engaged in less than 3 MET-hours per week of physical activity, the adjusted relative risk (RR) of death from breast cancer was 0.80 (95% confidence interval [CI], 0.60-1.06) for 3 to 8.9 MET-hours per week; 0.50… Three MET-hours is equivalent to walking at average pace of 2 to 2.9 mph for 1 hour… Physical activity after a breast cancer diagnosis may reduce the risk of death from this disease. The greatest benefit occurred in women who performed the equivalent of walking 3 to 5 hours per week at an average pace, with little evidence of a correlation between increased benefit and greater energy expenditure." – PubMed ID#15914748 (2005) [162]

The following study investigated physical activity and motility among women with breast cancer.

"Compared with women who were inactive both before and after diagnosis, women who increased physical activity after diagnosis had a 45% lower risk of death… women who decreased physical activity after diagnosis had a four-fold greater risk of death" – PubMed ID#18711185 (2008) [163]

The following paper highlighted some of the many studies that have shown the benefits of moderate exercise on cancer (prevention and outcomes). It may also show significant adjuvant benefits to immunotherapy.

"Exercise improves functional capacity and patient-reported outcomes across a range of cancer diagnoses. The mechanisms behind this protection have been largely unknown, but exercise-mediated changes in body composition, sex hormone levels, systemic inflammation, and immune cell function have been suggested to play a role… We recently demonstrated that voluntary exercise leads to an influx of immune cells in tumors, and a more than 60% reduction in tumor incidence and growth across several mouse models. Given the common mechanisms of immune cell mobilization in mouse and man during exercise, we hypothesize that this link between exercise and the immune system can be exploited in cancer therapy in particular in combination with immunotherapy. Thus, we believe that exercise may not just be "healthy" but may in fact be therapeutic… Exercise has also been shown to have a preventive effect on the risk of cancer, i.e., leisure-time exercise is associated with a lower cancer incidence… (in a mouse studies) voluntary exercise (wheel running) leads to a significant reduction in tumor size or incidence… exercise had a significant impact on tumor size in the transplanted lewis lung cancer and B16 melanoma models—the latter studied both as subcutaneous (s.c.) tumors, as well as lung metastases established upon intravenous administration of cancer cells… we could show an impact of exercise on tumor size and incidence on liver cancer using a diethylnitrosamine (DEN) induced liver cancer model, as well as the spontaneous melanoma model GrM1… recently pooled data from 12 prospective cohorts with self-reported physical activity for association with incidence of 26 types of cancer, and could demonstrate that leisure-time physical activity is significantly associated with a lower risk of cancer, e.g., cancers of the oesophagus, liver, lung, kidney, colon, breast, and as well as leukemia and myeloma" – PubMed ID#PMC5406418 (2017 – Creative Commons attribution available at the link) [164]

Idorn, Manja, and Per Thor Straten. "Exercise and cancer: from "healthy" to "therapeutic"? Cancer immunology, immunotherapy : CII vol. 66,5 (2017): 667-671. doi:10.1007/s00262-017-1985-z

Exercise has been shown to reduce the risk of contracting several cancers (probably all of those researched).

"A 2009 meta-analysis of 52 epidemiologic studies that examined the association between physical activity and colon cancer risk found that the most physically active individuals had a 24% lower risk of colon cancer than those who were the least physically active… a 2013 meta-analysis of 31 prospective studies, the average breast cancer risk reduction associated with physical activity was 12%… In a meta-analysis of 33 studies, the average endometrial cancer risk reduction associated with high versus low physical activity was 20%… In a study of over 1 million individuals, leisure-time physical activity was linked to reduced risks of esophageal adenocarcinoma, liver cancer, gastric cardia cancer (a type of stomach cancer), kidney cancer, myeloid leukemia, myeloma, and cancers of the head and neck, rectum, and bladder" – Cancer.gov [165]

❖ STRATEGY

It is clear from the research that sleep disruption, stress and lack of exercise can all worsen your odds with cancer. Ignoring any of these not only increases your odds of contracting cancer, but also worsens any existing cancer prognosis. Even minor changes in your daily routine may *Improve Your Odds*. Though you may not always be able to get more sleep, perhaps due to health issues, you should always try. Our bodies are tuned to the sun; we are controlled by circadian rhythms, and circadian rhythms are largely controlled by the sun. Follow the tips above to *Improve Your Odds* of a good night's sleep.

Updates at - https://improvingyourodds.com

Support at - https://www.facebook.com/groups/cancer.improving.your.odds

Dealing with stress is just as important, and there are well known strategies people can take to help deal with stress. Even if you are not in the mood, exercise always helps (even if you don't realize it at first). There are many self-help guides for dealing with stress; most of them work to some degree or another. You'll need to find what works best for you. Improving your health, exercise, regular sleep, quiet time, and giving up drinking all help and would be a great place to start.

Exercise seems daunting to many people. But the research shows that even moderate exercise, such as a 10-minute walk per day, has its benefits, and as little as 3 to 5 hours per week may be optimal. Don't feel you are wasting your time simply because you can't run, can't afford a gym membership, or don't have the time. None of these things matter; what matters is daily movement. Try increasing the amount you do a little at a time and find ways to make it interesting. Even volunteering to walk a neighbor's dog can help with that (and I guarantee you the dog will appreciate it). A moderately brisk walk seems to be one of the better forms of exercise when it comes to improving cancer outcomes.

Being overweight is also associated with an increased risk of many different cancers. Everything in this chapter has been associated with helping people lose weight; ketogenic diets also help overweight people lose weight. Because there are many books on weight loss, I have chosen not to cover it in this book. Just know that if you do what is advised in this book, you will be *Improving Your Odds* with cancer regardless of your weight.

Each of the subjects in this chapter deserves much more coverage, but there is simply way too much information to include here. I recommend joining online groups and following the conversation for a while. This will help you learn where your interests lie and help you form questions regarding your specific situation.

I will end this section with the advice not to ignore sleep, stress or exercise. Most of the other recommendations in this book depend on these not being existing issues. Any therapy will work far more effectively if these basics are not ignored.

◆ ❖ ◆

Updates at - https://improvingyourodds.com/

Support at - https://www.facebook.com/groups/cancer.improving.your.odds

--- The Remainder of This Page Intentionally Left Blank ---

Chapter 6
Cancer-Fighting Natural Supplements

"The doctor of the future will no longer treat the human frame with drugs, but rather will cure and prevent disease with nutrition." ~ Thomas Edison

While doing the research for this book, I was frequently amazed by how many different plants and natural substances affected the progression of human cancer. Some of these had dramatic effects on cancer, both in vitro (in the test tube) and in vivo (in the body). For many of the natural compounds, the research was clear: Some natural supplements can be as beneficial, or even more so, as many of the cancer drugs. This chapter is going to cover many different natural supplements and foods.

I would like to stress (yet again) that just because some natural compounds can help fight cancer, that doesn't mean you should avoid medical treatment. Just the opposite: Most of the natural compounds can be used as adjuvants to (alongside) medical treatments; in many cases the results will be synergistic (having an effect greater than the sum of the two individually). You're fighting cancer here, not a cold, so throw everything effective at it that you safely can.

I don't spend a lot of time evaluating which cancers a specific supplement affected and which it didn't. Most of these natural compounds are immunomodulating—that is, they improve or tweak the immune system to battle cancer. Most have been found in research to benefit many types of cancer. Because there is no profit motivation for studies of these botanicals, many simply have not been tested against all (or even many) forms of cancer.

Most of the natural anti-tumor botanicals are biological response modifiers (BRM). These are substances that can stimulate the immune system into doing a better job, and thus provide therapeutic benefits. Unlike some prescription drugs, most do not overstimulate the immune system. They provide what the immune system needs to identify their targets or build up the potential to attack cancer cells, meaning they strengthen the immune system to allow it to do a better job, rather than revving it up artificially and forcing it into action.

Because these therapies are based on natural products or extracts, most cannot receive a patent, at least not in the US and EU. This makes it very difficult for drug companies to make a profit. Without high profits, no company is going to spend the millions of dollars (some say billions!) to obtain FDA approval to utilize them as a medical treatment or prescription drug. To obtain FDA approval for human research studies, researchers must use standardized chemical isolates, not whole foods, herbs or even multiple natural compounds. Though most of these isolates show great promise, this misses the very likely possibility that utilizing the whole plant, or multiple isolates, might have an even greater, synergistic effect. In fact, some research has shown exactly that—the natural compounds are often better than the isolates.

This chapter is laid out first by the type of natural product, and then by compound or name. For instance, magnesium is found under Minerals. Of course, you mostly want to know what benefits your type of cancer. However, as I mentioned earlier, most of these natural products benefit many or all types of cancer. If you only want to see references to your particular type of cancer, you can use the Index and follow those page references. However, I would prefer that you get a highlighter, read through this entire chapter and highlight information that you think applies to you. If a compound greatly improves the immune system, your type of cancer may not be mentioned, but you can probably benefit from it. If a supplement benefits two or three distinctly different cancers (e.g., skin, liver and colon), you can be pretty sure it is going to benefit most cancer (quite possibly including yours).

The use of a combination of anticancer compounds that affect different functional pathways may possess the capacity to generate additive or synergistic activity. In theory, this is an attractive approach for the prevention and/or treatment of most cancers. I highly recommend the kitchen sink approach—taking several supplements that attack cancer in different ways.

I hope that as you read this section, you get as excited as I did as I researched it. Several of the botanicals and foods mentioned here have shown dramatic abilities to fight and prevent cancer—so much so that I think it is almost a crime that they haven't received more attention. My hope is this book will help change that.

Note

If you are on any medications or have other health issues, be sure to look up any herbals or botanicals that you plan to take for contraindications. One of the best ways to do this is on the Memorial Sloan Kettering "Herbs and Dietary Supplements" website. It is not uncommon for dietary supplements to interfere with certain medications. [166] Your doctor, and especially your oncologist, should also be told of any supplements you plan to take.

BETA-GLUCANS

Cancers: All
Body of Evidence: Large
Cost: Low to moderate

Beta-glucans (or β-glucans) occur in the cellular wall of some plants, bacteria, fungi, yeast, some grains and most types of seaweed. They are polysaccharides, a type of carbohydrate, made up of long chains of glucose molecules. Beta-glucans vary in makeup and physiological benefits depending on the source. Mushrooms, which contain beta-glucans, will be covered in another section in this chapter as they contain unique chemotherapeutic properties.

Researchers have taken great interest in the properties of beta-glucans and how they improve and modulate the immune system, the hope being that discoveries could lead to new, better, safer, and most importantly, patentable drugs.

> "more than 6000 publications investigating the immune-modulating effects of β-glucans, such as anti-inflammatory or antimicrobial abilities, have been published" – PubMed ID#PMC4012169 (2014) [167]

Each source of beta-glucan has differing physicochemical properties. Some of these properties are significant, and each can confer different health and chemotherapeutic properties. Beta-glucans are made up of complex long-chain molecules; what differentiates one type from another are their unique side-branching patterns. These unique branches must match those of cellular receptor sites, like a lock and key, in order to confer benefits. Therefore, it is important to obtain beta-glucans from a variety of sources. Some of the chemotherapeutic properties of mushrooms, found in the next section, are due to unique beta-glucans not found in grain sources. As you'll see in this section, and the next one on mushrooms, beta-glucans have a lot to offer, including anticancer properties, significant immune system improvements, anti-inflammatory and general health benefits.

> "Typically, β-glucans form a linear backbone with 1-3 β-glycosidic bonds but vary with respect to molecular mass, solubility, viscosity, branching structure, and gelation properties, causing diverse physiological effects in animals... Differences in molecular weight, shape, and structure of β-glucans dictate the differences in biological activity." – Wikipedia - Beta-glucan [168]

> "β-glucans are absorbed in the small intestine and taken up by macrophages. β-glucans are considered to be 'biological response modifiers' since they exhibit immunomodulatory, wound-healing, antiviral, antibacterial, anti-coagulatory and antitumoral activities... Our data indicate that β-D-glucan regulates breast cancer-relevant gene expression and may be useful for inhibiting endocrine-resistant breast cancer cell proliferation." – PubMed ID#PMC3977804 (2014) [169]

"Beta-glucan, a "specific" biologic response modifier that uses antibodies to target tumors for cytotoxic recognition by leukocyte complement receptor type 3 (CD11b/CD18)." – PubMed ID#10477568 (1999) [170]

"combined therapy of β-glucan with anti-tumor mAbs has achieved significant therapeutic efficacy in a variety of murine syngeneic tumors… as well as in human carcinoma xenograft models" -- PubMed ID#PMC2685877 (2009) [171]

There are two basic mechanisms of polysaccharide action against tumor cells:

- Indirect action (immunostimulation) – Indirect action has a stimulating, or modulating, effect on the immune system. This can include T and B lymphocytes, macrophages and natural killer (NK) cells. Mushroom beta-glucans can stimulate the production of interferons, interleukins and other cytokines. These are the body's natural cancer-killing mechanisms and are not toxic to healthy cells. Beta-glucans enhance the ability of these immune cells to recognize cancer cells. There is a lot to this, and though these mechanisms have been extensively studied, there is much left to be discovered. What is important here is that research studies have shown, both in vitro and in vivo, that these substances have very important cancer-fighting properties.

- Direct action (inhibition of tumor cell growth and apoptosis induction) – These unique bioactive polysaccharides can also directly inhibit cancer cell growth and enhance apoptosis. Again, these are non-toxic mechanisms that only affect the aberrant nature of cancer cells and have shown no negative effects on normal cells. Apoptosis is the body's natural way of initiating programmed cell death when a cell becomes damaged or isn't functioning correctly. Some cancers can turn off this process, so even if the immune system recognizes a cancerous cell, it may be unable to initiate apoptosis. These unique polysaccharides can help normalize this process and allow the immune system to turn apoptosis back on in cancer cells. This is correcting the cells' natural apoptotic programming and causes no damage to normal cells.

Because beta-glucans are not water soluble and are not a vitamin, mineral or calorie source, it was once thought that they served no role outside of the intestines. Due to their molecular size, researchers thought they couldn't pass through the intestinal wall. However, it turns out that beta-glucans are *allowed* to pass through the small intestine into the systemic environment. This is thought to occur when Bifidobacteria in our gut break up the beta-glucans into smaller soluble pieces and our immune system's macrophages further break these down. Dendritic cells will then transport this material to the spleen, lymph nodes and bone marrow (all key components of the immune system), where they help modulate our immune system's T cells. It is the job of dendritic cells to transport antigen material and present it on the cell surface to the T cells of the immune system in order to modulate an immune response. Some of what follows may sound like mumbo jumbo, but in reading over it you'll see that beta-glucans are an important part of our immune system's ability to fight cancer. This is the part you may want to show your oncologist if they've never heard of this before (again, they're taught medicine, not nutrition. But most are eager to learn).

> "Orally administered beta-1,3-glucans were taken up by macrophages that transported them to spleen, lymph nodes, and bone marrow. Within the bone marrow, the macrophages degraded the large beta-1,3-glucans into smaller soluble beta-1,3-glucan fragments that were taken up by the CR3 of marginated granulocytes. These granulocytes with CR3-bound beta-1,3-glucan-fluorescein were shown to kill iC3b-opsonized tumor cells" – PubMed ID#15240666 (2004) [172]

> "The induction of cellular responses by mushroom and other beta-glucans is likely to involve their specific interaction with several cell surface receptors, as complement receptor 3 (CR3; CD11b/CD18), lactosylceramide, selected scavenger receptors, and dectin-1 (betaGR). beta-Glucans also show anticarcinogenic activity. They can prevent oncogenesis due to the protective effect against potent genotoxic carcinogens... acts through the activation of macrophages and NK cell cytotoxicity, beta-glucan can inhibit tumor growth in promotion stage too." – PubMed ID#17895634 (2007) [173]

> "β-Glucans are potent immunomodulators that have multiple activities such as anti-tumor and anti-infective activities... binding of β-glucan to specific receptors in macrophages and dendritic cells can induce the production of various cytokines, indirectly activating other immune cells such as T cells and B cells under in vivo conditions. Systemic immunostimulation might be the main route in preventing the growth of cancer cells and infective microorganisms in the host. Several β-glucan receptors in macrophages and dendritic cells, such as dectin-1 and TLRs, might play a key role in the recognition of β-glucans" – PubMed ID#PMC3202617 (2011) [174]

> "Beta-glucans (β-glucans), naturally occurring polysaccharides, are present as constituents of the cell wall of cereal grains, mushrooms, algae, or microbes including bacteria, fungi, and yeast... As an immunomodulating agent, β-glucan acts through the activation of innate immune cells such as macrophages, dendritic cells, granulocytes, and natural killer cells. This activation triggers the responses of adaptive immune cells such as CD4(+) or CD8(+) T cells and B cells, resulting in the inhibition of tumor growth and metastasis. Reports have shown that β-glucans exert multiple effects on cancer cells and cancer prevention." – PubMed ID#23140352 (2013) [175]

"A well-functioning immune system is crucial for staying healthy… not all β-glucans are able to modulate immune functions. These properties mainly depend on the primary chemical structure of the β-glucans. Cellulose for example, a (1,4)-β-linked glucan, does not exhibit immune-modulatory effects… β-glucans derived from fungi and yeast, which consist of a (1,3)-β-linked backbone with small numbers of (1,6)-β-linked side chains, are essentially known for their immune-modulating effects" – Open Access License - Copyright © 2014 Stier et al.; licensee BioMed Central Ltd., doi: 10.1186/1475-2891-13-38 (2014) [176]

"beta-glucan enhances tumor killing through a cascade of events, including in vivo macrophage cleavage of the polysaccharide, dual CR3 ligation, and CR3-Syk-PI3K signaling. These results are important in as much as beta-glucan… may be used to amplify tumor cell killing and may open new opportunities in the immunotherapy of cancer." – PubMed ID#16849475 (2006) [177]

"Current data suggests that β-glucans are very potent immunomodulators with effects on innate and adaptive immunity… The antitumor effect of β-glucan can be attributed to cancer-preventing, immune-enhancing and direct tumor inhibition activities… Our results showed that new LMW beta-glucan from oat significantly decreased human melanoma and human epidermoid carcinoma viability… Our preliminary studies show strong anti-tumor properties of new low molecular weight beta-glucan from oat and at the same time no toxicity for normal cells." -- DOI: 10.1016/j.ijbiomac.2015.05.035, PubMed ID#26092171 (2015) [178]

"Glucans exert adjuvant activities through their capability to bind to specific surface carbohydrate receptors, such as CR-3 and Dectin-1, expressed on the monocyte-macrophage cell lineage and other antigen-presenting immunocompetent cells, i. e. dendritic cells. The attachment of glucan molecules to these receptors results in the activation of a cascade of pathways that subsequently increase the production of proinflammatory cytokines and chemokines inducing antigen presentation and cellular co-stimulation, which leads to enhancing of both humoral and cellular immunity." – PubMed ID#PMC4231372 (2014) [179]

As you can see, there are a lot of studies on the benefits of beta-glucans in fighting cancer. The importance of various sources, and types, of beta-glucans cannot stressed enough. Different beta-glucans appear to bind to different T cell receptors and modulate the immune response differently.

You should consume a variety of foods and supplements containing beta-glucans. Beta-glucans vary based on their molecular branching and mass, with each showing different benefits.

> "Mushroom β-glucans are structurally diverse molecules varying in branching, through 1,6 linkages, and in molecular mass (21, 22). β-Glucans with a degree of branching between 0.20 and 0.33 seem to be the most active" – PubMed ID#PMC5118454 (2016) [180]

Strategy

Good sources of beta-glucans include mushrooms (see the next main section), oats (though high in carbohydrates), nutritional yeast (this type of yeast is dead and cannot grow in the body) and the EpiCor® fermentate (discussed next). A good strategy is to consume lots of mushrooms/mushroom powders, add nutritional yeast to recipes and take an EpiCor fermentate supplement.

Another excellent source of beta-glucans is a supplement containing a phage complex to kill unwanted bacteria in the gut. The phages will kill unwanted bacteria that may be causing your gut issues or outcompeting beneficial bacteria. Phages are very specific in what they kill; at this time, I think the only commercially available phage products all kill unwanted strains of *E. coli*. When they do this, the dead *E. coli* cells feed beneficial bacteria throughout the gut, such as the highly valuable Bifidobacterium strains. These strains can greatly benefit the immune system and immunotherapy. See the research in Chapter 2. A supplement containing a phage complex and Bifidobacterium probiotic strains is a perfect combination.

❖ EPICOR FERMENTATE

EpiCor is a proprietary formulation that uses a stressed baker's yeast (*Saccharomyces cerevisiae*) to produce a prebiotic whole food. This yeast is then "deactivated" (kills the yeast) so it cannot cause any sort of intestinal yeast infection. It is essentially an enhanced version of nutritional yeast.

> "Beta glucans are simple extracts from the cell wall of yeast or grains like oats and cannot be considered a whole food. Because EpiCor is not highly processed or refined, it is a whole food yeast fermentate containing a complex range of nutrients and metabolites, in which beta glucan is only one of dozens. It's the whole, natural composition of EpiCor that makes it so beneficial and unique… specialized process begins with microorganism cells being deprived of oxygen, which causes them to produce immune supporting compounds and metabolites

such as proteins, peptides, antioxidants, polyphenols, organic acids, and nucleotides. This natural, unique fermentation complex also contains the beneficial yeast cell compounds such as 1-3 1-6 beta glucans and mannans." – EpiCor [181]

This specific formula has been the subject of several research studies. It has been shown to be anti-inflammatory, improve the immune response and produce the short-chain fatty acid butyrate (discussed later in this chapter).

"Treatment of inflammatory cells in vitro with dried fermentate resulted in reduced inflammatory responses. This was confirmed in vivo, suggesting that the dried fermentate facilitates the resolution of inflammatory responses... In contrast to pure beta-glucans and yeast cell wall preparations, complex fungal-derived products present a highly complex profile of bioactive compounds to the immune system. The dried fermentate tested in this study (EpiCor®) does not consist solely of yeast cells or yeast biomass... Furthermore, this dried fermentate inhibited ROS formation and chemotactic migration toward the inflammatory mediator Leukotriene B4 in human PMN cells... Among the known immuno-modulatory compounds from S. cerevisiae, various cell wall compounds have been studied. The primary compound of the inner layer of the cell wall is beta-1–3-glucan... The fermentate promoted probiotic bacterial strains capable of production of short-chain fatty acids, particularly butyrate, which was produced at higher levels than in the presence of the known prebiotics inulin and fructooligosaccharide." – PubMed ID# PMC4350453 (2015) [182]

The following two papers show the importance of controlling ROS (reactive oxygen species). ROS is an unstable molecule that can react with other cell molecules. This can cause damage to the cell's RNA, DNA and proteins and cause the death of the cell. They are a type of free radical often produced by cancer. ROS can cause a lot of damage to healthy tissue around tumors and promote additional tumor growth.

"Cancer cells including melanoma cells exhibit high levels of ROS... , emerging evidence from specific investigations of melanoma cells indicates that other cellular compartments and enzymes also contribute significantly to ROS generation, including the NADPH Oxidase (NOX) family, nitric oxide synthase (NOS) uncoupling, peroxisomes and melanosomes... melanoma is a ROS-driven tumor -- PubMed ID# PMC4209333 (2014) [183]

> Elevated rates of reactive oxygen species (ROS) have been detected in almost all cancers, where they promote many aspects of tumor development and progression. However, tumor cells also express increased levels of antioxidant proteins to detoxify from ROS, suggesting that a delicate balance of intracellular ROS levels is required for cancer cell function." – PubMed ID# PMC3880197 (2014) [184]

There is evidence that EpiCor provides benefits to the immune system that can help it identify and attack cancer cells. The evidence below is in vivo and placebo-controlled, but the study used a relatively small sample size. However, it is very promising research.

> "In this study we have shown evidence for rapid changes in serum antioxidant status, cytokine levels, and immune surveillance after consumption of a single dose of the immunogenic yeast product EP, compared with placebo… a single 500 mg dose of EP provides a rapid and transient effect on the trafficking and activation status of specific lymphocyte subsets, as well as increased antioxidant protection… The production of interferons (IFNs), combined with NK cell trafficking, is an important aspect of immune surveillance against viral infections. NK cells are also an important part of eliminating malignant cells,4,5 and reduced NK cell numbers and function are reported in many cancers… This is a direct extension of our previous publication showing direct activation of NK cells in vitro and in vivo. These combined data may help explain data from other clinical studies where reduced incidence and duration of cold/flu were observed." – PubMed ID#PMC3157306 (2011) [185]

Strategy

Adding EpiCor is an easy way to help *Improve Your Odds*. The evidence does not seem to be as strong as with some of the other recommendations, but it is likely not to be duplicative. Therefore, adding one to two 500 mg capsules per day has the potential to add yet another avenue of attack.

> *I myself take EpiCor. Because I take so many supplements, shooting for that multifaceted synergetic effect, I usually only take 1 capsule per day.*

MUSHROOMS

Cancers: All
Body of Evidence: Large
Cost: Moderate
Recommendation: High

When I first started studying mushrooms for this book, I was aware that many "medicinal mushrooms" could help our bodies fight disease and cancer. I thought this was fascinating but assumed at the time that the medicinal mushrooms were probably toxic and would have side effects (toxicity) towards human cells as well. As I know now, this is definitely <u>not</u> the case. The mushrooms covered in this section are exceedingly safe for humans, and most exhibit powerful chemotherapeutic benefits. Unlike most chemotherapy drugs, our bodies are designed to make use of the compounds found in mushrooms. These compounds are "immunomodulators," "immunologic adjuvants," and "adaptogens," meaning that they help our immune system recognize threats and/or provide it the raw materials for it to do its job. They do not overstimulate, or force, our immune system to do anything (which can be dangerous). This is a natural process and one that evolved, alongside mushrooms, over millions of years. Mushrooms created these substances for their own uses, and we have always consumed mushrooms (see the Brief History of Mushrooms that follows); we evolved to utilize the compounds that they create. Most of these compounds, interestingly, are no more than specially constructed complex sugars (polysaccharides); all have been extensively tested for safety (see the Safety section at the end of this section on Mushrooms).

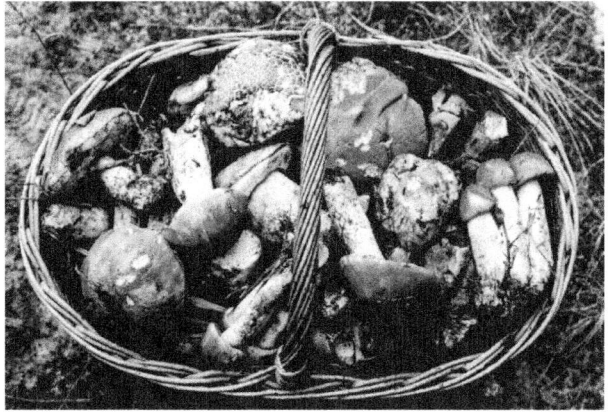

Several types of mushrooms have been studied extensively for their anti-tumor, immunomodulating and anti-metastasis properties. Others have more general immune enhancing/modulating properties. There are hundreds of research studies on medicinal mushrooms, and many of these are peer-reviewed in vivo (in the body) studies on human cancers. Some of the studies are done in conjunction with standard chemotherapy; these too have shown dramatic improvements compared to chemotherapy alone. Some of the studies have also shown diminished chemotherapy symptoms when mushrooms were given as adjuvant therapy. There are also thousands of research papers describing and analyzing these studies; there is clearly a great deal of interest in this topic.

Updates at - https://improvingyourodds.com

Support at - https://www.facebook.com/groups/cancer.improving.your.odds

Several types of mushrooms have been shown to encourage the growth of the Bifidobacterium species of bacteria in the gut. Some of the more popular medicinal mushrooms that encourage Bifidobacteria growth include reishi, turkey tail and various oyster mushrooms (including culinary varieties) (PubMed ID#PMC5618583 [186]). It is likely that every mushroom listed in this section supports Bifidobacterium spp. growth, but many simply haven't been tested yet. It is very important to cultivate the various species of probiotic bacteria under the Bifidobacterium genus, as several have been found to tune the immune system to fight cancer and improve immunotherapy outcomes (see Chapter 2 for more information). I consider consuming a good medicinal mushroom powder mix, chaga tea, mushroom fractions and whole mushrooms to be vitally important.

> *I personally consume a good medicinal mushroom powder mix daily. I brew this in our coffee in the morning and mix it into chaga tea in the afternoon. I also add some larch tree arabinogalactan fiber to both. In addition, we try to cook with mushrooms as often as possible. My wife and I grind them up into small pieces when cooking for the mushroom haters. They are not allergic—they just hate the texture; they seem to love the flavor.*

Like other natural products, obtaining FDA approval to utilize the mushroom isolates as a medical treatment or prescription drug is probably not going to happen. This approval process costs millions of dollars (some sources say billions!), and without the ability to obtain a patent for natural isolates, no company is going to invest that kind of money knowing there will be no return on their investment. Similar problems are faced in many countries around the world.

And yet, it is clear from the volume of research that utilizing medicinal mushrooms as adjuvant therapy is well worth considering. First, there is little to no downside. Side effects are usually non-existent. From what I've seen, there is no evidence that medicinal mushrooms conflict with other cancer drugs (but be sure to consult with your oncologist). They are also relatively inexpensive and can be incorporated into any diet.

Even though I will spend a lot of time on this topic, this is just scratching the surface. Whether it is for treatment or prevention, I would highly encourage you to add more mushrooms to your diet and take a high-quality multi-mushroom (medicinal) powder supplement (see the book's website for recommendations).

> "The functioning of the immune system may be impaired as a consequence of dietary deficiencies or imbalances and may thereby negatively impact health. Edible mushrooms are appreciated as health promoting food, notably having antitumor and immunomodulatory effects. Mushrooms contain compounds that stimulate the immune system as well as prevent or cure infectious diseases, cancer, allergies, autoimmune, and inflammatory disorders. Various compounds including polysaccharides, mainly α- and β-glucans, saccharopeptides, (glyco)proteins, and various low molecular weight compounds such as terpenes and phenols, contribute to these medicinal effects. Of these compounds the role of β-1,3-glucans with β-1,6 branches is best documented, although the role of

other compounds is increasingly appreciated" – PubMed ID#PMC5118454 (2016) (Open Access licensed, attribute at the link) [187]

The mushrooms mentioned in the following sections should be a part of any cancer fighting protocol. This research paper covers the various therapeutic fractions found in medicinal mushrooms.

"The therapeutic effects of medicinal mushrooms are due to the presence of lectin, β-glucan, ergosterol, arginine, and other bioactive substances in mushrooms…

Lectins have been shown to be therapeutic agents with anticancer properties in animals and in clinical studies. They cause cytotoxicity and apoptosis and inhibition of tumor growth by preferentially binding to cancer cell membranes. Lectins function by sequestering the body's polyamines, thereby inhibiting cancer cell growth. Lectins also alter the production of many interleukins, activate protein kinases, bind to ribosomes, and inhibit protein synthesis…

β-glucan is a glucose polymer present in medicinal mushrooms. It exhibits immunomodulatory effects as well as tumoricidal and antiproliferative activities in cancer patients through the stimulation of natural killer cells, neutrophils, monocytes, macrophages, and T-cells…

Ergosterol (or provitamin D2) is a precursor of ergocalciferol, an important substrate in vitamin D biosynthesis and is found in the lipid fraction of Agaricales extracts. This substance has antitumor, antiproliferation, and antimigratory effects on human cancer cells. It has also been shown to inhibit angiogenesis…

Arginine is a semi-essential amino acid used as a dietary supplement in cancer patients. It has been associated with a reduction of tumor growth and metastasis progression, and it is reported to have beneficial effects on the immune system, weight gain, and the time of survival of cancer patients."

– PubMed ID#PMC3226611 (Open Access license, attribute at the link) [188]

Novaes MR, Valadares F, Reis MC, Gonçalves DR, Menezes Mda C. The effects of dietary supplementation with Agaricales mushrooms and other medicinal fungi on breast cancer: evidence-based medicine. Clinics (Sao Paulo). 2011;66(12):2133–2139. doi:10.1590/s1807-59322011001200021

Mushrooms have a very diverse inventory of unique beta-glucans, and many have shown powerful anti-tumor properties. These properties complement each other. Medicinal mushrooms have a very large amount of research showing significant benefits in treating and preventing various cancers. They also improve the immune system and are very beneficial as adjunct therapy to traditional treatments. Because of the large body of evidence, I will be spending quite a bit of time on this subject.

"medicinal mushrooms contain biologically active compounds in fruit bodies, cultured mycelia, and cultured broth. Special attention has been paid to mushroom polysaccharides. Numerous bioactive polysaccharides or polysaccharide-protein complexes from MMs seem to enhance innate and cell-mediated immune responses, and they exhibit antitumor activities in animals and humans. While the mechanism of their antitumor actions is still not completely understood, stimulation and modulation of key host immune responses by these mushroom compounds seems to be central. Most important for modern medicine are polysaccharides and low–molecular weight secondary metabolites with antitumor and immunostimulating properties. More than 600 studies have been conducted worldwide, and numerous human clinical trials on MMs have been published. Several of the mushroom compounds have proceeded through phase I, II, and III clinical studies and are used extensively and successfully in Asia to treat various cancers and other diseases." – PubMed #28605319 (2017) [189]

The main chemotherapeutic properties of mushrooms, various beta-glucans/polysaccharides, are often bound up in the chitin (the insoluble fiber) of the mushroom. Because of this, simply eating raw mushrooms will not provide all the benefits. A hot water extraction is the easiest way to overcome much of this problem, and it is up to 5 to 10 times more effective at releasing the polysaccharides than oven cooking. Simply adding the mushrooms to hot water to make a tea can help. If you have a pressure cooker (either new- or old-style is fine), pressure cooking for 15 minutes will do an even better job. Pressure cooking allows greater extraction without a significant increase in heat; this method has been shown to improve extraction. You can also sweat mushrooms on low heat, simmering (using water or broth) in a covered pan.

"the data demonstrated that hot water mushroom extracts are more potent than ground mushroom products in activating TLR2 and inducing TNF-α. These data provide evidence that extraction methods may affect the biological activity of mushroom products" – PubMed ID#26559858 (2015) [190]

You can also purchase various tinctures that use a dual extraction method, first using a hot water extraction and then an ethanol extraction. This improves the concentration of beneficial compounds even more. However, as the study above points out, even ground encapsulated mushrooms will still have some benefit. Again, *Improve your Odds* and take a supplement that has been hot water extracted, or make your own using a pressure cooker.

Many of the research studies refer to mushroom extracts, usually either hot water or alcohol extracts. These studies are looking at fractional compounds of the mushroom. This helps narrow down what aspects of the mushroom are the most beneficial and makes it easy to standardize dosage. It also makes it easier to develop patentable prescription drug analogs (so that pharmaceutical companies can possibly make billions of dollars from a natural food). In some cases, the amount of the compound being studied exceeds the amount a person is likely to obtain when consuming whole mushrooms or a mushroom tea. It is sometimes unclear (due to a lack of research) if consuming the whole mushroom will have the same benefit. Keep in mind that these mushrooms came to the attention of researchers because they have been used to treat diseases, such as cancer, for thousands of years. There is also a huge amount of anecdotal evidence to support consumption of all these mushrooms.

The following research takes an in-depth look at the use of medicinal mushrooms in the treatment of breast cancer (though other cancers are also mentioned).

"Ingestion of oral β-glucans in medicinal mushrooms has been found to activate various immune system components, including macrophages, NK cells, DCs, and T helper lymphocytes, which affects tumor cell viability and potentiates the release of various mediators including lymphokines and interleukins (ILs)... The anticancer activities of mushrooms have been linked primarily to the modulation of the immune system by branched polysaccharides (glucans), sesquiterpenes, glycoproteins, or peptide/protein-bound polysaccharides... The purpose of this review was to critically evaluate the described effects of the edible G. frondosa (Maitake) and G. lucidum (Reishi) mushrooms in patients with BC (breast cancer)... Ingestion of oral β-glucans in medicinal mushrooms has been found to activate various immune system components, including macrophages, NK cells, DCs, and T helper lymphocytes, which affects tumor cell viability and potentiates the release of various mediators including lymphokines and interleukins" – PubMed ID#PMC5973856 (2018) [191]

Citation "B-glucans from Grifola frondosa and Ganoderma lucidum in breast cancer: an example of complementary and integrative medicine." Authors: Paola Rossi, Raffaele Difrancia, Vincenzo Quagliariello, Elena Savino, Paolo Tralongo, Cinzia Lucia Randazzo and Massimiliano Berretta. Oncotarget. ©2018 Rossi et al; 9:24837-24856. https://doi.org/10.18632/oncotarget.24984. Creative Commons Attribution License 3.0 (CC BY 3.0), which permits unrestricted use, distribution, and reproduction in any medium, provided the original author and source are credited.

Do not stop at just eating the mushrooms that have shown effectiveness against your type of cancer (although of course you should consume those). Often, scientists will simply follow the leads of previous research; when looking for gold, you first look in the area where someone else just found some. Since research dollars and time are scarce, there simply hasn't been research for all mushrooms against all cancers. A Japanese edible mushroom, *Hypsizygus tessulatus* (the common name is Buna shimeji), has one of the highest beta-glucan contents, and yet it is only mentioned in one research study. I'm sure there are uncommon mushrooms (probably tasteless and woody) that haven't been researched at all. So, try to consume a wide variety of mushrooms, making sure that you consume those that have proven to be beneficial against your type of cancer.

> *What are "medicinal" mushrooms? In short, they are edible mushrooms that also contain "biologically active compounds" that have health benefits beyond a vitamin, mineral or calorie source. Some, such as reishi, are also used in the culinary world. In fact, most of them are consumed in countries like Japan. So, they are considered a food and can be consumed that way.*

The following study was conducted in China with "1,009 female patients aged 20-87 years with histologically confirmed breast cancer." The outcome was quite startling: Women who consumed both mushrooms and green tea daily reduced their risk of cancer by 82% to 89%! Or, they could reduce their odds of contracting breast cancer by 64% simply by adding 10 grams of mushrooms per day to their diet. Those are significant numbers and clearly show a strong benefit to consuming medicinal mushrooms for breast cancer prevention!

> Compared with nonconsumers, the Odds ratios (Ors) were 0.36 (95% CI = 0.25-0.51) and 0.53 (0.38-0.73) for daily intake of >or=10 g fresh mushrooms and >or=4 g dried mushrooms, based on multivariate logistic regression analysis adjusting for established and potential confounders... An "inverse association was found in both pre- and postmenopausal women. Compared with those who consumed neither mushrooms nor green tea, the ORs were 0.11 (0.06-0.20) and 0.18 (0.11-0.29) for daily high intake of fresh and dried mushrooms combined with consuming beverages made from >or=1.05 g dried green tea leaves per day. The corresponding linear trends were statistically significant for joint effect ($p < 0.001$). We conclude that higher dietary intake of mushrooms decreased breast cancer risk in pre- and postmenopausal Chinese women and an additional decreased risk of breast cancer from joint effect of mushrooms and green tea was observed." – PubMed ID#19048616 (2009) [192]

It is my opinion that mushrooms and mushroom extracts may have the greatest potential for treating and preventing cancer of any natural product currently being researched. My advice would be to *Improve your Odds* and consume a variety of these mushrooms whenever possible.

"Beside the routine methods of surgery, radiotherapy and chemotherapy, traditional herb medicine is one of the major complementary and alternative medicines for treating various malignant diseases, including colorectal cancer" – PubMed ID#PMC4491205 (2015) [193]

"Natural products have gradually became one of the most productive strategies in the development of antitumor agents (6), which possess potent cytotoxic abilities with fewer adverse effects." – PubMed ID#PMC4878560 (2016) [194]

A Brief History of Mushrooms

Meet Ötzi, better known as "The Iceman." The mummified body of Ötzi (also spelled Oetzi) was found in 1991 by 2 German tourists at 3,210 meters (10,530 ft) on the east ridge of a mountain in the Ötztal Alps on the Austrian-Italian border. He was found frozen in ice, where he had been well preserved for over 5,000 years! Ötzi was so well preserved that scientists were able to count 61 tattoos on his skin and could identify what he ate for his last two meals!

Among Ötzi's possessions were two types of mushrooms; one was used as tinder for lighting fires, the other was a medicinal birch polypore. It is believed that he carried the birch polypore to treat intestinal parasites. An examination of his body showed that he had whipworms. The birch polypore also has very strong antibacterial properties and could have been used to ward off food poisoning. Even though humans at that time had a much stronger microbiome (gut) and (most likely) better adapted immune systems, food poisoning was likely fairly common in the days before refrigeration. Mushrooms may have played a medicinal role in treating such maladies. We do know food didn't kill Ötzi; he had been shot by an arrow. Since his stomach was full at the time he died, perhaps he had trouble outrunning his pursuers.

Research has also been done on the teeth of individuals found in El Mirón Cave in Cantabria, Spain. Researchers found that bolete mushrooms were a routine part of their diet. This evidence dates mushroom consumption back to the Upper Paleolithic period (10,000 to 50,000 years before present). In this cave they discovered the buried remains of a woman they dubbed the "Red Lady" (she was dubbed the "Red Lady" due to the fact that she was covered in a red ochre made from hematite, an iron oxide found in clay, at the time of burial approximately 18,500 years ago). When researchers examined hardened plaque from the Red Lady's teeth, they found spores from at least two types of mushrooms in the hardened tartar. The way in which she

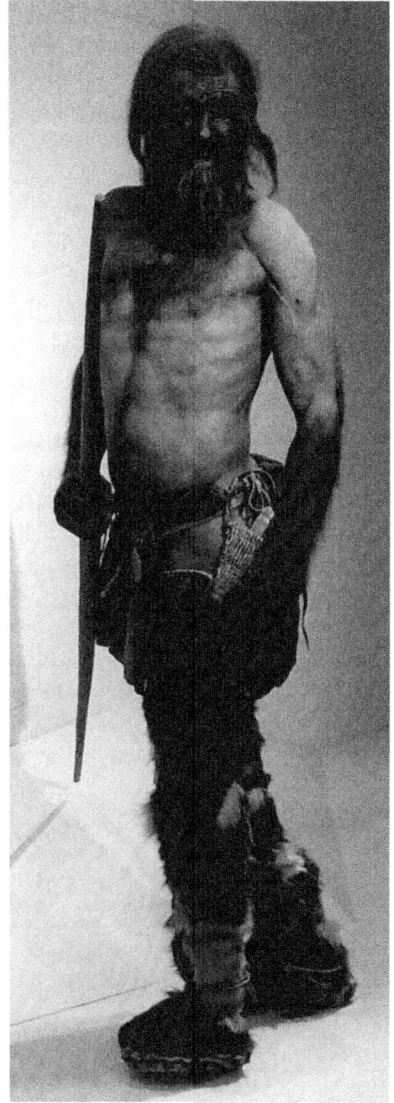

Figure 0-1 Ötzi at Museum Bozen by Andre, Schade, CC BY 3.0, https://commons.wikimedia.org/w/index.php?curid=57934493

was buried indicates that she may have been a spiritual leader or healer. Research from the Spy Cave in Belgium and the El Sidrón Cave in Spain showed that Neanderthals were consuming mushrooms on a regular basis 48,000 years ago. [195] There is every reason to believe that humans have been consuming mushrooms for as long as they've been on this planet, as mushrooms were readily available and the vast majority were non-toxic.

Evidence of mushroom consumption is difficult to come by; mushrooms are very delicate and weren't commonly the subject of cave art (that was usually reserved for great hunts, large animal kills and other macho endeavors). However, the evidence suggests that humans (and our humanoid ancestors) have been eating mushrooms for nearly as long as they've been on this planet. When a tribe would find an edible mushroom, this knowledge would get passed from person to person. Of course, when someone died from trying a poisonous mushroom, the rest of the tribe would know to avoid that type of mushroom as well (I envision a lot of "I double dog dare you" challenges). In a paper published in the Proceedings of the National Academy of Sciences (PNAS) in 2012, they discussed the discovery of burned plants and bones from 1 million years ago in South Africa's Wonderwerk Cave. Their findings suggest that *Homo erectus*, not *Homo sapiens* or Neanderthals, were the first to use fire, and most likely, to cook their food. It should surprise no one if these Paleolithic humans were cooking some mushrooms with their venison (just the thought of which makes me hungry).

In more modern times, mushrooms can be found mentioned throughout human history. Ancient Chinese, Greeks, Romans and Egyptians all consumed them. Egyptian pharaohs and Roman emperors often forbade commoners from eating mushrooms, strictly reserving them for nobility. There is even evidence that hallucinogenic mushrooms were first used over 10,000 years ago, and their use most likely goes back much further. Medicinal uses of mushrooms likely go back at least this far.

Humans evolved with mushrooms. We've most likely been consuming them for more than a million years. It would have been pretty easy to quickly figure out which ones made us sick and which ones didn't, and this information would have been passed down generation to generation. This process was used for other foods, such as wild berries—some make you sick, some don't. When you figure out which are which, you share this information with your children and tribe. When an animal evolves with something, the body makes good use of it. We try not to let anything go to waste (unless the energy involved in utilizing it is more than we get back after digesting it. This explains why we didn't evolve to utilize cellulose as an energy source). Because the mushrooms produced many complex polysaccharides to help the body ward off bacteria, parasites, cancers, etc., our bodies utilized this blueprint to evolve their own system for helping fight cancers, and this system is grounded in mushroom polysaccharides. Don't believe me? Maybe you will after reading the dozens of scientific research studies on just how beneficial these mushrooms are to us in fighting cancer—not attacking cancer, not poisoning cancer, but enabling our own immune system to better identify and tailor a response to cancer. Mushroom polysaccharides are primarily immunomodulators; they assist our immune system so that it can kill cancer the way it has evolved to do. It is all quite fascinating.

AGARICUS BLAZEI MURILL

Related Strains: *Agaricus brasiliensis*, *Agaricus subrufescens*, almond mushroom, Piedade mushroom, Himematsutake (in Japan), *Agaricus blazeri*

Agaricus blazei Murill is an edible mushroom grown in Brazil (thus the name) and Japan. It has been used to treat diabetes, arteriosclerosis, hepatitis, high cholesterol, dermatitis and cancer.

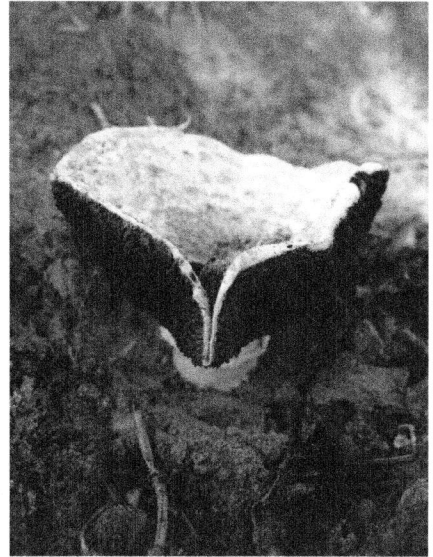

"Blazein was isolated from mushroom (Agaricus blazei Murrill) and identified by Mass and 1H-NMR as blazein. The effect of blazein on the DNA of human various cancer cells was investigated. DNA fragmentations by blazein to oligonucreosomal-sized fragments, a characteristic of apoptosis, were observed in the human lung LU99 and stomach KATO III cancer cells. The DNA fragmentations by blazein were observed from day 2 (KATO III cells) or day 3 (LU99 cells) after the addition of blazein to the culture cells. These findings suggest that growth inhibition by blazein results from the induction of apoptosis by the compound." – PubMed ID#19020714 (2008) [196]

Here researchers looked at the effects of *A. subrufescens* (*A. blazei*) on leukemia cells in vitro. They found that it had clear anti-tumor effects on leukemia (cancer) cells but had no negative effects on normal lymphatic cells. (Image Attribution [197])

"In this review we refer to the mushroom as A. subrufescens and treat results of studies on mushrooms named as A. blazei and A. brasiliensis as this species… The agaritine extracted from A. subrufescens exerts an in vitro anti-tumor activity in leukemic cells with no significant effects on normal lymphatic cells. The cytotoxicological effect of agaritine has been demonstrated on leukemic cell lines… A. subrufescens is a well-known medicinal mushroom used in many countries, and thus consumption of this mushroom is used as an alternative way to cure diseases. Various pharmaceutical activities have been found associated with A. subrufescens… Recent studies have been performed in vitro and in vivo to confirm the mushrooms therapeutic properties (Firenzuoli et al., 2008). Identification of (novel) immunomodulating bioactive compounds from the mushroom may also help in new treatments for patients suffering from cancer and immunodeficiency… Mushroom polysaccharides are thought to prevent oncogenesis, have shown an indirect anti-tumor activity against various allogeneic and syngeneic tumors, and prevent tumor metastasis… The major polysaccharide fraction of A. subrufescens extract is revealed as β-glucan" – PubMed ID#PMC3730566 (2012) [198]

A. brasiliensis (or *A. blazei*) was tested using 4 different extraction methods (including a regular water extraction), and researchers found that in all 4 different treatments the tumor sizes were significantly reduced. The study used Walker 256 rat breast cancer cells due to their similarity to human breast cancers, larger tumor volume and high metastasis abilities. Metastatic brain tumors are present in 22% to 30% of patients diagnosed with breast cancer.

"Agaricus brasiliensis is a mushroom native to São Paulo State, Brazil, that is studied for its medicinal proprieties… The results showed that all 4 treatments (pure powdered basidiocarp and aqueous, acid, and alkaline extracts) significantly reduced tumor size… The data collected from the W256 tumor-bearing rats revealed the beneficial effects of A. brasiliensis in tumor treatment" – PubMed ID#20130735 (2010) [199]

In this study they used a mouse model of human breast cancer. They found that *A. brasiliensis* reduced tumor growth and reduced mitotic cells (mitosis). They also found that apoptosis (the natural process where abnormal cells destroy themselves) increased. This process is often defective, or turned off, in cancer cells.

"Subcutaneous Ehrlich tumor-bearing mice were treated with in situ inoculation of a beta-glucan-rich extract of Agaricus brasiliensis (ATF), which reduced tumor growth. Histopathological analysis showed that the tumor masses of control mice (Ehr) presented giant tumor cells and many mitotic figures whereas the tumor tissue obtained from ATF-treated animals (Ehr-ATF) presented a lower frequency of both mitotic and giant cells, associated with a higher frequency of apoptotic cells than Ehr." – PubMed ID#19243740 (2009) [200]

"The Mushroom Agaricus blazei Murill Elicits Medicinal Effects on Tumor, Infection, Allergy, and Inflammation through Its Modulation of Innate Immunity and Amelioration of Th1/Th2 Imbalance and Inflammation" – PubMed ID#PMC3168293 (2011) [201]

CHAGA

AKA: *Inonotus obliquus*, clinker polypore

Chaga is not your typical "mushroom." From the outside it looks like a mass of burnt coal. When you cut into the chunks, it looks like wood on the inside. It is a fungus that grows primarily on wild birch trees in northern climates. Chaga is primarily found in colder regions of Russia and North America.

A quick search of PubMed (a US government-run index of research studies) shows over 800 research studies and scientific papers on chaga. This does not even include many studies from Japan, China, Russia and some northern European countries. Though there hasn't been a lot of in vivo (in the body) human research, the amount and quality of animal and in vitro research is very compelling.

Chaga can easily be made into a very tasty tea. My family is originally from Louisiana and I grew up drinking black iced tea. I tell people I was weaned on iced tea; it would not surprise me if this were true. I now mostly drink chaga tea; don't tell my family, but I actually like it better than traditional iced tea! Though you can purchase chaga teabags, I recommend making it from the chunks; one never knows what fillers or byproducts (in this case, tree bark) might be in the bags. Making it in bulk from chunks is also a lot less expensive than from teabags.

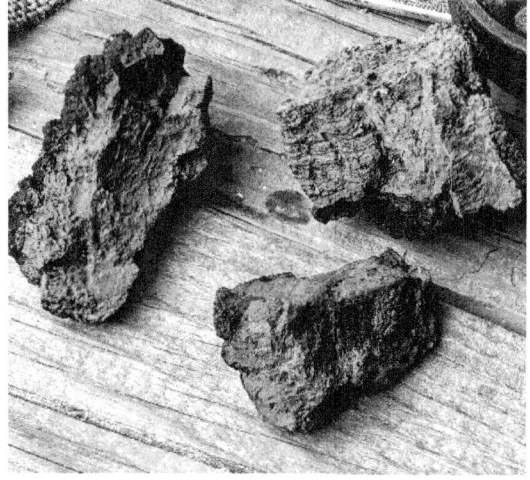

The chaga "mushroom" (actually a fungus, not technically a mushroom) has been used medicinally for generations. Only recently has science started to confirm its many benefits. What they're finding is that chaga has some amazing health benefits, especially in treating and preventing cancer. Using objective standards such as the ORAC (oxygen radical absorbance capacity) value (which is a measurement of antioxidant capacity), chaga surpasses nearly all other antioxidant foods (including acai, pomegranate, blueberries, etc.). Chaga also contains more SOD (superoxide dismutase) enzymes than any other mushroom. Both ORAC and SOD levels are very important objective measures used to quantify certain anticancer benefits. Chaga also contains at least 29 different polysaccharides; many have been found to have anticancer benefits. In addition to polysaccharides, chaga also contains beneficial sterols, polyphenols and a host of other super healthy antioxidant constituents, including melanin, superoxide dismutase triterpenes, botulin, inotodiol and lupeol.

Research

Many of the studies below looked at isolated fractions from chaga, rather than chaga as a whole. This is common in research as they are looking for something that can be turned into a pharmaceutical, and hopefully patented (otherwise there is no profit in it). Chaga contains many substances that have shown great promise in treating (and preventing) cancer. It is my recommendation that chaga be consumed as a tea so that you are consuming all of the fractions. Each of the fractions work synergistically, with the benefit exceeding the sum of their parts.

The following in vivo study used human lung cancer (xenographed onto mice). Researchers had mice drink an amount of chaga tea similar to what people commonly drink (per kg of body weight). After 3 weeks they found a 60% reduction in tumor size, and the number of metastatic nodules decreased by 25% compared to the control group.

> "Continuous intake of the Chaga mushroom (Inonotus obliquus) aqueous extract suppresses cancer progression… Anticancer activity of the I. obliquus extract was examined in mouse models of Lewis lung carcinoma growth and spontaneous metastasis after 3 weeks of continuous extract intake at the dose of 6 mg/kg/day, which corresponded to that ingested daily with Chaga infusion in Japan… The extract of I. obliquus caused significant tumor suppressive effects in both models. Thus, in tumor-bearing mice, 60% tumor reduction was observed, while in metastatic mice, the number of nodules decreased by 25% compared to the control group. Moreover, I. obliquus extract-treated mice demonstrated the increase in tumor agglomeration and inhibition of vascularization." – PubMed ID#PMC4946216 (2016) [202]

Here they researched chaga's anticancer effects against human lung carcinoma, colon adenocarcinoma and rat glioma cell cultures. They found that chaga had a number of different anticancer effects.

> "Chaga fraction elicited anticancer effects which were attributed to decreased tumor cell proliferation, motility and morphological changes induction. Of note is the fact that it produced no or low toxicity in tested normal cells. The data presented could open interesting paths for further investigations of fraction IO4 as a potential anticancer agent." – PubMed #22135889 (2011) [203]

All of the chaga subfractions tested in the study below showed "significant inhibitory activity against the proliferation" of 4 different human cancer cell lines (breast, lung, stomach and cervical). The subfractions were obtained from simple hot water extraction, so this would be comparable to making it at home. The amounts of the subfraction used were small (maximum

0.2 mg/day added to the mouse chow). This study shows that chaga, when consumed normally, may have significant benefits against a variety of human cancers. Because the goal of most research is to find an isolate that can be used to create a pharmaceutical drug, this research did not test a combination of all 4 fractions, nor did they test whole chaga (which would contain all 4 fractions, as well as other fractions not tested here). Further into the study you'll find Table 1, which shows that higher concentrates of the fractions exhibited up to a 72% inhibition of tumor growth. The chaga fractions also showed the ability to increase apoptosis of cancer cells (apoptosis is the natural function that most normal cells have to destroy themselves if something goes wrong with them, e.g., they become cancerous).

> "This is the first study to report an antitumor effect of three subfractions (3β-hydroxy-lanosta-8,24-dien-21-al, inotodiol, and lanosterol) from I. obliquus extracts in the Sarcoma-180-cell-bearing mice and various cancer cell lines… All of the subfractions showed significant inhibitory activity against the proliferation of the selected cancer cell lines (A549, AGS, MCF-7, and HeLa), but these subfractions have low cytotoxicity against normal cells… In *in vivo* results, subfraction 1 isolated from *I. obliquus* at concentrations of 0.1 and 0.2 mg/mouse per day significantly decreased tumor volume by 23.96% and 33.71%, respectively, as compared with the control… the hot water extract of Inonotus obliquus would be useful as an antitumor agent via the induction of the apoptosis and inhibition of the growth of cancer cells… the three subfractions (3β-hydroxy-lanosta-8,24-dien-21-al, inotodiol, and lanosterol) inhibited in vitro proliferation of various human cancer cell lines. The three subfractions also had in vivo antitumor effects" – PubMed ID#PMC2895696 (2010) [204]

In this 2015 study, published in the peer-reviewed *Journal of Ethnopharmacology*, researchers again found that chaga has powerful anticancer properties. Ergosterol peroxide is a component found in chaga and is being studied for its ability to suppress cancer growth. Here chaga was tested for its anticancer activities in 4 different human colorectal cancer (CRC) cell lines (HCT116, HT-29, SW620 and DLD-1). The research found that chaga inhibited cancer cells through downregulating β-catenin signaling (cell-cell adhesion and gene transcription), slowing proliferation and increasing cancer cell apoptosis. All are important mechanisms in fighting cancer tumors.

> "In this study, we examined the effect of different fractions and components of Chaga mushroom (Inonotus Obliquus) on viability and apoptosis of colon cancer cells… Ergosterol peroxide inhibited cell proliferation and also suppressed clonogenic colony formation in HCT116, HT-29, SW620 and DLD-1 CRC cell lines. The growth inhibition observed in these CRC cell lines was the result of apoptosis… Ergosterol peroxide down-regulated β-catenin signaling, which exerted anti-proliferative and pro-apoptotic activities in CRC cells. These properties of ergosterol peroxide advocate its use as a supplement in colon cancer chemoprevention." – PubMed ID#26210065 (2015) [205]

An "antimutagenic" is a substance that helps prevent cells from mutating—the underlying cause of normal cells becoming cancer cells. Here chaga was found to have both antimutagenic and antioxidant properties, thus preventing cancer formation.

> "Here, we evaluated the antimutagenic and antioxidant capacities of subfractions of Inonotus obliquus (Chaga) extract… At 50 μg/plate, subfractions 1 and 2 strongly inhibited the mutagenesis induced in Salmonella typhimurium strain TA100 by the directly acting mutagen MNNG (0.4 μg/plate) by 80.0% and 77.3%, respectively. They also inhibited 0.15 μg/plate 4NQO-induced mutagenesis in TA98 and TA100 by 52.6-62.0%. The mutagenesis in TA98 induced by the indirectly acting mutagens Trp-P-1 (0.15 μg/plate) and B(α)P (10 μg/plate) was reduced by 47.0-68.2% by the subfractions, while the mutagenesis in TA100 by Trp-P-1 and B(α)P was reduced by 70.5-87.2%… Thus, we show that the 3beta-hydroxy-lanosta-8, 24-dien-21-al and inotodiol components of Inonotus obliquus bear antimutagenic and antioxidative activities." – PubMed ID#18992843 (2009) [206]

The following study looked at one of the chaga isolates, IO4, and found that it decreased cancer cell proliferation and helped prevent normal cells from mutating into cancer cells. Preventing cells from mutating into cancer cells can help stop tumor growth. It also found that this isolate had "no or low toxicity" to normal cells.

> "The purpose of the present study was evaluation of in vitro anticancer activity of fraction IO4 isolated from I. obliquus. The effect on cell proliferation, motility and viability was assessed in a range of cancer and normal cells… Chaga fraction elicited anticancer effects which were attributed to decreased tumor cell proliferation, motility and morphological changes induction. Of note is the fact that it produced no or low toxicity in tested normal cells. The data presented could open interesting paths for further investigations of fraction IO4 as a potential anticancer agent." – PubMed ID#22135889 (2011) [207]

Here an ethanol extract of *I. obliquus* (chaga) was used. They found that a fraction not normally found in hot water extracts was able to induce cell cycle arrest and cancer cell proliferation. You can purchase chaga ethanol extracts, or there are instructions on the internet on how to do this yourself; you can then add a small amount of the extract to your normal chaga tea. Though hot water extracts have plenty of beneficial fractions, it never hurts to add another one.

> "Inonotus obliquus (I. obliquus, Chaga mushroom) has long been used as a folk medicine to treat cancer. In the present study, we examined whether or not

ethanol extract of I. obliquus (EEIO) inhibits cell cycle progression in HT-29 human colon cancer cells… These results demonstrate that fraction 2 is the major fraction that induces G1 arrest and inhibits cell proliferation, suggesting I. obliquus could be used as a natural anti-cancer ingredient" – PubMed ID#25861415 (2015) [208]

> *I purchase an ethanol extract from a man in Canada who makes it himself. The process to make it isn't that hard, but it is time consuming to do in small batches. I mix 1 tsp of this in with a normal glass of chaga tea. (It contains a small amount of alcohol.)*

Various chaga fractions show "strong anti-cancer effects." This is how they are researched, but they show even stronger benefits when used together. In this study chaga inhibited proliferation and metastasis.

> "Prior studies with various cells have reported that extract of I. obliquus from several types of solvents, including-water, ethanol, methanol, and hexane, prevents proliferation and metastasis of cancer cells… These results collectively show that both water and ethanol extracts of I. obliquus inhibit cancer cell proliferation in various cells through cell cycle arrest… the compounds contained in EEIO and the dichloromethane fraction showed strong anti-cancer effects" – PubMed ID#PMC4388940 (2015) [209]

The following study shows that chaga is a useful anti-tumor food that should be considered in complementary treatment. It also shows that a simple hot water extract is enough to release the beneficial constituents from the mushrooms' chitin (fiber).

> "In the current study, it was demonstrated that the hot water extract of I. obliquus (IOWE) exerts inhibitory activity against the proliferation of human colon cancer cells (HT-29)… The results suggest that IOWE would be useful as an antitumor agent via the induction of apoptosis and inhibition of the growth of cancer cells through up-regulation of the expression of proapoptotic proteins and down-regulation of antiapoptotic proteins." – PubMed ID#19367670 (2009) [210]

The following study examines the use of chaga extract on hepatocellular carcinoma (liver cancer).

> "Chaga extract inhibited the cell growth in a dose-dependent manner, which was accompanied with G0/G1-phase arrest and apoptotic cell death. In addition, G0/G1 arrest in the cell cycle was closely associated with down-regulation of p53, pRb, p27, cyclins D1, D2, E, cyclin-dependent kinase (Cdk) 2, Cdk4, and Cdk6 expression… CONCLUSION: Chaga mushroom may provide a new

therapeutic option, as a potential anticancer agent, in the treatment of hepatoma."
– PubMed ID#PMC2681140 (2008) [211]

The following study looked at 6 different isolates from chaga and found "obvious" anticancer activity against prostate and breast cancers (in vitro).

"fractions were found to have significant inhibition effects on NO production and NF-κB luciferase activity in macrophage RAW 264.7 cells and cytotoxicity against human prostatic carcinoma cell PC3 and breast carcinoma cell MDA-MB-231… Compound ergosterol, ergosterol peroxide and trametenolic acid showed anti-inflammatory activities and ergosterol peroxide and trametenolic acid showed obviously cytotoxicity on human prostatic carcinoma cell PC3 and breast carcinoma MDA-MB-231 cell." – PubMed ID#23561137 (2013) [212]

"The *I. obliquus* extract sharply decreased the expression of Bcl-2 but dramatically increased the expression of caspase-3. This function was gradually enhanced with increased drug concentration and prolonged treatment duration. The *I. obliquus* extract can inhibit the proliferation of tumor cells. This inhibition function is closely related to the downregulation of Bcl-2 and the upregulation of caspase-3." – DOI: 10.1615/IntJMedMushr.v16.i1.30 (2014) [213]

The following study, which is available in full online, contains a lot of information. It discusses various cancer research studies that looked at chaga (*I. obliquus*).

"The current anti-cancer… have been demonstrated to pose several side-effects and complications as compared with natural anticancer materials… As a medical mushroom, Inonotus obliquus for containing myriad bioactive components known to exhibit potent effects of scavenging free radicals, antioxidant, hypoglycemic, antiviral, anti-inflammatory and antitumor, etc., has become an important resource of developing nutraceutical and natural drugs for anticancer… Having an obvious inhibit effect on a variety of tumor cells, I. obliquus prevents the metastasis and recurrence of cancer cells… Besides, the anti-proliferation effect of IWE on melanoma B16-F10 cells by Youn et al. (2009) suggested that it not only inhibited the growth of cancer cells by causing cell cycle arrest at G0 /G1 phase and apoptosis, but also induced cell differentiation… When an alien substance enters into the body, the immune system will see it as an antigen frstly and attack it to eliminate this potential dangerous invader. I. obliquus polysaccharides may contain some antigen fragments of or the structure of which may alike some component of cancer cells, bridging the cancer cells with immunocytes and facilitating the immunocytes to discriminate cancer cells with more precision." -- "Progress on Understanding the Anticancer Mechanisms of Medicinal Mushroom: Inonotus Obliquus" – APOCP Full Paper (2013) (Creative Commons Attribution Licensed - Attribution) [214]

The following study from the journal *BioFactors* (an international biochemistry journal) found that chaga can protect human DNA from damage. This can be very import during chemotherapy, radiation treatments and even antibiotic treatments (all of which are known to damage DNA).

"Using image analysis, the degree of DNA damage was evaluated as the DNA tail moment. Cells pretreated with Chaga extract showed over 40% reduction in DNA fragmentation compared with the positive control (100 micromol H_2O_2 treatment). Thus, Chaga mushroom treatment affords cellular protection against endogenous DNA damage produced by H_2O_2." – PubMed ID#15630179 (2004) [215]

The following study showed similar results with chaga protecting cells from free radical damage.

"As early as in the sixteenth century, I. obliquus was used as an effective folk medicine in Russia and Northern Europe to treat several human malicious tumors such as breast cancer, liver cancer, uterine cancer and gastric cancer and other diseases like hypertension and diabetes, with little toxic side effects… their protective effects on H_2O_2-induced PC12 cell death were explored. Results indicated that I. obliquus polysaccharides possess multiple radical scavenging activities in a dose-dependent manner and protect PC12 cells from H_2O_2-induced death. These antioxidant activities might account, at least in part, for the pharmaceutical effects of I. obliquus." – PubMed ID#PMC3430291 (2012) (Open Access attribution available at the link) [216]

Chaga was shown in this study (both in vitro and in vivo) to significantly inhibit melanoma cells' growth, morphology (the cellular change from benign to malignant) and proliferation in mice, in a dose-dependent manner. After treatment for 48 hours, cancer cell viability went from 100% in the control to 35% in the highest dosage group. Apoptosis and cell differentiation were also increased.

"The water extract of Inonotus obliquus (chaga) was studied for anti-proliferative effects on the growth and morphology of B16-F10 melanoma cells and for anti-tumor effect using in vivo in Balb/c mice… Inonotus obliquus extract not only inhibited the growth of B16-F10 cells by causing cell cycle arrest at G(0)/G(1) phase and apoptosis, but also induced cell differentiation… Inonotus obliquus extract significantly inhibited the growth of tumor mass in B16-F10 cells implanted mice, resulting in a 3-fold inhibit at dose of 20mg/kg/day for 10 days… This study showed that the water extract of Inonotus obliquus mushroom exhibited a potential anticancer activity against B16-F10 melanoma cells in vitro and in vivo through the inhibition of proliferation and induction of differentiation and apoptosis of cancer cells." – PubMed ID#19041933(2009) [217]

Safety

Chaga is extremely safe, but like any other food, a rare minority of consumers can have issues with it. If you are allergic to mushrooms and other fungi, it might be best to avoid chaga.

If you have been told to avoid high-oxalate foods (such as spinach, beets and rhubarb), then you may want to avoid chaga. There is one case study from Japan involving a 72-year-old woman with liver cancer, who developed kidney issues after 6 months of consuming a large amount of concentrated chaga powder each day. There was no direct evidence that her kidney issues were actually caused by chaga. [218]

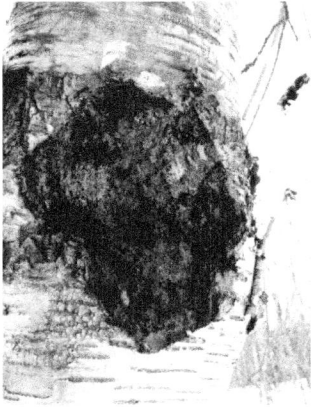

Anecdotal evidence suggests that chaga appears not to contribute to gout symptoms (as people with gout are often told to avoid mushrooms, though this recommendation appears to be overblown), and chaga may actually have benefits for gout sufferers (evidence is lacking here).

No toxins have been reported in chaga, and it has been well studied. It is also commonly consumed in many areas of the world (e.g., Russia and Japan are two of the biggest consumers, but it is widely consumed in many countries). (This image shows chaga growing on a birch tree. Image attribution [219])

Usage Instructions

Chaga makes a very good-tasting, caffeine-free tea. It tastes a lot like regular black tea; some people like it even better. The recipe I use makes a 2:1 concentrate; just mix the chaga concentrate with the same amount of water. Since you need to refrigerate the concentrate, it's ready to make iced tea. I avoid sugar, so I use monk fruit sweetener or stevia to sweeten.

If you have a pressure cooker, that is the best way to extract the goodness from chaga, but you can also make it on a stovetop. You can find the recipe I use to make chaga on *The Gut Health Protocol* website. [220] This is something I continue to drink daily, and it tastes delicious.

Once you've made the chaga tea concentrate, it can be used in various ways:

- Drink it by itself 1 to 2 times per day, diluting 1:1 with water. Sweeten with stevia or monk fruit powder to taste. You can also add lemon if you wish.
- Use it in smoothies as your liquid.
- Mix in other beneficial powders. I mix in ½ tsp of medicinal mushroom powder, ¼ tsp of beta-glucan powder and ½ scoop of larch tree fiber. Sweeten with stevia to taste.
- Use the tea (unsweetened) to replace some of the water in soups and stews. Nobody will even know.

Perhaps one of the best chaga supplement products on the market is Oriveda's dual extraction powder. This company uses special techniques to extract the most beta-glucans from chaga; it also uses an ethanol extraction process to liberate components that are not water soluble: betulinic acid, polyphenols and triterpenes. This is the only company I know that tests and guarantees the potency of these components in their product. This is an excellent product that is very easy to use (½ tsp mixed in hot water makes a great tea), but it is more expensive ($1 to $2 per day if you drink 1 or 2 cups per day). I use this if I'm traveling.

Strategy

I would drink at least one glass per day (50% concentrate, 50% water). I personally drink 2 glasses sweetened with a little stevia on most days, and use this as a base for mixing in other mushroom powders. If you have gut issues or are not used to soluble fibers in your diet, you might have to start slow (e.g., one glass per day, diluted a little more) as the fiber can give some people intestinal issues at first. Any such issues are a sign your gut is not in good order and you need to work on that.

I also purchase a dual extracted powder and a liquid tincture concentrate to mix with my chaga (by the glass). Very little is needed, and I rotate between the powder and the tincture.

CORDYCEPS

AKA: *Ophiocordyceps sinensis,*
Cordyceps militaris, **Dong Chong Yia**
Cao

Cordyceps contains several bioactive compounds, including polysaccharides, peptides, cordycepin, cordycepic acid, ergosterols and nucleosides. Studies have shown a wide variety of pharmacological benefits, including anti-inflammatory, antioxidant, anti-tumor, restoring apoptosis in tumors, immune-modulatory, nephroprotective, hepatoprotective and anti-hyperglycemic properties. With over 2,800 research studies or scientific papers indexed in PubMed (part of the US government's National Institutes of Health) that include both the words "cancer" and "Cordyceps," the body of evidence for this mushroom is very high.

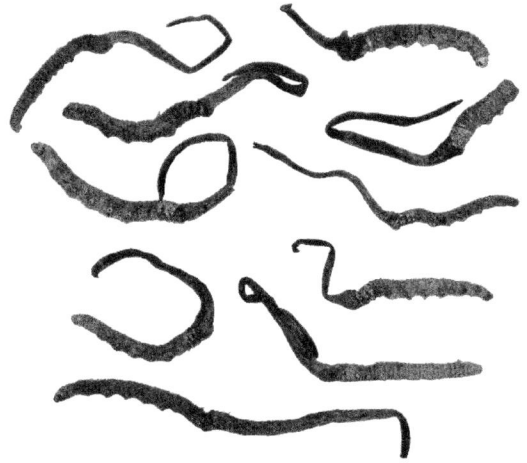

Cordyceps sinensis choice specimens, mostly whole. Created by William Rafti of the William Rafti Institute, via WikiMedia

During the 1993 Olympics, 3 female Chinese runners broke 5 world records. This was an outstanding feat, but officials at the time immediately suspected doping or anabolic steroids. When tests came back, officials were stunned that the entire team tested negative for banned substances. Officials then thought that perhaps the Chinese had developed a new drug, one for which there wasn't a test, and an investigation was begun. When investigators couldn't find any evidence of a new drug, they interviewed the team's coach, asking what foods and nutrients the team had been using that could explain these outstanding achievements. The coach credited Cordyceps mushrooms. Cordyceps is well known in China for its physical performance boosting properties, antifatigue properties, use in combating sexual dysfunctions, immune supplementation and even anticancer benefits. It is even described in 2,000-year-old medical texts. Though many called for the Cordyceps use to be banned in Olympic competition, the US Olympic Committee has officially ruled that Cordyceps can be used legally, basing this decision on its strong safety record, outstanding health benefits, and thousands of years of being used as a food product.

A "xenograft" model is where human cancer cells are grafted (or transplanted) onto those of an animal (often mice). Many tumors will continue to grow much like if they were in a human body. This allows in vivo (within the body) studies without jeopardizing humans; studies can be double-blind, and the test subjects are otherwise healthy (not immunocompromised by other, conventional, cancer therapies). In this study, Cordyceps interfered with both cancer cell development and induced apoptosis (programmed cell death, a normal process where abnormal cells basically commit suicide. This process often does not work properly in cancer cells).

> "Ethanol extract of Cordyceps militaris was highly cytotoxic to human colorectal carcinoma RKO cells and inhibited the growth of tumor in xenograft model. The anti-tumor effect of Cordyceps militaris was associated with an induction of cell cycle arrest and mitochondrial-mediated apoptosis… Different types of extracts of Cordyceps militaris have been reported to exert immunomodulatory, anti-inflammatory, anti-microbial and antitumor effects… Cordyceps extract has been reported to have a potent cytotoxic effect on various human cancer cells, including human lung carcinoma cells" – PubMed ID#PMC4491205 (Open Access licensed, attribute at the link) [221]

This study investigated using Cordyceps against liver and breast cancer cells (in vitro and in vivo). It too found strong anti-tumor effects of hot water extracted Cordyceps in both liver and breast cancer cells.

> "Cordyceps militaris (CM), an entomopathogenic fungus belonging to the class ascomycetes, possesses various pharmacological activities, including cytotoxic effects, on various types of human tumor cells… The present study investigated the anti-hepatocellular carcinoma (HCC) and anti-breast cancer effects of CM in in vitro and in vivo models. CM aqueous extract reduced cell viability, suppressed cell proliferation, inhibited cell migration ability… and enhanced apoptotic rates in MCF-7 and HepG2 cells… the migratory abilities of the MCF-7 and HepG2 cells were significantly inhibited following CM treatment… Collectively, CM induced intracellular toxicity, which was associated with its regulation of mitochondrial function and the expression of pro-apoptotic proteins… In conclusion, the present study confirmed the anti-HCC and anti-breast cancer effects of CM aqueous extract in in vitro and in vivo experiments… These findings provide pharmacological evidence that CM possesses antitumor effects in HCC and breast cancer, offering potential as a chemotherapeutic agent." – PubMed ID#PMC4878560 (Open Access licensed, attribute at the link) [222]

A 2018 study using water extracts of Cordyceps showed "potent anti-metastasis activity." This can significantly help slow (or stop) the spread of cancer from one location to another.

> "Treatment with WECS (water extracts of Cordyceps sinensis) (0.10-0.40mg/ml) significantly inhibited 4T1 cell viability in vitro. In animal studies, 50mg/kg WECS significantly reduced the number of metastatic lung nodules… WECS increased the survival rate of 4T1 tumor bearing mice in a dose dependent manner, and at high dose, WECS (50mg/kg) significantly increased the life span of the mice compared to untreated control group… CONCLUSION: Our results demonstrated that WECS has potent anti-metastasis activity in a mouse breast

cancer metastasis model possibly by down-regulation the expression of several metastasis-related cytokines." – PubMed ID#29253616 (2018) [223]

The following study used mice with human melanoma cells xenografted onto them. These types of studies use actual human cancer cells and produce outcomes very similar to human in vivo studies. Most cancer cells depend on the ability to make new blood vessels; this is known as angiogenesis (VEGF = vascular endothelial growth factor; VEGF induces angiogenesis). This study shows that Cordyceps interferes with the cancer cells' ability to produce VEGF, as well as inducing apoptosis in cancer cells.

"We demonstrated that Cordyceps militaris extract remarkably suppressed tumor growth via induction of apoptotic cell death in culture that links to the abrogation of VEGF production in melanoma cells. This was followed by mitigation of Akt1 and GSK-3β activation, while p38α phosphorylation levels were increased. Extract treatment in mouse model xenografted with human melanoma cells resulted in a dramatic antitumor effect with down-regulation of VEGF expression. The results suggest that suppression of tumor growth by Cordyceps militaris extract is, at least, mediated by its anti-angiogenicity and apoptosis induction capacities. Cordyceps militaris extract may be a potent antitumor herbal drug for solid tumors." – PubMed ID#24789042 [224] Full Study - International Journal of Oncology doi:10.3892/ijo.2014.2397 (2014) [225]

Metastasis is how cancer spreads from one area of the body to another. Being able to stop or slow this process is very important to survival. For example, malignant melanoma (the most dangerous form of skin cancer, and the type of cancer I had) rarely kills at the site of the original tumor. It is when the cancer spreads to the brain or other vital organs that it becomes problematic. Cordyceps can help slow this process, hopefully to the point where the body's immune system can kill off the remaining migrating cancer cells.

"We investigated the anti-metastatic activity of a water extract of Cordyceps sinensis (WECS)… WECS reduced HGF-accelerated B16-F0 cell invasion in a concentration-dependent manner. These findings suggest that WECS exerts an anti-metastatic action, in part by inhibiting the HGF-accelerated tumor invasiveness of mouse melanoma cells." – PubMed ID#20944118 (2010) [226]

Cordyceps improves the immune response against various cancers (as it is immunopotentiating and chemotherapeutic), even if a person has been left immunodeficient by other, conventional, cancer treatments.

> "This paper reports the study on the effects of the ethanol extract of Cordyceps sinensis (CS-II), a potent herbal tonic, on murine and human in vitro natural killer cell (NK) activities and on murine in vivo NK activity… This study indicates that CS-II may be used as an immunopotentiating agent in treating cancer and immunodeficient patients." – PubMed ID#1597083 (1992) [227]

The following study shows that it is often better to use hot water extracted whole mushrooms rather than isolated compounds from the mushroom. There is much to be learned about medicinal mushrooms, and not all of the active compounds in these mushrooms have been discovered. Many of the compounds work synergistically with each other, though this is rarely studied as research is usually done on single isolates.

> "We investigated the effect of the water extract of Cordyceps sinensis (WECS) on liver metastasis of Lewis lung carcinoma (LLC) and B16 melanoma (B16) cells… WECS showed a strong cytotoxicity against LLC and B16 cells, while cordycepin, an active component of WECS, was not cytotoxic against these cells. These findings suggest that WECS has an anti-metastatic activity that is probably due to components other than cordycepin." – PubMed ID#10230862 (1999) [228]

The following in vitro (in the test tube) study examined an extract isolated from Cordyceps mycelium (similar to the roots of a plant). This shows that we should consume both the fruiting body and the mycelium of mushrooms when possible. This extract was studied for its effects on melanoma cells.

> "We examined the anticancer effect of CME-1, a novel water-soluble polysaccharide fraction, isolated from Cordyceps sinensis mycelia on B16-F10 melanoma cells… These results indicate that CME-1 inhibited MMP-1 expressions in B16F10 melanoma cells through either NF-kB or ERK/p38 MAPK down regulation thereby inhibiting B16F10 cell migration. Therefore, we proposed that CME-1 might be developed as a therapeutic potential candidate for the treatment of cancer metastasis." – PubMed ID#24762485 (2014) [229]

Cordyceps is considered to be extraordinarily safe. However, you can always find someone allergic to anything, and people allergic to mushrooms should avoid consuming them, and their extracts, unless under direct supervision of a medical doctor. Never take anything intravenously unless prescribed by your doctor.

> "Cordyceps is one of the best medicinal fungi known for numerous positive aspects in terms of pharmacological effects and considered to be safe. Some reports are published on its adverse gastrointestinal behaviors like dry mouth, nausea and diarrhea. In some patients, allergic response has been seen during treatment with a strain of Cordyceps, i.e., CS-4 (Xu 1994). Patients, who suffer

> from autoimmune diseases such as rheumatoid arthritis, systemic lupus erythematosus and multiple sclerosis, are generally suggested to avoid its use. Reports are still lacking on pregnant and lactating women but some animal studies in mice have revealed that Cordyceps have effects on plasma testosterone levels (Huang et al. 2004; Wong et al. 2007)… Cordyceps is relatively considered to be a non-toxic medicinal mushroom." – PubMed ID#PMC3909570 [230]

Cordycepin, an extract from Cordyceps, has been studied for its anti-tumor effects for over 60 years. Research shows that cordycepin "may greatly reduce the risk of cancer cell metastasis of all types." Metastasis is the spread of cancer from one location to another, which very often and for many cancers is the cause of death for patients.

> "Cordycepin, a 3-deoxyadenosine, is the predominant functional component of the fungus Cordyceps militaris, a traditional Chinese medicine… Cancer is caused by an imbalance between cell cycle progression and apoptosis… cordycepin was shown to induce antitumor effects or apoptosis in human head and neck squamous cell carcinoma, bladder cancer, thyroid carcinoma, breast cancer, multiple myeloma, leukemia, lymphoma and mouse leydig tumor cells. Additionally, the inhibitory effect of cordycepin was observed in hematogenic metastasis of mouse melanoma and lung carcinoma cells… Cordycepin induces cell apoptosis through three signaling pathways: PKA/TdT signaling pathway, caspase signaling pathway and p38/JNK signaling pathway… cordycepin may greatly reduce the risk of cancer cell metastasis of all types. The significance of cordycepin as a natural medicine is that may be used to treat or prevent cancer progression in the future" – PubMed ID#PMC4509066 (2015) [231]

I've only included a small, representative sample of the studies and medical research papers examining Cordyceps' use in treating or preventing cancer. By my count there are over 2,700 such entries listed in PubMed. As you can see, Cordyceps should be a part of anyone's protocol to fight or prevent cancer.

ENOKI

AKA: *Flammulina velutipes*, velvet foot, velvet shank, winter mushroom, winter fungus, *Flammulinavelutipes*, Enokitake, Enokidake Futu, golden needle mushroom, futu mushroom, *Basidiomycotina, Agaricales*, Tricholomataceae and lily mushroom

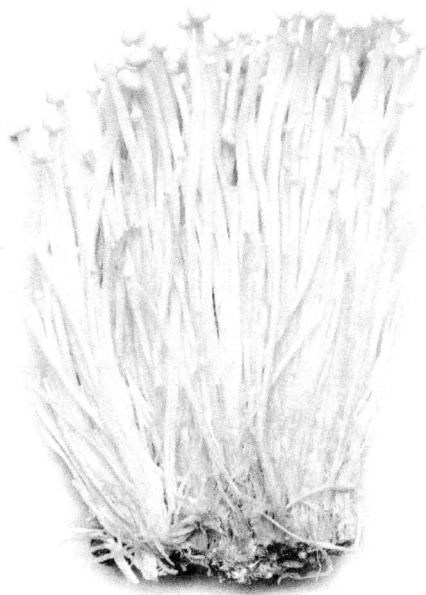

Enoki mushrooms are a tasty edible mushroom that grows wild in Europe, Asia and a large chunk of the United States. The wild variety can be found September through March, thus the name "winter mushroom." In the wild it is often a golden-brown color. The cultivated variety found in specialty grocery stores is a pale white color, as it is grown without being exposed to light. Since the research studies used the cultivated variety, either variety should have medicinal value.

According to the book *Edible Mushrooms and Their Cultivation*, enoki has no toxic effects on the human body. It has also been shown to have benefits for hypertension, high blood sugar and high cholesterol, and it has antithrombotic properties in people prone to venous thrombosis (and other thromboembolic diseases). This is in addition to its well-studied anticancer and immunomodulating properties.

> "FVE is a documented immunomodulatory protein purified from Enoki mushroom (Flammulina velutipes) and known as an activator for human T lymphocytes... Oral administration of FVE (10mg/kg) significantly increased the life span and inhibited the tumor size of BNL 1MEA.7R.1 (BNL) hepatoma-bearing mice. Taken together, oral administration of FVE displayed anti-tumor activity through activating both innate and adaptive immunity of the host to prime a cytotoxic immune response and IFN-gamma played a key role in the anti-tumor efficacy of FVE." – PubMed ID#19909827 (2010) [232]

> "the fruiting bodies of the mushroom Flammulina velutipes... inhibits proliferation of leukemia L1210 cells with an IC50 of 13 microM" – PubMed ID#16894961 (2006) [233]

Enoki (FVE below) was tested against two common breast cancer cell lines (in vitro) and "induced an exceptionally rapid apoptosis." Tumor growth was inhibited by 99%. This speaks very loudly for including enoki mushrooms in a breast cancer prevention or treatment protocol. (FVE = *Flammulina velutipes*)

C a n c e r : I m p r o v i n g Y o u r O d d s

"mushroom extracts CME and FVE induced an exceptionally rapid apoptosis on MCF-7 and MDA-MB-231 detected by Annexin V-FITC within 2 h of treatment and DNA fragment end-labeling assay (TUNEL) in 5 h of treatment. Anchorage-independent growth assays indicated that the MCF-7 tumor colony formation rate was reduced by 60% in CCE- and CME-treated cells and nearly completely inhibited (99%) by FVE treatment… These results suggest that mushroom species Coprinus comatus, Coprinellus sp. and Flammulina velutipes contain potent antitumor compounds for breast cancer. Our finding is important due to the lack of chemotherapeutic and chemopreventive agents for ER- human breast cancer." – PubMed ID#16391863 (2006) [234]

This paper outlines the evidence from dozens of research studies that show anti-tumor and anticancer properties of the enoki mushroom. Though it seems especially effective against certain breast cancers, it has also shown strong benefits against several other cancers (stomach, lung, liver, melanoma, sarcoma, fibrosarcoma, leukemia, colorectal, cervical, glioma, etc.) and is likely to show benefits with most cancers. As with other natural biologics, there just isn't the research money available to properly study enoki against every cancer. However, the research clearly indicates that enoki contains various anti-tumor and anticancer properties, making it very likely to have a broad-spectrum action against a variety of cancers.

"F. velutipes has been reported to have multiple beneficial effects on human health. They include antitumour, anticancer and anti-atherosclerotic activity, thrombosis inhibition, antihypertensive and cholesterol lowering effects, anti-aging and antioxidant properties, ability to restore neurotransmitters associated with memory and learning, anti-inflammatory, immunomodulatory and anti-bacterial activities… proflamin, a glycoprotein enzyme with anticancer activity, and asparaginase were also discovered in the mycelium of the mushroom… Beta-glucan is one of the many interesting polysaccharides found in F. velutipes, having demonstrated anticancer properties… F. velutipes possess antiproliferative activity against several cancer cell lines and have the potential to be developed as chemotherapeutic agents… various novel sesquiterpenes and norsequiterpenes were also identified from the extract of F. velutipes. These compounds exhibited several bioactivities such as anticancer, antibacterial and antioxidant activity… In 2003, Ikekawa (2001) presented an epidemiological study spanning 15 years (1972–1986) which showed that the cancer related death rates of farmers who grew F. velutipes mushroom—assuming that they would have eaten some of the mushrooms they farmed—were lower by 39% when compared to comparable populations not involved in mushroom farming… F. velutipes extract possesses anticancer properties, and several anticancer compounds have been isolated from

Updates at - https://improvingyourodds.com

Support at - https://www.facebook.com/groups/cancer.improving.your.odds

F. velutipes in recent decades… anticancer potential of fruiting bodies extract from F. velutipes, which was particularly effective against breast cancer cell lines… the extract induced apoptosis in the breast cancer cells and also caused 99% inhibition of colony formation of MCF-7… These isolactarane-related norsesquiterpenes (15 to 17, 19 to 21) extracted from the solid culture of F. velutipes were found to possess cytotoxic effect against several cancer cell lines… sesquiterpenes (22 to 24, 30) were reported to have moderate cytotoxicity against human tumor cell lines: HepG2 (liver cancer cells), MCF-7 (breast cancer cells), SGC7901 (stomach cancer cells), and A549 (lung cancer cells)" – PubMed ID#PMC5141589 (2016) [235]

A protein isolated from enoki modulates the immune system, is anti-inflammatory and inhibits cancer cell migration. Immunomodulators help the immune system identify targets, including cancer cells, but they do not overstimulate the immune system.

"FIP-fve is an immunomodulatory protein isolated from Flammulina velutipes that possesses anti-inflammatory and immunomodulatory activities… In conclusion, FIP-fve inhibits lung cancer cell migration via RacGAP1 and suppresses the proliferation of A549 via p53 activation pathway." – PubMed ID#24274472 (2013) [236]

TNF-alpha (or tumor necrosis factor alpha) is produced by our macrophages, lymphocytes, NK (natural killer) cells and other immune cells. One of its main jobs, as the name implies, is to inhibit tumorigenesis. Dysregulation of TNF-a is also linked to Alzheimer's disease, major depression, psoriasis and inflammatory bowel disease (IBD). TNF-a is best produced and regulated by the body (where it can focus it on the tumor), rather than by medicines that cause a systemic overstimulation of TNF-a. Prolonged exposure to artificially raised TNF-a can also lead to cachexia, a wasting syndrome often seen in advanced cancer patients. The immunomodulating effects of medicinal mushrooms, such as enoki, help the immune system focus on the tumor, rather than stimulating compounds like TNF-a, throughout the body.

"FVP (200, 100, 50 microg/mL) could promote the metabolic activity of murine splenocytes and peritoneal exudate cells (PEC) and increase the amounts of TNF-alpha, INF-gamma and IL-2 in the supernatants of splenocyte cultures, and the amount of TNF-alpha in PEC cultures, with the most marked increase on TNF-alpha level. FVP (100, 50, 25 mg/kg) could raise the serum levels of TNF-alpha and INF-gamma in S180 tumor-bearing mice." – PubMed ID#19645242 (2009) [237]

Here the FVP compound in enoki "significantly prolonged survival time and reduced tumor size" by enhancing the body's own innate and adaptive immune response.

> "The study reported a glycoprotein (FVE) with immunomodulatory properties from Flammulina velutipes. In hepatoma-bearing mice, the oral treatment of FVE (10 mg/kg) significantly prolonged survival time and reduced tumor size, through inducing cytotoxic immune response by enhancing innate and adaptive immunity." – PubMed ID#PMC4808884 (2016) [238]

Safety

It should be noted that one study showed mild myotoxic (poison) effects (increased activities of plasma creatine kinase, DOI:10.1177/1535370218762340) from consuming over 200 grams (7 ounces) per day of uncooked wild enoki mushrooms over an extended period. As this mushroom weighs very little, this would require the consumption of a whole lot of enoki each day (an amount few people would try). Consuming this mushroom raw is not recommended, and cooking gets rid of most of the myotoxin risk. Though it is unknown if cooking will neutralize the myotoxins in question, the full study has this to say on the topic: "If the myotoxic substance in F. velutipes was a protein or a shorter peptide, it could be assumed to be at least partly inactivated or destroyed by cooking." Still, it is best to limit your intake to under 100 grams (3.5 ounces) per day of cooked enoki (this is still a lot of enoki!). This most likely applies to most edible mushrooms: Cooking is always best, and moderation is key (under 100 grams per day of any cooked mushroom, or 25 grams (1 ounce) of uncooked mushrooms for those that are meant to be consumed raw). My wife and I consume this mushroom and most of the other ones in this chapter.

LION'S MANE

AKA: *Hericium erinaceus,* **monkey head, bearded hedgehog, hedgehog, hog's head fungus, white beard, satyr's beard, old man's beard, pom pom, bearded tooth, Yamabushitake (Japanese), Houtou (Chinese)**
(Image Footnote [239])

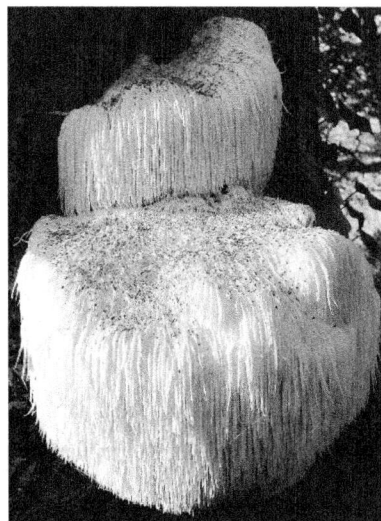

Lion's mane is one of the more unique looking mushrooms, looking like a white beard hanging off a hardwood tree. It is an edible mushroom with many medicinal properties. Though not all neighborhood grocery stores carry it, you can often find it at gourmet stores, farmer's markets and sometimes, Whole Foods. If you find it in dried form, it will still have its medicinal properties; you will just want to rehydrate it before consuming. Some people take the dried mushrooms, run them through a food processor and use the powder as a seasoning in dishes prior to cooking. In order to get the most benefits from any mushroom, they should be moist cooked.

Lion's mane has become a popular supplement in large part due to its nootropic benefits (cognitive enhancement). It has also been shown in research studies to have chemotherapeutic, antidiabetic, antihypertensive and heart protective effects, and it has been shown to benefit anxiety and depression. It is quite an amazing superfood. Lion's mane contains several medicinal polysaccharides, including beta-glucans, HEP1 and HEPF3 (two hetero-polysaccharides). Over 35 polysaccharides in total have been extracted from lion's mane; most seem to be bioactive.

Cooking lion's mane couldn't be easier. It is a large mushroom; purchase one about the size of a head of cauliflower. Cut off the "foot," the part that was attached to the tree. Brush off any dirt or particles; usually there is no need to rinse it as it grows on wood, not dirt. Slice it like steak, about ½ inch thick, and then fry it in a dry non-stick pan for 5 to 7 minutes per side. When it starts to brown, add 2 Tbsp of butter to the pan and gently coat both sides. Add salt and pepper. Turn heat to low and cook until both sides are golden brown. There are many more recipes online.

> "a total of more than thirty-five polysaccharides have been isolated from H. erinaceus. Studies on pharmacological activities have revealed that H. erinaceus polysaccharides possess the potential to help prevent, alleviate, or treat major diseases including cancer, gastric ulcer, diabetes, hyperlipidemia, hepatic injury, and neurodegenerative diseases… "This mushroom is rich in some physiologically important components, especially ˇ-glucan polysaccharides, which are responsible for anti-cancer, immuno-modulating, hypolipidemic, antioxidant and neuro-protective activities of this mushroom" --
> doi:10.1016/j.ijbiomac.2017.01.040 (2017) [240]

The lion's mane extract showed strong anti-metastatic potential, stopping the colon cancer from spreading to the lungs and inhibiting it by up to 69%.

> "H. erinaceus strongly elicited cancer cell death through apoptosis and inhibited metastasis of cancer cells to the lungs by 66% and 69%, respectively... down-regulated extracellular signal-regulated kinase (ERK), c-Jun N-terminal kinase (JNK), and p38 mitogen-activated protein kinase (MAPK) phosphorylations. The reduced phosphorylations seem to cause reduction of activity of the MMPs, thereby blocking migration and invasion of cells." – PubMed ID#23668749 (2013) [241]

The following study was done in mice (in vivo). This study also included a lot of the biomarker tests for tumor improvement. These markers are very similar in humans and mice, though the degree of improvement may vary.

> "significantly reduced tumor weights by 38 and 41%. Tumor regressions were associated with changes in the following cancer biomarkers as compared to phosphate buffer (PBS)-treated control mice: 2.7- and 2.4-fold increases in cytolytic activity of splenic natural killer (NK) cells; restored nitric oxide production and phagocytosis in peritoneal macrophages to 95-98% of normal levels; ~2-fold increase in released pro-inflammatory cytokines tumor necrosis factor-α, interleukin-1β, and interleukin-6 from macrophages; and ~56 and ~60% reductions in the number of blood vessels inside the tumor... Reduced COX-2 and 5-LOX expression down-regulated VEGF expression, resulting in inhibition of neo-angiogenesis inside the tumors. The results indicate that induction of NK activity, activation of macrophages, and inhibition of angiogenesis all contribute to the mechanism of reduction of tumor size." – PubMed ID#21846141 (2011) [242]

Lion's mane also improves the immune system, which is important for people undergoing any traditional cancer treatment.

> "These results suggest that the mushroom extract activities against bacterial infection in mice occur through the activation of innate immune cells." – PubMed ID#22624604 (2012) [243]

The following shows the anticancer effects of lion's mane on liver and intestinal cancers. In the below study, 5-FU is Fluorouracil, a chemotherapy drug. In this study lion's mane was compared to 5-FU and found to be more effective and less toxic.

> "Hericium erinaceus (HE) possesses many beneficial functions such as anticancer, antiulcer, antiinflammation and antimicrobial effects, immunomodulation and other activities… HE extracts (HTJ5 and HTJ5A) are active against liver cancer HepG2 and Huh-7, colon cancer HT-29 and gastric cancer NCI-87 cells in vitro and tumor xenografts bearing in SCID mice in vivo. They are more effective and less toxic compared to 5-FU in all four in vivo tumor models. The compounds have the potential for development into anticancer agents for the treatment of gastrointestinal cancer used alone and/or in combination with clinical used chemotherapeutic drugs." – PubMed ID#24631140 (2014) [244]

This 2016 research study goes into a lot of detail on how lion's mane works to fight cancers and describes the work of dozens of other studies. Like other mushrooms, it has been found that this mushroom has several compounds that all fight cancer without harming human cells.

> "Hericium erinaceus (HE) is an edible mushroom that has been shown to exhibit anticancer and anti-inflammatory activities… Our findings conclude that antiangiogenic and anti-inflammatory activities of H. erinaceus may contribute to its anticancer property through modulation of MMP-9/NF-κB and Nrf2-antioxidant signaling pathways… Many medicinal mushrooms and herbs have been shown to be the rich source of phytochemicals with chemoprevention potential for various human cancers and inflammatory diseases. The results demonstrate that H. erinaceus markedly inhibited the TNF-α-induced angiogenesis in human EA.hy926 endothelial cells through downregulation of MMP-9/NF-κB signaling and upregulation of Nrf2-mediated antioxidant genes (Figure 8). These findings added some novel information on the biological activities of H. erinaceus, in relevance to suppression of toxic ROS and upregulation of antioxidant genes… In our study, release of MMP-9 upon TNF-a-stimulation was found to be suppressed by HE treatment in endothelial cells. This phenomenon implies that antiangiogenic property of HE is closely associated with decreased endothelial cell MMP-9 activity. Both *in vivo* and *in vitro* studies clearly demonstrated that absolute lack/inhibition of MMP-9 can reduce the cell-cell interaction and prevent the formation of new capillary network" – PubMed ID#PMC4707368 (Open Access attribute at the link) (2016) [245]

Lion's mane can also provide a strong synergistic anti-tumor activity in combination with chemotherapy.

> "One feature that cytotoxic treatments of cancer have in common is their activation of the transcription factor NFjB, which suppresses the apoptotic potential of chemotherapeutic drugs and contributes to resistance… Apoptosis, or programmed cell death, is an important physiological process of cell death and occurs during tissue remodeling, immune regulation, and tumor regression."

Apoptotic potential means a cell's "apoptosis" ability, or programmed cell death. Apoptosis is the body's way of killing off old and damaged cells, including cancer cells, when things are no longer working properly. It is a highly regulated process that in a healthy adult normally kills between 50 to 70 billion cells per day. When the process of regulated apoptosis breaks down, too much inappropriate apoptosis will lead to atrophy, and too little can lead to uncontrolled cell proliferation, including diseases such as cancer. Supporting the body's ability to maintain regulated apoptosis is essential to helping it fight cancer. The next paragraph is an important one.

> "Inhibition of NF-jB translocation has been implicated in enhanced chemosensitivity of chemotherapeutic drugs. Using Western blot analysis we found that combination treatment with HE and Dox could inhibit NF-jB nuclear translocation, whereas Dox increased it.

In other words, chemotherapy drugs (such as Doxorubicin, or Dox) suppressed apoptosis. HE (*Hericium erinaceus*, or lion's mane) inhibited NF-jB translocation, thus maintaining proper apoptosis. In this study the combination increased the apoptotic rate from 15% in the control group to 40% in the combined lion's mane/Dox group. This is very exciting, especially considering the apoptotic rate was virtually unchanged when either lion's mane or Dox was given individually!

> … the combination of low doses of HE and 1 lg/ml of Dox had a significantly ($p < 0.05$) greater dose-dependent inhibitory effect than that of HE or Dox alone at comparable concentrations" – PubMed ID#20554107 (2010) [246] doi:10.1016/j.canlet.2010.05.006.

Many people reading this are on, or are considering, chemotherapy drugs, and you may want to consider adding this mushroom for its synergistic effect with chemotherapy.

As discussed elsewhere, natural treatment options receive very little research funding (due to the inability to patent them). Though lion's mane does have several studies showing its strong anticancer activity, researchers are continuing to identify additional isolates as research dollars allow. This 2015 study identified yet another cancer-fighting substance in lion's mane (*H. erinaceus*). This simply goes to show that we don't always need to know exactly why a food fights cancer in order to utilize it.

"cerebroside E was found to have beneficial effects in cancer treatment, not only by inhibiting angiogenesis, but also by attenuating anticancer drug-induced side effects… In conclusion, we isolated and identified a new cerebroside, cerebroside E (1), which was isolated from the fruiting bodies of H. erinaceus and its various biological activities were evaluated for the identification of its medicinal applicability… This study suggests beneficial effects of the cerebroside isolated from H. erinaceus in cancer treatment." – PubMed ID#26547693 (2015) [247], doi: 10.1016/j.bmcl.2015.10.092 (quotes from the full study)

Immunomodulating Effects

HEP-S "was extracted and isolated from the fruiting bodies of Hericium erinaceus… The immunomodulatory assay indicated that HEP-S could significantly enhance the pinocytic and phagocytic capacity and promote the secretion of nitric oxide and pro-inflammatory cytokines by activating the corresponding mRNA and protein expression in RAW 264.7 cells involving a toll-like receptor 2 membrane receptor. Besides, HEP-S was also found to improve the adaptive immune function by enhancing T and B lymphocyte proliferation and increasing the interleukin-2, interleukin-4 and interferon-γ secretion in spleen lymphocytes. These results suggested that HEP-S could be used as a potential immunoregulatory agent in functional foods." – PubMed ID#29168863 (2018) [248]

"Here, we report that HEP improves immune function by functionally enhancing cell-mediated and humoral immunity, macrophage phagocytosis, and NK cell activity. In addition, HEP was found to upregulate the secretion of SIgA and activate the MAPK and AKT cellular signaling pathways in the intestine. In conclusion, all these results allow us to postulate that the immunomodulatory effects of HEP are most likely attributed to the effective regulation of intestinal mucosal immune activity." – PubMed ID#28266682 (2017) [249]

MAITAKE

AKA: *Grifola frondosa*, hen-of-the-woods, sheep's head, ram's head, shelf mushroom, dancing mushroom, king of mushrooms, monkey's bench

Maitake is a mushroom that has been used medicinally for thousands of years. In medieval Japan it was so prized it was worth its weight in silver.

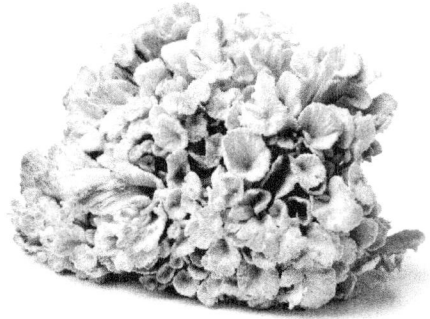

The maitake mushroom is a polypore, meaning that it has no gills like most mushrooms; it releases spores through small pores. It is found mainly on the bases of oak trees but is occasionally found on maples and elms. They're common in the northeastern United States and Canada, and in hardwood forests of China, Japan and Europe. The fruiting body can grow quite large, up to a few feet across, weighing as much as 40 or 50 pounds (about 18 to 23 kg), though they can occasionally grow to twice this weight.

Maitake mushrooms are edible, with a stronger—but delicious—flavor, especially compared to button mushrooms. They can replace button mushrooms in any recipe and can be stir-fried, sautéed, baked or even made into a tea. Though not found in your average neighborhood grocery, they can be found in specialty stores and sometimes at farmers markets in the northeastern US states. Dried maitake can easily be found online (simply rehydrate them and use as normal). If you're feeling adventuresome you can purchase maitake spore-infused plugs and grow your own in a log! Simply drill holes in the log and push in the plugs, and in a couple of years you'll have lots of mushrooms.

Of course, you're here to find out about the anticancer properties of maitake. This is one of the more important mushrooms to include in your treatment protocol. Because it is a powerful immunomodulator, it shows benefits against most cancers, with research studies showing treatment benefits for several different forms of cancer.

"Maitake D-Fraction, extracted from maitake mushroom, has been reported to exert its antitumor effect in tumor-bearing mice by enhancing the immune system through activation of macrophages, T cells, and natural killer (NK) cells… After administration of D-Fraction, dramatic increases in NK cell activity were seen… D-Fraction has been shown to enhance the activity of immune-competent cells such as macrophages, helper T cells, cytotoxic T cells, and NK cells, resulting in reduced tumor size in mice, without causing unwanted side effects… D-Fraction therapy was administered to 10 patients with stage II–IV lung or breast cancer… In conclusion, D-Fraction may inhibit cancer progression even without adjunct

> therapies… D-Fraction reverses the decrease in T cell number and activity seen in cancer, and is capable of enhancing and maintaining peripheral blood NK cell activity in patients with lung and breast cancer. Oral administration of D-Fraction… may be an effective method of stimulating the immune system to fight cancers" – PubMed ID#14977447 (2003) [250]

Simply by adding the maitake mushroom, MD-fraction has been shown to improve various cancers in up to 68.8% of patients. These types of research studies almost always study one treatment at a time. I would love to see a study look at a more broad-spectrum approach, such as administering 5 or 6 different medicinal mushrooms to patients (with each mushroom containing several anticancer isolates). I'm sure the results would be amazing.

> "Maitake mushroom (Grifola frondosa) MD-fraction containing beta-1,6 glucan with beta-1,3 branched chains has previously exhibited strong anticancer activity by increasing immune-competent cell activity… Cancer regression or significant symptom improvement was observed in 58.3 percent of liver cancer patients, 68.8 percent of breast cancer patients, and 62.5 percent of lung cancer patients. The trial found a less than 10-20 percent improvement for leukemia, stomach cancer, and brain cancer patients. Furthermore, when maitake was taken in addition to chemotherapy, immune-competent cell activities were enhanced 1.2-1.4 times, compared with chemotherapy alone. Animal studies have supported the use of maitake MD-fraction for cancer." – PubMed ID#12126464 (2002) [251]

As mentioned earlier in this book, inhibiting metastasis is very important to improving survival rates. For instance, if malignant melanoma didn't move to the organs (metastasize), it would rarely cause death. The tumor would simply be surgically removed, and that would be that. But of course, human cancers do metastasize; that is what makes them so fatal. So, seeing a metastasis inhibition rate of 92.1% is spectacular. The D-Fraction isolate, found in fresh maitake mushrooms, is commercially available in a purified form. Of course, it is also found in the whole mushroom and mushroom powders.

> "tumor metastasis was inhibited by 92.1% in mice given D-fraction compared to the control group, and tumor recrudescence was also inhibited by 91.9%... D-fraction is effective against the metastasis of liver cancer (MM-146 liver carcinoma) with 91.3% inhibition… Mitomycin C (MMC) is an anti-cancer drug widely used both in Japan and the United States… Rate of inhibition of metastasis by MMC alone was 51.3%, but increased to 87.5% when D-fraction was added… These results indicate that Maitake D-fraction potentiates the activity of cellular immune-competent cells and is effective in inhibition of cancer metastasis/recrudescence as well as carcinogenesis" – 10.1111/j.1749-6632.1997.tb48611.x, PubMed ID#9616756 (from the full report) (1997) [252]

The following study looked at prostate cancer cells (in vitro) and found that maitake D-Fraction was as effective as interferons in reducing prostate cancer cell growth. A combination of the two was even more effective, and adding maitake D-Fraction allowed the use of 1/5 the amount of interferon while achieving the same results.

> "The D-fraction (PDF), the unique proteoglucan extracted from maitake mushroom (Grifola frondosa), is the acid-insoluble, alkali-soluble and hot water-extractable fraction… It has been shown in an animal model that PDF was capable of activating immune-competent cells such as natural killer cells and cytotoxic T-cells with a concomitant increase in interleukin-1 production [11], indicating stimulation of immune responses. A preventive or inhibitory activity of PDF on carcinogenesis and metastasis has also been demonstrated… Possible immunotherapeutic potentiation with D-Fraction in prostate cancer cells… ~65% growth reduction was seen at 1,000 µg/ml… The combination of IFN-α2b (10 K IU/ml) and PDF (250 µg/ml) is capable of inducing a ~65% reduction in PC-3 cell growth." -- Journal of Hematology & Oncology 2008, 1:25 doi:10.1186/1756-8722-1-25 (An OpenAccess paper, attribution at the link) (2008) [253]

The following phase I/II trial involved 34 breast cancer patients (12 stage I, 16 stage II, 6 stage III). Patients were given a polysaccharide extract from maitake mushrooms (most likely beta-glucans). As with many of these studies, the maitake mushroom extract showed multiple types of benefits. Considering that one mushroom may have many beneficial isolates, multiply that times consuming several different kinds of mushrooms, and you can see that mushrooms are broad-spectrum cancer fighters.

> "A phase I/II trial of a polysaccharide extract from Grifola frondosa (Maitake mushroom) in breast cancer patients: immunological effects: The largest phenotypical changes were seen with CD3+ CD56+ NK T cell and CD4+ CD25+ T cell (50% higher than baseline), both at a high dose of Maitake extract (10 mg/kg per day)" -- DOI: 10.1007/s00432-009-0562-z, PubMed ID#19253021 (2009) [254]

In the following study, maitake mushrooms were shown to increase TNF-a and NK levels, both of which are vitally important in tumor suppression. Maitake was also shown to increase interleukin (IL)-12 levels. Human in vivo use found that D-Fraction enhanced NK cell activity by 1.2 to 2.7 times in various types of cancers. Other immune system activity also improved.

"Natural killer (NK) cells are directly cytotoxic for tumor cells and play a primary role in regulating immune responses. We monitored levels of NK cell cytotoxic activity in cancer patients receiving D-Fraction extracted from maitake mushrooms (Grifola frondosa). Elevated levels of cytotoxic activity were maintained for one year… D-Fraction markedly suppressed tumor growth, corresponding with increases in TNF-a and IFN-g released from spleen cells and a significant increase in TNF-a expressed in NK cells. This suggests that the D-Fraction activates NK cells even on the 20th day after treatment. Furthermore, D-Fraction increased macrophage-derived interleukin (IL)-12, which serves to activate NK cells. These results suggest that NK cells are not only responsible for the early effects of D-Fraction on tumor growth, but also for the long-term tumor-suppressive effects of D-Fraction through increased IL-12 released from macrophages… In conclusion, D-Fraction represents an important BRM for NK cells by enhancing IL-12 release from macrophages. In immunotherapy using D-Faction for cancer patients, NK cells are responsible for early anti-tumor responses, while both NK and T cells are responsible for long-term anti-tumor responses." – PubMed ID#12499658 (2002) [255] Full Study free access [256]

Safety

Maitake mushrooms have been found to be extremely safe; when consumed orally, no serious adverse effects have been noted, regardless of dosage. It is a common food ingredient, especially in Japan. However, some people are allergic to mushrooms, and those people, of course, will need to avoid them.

"No serious adverse event was observed during the study period in any study subject. No dose-limiting toxicity was encountered." -- DOI: 10.1007/s00432-009-0562-z, PubMed ID#19253021 (2009) [257]

Usage

Consuming maitake mushrooms, and even cooking with them, is a good way of obtaining D-Fraction. Like most mushrooms, to obtain the most benefit it should be cooked or hot water extracted, in order to release the polysaccharides from the chitin (mushroom fiber). Eating maitake mushrooms raw means that some of the beta-glucans will not be available to us and will simply pass though the digestive system. If you dry cook mushrooms, they should be sweated, or steamed, first.

Obviously, this is a mushroom you want to be consuming.

MESIMA

AKA: *Phellinus linteus*, **Song Gen (Chinese), Sanghwang, Sang-Hwang or Sangwhang (Korean), Meshimakobu (Japanese), Meshima, black hoof**

This mushroom grows on mulberry trees and is shaped like a hoof. The color is usually dark brown to black. Mesima has been used in the traditional medicine in China, Japan and Korea for centuries. It has traditionally been used to treat ailments such as wrinkles, aging, gastritis, intestinal dysfunction, inflammatory bowel disease, inflammation, diarrhea and cancers. In recent times these countries were also the first to explore the benefits of this mushroom scientifically. In Korea this mushroom is commonly used in adjunct treatment alongside chemotherapy for cancer.

Nine different beneficial fractions have been isolated from the fruiting body. These include hispidin, caffeic acid, ellagic acid, protocatechuic acid, protocatechualdehyde, davallialactone, hypholomine B, interfungins A and inoscavin A. Of these interfungins, A is a potent inhibitor of protein glycation.

In this study out of Taiwan, the researchers evaluated the hispolon fraction from Mesima (*P. linteus*) and found that it had an antiproliferation effect on both breast and bladder cancer cells. It also led to apoptosis in gastric cancer cells.

> "Hispolon from Phellinus linteus has antiproliferative effects via MDM2-recruited ERK1/2 activity in breast and bladder cancer cells… Hispolon extracted from Phellinus species was found to induce epidermoid and gastric cancer cell apoptosis… hispolon inhibited breast and bladder cancer cell growth, regardless of p53 status… hispolon may be a potential anti-tumor agent in breast and bladder cancers." – PubMed ID#19477214 (2009) [258]

Glioblastoma refers to an aggressive brain cancer that can also spread to the spine. It is also known as glioblastoma multiforme (GBM). The following study shows that Mesima may help people live longer and better lives, especially in conjunction with more traditional treatments, such as radiation, chemotherapy and surgery. But, again, this is a very aggressive form of cancer, so all you can do with Mesima is *Improve Your Odds*.

> "Hispolon is a polyphenolic compound isolated from Phellinus linteus which exhibits antitumor activity… Hispolon treatment was effective on U87MG cells in inhibiting cell viability and inducing cell apoptosis. Our results indicate that hispolon inhibits the cell viability, induces G2/M cell cycle arrest and apoptosis in glioblastoma U87MG cells, and p53 should play a role in hispolon-mediated antitumor activity." – PubMed ID#28618133 (2017) [259]

Updates at - https://improvingyourodds.com

Support at - https://www.facebook.com/groups/cancer.improving.your.odds

Immunotherapy is where medicinal mushrooms shine. Though no one can make any guarantees mushrooms will help, and in vivo research is lacking, a good mix of various mushrooms (and mushroom powders), including Mesima, is certainly worth considering.

> "Treatment advances for patients with glioblastoma, an aggressive form of brain cancer, have been rare. But recent studies have raised hopes that immunotherapy, which has recently established itself as a proven therapy for several types of cancer, may be able to reverse this trend." – Cancer.gov [260]

Hispolon (extracted from Mesima mushrooms for research use) has similar effects on lung cancer cells.

> "The anticancer effects of hispolon on lung cancer cells… Hispolon decreased cell viability in a dose- and time-dependent manner… Moreover, hispolon induced cell apoptosis through activation of the mitochondrial pathway… Additionally, hispolon enhanced the expression of p53, specific silencing of which almost completely reversed hispolon-mediated antitumor activity" – PubMed ID#25268766 (2014) [261]

When non-cancerous cells become damaged, get too old, etc., they initiate a process called apoptosis, or programmed cell death. They basically commit suicide. Cancer cells turn off this normal cellular function. Turning this process back on in cancer cells is very beneficial to treatment.

> "Hispolon (a phenolic compound isolated from Phellinus linteus) has been shown to possess strong antioxidant, anti-inflammatory, anticancer, and antidiabetic properties. In this study, we investigated the antiproliferative effect of hispolon on human hepatocellular carcinoma NB4 cells… We conclude that hispolon induces both of extrinsic and intrinsic apoptotic pathways in NB4 human leukemia cells in vitro." – PubMed ID#24228611 (2013) [262]
>
> "This study investigated the antiproliferative effect of hispolon on human hepatocellular carcinoma Hep3B cells… These findings establish a mechanistic link between the MAPK pathway and hispolon-induced cell cycle arrest and apoptosis in Hep3B cells." – PubMed ID#21630638 (2011) [263]

Here hispolon was isolated from a tree fungus, but the compound benefits would apply to Mesima as well. This study also shows that apoptosis is restored, and it noted that hispolon inhibited the spread of cancer (through metastasis) and modulated the immune system to improve its ability to fight the cancer.

"Hispolon, a phenolic compound isolated from Phellinus igniarius, induces apoptosis and anti-tumor effects in cancers… treatment with hispolon inhibited cell metastasis in two cervical cancer cell lines… Moreover, hispolon induced autophagy, which increased LC3 conversion and acidic vesicular organelle formation… Our results indicate that autophagy is essential for decreasing CTSS activity to inhibit tumor metastasis by hispolon treatment in cervical cancer" – PubMed ID#28981104 (2017) [264]

The following research looked at Cambodian *Phellinus linteus* (CPL), which shares 99% of the DNA and function of *Phellinus linteus* (PL, or Mesima). Other studies on PL have shown very similar results, and the following research on CPL most likely applies, or the results would be similar. This still goes to show how important it is to consume a variety of fungi. B16BL6 is a melanoma cell line capable of metastasizing to the lungs. The first study below indicates that a simple hot water extract is enough to obtain the benefits of *P. linteus*.

"Phellinus linteus (PL) is a fungus mainly found in tropical America, Africa and Asian countries including Korea, Japan and China… in the present study, the anti-metastatic mechanism of aqueous extract of Cambodian Phellinus linteus (CPL) was evaluated. Cambodian mushroom was identified as a Phellinus species with 99% homology of Phellinus linteus by DNA sequence analysis… Overall, PL was reported to be a medicinal mushroom with anti-tumor activity, protective effect on liver damage, immunomodulatory action, anti-angiogenic and antioxidant activity. The hot aqueous extract of PL inhibited the growth of sarcoma 180 to about 96.7% of untreated control in ICR mice… In summary, aqueous extract of Camboidan Phellinus linteus may inhibit experimental metastasis of B16BL6 cells" – PubMed ID#15635158 (from the full study which is available at the link) [265]

"Polysaccharide from Phellinus linteus induces S-phase arrest in HepG2 cells by decreasing calreticulin expression and activating the P27kip1-cyclin A/D1/E-CDK2 pathway…. Both the volume and the weight of solid tumors were significantly decreased in P1-treated mice (200mg/kg) compared with the control. The HepG2 cells in the P1-treated tumors were significantly decreased, irregularly shaped, and smaller." – PubMed ID#24001891 (2013) [266]

This research study out of South Korea showed that Mesima has a direct antiproliferation effect on human colon cancer cells. This occurs by 4 different mechanisms: 1) stimulates the immune system's T lymphocytes, 2) induces the secretory and cellular macrophage immune response, 3) through an immunomodulatory mechanism, it inhibits metastasis and tumor growth, 4) it may, through some yet-to-be-identified method, have a direct action on tumor cells (without causing any harm to normal cells).

> "The cytotoxic mechanism of protein-bound polysaccharide isolated from Phellinus linteus (PL, Mesima) has been investigated. PL inhibited the proliferation and colony formation of SW480 human colon cancer cells... These results suggest that PL has a direct antitumor effect through apoptosis and cell cycle blockade in certain cancer cells." – PubMed ID#15533593 (2004) [267]

Mesima shows anticancer benefits from several different mechanisms. Though many of the medicinal mushrooms show such properties, it is clear that Mesima should be one we want to include in our protocol. It is not commonly found in medicinal mushroom mixes, but it can be ordered separately.

> "Polysaccharides extracted from the Phellinus linteus (PL) mushroom are known to possess anti-tumor effects... PL (125-1000 µg/mL) significantly inhibited cell proliferation and decreased β-catenin expression... tumor tissues from treated animals showed an increase in the apoptotic index and a decrease in β-catenin expression. Moreover, the proliferation index and microvessel density were significantly decreased... These data suggest that PL suppresses tumor growth, invasion, and angiogenesis through the inhibition of Wnt/β-catenin signaling in certain colon cancer cells... suppressed proliferation of lung cancer cells... apoptosis of prostate cancer cells... inhibition of tumor growth and invasive behavior of breast cancer cells... The key enzymes that have been shown to be closely associated with invasive and metastatic potential are MMPs and uPA. Several studies have shown that PL inhibits cancer cell invasion and metastasis by activating host immunity. Recently, PL was shown to suppress invasiveness through the inhibition of uPA secretion in mouse melanoma cells and breast cancer cells" – PubMed ID#PMC3154178 (2011) [268]

The following study showed that hispolon, found in the Mesima mushroom, clearly suppressed melanoma cell growth and induced apoptosis in those cancer cells.

> "we analyzed the functions of hispolon on melanogenesis and apoptosis in B16-F10 melanoma cells. The results demonstrated that hispolon is not an enzymatic inhibitor for tyrosinase; rather, it represses the expression of tyrosinase and the microphthalmia-associated transcription factor (MITF) to reduce the production of melanin in α-melanocyte-stimulating hormone (α-MSH)-stimulated B16-F10 cells at lower concentrations (less than 2 µM). In contrast, at higher concentration (greater than 10 µM), hispolon can induce activity of caspase-3, -8 and -9 to

trigger apoptosis of B16-F10 cells but not of Detroit 551 normal fibroblast cells. Therefore, we suggest that hispolon has the potential to treat hyperpigmentation diseases and melanoma skin cancer" – PubMed ID#PMC3907864 (2014) [269]

"The roles of ERK1/2 and p38 MAP kinases in the preventive mechanisms of mushroom Phellinus linteus against the inhibition of gap junctional intercellular communication by hydrogen peroxide… These inhibitors were also found to prevent the inhibition of GJIC induced by H(2)O(2), which suggests that PL may act as a natural anticancer product by preventing the inhibition of GJIC through the inactivation of ERK1/2 and p38 MAP kinases. In addition, our results indicate that the p38 kinase signaling pathway may be closely related functionally to the gap junction in rat liver epithelial cells." – PubMed ID#12117774 (2002) [270]

Recommendations

The Mesima mushroom shows strong anticancer and immunomodulating benefits across a wide range of cancers. Its benefits extend to helping the immune system fight all cancers. Because of this I would try to include this mushroom in your treatment protocol if possible (and it can certainly show benefits in prevention as well). If consuming many different mushrooms, taking as little as 1/8 tsp per day (of a concentrated Mesima powder) can be beneficial.

Nameko

AKA: *Pholiota* microspore, *Pholiota nameko,*
butterscotch mushroom

Nameko is a popular mushroom in Japanese and
Chinese foods and is one of the ingredients in miso
soup. It is also often used in stir-fries. It is one of
the most popular cultivated mushrooms in Japan.
It can have a slightly slimy or thin gelatinous
coating; this can help thicken soups. It is very tasty,
with a nutty, slightly earthy flavor.

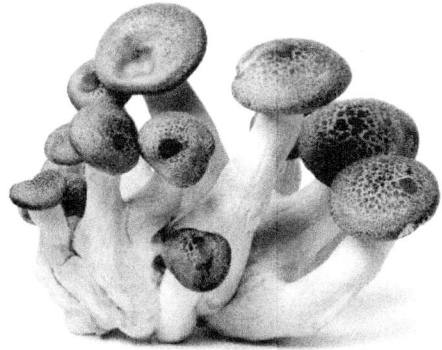

Many of the anticancer benefits from mushrooms
are derived from polysaccharides (basically very complex sugars with special structures). In this
study, a water-soluble protein (PNWSP) in nameko was identified and studied. They found that
this protein (a proteoglycan) was able to induce apoptosis in human breast cancer cells.
Combining a water-soluble protein with anticancer capabilities together with anticancer
polysaccharides should show strong synergy.

> "Pholiota nameko water-soluble protein (PNWSP), isolated from the dried
> fruiting bodies of Pholiota nameko… It showed potential antioxidant activities in
> scavenging free radicals, reducing power and chelating effect on Fe(2+), and had
> a protective effect against DNA damage. Moreover, it inhibited the proliferation
> of MCF7 cells by inducing apoptosis… The results showed that PNWSP could
> be a natural antioxidant and developed as a potential chemotherapeutic agent
> candidate against human breast cancer." – PubMed ID#25827476 (2016) [271]

> "PNWSP is an inhibitor of tumor cell proliferation in the micromolar
> concentration range (Table 4). After 24 h treatment, it exhibited the ability to
> inhibit cell viability in all tested cancer cell lines" -- 10.1002/jsfa.7194 (from the
> full study of the above extract)

> "A polysaccharide purified from Pholiota nameko (PNPS-1) was found to have
> anticancer and anti-inflammatory activity. This study investigated the effect of
> PNPS-1 on the nuclear factor (NF)-$\varkappa$B signaling pathway… A Polysaccharide
> from the Culinary-Medicinal Mushroom Pholiota nameko (Agaricomycetes)
> Inhibits the NF-$\varkappa$B Pathway in Dendritic Cells Through the TLR2 Receptor." –
> PubMed ID#28008810 (2016) [272]

This research indicates that PNAP protein from nameko mushrooms was able to return normal
apoptosis to tested human breast cancer cells. Cancer cells often turn off the apoptosis (the
process whereby the cell destroys itself if it becomes damaged or can no longer function properly,

e.g., it becomes cancerous). Turning normal apoptosis back on in cancer cells can help the body get rid of cancer naturally.

> "A novel antitumor protein from the edible mushroom Pholiota nameko (PNAP)… Human breast cancer MCF7 cells treated with PNAP produced typical apoptotic morphological changes including chromatin condensation, accumulation of sub-G1 cells and alternation of mitochondrial permeability. The PNAP induced apoptosis of MCF7 cells entailed loss of mitochondrial membrane potential" – PubMed ID#24189312 (2014) [273]

There isn't a great deal of information on this mushroom, at least not information published in English.

OYSTER MUSHROOM

AKA: *Pleurotus ostreatus, Pleurotus populinus*

Oyster mushrooms are one of the more common mushrooms and are found in many countries around the world. They tend to grow on dead, decaying trees, but they can be found on the bark of living trees as well. The caps can grow up to 10 inches, and as they grow, the caps flatten and resemble a fan or oyster. They are one of the few carnivorous mushrooms, in that their mycelia (rootlike system) can consume nematodes (small roundworms) and bacteria. Besides being medicinal, the oyster mushroom is a very common culinary delicacy.

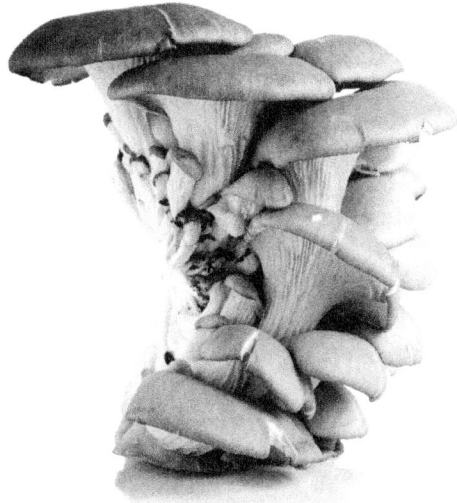

There are numerous studies verifying the cancer-fighting properties of oyster mushrooms. These mushrooms contain several compounds that help our bodies fight cancer, and the evidence is deemed very strong. One of those compounds is an insoluble beta-glucan (a polysaccharide, basically a specially formed complex sugar) called pleuran. Medicinally it falls into the category of an "immunologic adjuvant" or an "immunomodulator." This means that it is not toxic to either our cells or cancer cells. Instead it helps our immune system know what to attack, and/or it helps stimulate it to do so.

Oyster mushrooms are also a delicious food. There are tens of thousands of free recipes online that include oyster mushrooms as an ingredient! They are tender, delicate and cook quickly compared to some mushrooms. This makes them great for stir-fries. If using them in a dish that requires long cooking times, they should be added in the last stage of cooking. I prefer to sweat my mushrooms in a covered pan; moist heat helps release the beta-glucans from the chitin (mushroom fiber that keeps the beta-glucans bound up and unavailable to us). If my dish requires onions, I sauté them first, then add some water or broth to deglaze the pan, and then I add the mushrooms. I might also add garlic, pepper, salt, etc., depending on the recipe. Then I turn the heat to simmer, cover and simmer for 15 to 30 minutes, depending on the density of the mushroom (e.g., oyster and fresh enoki would get 15 minutes). Then I add this mix to whatever dish I'm cooking. Though they can be batter fried, you are more likely to get the full benefits from this, and any mushroom, if they are moist cooked.

In the following study, the authors describe oyster mushrooms as one of the more potent mushrooms in fighting breast and colon cancer. This may be; however, I want to consume some of each of those described (thus why I supplement with a powdered mix). These mushrooms have a synergistic effect with each other. The oyster mushroom is certainly one that breast and colon cancer patients should be consuming. Since many of these mushrooms have studies showing that they improve symptoms from chemotherapy and radiation, all the more reason to consume them.

"edible mushrooms Agaricus bisporus (portabella), Flammulina velutipes (enoki), Lentinula edodes (shiitake) and Pleurotus ostreatus (oyster) affect the growth of breast and colon cancer cells. Here, we identified as the most potent, P. ostreatus (oyster mushroom) which suppressed proliferation of breast cancer (MCF-7, MDA-MB-231) and colon cancer (HT-29, HCT-116) cells, without affecting proliferation of epithelial mammary MCF-10A and normal colon FHC cells. Flow cytometry revealed that the inhibition of cell proliferation by P. ostreatus was associated with the cell cycle arrest at G0/G1 phase in MCF-7 and HT-29 cells... In addition, P. ostreatus also up-regulated expression of p21 and inhibited Rb phosphorylation in HT-29 cells, suggesting that that P. ostreatus suppresses the proliferation of breast and colon cancer cells via p53-dependent as well as p53-independent pathway. In conclusion, our results indicated that the edible oyster mushroom has potential therapeutic/preventive effects on breast and colon cancer." – PubMed ID#19020765 (2008) [274]

When compared to other mushrooms, oyster mushrooms also seem to have the most benefit against prostate cancer cells. But again, that synergistic effect should be considered, and you should consume a wide variety of beneficial mushrooms. Many of the other mushrooms have also shown strong benefits (through other mechanisms against prostate, breast and colon cancers, along with other cancers). This study shows that oyster mushrooms improved apoptosis, or the body's natural ability to cause cancer cells to kill themselves. Apoptosis occurs all the time in the body; it is when cancer cells turn off this function that they're allowed to grow out of control. Oyster mushrooms, and many other mushrooms, simply turn the cancer cells' apoptosis ability back on again. This study looked at a hot water extract of fresh oyster mushrooms. Though they wanted a standardized preparation for research purposes, this is the same process you will use at home when you sweat, and then cook, your mushrooms.

"Cytotoxic effect of oyster mushroom Pleurotus ostreatus on human androgen-independent prostate cancer PC-3 cells." "A water-soluble extract (POE) prepared from the fresh oyster mushroom Pleurotus ostreatus produced the most significant cytotoxicity on PC-3 cells among the mushroom species tested... Induced apoptosis was also confirmed" – PubMed ID#16822205 (2006) [275]

What is most interesting about this study is that they used dried oyster mushrooms in the diets of rats, rather than extracts, and yet there was still a significant reduction in the number of tumors.

"The effect of 5% of dried oyster mushroom (Pleurotus ostreatus) in the diet on the dimethylhydrazine (DMH)-induced colon carcinogenesis was studied in male

> Wistar rats… Mushroom diet reduced significantly the incidence of lymphoid hyperplasia foci when mushroom was supplemented during the whole experiment. Tumour lesions could be characterized either as carcinoma in situ, or as infiltrating adenocarcinoma. Mushroom diet did not affect significantly the incidence of tumours. Nevertheless, a reduction in total number of tumours was observed in both groups of animals fed mushroom diet. A significant reduction of the number of tumour foci of the type carcinoma in situ was observed in animals fed the oyster mushroom during the whole experiment." – PubMed ID#9538185 (1998) [276]

This study also used a hot water extract. The study showed that the oyster mushroom "induces anti-proliferative and pro-apoptotic effects" on colon cancer cells.

> "An aqueous polysaccharide extract from the edible mushroom Pleurotus ostreatus induces anti-proliferative and pro-apoptotic effects on HT-29 colon cancer cells… Here, we describe a newly identified low-molecular-weight alpha-glucan with promising anti-tumorigenic properties, and demonstrate its direct effect on colon cancer cell proliferation via induction of programmed cell death." – PubMed ID#16413114 (2006) [277]

Lectin is an additional component of mushrooms, and it is separate from beta-glucans and other polysaccharides. The lectin described here has "potent antitumor and mitogenic" (prevents mitosis, or the cancer's ability to spread from one location to another) properties. This is why consuming whole mushrooms is better than consuming single-compound extracts.

> "A novel lectin with potent antitumor, mitogenic and HIV-1 reverse transcriptase inhibitory activities from the edible mushroom Pleurotus citrinopileatus." This is the Golden Oyster Mushroom "The lectin exerted potent antitumor activity in mice bearing sarcoma 180, and caused approximately 80% inhibition of tumor growth when administered intraperitonealy at 5 mg/kg daily for 20 days. It elicited a mitogenic response from murine splenocytes in vitro with the maximal response at a lectin concentration of 2 microM." – PubMed ID#17961926 (2008) [278]

In the following study, mice were given a bladder cancer-inducing chemical, BBN, for 8 weeks. In the group of 10 mice that were given only BBN, all 10 contracted bladder cancer. In the group that were given oyster mushrooms as well, only 65% contracted cancer. However, in this group (as well as the other two mushroom groups) their immune system measurements were much stronger than the control group (BBN only). Those receiving the mushrooms in their diet had a normal blastogenic response, as well as a normal NK (cancer killing cells, a type of lymphocyte—that is, a white blood cell) response, whereas those only receiving BBN had a "significant depression of NK cell activity." These are two very important immune system measures that show how well the immune system can fight cancer.

> "mice were treated with a carcinogen, N-butyl-N'-butanolnitrosoamine (BBN), every day for 8 consecutive weeks and the effects of oral administration of edible mushrooms on the induction of urinary bladder carcinoma and on the activities of macrophages and lymphocytes were studied. Bladder carcinoma were found in all 10 mice (100%) treated with BBN alone, while we observed carcinoma only in 9 of 17 mice (52.9%), in 7 of 15 mice (46.7%) and 13 of 20 mice (65.0%) treated with Lentinus edodes, Grifola frondosa and Pleurotus ostreatus, respectively. Chemotactic activity of macrophages was suppressed in mice treated with BBN alone but maintained almost the normal level in mice treated with BBN plus Lentinus, Grifola or Pleurotus. Lymphocytes collected from mice treated with BBN plus each mushroom showed almost normal blastogenic response against concanavalin A, although those from mice treated with BBN alone completely retarded their response... Significantly higher cytotoxic activity against P-815 cells was observed in lymphocytes from mice treated with BBN plus each mushroom than that in lymphocytes from normal mice or mice treated with BBN alone." – PubMed ID#9130004 (1997) [279]

The following study investigated an extract from oyster mushrooms called CBAEP (cibacron blue affinity purified protein). It showed that this extract can improve the immune system's ability to activate macrophages and NK cells (again, anticancer "natural killer" cells).

> "In the present study, we investigated the in vivo antitumor potential of CBAEP in different tumor-bearing mice models... The in vivo CBAEP treatment showed an apoptotic feature as demonstrated in morphological study and sub-G0/G1 population in cell cycle and Western blot of DL cells. CBAEP also activated immunosuppression condition in DL tumor-bearing host. It also stimulated immune cells in the presence of nonspecific immunostunulator (LPS and ConA) ex vivo as well as enhanced Th1 response with production of TNF-α, IFN-γ, and IL-2. Moreover, it activated tumor-associated macrophages and NK cells. The present findings revealed the potent antitumor property of CBAEP" – PubMed ID#22324408 (2011) [280]

Here we find three more polysaccharides in oyster mushrooms that improve the immune system's response to cancer.

"Three neutral fractions were found, which had polysaccharide to protein ratios 14.2, 26.4 and 18.3, respectively. These fractions were tested for in vitro and in vivo immunomodulatory and anticancer effects... All of the three proteoglycans elevated mouse natural killer (NK) cell cytotoxicity and stimulated macrophages to produce nitric oxide... the three neutral proteoglycans derived from the mushroom (P. ostreatus) mycelia could be used as immunomodulators and anti cancer agents." – PubMed ID#16782541 (2006) [281]

The following study evaluated an oyster mushroom extract against human gastric cancer (with mice, in vitro and in vivo). The extract used was *Pleurotus ostreatus* mycelium polysaccharides 2 (or POMP2 below).

"MTT assay indicated that POMP2 had a marked inhibitory effect on the BGC-823 human gastric cancer cell line; when administered at a concentration of 400 mg/l for 72 h, the rate of inhibition was 35.6%. In addition, the colony forming capacity of the BGC-823 cells was significantly reduced following treatment with POMP2. A migration assay indicated that the invasive capabilities of the BGC-823 cells were also significantly inhibited by POMP2. Furthermore, in vivo tests of mice engrafted with BGC-823 cancer cells demonstrated that both tumor weight and volume were markedly reduced following two weeks of treatment with POMP2. The results of the present study suggested that the polysaccharide POMP2 may have a potential application as a natural antitumor treatment for gastric cancer." – PubMed ID#25892617 (2015) [282]

"both intracellular and extracellular polysaccharides exhibited antitumour activity towards several tested human carcinoma cell lines in a dose-dependent manner... The polysaccharides of P. ostreatus exhibited high SOD-like activity, which strongly supports their biological effect on tumour cell lines. The extracellular polysaccharides presented the highest antitumour activity towards the RL95 carcinoma cell line and should be further investigated as an antitumour agent." – PubMed ID#22234986 (2012) [283]

Obviously, this is a mushroom you want to make sure you are consuming. I would consume it both in a powdered mix and use it in food recipes. This mushroom has a lot of anticancer benefits and, as with other mushrooms, it does not harm normal cells.

REISHI

Ganoderma lucidum, lingzhi mushroom, medicine of kings

The reishi mushroom has been used medicinally in China for over 2,500 years. It is known as the "divine fungus" or "the mushroom of immortality." In modern times this mushroom has been shown to boost the immune system, fight heart disease, benefit allergies and calm inflammation. These aren't simply wild boasts; there are over 2,000 research papers on reishi indexed on the US government's PubMed and MedLine systems.

The reishi mushroom can improve overall immunity and has been shown to reduce tumor size. It can also help prevent invasion, increase apoptosis, etc. in a wide variety of cancers. Improvements to the immune system are very important after chemotherapy or radiotherapy as these can weaken the immune system. My wife and I personally know a woman who was fighting ovarian cancer. She had her ovaries removed and was, by all accounts, doing well. Within two weeks she was dead. She wasn't killed by the cancer; she died from an opportunistic infection of the lungs, pneumonia. Her immune system was severely impacted by the chemotherapy (and most likely by the antibiotics she was on). This left her wide open to any pathogenic bacteria or virus that she encountered (and you encounter a lot when visiting hospitals). Anything that can benefit and nourish the immune system can *improve your odds* of surviving treatment.

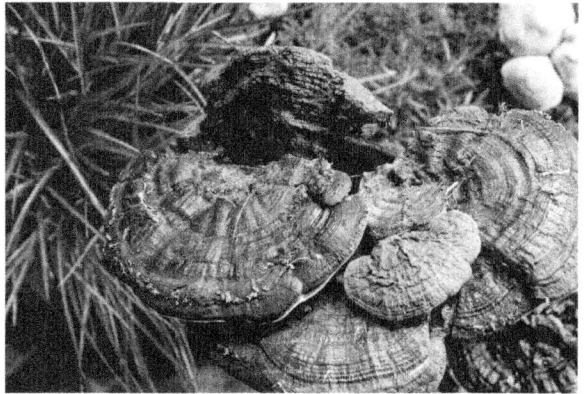

> "As chemotherapy medicines damage the bone marrow, the marrow is less able to produce enough red blood cells, white blood cells, and platelets. Typically, the greatest impact is on white blood cells. When you don't have enough white blood cells, your body is more vulnerable to infection." – BreastCancer.org [284]

In the following study, reishi was shown to directly inhibit breast and prostate cancer cell adhesion and migration. This means it can help prevent the cancer from spreading. Though only two cancers were tested, this benefit may apply to other cancers as well (but the tests haven't been conducted).

> "Ganoderma lucidum inhibits constitutively active transcription factors nuclear factor kappa B (NF-kappaB) and AP-1, which resulted in the inhibition of

expression of urokinase-type plasminogen activator (uPA) and its receptor uPAR. Ganoderma lucidum also suppressed cell adhesion and cell migration of highly invasive breast and prostate cancer cells, suggesting its potency to reduce tumor invasiveness. Thus, Ganoderma lucidum clearly demonstrates anticancer activity in experiments with cancer cells and has possible therapeutic potential as a dietary supplement for an alternative therapy for breast and prostate cancer." ~ PubMed ID#14713328 (2003) [285]

The below study shows the various ways that reishi compounds can serve as a "natural therapeutic for breast and other cancers" without doing harm to human cells. The study specifically examined "inflammatory breast cancer (IBC)," which "is a rare, aggressive and lethal type of breast cancer." The results suggest that the benefits could be applicable to other forms of cancer as well.

"G. lucidum extract (GLE), containing polysaccharides and triterpenes, was reported to suppress growth and metastatic potential of human MDA-MD-231 breast cancer cells by inhibiting the activity of Akt and transcription factors AP-1 and NF-$\varkappa$B, resulting in the downregulation of expression of cyclin D1 [6], [7], [8]. Moreover, we recently reported that Reishi selectively inhibits SUM-149 IBC cell viability and invasion, while not affecting non-cancerous mammary epithelial (MCF10A) cell viability, making it a potential anti-cancer therapeutic… Using the established IBC cell model, SUM-149 cells, we previously published that Reishi selectively reduced cancer cell viability and invasion… Our in vivo studies show that Reishi treated mice have statistically significantly reduced tumor growth and tumor weight… Based on our findings, we conclude that Reishi is an anti-cancer agent that selectively affects gene and protein expression and therefore, activity of molecules involved on cancer cells and shows tumor inhibitory effects." – PubMed ID#PMC3585368 (2013) (Open Access license, see link for attribute) [286]

The following study, using a commercially available reishi extract, shows that reishi mushrooms are toxic to cancer cells, yet completely harmless to noncancerous cells (while other studies also showed significant benefits to the immune system). Reishi induced apoptosis in cancerous cells and inhibited them from invading nearby tissue. Inhibiting metastasis (spreading to other parts of the body) while inducing (natural) cancer cell death is exactly what you're looking for in any cancer treatment.

"Reishi contains biological compounds that are cytotoxic against cancer cells. We report the effects of Reishi on viability, apoptosis, invasion, and its mechanism of action in IBC cells (SUM-149). Results show that Reishi selectively inhibits cancer cell viability although it does not affect the viability of noncancerous mammary epithelial cells. Apoptosis induction is consistent with decreased cell viability. Reishi inhibits cell invasion and disrupts the cell spheroids that are characteristic of the IBC invasive pathology." – PubMed ID#21888505 [287] Full Study PubMed ID#PMC3201987 [288] (2011)

In the following study, reishi (GLE) was studied to see if it would have an effect on larger breast cancer tumors. They "found statistically non-significant inhibition of tumor growth" of over 50% (in vivo) and a significant reduction in breast-to-lung cancer metastases, from 33.9 ± 15.2 in the control to 10.2 ± 5.4 in reishi-treated animals.

"Our study suggests that an oral administration of GLE can inhibit breast-to-lung cancer metastases through the downregulation of genes responsible for cell invasiveness… In conclusion, the chemically characterized dietary mushroom extract GLE inhibits breast-to-lung cancer metastasis of highly invasive human breast cancer cells implanted in mouse mammary tissue. In addition, GLE suppresses the expression of genes involved in the invasive behavior of cancer cells." – PubMed ID#PMC4735696 (2014) (An Open Access study, attribute at the link) [289]

When research studies on cancer refer to an ability to "modulate" the immune system, they are referring to small tweaks that help the immune system identify and attack cancer cells. The nice thing about immunomodulators is that they do not overstimulate the immune system (which can damage healthy cells or overall health). Instead they help the immune system focus on, and attack, cancer cells.

"Large numbers of studies have shown that G lucidum modulate many components of the immune system such as the antigen-presenting cells, NK cells, T and B lymphocytes. The water extract and the polysaccharides fraction of G lucidum exhibited significant anti-tumor effect in several tumor-bearing animals mainly through its immunoenhancing activity." – PubMed ID#15525457 (2004) [290]

Reishi has been shown in several studies to be highly effective against breast and prostate cancers. Though most of the studies have been done in vitro (in the test tube), the markers they watch for have all been very promising and normally carry over very well to in vivo (in the body) testing.

"we investigated the effect of G. lucidum on highly invasive breast and prostate cancer cells. Here we show that spores or dried fruiting body of G. lucidum inhibit constitutively active transcription factors AP-1 and NF-kappaB in breast MDA-MB-231 and prostate PC-3 cancer cells. Furthermore, Ganoderma inhibition of expression of uPA and uPA receptor (uPAR), as well secretion of uPA, resulted in the suppression of the migration of MDA-MB-231 and PC-3 cells. Our data suggest that spores and unpurified fruiting body of G. lucidum inhibit invasion of breast and prostate cancer cells by a common mechanism and could have potential therapeutic use for cancer treatment." – PubMed ID#12408995 (2002) [291]

In this 2017 study, reishi was found to be effective against melanoma and several types of breast cancer. Again, I would like to remind you that simply because a study (or all studies) only mentions certain cancers, that does not mean that reishi's benefits are limited to just those types of cancer. It simply means there are not the research dollars to test it against all cancers. The fact that this study looked at two very different types of cancer (melanoma and breast cancer) may mean the researchers were trying to point this out.

"Our study demonstrates, for the first time, how Ganoderma lucidum extracts can significantly inhibit the release of IL-8, IL-6, MMP-2 and MMP-9 in cancer cells under pro-inflammatory condition. Interestingly, Ganoderma lucidum extracts significantly also decrease the viability of both cancer cells in a time- and concentration-dependent manner, with abilities to reduce cell migration over time, which is correlated with a lower release of matrix metalloproteases. Taken together, these results indicate the possible use of Ganoderma lucidum extract for the therapeutic management of melanoma and human triple-negative breast cancer." – PubMed ID#28264501 (2017) [292]

Reishi mushrooms were tested against human breast cancer cells, where they were shown to inhibit hyper-proliferation and cell migration (which would otherwise lead to metastasis).

"Here we investigated the effect of Reishi on Wnt/β-catenin signaling pathway and elucidated the molecular mechanism of its function in inhibiting breast cancer cells… Reishi inhibited Wnt-induced hyper-proliferation of breast cancer cells and MDA-MB-231 cell migration. Our results provide evidence that Reishi suppresses breast cancer cell growth and migration through inhibiting Wnt/β-catenin signaling, indicating that Reishi may be a potential natural inhibitor for breast cancer." – PubMed ID#28427938 (2017) [293]

SHIITAKE

AKA: *Lentinula edodes, Lentinulaedodes, Lentinus edodes,* **oakwood mushroom, golden oak mushroom, sawtooth oak mushroom, black mushroom, black forest mushroom, dongo, shanku, koshin**

Shiitake mushrooms are one of the most popular of the edible mushrooms. Some reports list shiitake mushroom cultivation as accounting for 25% of the world's production of cultivated mushrooms, and they are the second most cultivated. This mushroom is native to East Asia and is cultivated in many Asian countries. Like nameko, shiitake is often used in miso soup. It is also frequently used to make the broth for Asian soups (a vegetarian dashi). Shiitake mushrooms are often steamed, simmered or sautéed to be used in a variety of dishes.

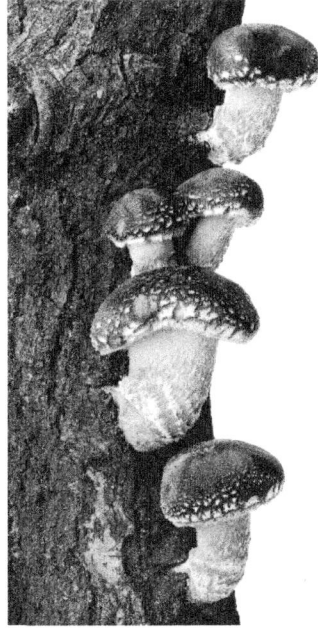

The shiitake mushroom has been used medicinally in Asia for hundreds of years. Shiitake mushrooms have a high beta-glucan content, averaging 26% to 30% in dried mushrooms. The unique beta-glucans account for much of the anticancer properties and immune system benefits. Shiitake mushrooms have also been shown to inhibit the development of intestinal ulcers, normalize high cholesterol levels, and treat hypertension, infectious diseases, diabetes and inflammation. Shiitake mushrooms are also antioxidants. The number of research studies showing general health benefits from shiitakes increases every year. Here we will focus on the anticancer, anti-tumor and immunomodulating benefits of this important mushroom.

> "The shiitake mushroom, Lentinula edodes, is one of most important edible mushrooms cultivated in the world…. β-Glucans bind to lymphocyte surfaces or serum-specific proteins, that activate macrophages, helper T-cells, natural killer cells, and other effector cells. The activation of these effectors results in an increase in the production and release of antibodies, interleukins, and interferon"
> – PubMed ID#PMC4206800 (2014) [294]

The following study was carried out on various breast cancer cells and two malignant plasma cell (myeloma) cell lines. Due to the major differences between these two types of cancers, it is likely that the shiitake fraction (extract) would benefit many other types of cancers as well.

> "The activities of an ethyl acetate fraction were evaluated… analysis using two human breast carcinoma cell lines (MDA-MB-453 and MCF-7), one human nonmalignant breast epithelial cell line (MCF-10F), and two myeloma cell lines (RPMI-8226 and IM-9)… Concentration-dependent antiproliferative effects of the fraction were observed in all cell lines using the MTT assay. Approximately 50 mg/L concentration of the fraction induced apoptosis in 50% of the population of four human tumor cell lines and the fraction-induced apoptosis may have been mediated through the pro-apoptotic bax protein which was up-regulated… A 51% anti-proliferative effect occurred at the highest concentration of the fraction… These data suggest that inhibition of growth in tumor cells by "mycochemicals" in shiitake mushrooms may result from induction of apoptosis." – PubMed ID#16566671 (2006) [295]

Here, lentinan extracted from shiitake mushrooms helped restore levels of two very important immune system cancer-fighting cells, killer T cells and NK (natural killer) cells. It also helped lower inflammation (which is often caused by cancer and can be serious).

> "Lentinan purified from Shiitake mushrooms has two β-(1, 6) side chains every five β-(1, 3)–linked backbone residues (beta-glucans)… In cancer patients, it is well known that DCs (dendritic cells) are functionally defective and T-cell function as well as NK activity are also down-regulated. Mushiake et al described lentinan as activating DC function by increasing the number of tumor-infiltrating CD86+ cells in cancer-bearing mice. The administration of lentinan was reported to stimulate the generation of both killer T cells and NK cells and then restore the ratio of killer/suppressor T cells. Lentinan up-regulated NK cell-mediated killing of tumor cells… Regular L. edodes consumption resulted in improved immunity, as seen by improved cell proliferation and activation and increased sIgA production." – PubMed ID#PMC3664515 (2013) [296]

For many years it was assumed that beta-glucans, such as lentinan, would not make it into the bloodstream and reach cancer cells. I've actually seen references to this in a recent medical database used by doctors (including oncologists). This assumption was made due to the molecular size of beta-glucans. Recently, however, dozens of studies have shown the beta-glucans do indeed reach cancer cells if consumed orally. The following is one of those studies.

> "Unlike previous reports whereby the lentinan was given parenterally, in this study the emphasis was on the oral administration of lentinan. The goal is to document whether the efficacy of the antitumor property is still expressed through this route of administration… Significant regression in tumor formation was observed in prefed mice compared to control (unfed) mice when K36 or human colon-carcinoma cells were used. Significant reductions in the size of the

tumors were observed in mice prefed with lentinan… inoculation of the human colon-carcinoma cell lines into these mice. Much smaller tumors were formed in nude mice inoculated with lymphocytes, in contrast to the larger tumor formed in nude mice without lymphocytes inoculation. This study showed that the antitumor property of lentinan was maintained with oral administration." – PubMed ID#12470439 (2002) [297]

Lentinan is a beta-glucan unique to the shiitake mushroom; it is found in both the fruiting body and the mycelium (basically, the root system) of the mushroom.

"Shiitake mushroom, Lentinulaedodes produces lentinan, a β-glucan known to suppress leukemia cell proliferation. The ethanol extract of this mushroom significantly decreased cell proliferation of CH72 cells" – PubMed ID#PMC3339609 (2012) [298]

"Human neutrophils," below, are human white blood cells, important to the innate immune system. You want IL-1 and apoptosis to be low in normal cells (such as white blood cells) and high in cancer cells. U937 is a cancer cell line used in research.

"Effects of shiitake (Lentinus edodes) extract on human neutrophils and the U937 monocytic cell line… The aqueous extract of the shiitake mushroom was found to decrease IL-1 production and apoptosis in human neutrophils, as measured by ELISA and flow cytometry respectively. It was found to increase IL-1 production and apoptosis in the U937 monocytic cell line." – PubMed ID#10190187 (1999) [299]

The following **in vivo study on humans** used 5 to 10 grams of whole shiitake mushrooms. Participants consumed these mushrooms for 4 weeks. Blood, saliva and serum were taken before and after the 4-week period. Consumption of shiitake mushrooms resulted in improved immune function, including "increased interleukin (IL)-4, IL-10, tumor necrosis factor (TNF)-α, and IL-1α levels, a decreased macrophage inflammatory protein-1α/chemokine C-C ligand 3 (MIP-1α/CCL3) level." This can enhance most any anticancer protocol you may be on.

"Eating L. edodes for 4 weeks resulted in increased ex vivo proliferation of γδ-T (60% more, p < 0.0001) and NK-T (2-fold more, p < 0.0001) cells. Both cell types also demonstrated a greater ability to express activation receptors, suggesting that consuming mushrooms improved cell effector function. The increase in sIgA implied improved gut immunity. The reduction in CRP suggested lower inflammation. The pattern of cytokines secreted before and after mushroom consumption was significantly different; consumption resulted in increased interleukin (IL)-4, IL-10, tumor necrosis factor (TNF)-α, and IL-1α levels, a decreased macrophage inflammatory protein-1α/chemokine C-C ligand 3 (MIP-1α/CCL3) level, and no change to IL-6, IL-1β, MIP-1β, IL-17 and interferon (IFN)-γ levels." – PubMed ID#25866155 (2015) [300]

The following study used a hot water extract from shiitake mushrooms to yield an extract high in polysaccharides (as usual, this is to produce a standardized extract so that study results can be replicated). Cancer proliferation was inhibited by 18% to 43% against 6 different cancers. This is a significant (in vitro) reduction and does not even consider improvements to the human immune system that occur in vivo (in the body).

"a high yield of crude polysaccharide (16.73 ± 0.756%) was extracted from the spent mushroom substrate of Lentinus edodes… MTT assays with refined polysaccharide doses of 25, 50, 100, 200, and 400 µg/mL suggested that both of the polysaccharide fractions exhibited antiproliferative activity against 6 tested human tumor cell lines in a concentration-dependent manner, and LSMS-2 had better anticancer capacity in vitro than LSMS-1. The inhibition ratio of LSMS-2 against A549 human lung cancer cells, the SGC7901 gastric cancer cell line, MCF-7 breast cancer cells, the U937 histiocytic lymphoma cell line, and the MG-63 human osteosarcoma cell line reached 43.55%, 29.97%, 19.63%, 18.24%, and 17.93%, respectively, at a concentration of 400 µg/mL." -- PubMed ID#28845769 (2017) [301]

The below study included 78 people with hepatocellular carcinoma (a form of liver cancer). The combination treatment below included lentinan, radiation (RFA) and chemotherapy (TACE). Those who received the combination therapy had much better results and a much longer average survival time. This shows that mushroom beta-glucans can be used as an adjuvant (adjunct) therapy to traditional cancer treatments.

"Hepatocellular carcinoma (HCC) is one of the most common cancer-related causes of death worldwide… Seventy-eight patients with HCC confirmed by pathology and iconographical checks were used in this study. A total of 136 tumours with a mean diameter of 6.5 cm were detected… The tumour necrosis was significantly higher in the combination group (88.6%), compared to the TACE (transcatheter arterial chemoembolization) group (37.5%)… mean survival duration was significantly higher in the combination group… Combination therapy involving lentinan, RFA and TACE was beneficial in terms of increasing mean survival duration, tumour necrosis and reducing the recurrence rate. Lentinan may therefore be of benefit to HCC patients." – PubMed ID#18670743 (2008) [302]

Cautionary Note

Consumption of <u>raw</u> shiitake mushrooms can cause a rare, temporary condition called "shiitake dermatitis." It appears as a rash about 24 hours after consumption. Cooking shiitakes appears to completely eliminate this slight risk. The rash usually occurs 2 to 3 days after the ingestion of raw or undercooked shiitake mushrooms, and it resolves by itself in about 10 days. It is estimated that only about 2% of people get this reaction, and only from consuming raw shiitake mushrooms. The takeaway point here is to cook (sweat, simmer, sauté, etc.) your shiitake mushrooms.

TURKEY TAIL

AKA: *Coriolus versicolor, Trametes versicolor, Polyporus versicolor,* Yun Zhi

Turkey tail, or Yun Zhi, was first mentioned around 200 BCE (during the Han Dynasty) in written texts about its medicinal properties. In the 15th century, it was thought that taking Yun Zhi for a long time would make one vigorous and cause a person to live longer.

Turkey tail has been studied in phase I, II and III randomized clinical trials in stomach, colorectal, esophageal and breast cancer patients. (Tv = *Trametes versicolor*, or turkey tail)

> "There have been many peer-reviewed publications on the Tv in cancer, including 37 in vitro articles, 55 animal studies, 43 published human clinical studies, and 11 review articles in gastrointestinal, breast, and lung cancer. In the last 2 years, five more Krestin (PSK) trials in colorectal cancer have been published, including one meta-analysis in 1,094 colorectal cancer patients, all showing a positive impact on clinical outcomes… It has been hypothesized that Tv's immunologic activity is the underlying mechanism responsible for its antitumor effects and its impact on survival rates." – PubMed ID#PMC2845472 (2008) [303]

Our immune system is very important in the fight against cancer. In fact, many small cancers are defeated by our immune system without any medical intervention, even without our knowledge. Our immune system is also vitally important to achieving positive outcomes from chemotherapy, radiation and other medical treatments. It is also well known that the strong chemotherapy drugs and radiation therapy take a heavy toll on our immune system, partially defeating the benefits of these therapies. Being able to protect our immune system during these treatments is vitally important. These medical treatments generally do not kill metastasizing cells; that is left to the immune system. Even without these treatments, improving the immune system is always beneficial.

In this study, special white blood cells, called lymphocytes and natural killer cells (phagocytes), were measured in women undergoing treatment for stage I to stage III breast cancer. This was a relatively small study, but it showed significant improvements in the participant groups. For the groups given turkey tail, improvements to lymphocytes were approximately 50% higher from post-radiation therapy compared to the control group. Improvements to natural killer cells were up to 300% higher than the control group, depending on when the measurements were taken (greater benefits were seen soon after radiation therapy). Large improvements were also seen in CD19+ B cell counts.

> "Here, we show that RT reduces NK cell activity per NK cell. Higher oral doses of Tv at 6 and 9 grams/day were associated with faster recovery of lymphocytes and NK cell activity, as well as increased numbers of CD8+T cells and CD19+ B cells." – PubMed #PMC3369477 (2012) [304]

Turkey tail, like most of the other medicinal mushrooms, shows broad chemotherapeutic benefits. Besides the already discussed role in treating breast, colon and lung cancers, the following study shows strong anticancer benefits with melanoma (in vitro and in vivo).

> "In vivo methanol extract treatment (i.p. 50 mg/kg, for 14 days) inhibited tumor growth in C57BL/6 mice inoculated with syngeneic B16 tumor cells. Moreover, peritoneal macrophages collected 21 days after tumor implantation from methanol extract-treated animals exerted stronger tumoristatic activity ex vivo than macrophages from control melanoma-bearing mice. Taken together, our results demonstrate that C. versicolor methanol extract exerts pronounced anti-melanoma activity, both directly through antiproliferative and cytotoxic effects on tumor cells and indirectly through promotion of macrophage anti-tumor activity… The prevention of tumor growth was exerted through diverse mechanisms, including cell cycle arrest, induction of tumor cell death by apoptosis and secondary necrosis, together with stimulation of the anti-tumor activity of macrophages." – PubMed ID#18313195 DOI: 10.1016/j.fct.2008.01.027 [305] (2008) [306]

The full study above is fascinating, showing in vivo (mice) melanoma tumor reduction of 300% to 400% compared to controls (tumors ended up ⅓ the weight and ¼ the volume after 21 days). The study used a methanol extract from the cultivated fruiting bodies of C. versicolor. It is known that some beneficial chemicals in mushrooms are not alcohol soluble and need to be hot water extracted. Both PSP and PSK, two well researched turkey tail mushroom constitutes that have chemotherapeutic properties, are insoluble in methanol (they are hot water soluble, but the study above used a methanol extract). So, whole mushrooms may provide even more benefits.

Turkey tail extracts have also shown very promising chemotherapeutic properties towards prostate cancer.

> "Recent evidence suggested that prostate cancer stem/progenitor cells (CSC) are responsible for cancer initiation as well as disease progression… Unfortunately, conventional therapies are only effective in targeting the more differentiated cancer cells and spare the CSCs… PSP, an active component extracted from the mushroom Turkey tail (also known as Coriolus versicolor), is effective in targeting prostate CSCs… transgenic mice (TgMAP) that spontaneously develop prostate tumors were orally fed with PSP for 20 weeks. Whereas 100% of the mice that fed with water only developed prostate tumors at the end of experiment, no tumors could be found in any of the mice fed with PSP, suggesting that PSP treatment can completely inhibit prostate tumor formation.

Our results not only demonstrated the intriguing anti-CSC effect of PSP, but also revealed, for the first time, the surprising chemopreventive property of oral PSP consumption against prostate cancer… These findings strongly suggest that oral intake of PSP may be a safe and effective chemopreventive agent against prostate cancer." – PubMed ID#21603625 [307], full study [308] (Open Access, information at the link)

The two primary anti-tumor extracts being studied in turkey tail are polysaccharide-Kureha (PSK) and polysaccharide-peptide (PSP). These compounds are not available medically in the US except in FDA-approved trial studies. However, there have been many studies (most done in Japan and China) that show simply consuming turkey tail mushrooms, or a hot water extract of them, has similar benefits. Because these are natural substances and cannot receive a patent, no drug companies are willing to spend the billions of dollars it takes to get FDA approval and bring these substances to market as an approved drug. Therefore, your oncologist has most likely never heard of them. However, turkey tail is commonly used in Japan for cancer treatment. In Japan, turkey tail extracts were first approved in 1977 for oncological use and by 1987 represented up to 25% of the national insurance system's cancer treatment costs.

Several of the research studies have used turkey tail in conjunction with conventional chemotherapy therapies. The following meta-analysis study looked at 13 clinical research studies.

"This meta-analysis of randomized controlled trials shows that Yun Zhi results in a significant survival advantage compared with standard conventional anti-cancer treatment alone… there was a 9% absolute reduction in 5-year mortality, resulting in one additional patient alive for every 11 patients treated. Further subgroup analysis showed that the overall 5-year survival rate in patients with breast cancer, gastric cancer or colorectal cancer treated with the combination of Yun Zhi preparation and standard anti-cancer treatment was more evident… This meta-analysis has provided strong evidence that Yun Zhi would have survival benefit in cancer patients, particularly in carcinoma of breast, gastric and colorectal." – PubMed ID#22185453 [309] DOI: 10.2174/187221312798889310

In this 2017 paper appearing in the *Frontiers in Immunology,* the authors found turkey tail (*C. versicolor*) showed numerous benefits in halting several types of cancers. This paper also looked at the turkey tail isolate polysaccharopeptide (PSP).

"Coriolus versicolor extracts are used as adjunct therapy for cancer in many Eastern countries… demonstrated reduced proliferation by disruption of their cell cycle, induction of apoptosis, and sensitization to various chemotherapeutics such as camptothecin, doxorubicin, and etoposide… Treating human PBMCs with PSP using conditioned media to grow HL-60 or U937 showed significant tumoricidal activity that could be inhibited by antibody blockade of either of TNF-α or IFN-γ… studies on the immunomodulatory effects of CV extract indicate increased NK cells activity… studies on the immunomodulatory effects of CV extract indicate increased NK cells activity… PSP promotes immune responses *via* induction of immunoglobulin production and engagement of various pattern-recognition molecules… PSP promotes immune responses *via* induction of immunoglobulin production and engagement of various pattern-recognition molecules… it can interrupt the cell cycle, induce apoptosis, and sensitize tumor cells to other chemotherapeutic agents." – PubMed ID#PMC5592279 (2017) [310]

Usage

If you can find a "hot water extract" supplement or powder, then it can be used "as is." Otherwise you'll need to make a hot water tea from the mushrooms (or mushroom powder if that is what you purchased). You can also cook with the mushrooms in soups or stews. The polysaccharides need to be released from the chitin (a mushroom fiber similar to cellulose); otherwise they will not be usable in the body. This is why it needs to be hot water extracted.

WHITE BUTTON MUSHROOMS

AKA: *Agaricus bisporus,* crimini, portobello, baby bella

Portobello mushrooms are simply mature button mushrooms (*Agaricus bisporus*), so what applies to one applies to the other. This very common mushroom should be cooked or hot water extracted; it should not be consumed raw. It contains a very small amount of a natural chemical that has been linked to cancer. However, cooking completely neutralizes this chemical; moist cooking can also improve the bioavailability of its anticancer properties. Nothing to be afraid of, but just to be safe, don't consume this mushroom raw (PubMed ID#8008044, [311] PubMed #7737599 [312]). If I find raw button mushrooms on a salad, I don't freak out about it; I just eat them. But at home we consume cooked mushrooms.

The following study used both in vitro and in vivo methods to test button mushrooms against prostate cancer cells.

> "White button mushrooms are a widely consumed food containing phytochemicals beneficial to cancer prevention. The purpose of this research was to evaluate the effects of white button mushroom extract and its major component, conjugated linoleic acid (CLA) on prostate cancer cell lines in vitro and mushroom extract in vivo. In all cell lines tested, mushroom inhibited cell proliferation in a dose-dependent manner and induced apoptosis within 72 h of treatment. CLA inhibited proliferation in the prostate cancer cell lines in vitro… DU145 and PC3 prostate tumor size and tumor cell proliferation were decreased in nude mice treated with mushroom extract, whereas tumor cell apoptosis was increased compared to pair-fed controls… this study illustrate the anticancer potential of phytochemicals in mushroom extract both in vitro and in vivo" – PubMed ID#19005974 (2008) [313]

The following study was conducted on breast cancer cells, again in vitro and in vivo, with much the same results (though lacking apoptosis).

> "we evaluated the activity of mushroom extracts in the estrogen receptor-positive/aromatase-positive MCF-7aro cell line in vitro and in vivo… The in vivo action of mushroom chemicals was shown using nude mice injected with MCF-7aro cells. The studies showed that mushroom extract decreased both tumor cell proliferation and tumor weight with no effect on rate of apoptosis. Therefore, our studies illustrate the anticancer activity in vitro and in vivo of mushroom extract and its major fatty acid constituents." – PubMed ID#17178902 (2006) [314]

Two unique polysaccharides were isolated from *A. bisporus* (white button mushroom, or WBM): ABP-1 and ABP-2. These two polysaccharides were tested in mice against human cancer cells.

The study found that these two polysaccharides have the ability to inhibit the growth of human breast cancer cells and sarcoma cells.

> "both fractions stimulated the production of nitric oxide, interleukin-6, and tumor necrosis factor-α. Modulation of macrophage function by A. bisporus polysaccharides was mediated in part through activation of nuclear factor-κB with the production p50/105 heterodimers. Both ABP-1 and ABP-2 had the ability to inhibit the growth of human breast cancer MCF-7 cells… our data provide a molecular basis to explain in part the reported beneficial therapeutic effects of A. bisporus WBM intake and suggest that macrophages likely contribute to the antitumor effects of Agaricus polysaccharides." – PubMed ID#22217303 (2012) [315]

Breast Cancer Prevention

> "The white button mushroom (species Agaricus bisporus) suppressed aromatase activity dose dependently. Enzyme kinetics demonstrated mixed inhibition, suggesting the presence of multiple inhibitors or more than one inhibitory mechanism. "In cell" aromatase activity and cell proliferation were measured using MCF-7aro, an aromatase-transfected breast cancer cell line. Phytochemicals in the mushroom aqueous extract inhibited aromatase activity and proliferation of MCF-7aro cells… diets high in mushrooms may modulate the aromatase activity and function in chemoprevention in postmenopausal women by reducing the in situ production of estrogen." – PubMed ID#11739882 (2001) [316]

Studies indicate that consuming whole mushrooms, rather than just an isolate, will most likely produce even better anti-tumor results. However, there are very few research studies using whole mushrooms or whole mushroom extracts. There are several reasons for this, and probably the primary reason is the need to standardize their tests. Study results need to be reproducible. Mushrooms from one area of the country, or different soil, are likely to contain different properties. Since properties can vary from mushroom to mushroom, this can skew results. The goal of looking for a possible prescription medication would also prohibit the use of whole mushroom extracts.

> "It is likely that mushrooms possess multiple immunoregulatory components including the selenium, B vitamins and polysaccharides that when ingested together or mixed *in vitro* together would have effects that differed from the isolated components. *In vitro* WB, crimini, shiitaki, and oyster extracts reduced IL-

10 production and increased IL-1β, and TNF-α production by macrophage. The activation of the macrophage with the mushroom extracts preferentially stimulated T cell production of TNF-α and IFN-γ and very little IL-10. This pattern of immuno-regulation by mushrooms is consistent with a model whereby whole mushroom consumption would induce a modest but important boost in immune responses that would improve anti-cancer immunity… Whole mushrooms have a number of components that are potentially immuno-modulatory. The in vitro data show that whole mushroom extracts regulate macrophage and T cell production of cytokines in a way that is predicted to be beneficial for boosting anti-tumor immunity." – PubMed ID#PMC2649035 (Open Access article) [317]

White button mushrooms have also shown benefits in prevention and treatment of estrogen-dependent breast cancers.

"Phytochemicals in the mushroom aqueous extract inhibited aromatase activity and proliferation of MCF-7aro cells. These results suggest that diets high in mushrooms may modulate the aromatase activity and function in chemoprevention in postmenopausal women by reducing the in situ production of estrogen… The data from our study suggest that the white button mushroom may have potential therapeutic benefit as a functional food by reducing the activity of aromatase, the putative enzyme for converting androgens to estrogens." – The Journal of Nutrition DOI: 10.1093/jn/131.12.3288 (2001) [318]

❖ SAFETY

Mushrooms are a food consumed all over the world. Culinary and medicinal mushrooms are exceptionally safe. There are a couple of minor cautionary notes concerning specific mushrooms, and those are mentioned at the end of the sections where they apply. I do not worry about consuming any of the mushrooms mentioned here.

❖ STRATEGY

It is my hope that after reading all this information about medicinal edible mushrooms, you have decided to include more of these mushrooms in your diet. Before I was diagnosed with melanoma, I occasionally consumed mushrooms, but only a couple of times per month. Now we try to put mushrooms in nearly every savory dish that we cook. They're delicious and add a complexity to foods. If you don't want the texture of mushrooms in a dish, no problem: Sweat the mushrooms first, then purée them; add this purée to your dish and no one will even know.

Consume as many of these mushrooms in your diet as possible; variety is best. Most are delicious and easy to prepare. I sweat mushrooms in a mixture of butter and water, covered, at low heat for 15 to 30 minutes, often sautéing onions with them in the same pan. This step is needed to release the polysaccharides (such as beta-glucans) from the mushroom fiber (chitin). If the mushrooms are not hot water cooked, the beneficial compounds will simply pass through you unutilized. Once the mushrooms are properly prepared, they can then be used in whatever recipe you wish.

You can also purchase prepared powders. These powders can then be used to make a tea, mixed in with your morning coffee, or used in soups or other recipes. Look for powders that list "hot water extracted" (for the same reasons as above) on the label and are made from the "fruiting body." Though the mycelium (the underground root system) of many of these mushrooms also contains beneficial compounds, the fruiting body usually contains the most. These powders are not inexpensive, but the good news is that you only need to use 1 to 2 tsp per day. The mix that I use includes reishi, maitake, Cordyceps, shiitake, lion's mane, turkey tail and chaga extracts. See the book's website for recommendations. I also add extra Cordyceps powder to what I consume every day. You can find a list of most of the supplements in this book, and links to their Amazon page, on the book's website.

Chaga is prepared differently, and this is explained at the end of its section. I make chaga tea concentrate and have 1 or 2 tall glasses of chaga tea per day. Besides having health benefits, it is delicious and can easily replace iced black tea. I often mix ½ to 1 tsp of the medicinal mushroom powder in with the chaga tea. This gives the tea a little more character without a strong mushroom flavor.

Even if you consume prepared powder mixes, I would recommend adding fresh mushrooms to your diet; they are delicious and allow you to add mushrooms not in your mix (e.g., oyster and button/portobello mushrooms). Culinary mushroom powders can add flavor to almost any savory dish and are excellent as a soup or stew base. Though they won't have all the medicinal benefits, they will still have some unique beta-glucans. I use a mushroom powder (made from unidentified mushrooms) and an oyster mushroom powder in cooking.

If you cannot find fresh mushrooms at your supermarket, dehydrated mushrooms maintain most (if not all) of the health benefits of fresh mushrooms. They are excellent for cooking; they just need to be rehydrated first. If your dried mushrooms didn't come with rehydration instructions, it's pretty easy to do. Simply pour boiling water over them and let them soak for 20 to 30 minutes. They should then be ready to add to any recipe calling for fresh mushrooms.

If you're not used to cooking with mushrooms, you can find plenty of recipes on the internet. Say you're wanting to make a chicken casserole; go to your favorite search engine and look for "chicken and mushroom casserole recipe," and you'll find thousands. You can even search for how to cook with a specific mushroom, such as "chicken and shiitake mushroom recipe." This search still turned up hundreds of recipes. If the recipe uses plenty of liquid (soups, stews, etc.), you can use the mushrooms as is; if the recipe doesn't use much liquid, you'll need to sweat them first (as described above). Don't be afraid to substitute one mushroom for another. If the recipe calls for button mushrooms, use shiitake instead. If you used dehydrated mushrooms and your recipe needs water, use the water from rehydrating the mushrooms. You'll add a little more flavor and may get some more beneficial polysaccharides that dissolved into the water.

Nature thrives on variety, and so do natural cures. Feel free to try all of the mushrooms in this section. I also highly recommend taking a powdered mushroom supplement. Though their benefits are difficult to quantify (at this time), medicinal mushrooms may be one of the best things you can do to "*Improve Your Odds*" at beating or preventing cancer! Besides directly helping your immune system, they also feed the beneficial bacteria that have been found to improve your immune system. Sort of like getting a 2-for-1 deal! They also taste great!

Updates at - https://improvingyourodds.com/

Support at - https://www.facebook.com/groups/cancer.improving.your.odds

MINERALS

I'm not going to spend a lot of time on this subject. This isn't because minerals are not important; they are. Minerals are important to every aspect of our biology; if you aren't consuming proper levels, you will have health issues and a poorly functioning microbiome. However, most minerals are not considered to be "cytotoxic"; in other words, they do not have the ability to kill cancer cells (at least at levels that won't also harm normal cells). There is some research showing that higher-than-normal amounts of a couple of minerals may kill some cancer cells, but this evidence is not very strong, and consuming minerals at these levels may have other health drawbacks— I'll cover these below. Mega-doses of minerals also have not been shown to improve the immune response. You need what you need, with or without cancer.

Therefore, the recommendation here is simple: Consume healthy foods containing the minerals we need. The FDA-recommended daily amount is probably sufficient for most minerals; the exceptions are covered below. We also need to make sure our gut is in good shape to absorb and utilize the minerals properly; you can consume all the minerals you need, but if the gut doesn't absorb them, they won't help you. In prosperous countries people have access to healthy foods; they either choose not to eat healthy, or they do not properly absorb nutrition. Though modern farming techniques may have reduced some minerals in the soil, this has not been found to be a significant issue. Nutritional deficiency, or at least insufficiency, of many minerals is still commonplace, but this is mostly due to poor dietary habits. This does not mean "more is better" for most minerals—consuming much more than the government recommendation provides no additional benefit.

There are a few minerals that I will call out as especially important. They have research showing that a deficiency of them is associated with cancer.

❖ IODINE

Iodine is a somewhat controversial topic, especially when it comes to breast cancer and thyroid disease (such as Hashimoto's disease). I think most experts agree that an iodine deficiency can increase the risk of breast cancer and thyroid conditions; the disagreement is about how to treat these conditions after they've been established.

There is a lot of information online about taking large amounts of iodine for both the prevention and treatment of breast cancer. However, the scientific research does not support the idea of taking mega-doses of iodine to treat or prevent cancer. Again, you need what you need, regardless of whether you have cancer. In fact, too much iodine has been associated with thyroid cancer and autoimmune thyroiditis (PubMed ID#PMC3976240 [319]).

Iodine is used in the body to make thyroid hormones. When we don't get enough iodine, we don't produce enough thyroid hormones. However, taking too much iodine can cause us to produce too much thyroid hormone, or paradoxically, can cause some people to produce too little. This is known as the "Goldilocks Zone"—you need to take enough so it is "just right." Luckily there is a fairly large margin of error.

It has become obvious that there is a cause-and-effect link between iodine insufficiency and breast cancer. Women with the worst insufficiency suffer higher rates of breast cancer and greater risk of metastasis. What is not clear is how much iodine can benefit a person who already has breast cancer, how much is too much, and whether someone with autoimmune Hashimoto's (or other thyroid conditions), or prone to it, should supplement iodine at all.

This last question is something I will not be addressing here; it is too complicated for this discussion and depends too much upon individual patients' health concerns (there are already several books on Hashimoto's). You will need to work with your endocrinologist and oncologist to figure out what is appropriate for you. If you do not currently have a thyroid condition and follow the recommendations to supplement iodine, you should be aware that if you are prone to Hashimoto's, adding iodine might cause it to manifest itself. I recommend that you have your thyroid levels checked if you have any doubts. You can find a list of Hashimoto's symptoms on the Mayo Clinic's Hashimoto's page. [320] Autoimmune diseases such as Hashimoto's involve the person's own immune system attacking itself; it is not the fault of any natural substance that is required for human life, such as iodine (so iodine is the cause, but it might trigger the preexisting condition). There are some theories that Hashimoto's sometimes may be caused by a lack of iodine earlier in life, but if you have it, you will need to work with your doctor on what is best for you.

Proper iodine levels are important for general health, immune system health, thyroid health and breast cancer prevention. Deficiency and insufficiency are common in many countries. This is in part due to poor iodine levels in the soil (especially for crops grown inland, away from the ocean). People today are also not consuming a lot of sea vegetables, which are very high in iodine. A small amount of iodine is added to some refined salt in this country, but many people are eating unfortified salt and are consuming much less of it. The salt found in processed foods is generally unfortified and provides no iodine.

> "The incidence of breast cancer with distant involvement at diagnosis is increasing in young women, age 25-39, possibly at an accelerating rate… This disturbing trend was also observed in women age 40-54… In animal models of breast cancer, iodine in supplement or seaweed form, has demonstrated beneficial effects in suppressing breast cancer cell and tumor growth… Iodine deficiency is an important cause of thyroid deficiency; the potential linkage between thyroid disease and breast cancer has been a matter of considerable interest and has been extensively reviewed… Since iodine deficiency is a major cause of hypothyroidism, breast cancer with distant metastasis may be promoted in part by reduced thyroid function, where slower tumor growth (precluding earlier diagnosis), yet increased invasiveness could be consequential. Iodine deficiency, therefore, may contribute to breast cancer and its progression directly within

breast tissue, and secondarily by decreased thyroid function leading to metastasis… Iodine deficiency is associated with fibrocystic breast disease, which can be effectively treated or prevented with iodine supplementation 24. Fibrocystic breast disease affects at least 50% of women of child-bearing age and is associated with an increased risk of developing breast cancer… Females showed a higher frequency of iodine deficiency than males (15.1 versus 8.1%)… For young women of child bearing age, age 15-44, there was a 3.8-fold increase in iodine insufficiency, with a 6.9-fold increase in the number of pregnant women also fitting this definition… dietary iodine insufficiency represents a plausible explanation for the increasing incidence of breast cancer in young women with distant metastasis. In view of the established reduction in iodine levels in US women of childbearing age since the mid 70s, this group would be most vulnerable to increased breast cancer risk". – PubMed ID#PMC5327366 (© 2017 Ivyspring International Publisher – Open Access / Creative Commons Attribution (CC BY-NC), further attribution available at the link) [321]

Rappaport, Jay. "Changes in Dietary Iodine Explains Increasing Incidence of Breast Cancer with Distant Involvement in Young Women." Journal of Cancer vol. 8,2 174-177. 13 Jan. 2017, doi:10.7150/jca.17835

There has been a lot of discussion about the recommended dietary amounts of iodine in Western countries. Most of these discussions have centered around the average consumption of iodine in Japan when compared to countries like America, and the cancer rates in each. It is well known that the Japanese consume far more iodine due to seaweed and seafood consumption. However, these estimates have usually significantly overestimated the Japanese consumption of seaweed, and thus iodine. With cancer rates, and especially breast cancer rates, much lower in Japan (about ⅓ the rate seen in America), knowing the Japanese's iodine consumption rates could be very important in understanding the difference in cancer rates. Due to modernization and Westernization of the Japanese diet, their rates of seaweed consumption have fallen significantly in many areas of the country over the past 60 to 70 years. During this period nearly all cancer rates have increased. Where the Recommended Daily Intake (RDI) of iodine in the US is 150 mcg (this is 0.150 mg, and most Americans do not get that much), it is now believed that the Japanese daily intake (in the 2000-2010 timeframe) averaged about around 1,000 to 3,000 mcg (3 mg) per day. Though this is about 20 times more than the RDI for America, it is still far less than what some alternative health books and websites are recommending. I've seen several recommendations for 50 mg (50,000 mcg)! These very high doses of iodine are not supported in peer-reviewed research for either prevention or treatment of any cancer, and they are not something I would recommend.

I have reviewed several studies that have tried to estimate the iodine consumption of the Japanese population, and I think most of them used far too simplistic of an approach. Some of these studies would use one type of seaweed that is very high in iodine (when the Japanese eat a diverse diet of seaweed), estimating that this one seaweed was consumed in very high amounts on a daily basis, etc. The following meta-study looked at many different Japanese research studies on the local diet, as well as research that analyzed iodine levels from 24-hour urine collection studies (an excellent method of judging iodine consumption). These studies were averaged out to reach the following conclusion.

> "We estimate that the average Japanese iodine intake, largely from seaweed consumption--based on dietary records, food surveys, urine iodine analysis and seaweed iodine content--is 1,000-3,000 µg/day (1-3 mg/day)." – PubMed ID#PMC3204293 (2011) [322]

Some individual Japanese undoubtedly consume larger amounts of iodine-rich seaweed, and thus have a higher iodine intake. However, it is doubtful that very many individuals consume more than twice this amount (6 mg). It is also possible that these outliers who do consume amounts greater than 6 mg have unrecognized health consequences from this more extreme diet. For this reason, I think it is best to use the average, especially since we are looking at the "average rates" of cancer across the populations. If the average rate of cancer in Japan is much less than in (say) America, then the average rate of iodine consumption should be utilized as the comparator, not the extreme. For this reason, I have chosen to use the 1 mg number as the maximum recommendation for a cancer prevention regime (see the Strategy section below). If you see recommendations for much more than this, I would consider those recommendations to be extreme and not justifiable by science.

Generally, most of the research agrees, high dietary intake of iodine does not <u>cause</u> positive thyroid antibodies (such as with Hashimoto's); however, it can worsen existing autoimmune thyroid conditions in susceptible individuals. So, if you have Hashimoto's, you should consult with your doctors before supplementing with iodine or consuming a high-iodine diet. The following two studies, and several others, agree that high levels of iodine consumption do not cause thyroid autoimmune disease, but they can worsen it in people predisposed.

> "Urinary iodine and thyroid antibodies in Okinawa, Yamagata, Hyogo, and Nagano, Japan: the differences in iodine intake do not affect thyroid antibody positivity... The differences in dietary iodine intake do not affect TGAb and/or TPOAb positivity." – PubMed ID#10395237 (1998) [323]

> "Although excess iodine exposure generally does not result in any apparent clinical consequences, thyroid dysfunction can occur in vulnerable patients with specific risk factors, including those with pre-existing thyroid disease, the elderly, fetuses and neonates. As iodine-induced hypothyroidism or hyperthyroidism might be either subclinical or overt, excess iodine exposure should be suspected if the aetiology of thyroid dysfunction is not discernible." – PubMed ID#PMC3976240 (2014) [324]

Iodine's benefits associated with cancer prevention have been mostly limited to breast, thyroid, prostate, gastric, ovary and endometrium cancers. This doesn't mean it is limited to those types of cancer, but that is primarily where the research is at. Iodine is an essential mineral, and deficiencies of any essential mineral may eventually be linked to increased rates of cancers. For instance, a well-functioning thyroid is essential for good health and our immune system; a deficiency of iodine will lead to a poorly functioning thyroid, and thus increased rates of cancer or poorer cancer outcomes.

> "given the geographical distribution of iodine deficiency, there is low incidence of cancers of the prostate, endometrium, ovary and breast in populations consuming diets with high iodine content (Stadel 1976)… Iodine deficiency is associated with a higher rate breast cancer. Similarly, higher dietary Iodine intake is associated with less goiter and breast cancer… in countries such as Japan and island that has the highest dietary intake of iodine lowest rates for goiter and breast cancers have reported… In Japan, where the incidence of breast cancer and infant mortality is very low… It is proven that iodine deficiency can lead to fibrocystic breast disease and/or ovarian cysts. Iodine can similarly reduce uterine fibroids and one of the first conventional medical treatments for severe fibroids was to paint the uterus with iodine (Lungo et al., 2000; Venturi 2001; Jang et al., 2013)." – PubMed ID#PMC5464505 (2017) [325]

The following study looked at iodine in prostate cancer. They found that iodine did <u>not</u> inhibit or delay the onset of prostate cancer.

> "The present study was designed to explore if continued supplementation with iodine inhibits or delays the development of prostate cancer in the TRAMP model. Our data showed that, although cancerous prostate takes up both I− and I2, supplementation with a mixture of the two species of iodine for 12 or 24 wks does not reproduce the antitumor effects previously reported in an in vitro model of prostate cancer… The inability of iodine to induce cell arrest or apoptosis could be explained by continued and exacerbated expression of TAG-oncoprotein (inhibitor of p53 and Rb) in the TRAMP model." – PubMed ID#PMC3883964 (2013) [326]

Recommendations

Iodine has a strong neutralizing effect on radical oxygen species (ROS) and thus may have the same negative effect on tumors as high-dose vitamins C and E. Though ROS can be damaging to normal cells, they can be even more damaging to cancer cells. Neutralizing ROS can actually protect cancer cells from apoptosis (programmed cell death). This can make it a poor choice for treating existing cancers.

Iodine deficiency has been linked to high risks of several cancers, but more is not necessarily better. High-dose iodine should not be used to treat existing cancers without your oncologist's approval. The recommended daily intake (RDI) for iodine is 150 mcg (this is 0.150 mg). This is generally considered the minimum needed to prevent goiter, but probably is not enough for optimal health or cancer prevention.

The best form of iodine is from seaweed and some seafood. It is bioavailable, and this is how our ancestors obtained it. The amount of iodine needed varies considerably depending on the type of seaweed and its preparation. Kelp flakes can contain over 8 mg (8,000 µg) per gram of the flakes. This is a tremendous amount of iodine.

> "Dried iodine contents range from 16 µg/g in nori to over 8,000 µg/g in kelp flakes" – PubMed ID#PMC3204293 [327]

Prevention – The ROS-neutralizing effect is probably not relevant to prevention (when a person doesn't yet have cancer). Therefore, taking slightly higher doses is probably not problematic (at least according to current research). However, there is no clear evidence that mega-doses of iodine are going to be beneficial. For this reason, I would stick to the Japanese consumption levels as your cap and would recommend a maximum of 1 mg per day for cancer prevention. It is not hard to obtain 1 to 3 mg per day from food if consuming seaweed products.

Treatment – If you already have cancer, including breast cancer, iodine might make it worse due to the ROS-neutralizing effect. This is a real issue, and supplementing even a little too much might make your cancer worse. Please do not be swayed by the popular media on this topic without discussing it with your oncologist. I would discuss your plans to start any iodine supplements with your oncologist before starting. I would also make sure that your current diet does not contain more than 1 mg (1,000 mcg) of iodine.

Note: Japan's Fukushima Nuclear Accident

The March 2011 tsunami and subsequent nuclear reactor accidents at Fukushima, Japan released radioactive iodine-131 into the environment. Some of this radioactive iodine entered the ocean and was taken up by seaweed off the east coast of Japan. This type of radiation has a half-life of just over 8 days. This makes it very radioactive, but only for a short period of time. Radioactive iodine from the Fukushima accident is no longer a threat. Iodine and cesium from Fukushima were detected in March 2011 (at levels below those of total background radiation levels) but were gone a month later.

Though seaweed does not take it up at nearly the levels it does iodine, seaweed can concentrate cesium-137 as well, and some of this was released by Fukushima. Cesium-137 stays in the environment much longer than radioactive iodine, having a half-life of over 30 years. In fact, cesium-137 is still detectable in the Pacific Ocean from Cold War nuclear bomb testing. However, even with Fukushima, radiation levels are still far below levels of concern. Because of this long half-life and how cesium-137 is utilized in the body, it is also far less dangerous than iodine-131. The following quote is very telling.

> "While elevated, these levels are still well below regulatory limits of 7,400 Bq/m3 set for drinking water (U.S. EPA). By our calculations, even if levels increase Bq/m3, swimming eight hours every day for an entire year would only increase one's annual dose by an amount, 1000 times less than a single dental X-ray." -- Center for Marine and Environmental Radiation, Woods Hole Oceanographic Institution [328]

Experts now agree that other than a few hotspots very near the reactors, there is no longer any current threat remaining from the Fukushima reactors (though this can change if someone screws something up during the cleanup process). In fact, the risk from radiation from living in Denver, Colorado is far greater (with radiation levels of 1.3 microsieverts per hour) than that from living in the city of Fukushima city today (0.14 microsieverts per hour)—in other words, Denver's radiation levels are 10 times worse than those in Fukushima! Though there have been 85 suicide deaths linked to the evacuation and fear from Fukushima, there has only been one death attributed to the radiation (a worker at the nuclear plant). The worry and fear about radiation has been far more harmful than the event itself.

In short, ocean seaweed is now as safe from radiation as it ever has been, and though there are many things we should be concerned about, this is not one of them.

❖ MAGNESIUM

Magnesium is an important mineral in the prevention of cancer, most likely due to its effect on the enzymatic processes in the body. Though we need all the essential minerals to stay healthy, this one is being called out, as it has been shown that even a small deficiency can increase the risk of cancer. Though there have been few studies on using magnesium to treat cancer, it almost goes without saying that a magnesium deficiency will impact the body's ability to fight cancer. Put another way, magnesium is not cytotoxic, so it cannot kill cancer cells; however, a deficiency of magnesium can impede the body's ability to fight cancer. So, taking much more than the government's recommended Daily Value (DV) will not have additional benefits for either cancer prevention or treatment.

On this topic I will simply let the studies speak:

> "Magnesium is an essential element required as a cofactor for over 300 enzymatic reactions and is thus necessary for the biochemical functioning of numerous metabolic pathways… evidence confirms that nearly two-thirds of the population in the western world is not achieving the recommended daily allowance for magnesium, a deficiency problem contributing to various health conditions… A decrease in Mg intake reduces intracellular Mg, thus reducing Mg-ATP, in turn increasing cell proliferation by activating Ca channels (TRPM7) which can provide the milieu for development of cancer. A higher ratio of calcium to Mg may increase the risk of postmenopausal breast cancer. Dietary Mg intake appears to be inversely related to a lower risk of developing colorectal adenomas and colorectal cancer. One study showed a 13% reduction in colorectal adenomas for every 100 mg/day increase in Mg intake. Other studies also show a modest 7% risk reduction with 100 mg/day increase in Mg intake" – PubMed ID#PMC5637834 (2017 – Open Access attribution available at the link) [329]

In this well-run study, they controlled for both vitamin D and calcium levels; they found that higher levels of dietary magnesium intake were associated with lower risk of "all-cause" mortality. However, this study also found no association with breast cancer mortality.

> "After adjustment for known prognostic factors, and intakes of energy, total vitamin D and total calcium, higher dietary intake of magnesium was inversely associated with risk of all-cause mortality… On the other hand, dietary and total Ca intake was not significantly associated with all-cause mortality. There were no associations between Mg and Ca intakes and breast cancer-specific mortality in our study." – PubMed ID#PMC4759402 (2016) [330]

When comparing high dietary intake of magnesium (Mg) to low intake, they found that DNA repair in lung cancer patients was 200% to 300% better in the high dietary magnesium group. They also found that lung cancer risk decreased by 17% to 53%, depending on a person's magnesium consumption. These are huge numbers—who wouldn't want to lower their risk of cancer by 53%? Though this may vary between types of cancer, there is reason to believe that this magnesium benefit would be seen in most types of cancer. Our bodies are very dependent on DNA repair in preventing the onset of cancer. This study explored whether additional benefits were seen when taking more than the recommended DV.

> "Low dietary Mg intake was associated with poorer DRC {DNA repair capacity} and increased risk of lung cancer. In joint effects analyses, compared with those with high dietary Mg intake and proficient DRC, the OR (95% CI) for lung cancer in the presence of both low dietary Mg and suboptimal DRC was 2.36 (1.83–3.04)… Increased Mg intake was associated with a monotonically

decreasing risk of lung cancer with 17, 36 and 53% reductions in risk by increasing quartile of intake… increasing dietary intake of Mg was associated with reduced lung cancer risk ranging from 17 to 53%." – PubMed ID#PMC2902380 (2008) [331]

Within the range of magnesium intake studied, each 100 mg less of magnesium consumed resulted in an additional 24% increase in the incidence of pancreatic cancer. Again, who wouldn't want to lower their risk of pancreatic cancer by 48% (or more) simply by adding more magnesium-rich foods to their diet? This shows that consuming at least the RDA (or DV) of magnesium each day is vitally important.

"Compared with those who met the recommended dietary allowance (RDA) for magnesium intake, the multivariable-adjusted HRs (95% CIs) for pancreatic cancer were 1.42 (0.91, 2.21) for those with magnesium intake in the range of 75–99% RDA and 1.76 (1.04, 2.96) for those with magnesium intake <75% RDA. Every 100 mg per day decrement in magnesium intake was associated with a 24% increase in the incidence of pancreatic cancer" – PubMed ID#PMC4705892 (2015) [332]

Recommendations

The US government recommends a magnesium consumption of 310 to 400 mg per day from all sources—that is, through a combination of food and supplements. This amount will be rather difficult to get just from food, so I do recommend a good supplement.

Foods high in magnesium include:

- Beans/legumes – Black beans (120 mg/cup), kidney beans (74 mg/cup), lima beans (84 mg/cup)
- Green leafy vegetables – All kinds. These are some of the best sources; as you can see, the currently popular kale does not stack up as well (but is still a good choice): Swiss chard (150 mg/1 cup chopped), spinach (157 mg/1 cup cooked), kale (23 mg/1 cup cooked), collard greens (38 mg/1 cup chopped and cooked)
- Grains – Oatmeal (57 mg/cup), Cream of Wheat (14 mg/cup)
- Nuts – Almonds (420 mg/cup), cashews (355 mg/cup), peanuts (150 mg/cup), whole pecans/walnuts (160 mg/cup), sunflower seeds (510 mg/cup)
- Vegetables – There are some very good choices in this category: asparagus (35 mg/cup), beets (63 mg/cup), broccoli (102 mg/cup), squash (22 mg/1 cup mashed)

- Tubers/rice – White potato (32 mg/cup cubed), sweet potato (59 mg/1 cup mashed), yam (24 mg/cup), white rice (24 mg/cup), brown rice (86 mg/cup)

- Fruit – Fruit is not a great choice for magnesium, especially considering the sugar content. Avocado is by far the best choice here: avocado (43 mg/cup cubed), banana (33 mg/1 medium), orange (13 mg/1 medium), strawberries (16 mg/cup), tomatoes (14 mg/1 medium)

- Meat – Meat is not a great choice for magnesium, but it is still a good choice for other vitamins and minerals: beef (7 mg/1 ounce), chicken liver (7 mg/1 ounce), chicken thigh (6 mg/1 ounce)

As you can see above, the best choices are also very healthy for other reasons; these include beans, green leafy vegetables, oatmeal, nuts, sweet potatoes and avocados. There is a lot of variety to be had within these groups and a lot of ways to cook or consume them. Cooked vegetables are far better than raw sources, as cooking unbinds minerals from the fiber, allowing the minerals to be absorbed by the body. Otherwise the minerals may simply go right through you, not getting unbound in time to be absorbed in the small intestine.

Nutritional Supplements – There is a huge difference in the bioavailability of magnesium supplements (something you don't have to worry about with food sources). I recommend a liquid ionic form, magnesium oils/lotions, magnesium malate and magnesium threonate. Epsom salt soaks are also an option. See the book's Amazon store for more specific recommendations.

❖ MANGANESE

Manganese is another mineral that can be difficult to obtain from modern diets. Luckily it is found in pretty much the same foods as magnesium: nuts, beans, legumes, oatmeal, brown rice, green leafy vegetables, cabbage and sweet potatoes. Retrospective studies show a clear link to poor manganese intake (in the diet) and several cancers, especially breast cancer.

The following meta-study looked at 11 research studies of manganese and breast cancer. They found a "significant association" between low manganese levels and breast cancer.

> "Eleven eligible studies involving 1302 subjects were identified. Overall, pooled analysis indicated that subjects with breast cancer had lower Mn levels than the healthy controls… The random-effects meta-analysis results indicated that subjects with breast cancer had lower Mn levels in serum and hair than healthy controls… In summary, this meta-analysis supports a significant association between deficient Mn concentration and breast cancer." – PubMed ID#PMC4443096 (2015) [333]

I find the following study very interesting. Rather than just looking at one mineral, such as manganese, it looked at 13. What they found was women with breast cancer had lower levels of all 13 minerals when compared to women without breast cancer! They were especially deficient in cadmium (Cd), manganese (Mn), iron (Fe), chromium (Cr) and zinc (Zn).

"In conclusion, there was a significant difference in concentrations of all 13 elements in serum between breast cancer patients and controls. A combination among Cd, Mn, Fe, Cr, and Zn might be important to determine a differentiating reference for breast cancers if a long-term followed-up study is to be conducted." – PubMed ID#17114811 (2006) [334]

The following study found that high chromium levels (usually from industrial pollution) and low manganese levels were correlated with higher breast cancer rates.

"results showed that the Cr content in the hair of the patients with breast cancer was much higher than that of the control... a clear negative correlation Cr and Mn in Hair of Cancer Patients between Mn content and breast cancer was observed. A low concentration of Mn clearly indicated that Mn might share the similar anticarcinogenic properties, as does the other anticarcinogenic elements Mg and Zn." – PubMed ID#15621924 (2004 – from the full study) [335]

❖ MOLYBDENUM

The connection between molybdenum and cancer is not as strong as the connection with some of the other minerals, but it shows that all the minerals are important. Many of the foods high in molybdenum are the same as the ones that are rich in magnesium and manganese: kidney beans, lima beans, navy beans, almonds, cashews, walnuts, peanuts, tofu, cheese, yogurt, tomatoes, green leafy vegetables (what are they not high in?), eggs and oatmeal. Yet again, eating properly and good gut health are important for proper absorption.

Molybdenum has many health benefits, but we're focusing on cancer and immune health. The connections here seem to be more in prevention of cancer, rather than treatment. Once again, there is also no evidence that consuming more than the recommended Daily Value will produce additional benefits. The increase in cancer risk seems only to be associated with a deficiency of this mineral.

Here are a few of the studies showing a correlation between low molybdenum levels and cancer.

"A negative correlation existed between soil available molybdenum content and mortality rate of gastric cancer... Deficiency of molybdenum may be one of the risk factors in gastric cancer." – PubMed ID#11819232 (1998) [336]

"A negative correlation existed between soil available molybdenum content and mortality rate of gastric cancer (r = -0.285, P < 0.05); hair molybdenum contents of gastric cancer cases were lower than those of healthy controls... serum molybdenum contents of patients were also lower than those of healthy controls... Deficiency of molybdenum may be one of the risk factors in gastric cancer." – PubMed ID#PMC4767765 (1998) [337]

"deficiency of Zn & Mo in food grains can be correlated to the deficiency of those elements in hair of RSA population. The deficiency of Zn & Mo can be correlated to the development of EC." – PubMed ID#22980353 (2012) [338]

❖ SELENIUM

There is a lot of controversy regarding the anticancer benefits of supplementing selenium. Several older studies seemed to show very clear benefits. Some later studies showed no benefits, especially for treating cancer. The hype surrounding selenium started in 1996 after the Dr. Larry C. Clark study was released. This was a randomized, placebo-controlled, double-blind study published in the *Journal of the American Medical Association* (*JAMA* 1996; 276:1957-1963). This study showed that 200 micrograms of selenium yeast cut participants' lung cancer death rate in half, and prostate cancer was cut by 63%. Total cancer incidence was reduced by 37% in the group studied. These were dramatic improvements! However, multiple, more recent studies do not confirm these dramatic results.

Newer and better run research studies have shown that selenium does not prevent skin, lung, prostate, stomach or esophageal cancer. High doses may even increase the likelihood of a skin cancer called squamous cell carcinoma and may lead to an increased risk of diabetes.

The following study used high oral doses and found selenium to be "selectively toxic" to melanoma cells. The amounts used are too high to DIY without doctor supervision. However, after reviewing the study, lower amounts appear to have benefits as well.

"MeSeH prodrug MSA is selectively toxic to melanoma cells, and our in vivo results (with a dose equivalent to 6.9 mg Se/day for a 70 kg human) demonstrate decreased growth of xenografted tumors. These results make MSA an excellent candidate for use as an oral agent in the adjuvant setting, where prevention of recurrence or development of a second primary tumor is the therapeutic goal, and the tolerance for potential side-effects are higher. However, the high dose required for the beneficial effects observed clearly moves MSA from the role of a nutritional selenium supplement to that of a drug" – PubMed ID#PMC3705316 (2013) (Open Access full study) [339]

Though this meta-analysis study was later superseded by the Cochrane study (see below under "Harmful Findings"), I felt it was important to include it. The study looked at 55 observational studies and 8 randomized control trials. The conclusion at the time was that selenium could help prevent certain types of cancer.

> "We included 55 prospective observational studies (including more than 1,100,000 participants) and eight RCTs (with a total of 44,743 participants). For the observational studies, we found lower cancer incidence (summary odds ratio (OR) 0.69, 95% (CI) 0.53 to 0.91, N = 8) and cancer mortality (OR 0.60, 95% CI 0.39 to 0.93, N = 6) associated with higher selenium exposure… The most pronounced decreases in risk of site-specific cancers were seen for stomach, bladder and prostate cancers." – PubMed ID#24683040 (2014) [340]

This study out of Malaysia showed a strong association between low selenium levels and breast cancer.

> "Breast cancer risk decreased with the increasing quartiles of selenium intake… Selenium intake and status was associated with breast cancer risk. Thus, it is essential for Malaysian women to achieve a good selenium status by consuming good food sources of selenium as a chemopreventive agent." – PubMed ID#19352569 (2009) [341]

> "Se supplementation exhibited beneficial effects on lung, bladder, colorectal, oesophageal, gastric cardia, and thyroid cancers… there is credible evidence of beneficial effects of Se supplementation in reducing cancer risks" – PubMed ID#PMC3705340 (2013) [342]

Here, selenium supplementation was shown to be beneficial when baseline selenium levels were very low. This is one of the few studies that showed a benefit for treating existing cancers, but benefits appeared only if the patient was selenium-deficient.

> "the results of many studies suggest that inorganic and organic forms of Se negatively affect cancer progression… In 1985, Clark et al. reported an inverse correlation between the Se content in forage crops in the United States and overall cancer mortality… It is also noted that Se supplementation had the greatest impact in men with the lowest Se baseline… the results of some studies demonstrated that Se affected cell-cell attachment, migration, and angiogenesis in breast cancer… selenite could lessen the angiogenesis signals from melanoma

cells and affect primary and metastatic tumor development… At least two molecules involved in angiogenesis, metastasis, and tumor growth, HGF and OPN, were significantly reduced in Lewis lung cancer… epidemiological data and clinical trial results do not fully agree on the benefits of Se supplementation, the results of many in vitro and animal studies have suggested that Se is a promising chemopreventive and anti-cancer agent." – PubMed ID#PMC3705340 (2013) (Open Access Study, attribution at the link) [343]

Below are the Dr. Larry C. Clark selenium studies. These studies are often cited in both medical literature and by alternative medicine proponents. Though not completely obsolete, both studies have been disputed, and newer studies do not seem to replicate these results. The first study is a double-blind study that found men with a history of non-melanoma skin cancers had a strong preventative association between selenium supplementation and prostate cancer. They found no association between selenium and non-melanoma skin cancers.

"the selenium-treated group had substantial reductions in the incidence of prostate cancer, and total cancer incidence and mortality" – PubMed ID#9634050 (1998) [344]

The following study was originally designed to look at "basal/squamous cell carcinomas of the skin." Though selenium supplementation showed no benefit in preventing a recurrence of basal/squamous cell cancer, it did find that selenium benefited "total mortality, mortality from all cancers combined, as well as the incidence of all cancers combined, lung cancer, colorectal cancer and prostate cancer."

"Se-treatment was associated with reductions in several secondary endpoints: total mortality, mortality from all cancers combined, as well as the incidence of all cancers combined, lung cancer, colorectal cancer and prostate cancer. The consistencies of these associations over time, between study clinics and for the leading cancer sites strongly suggests benefits of Se-supplementation for this cohort of patients, supporting the hypothesis that supplemental Se can reduce cancer risk." – PubMed ID#9315315 (1997) [345]

Again, more recent—and arguably, better run—studies did not show these benefits.

Harmful Findings

In this 2018 meta-study, the conclusion was that selenium does not lower the risk of cancer. RCT below stands for "randomized controlled trial." However, this type of study mixes in all types of cancers and all stages (preventative to stage IV). Each study also used different methods (or no methods) to adjust for confounders (e.g., smoking, drinking, medications). There are many other studies that were much more selective (e.g., they focused only on prevention, or only on reoccurring risk) and did show benefits. Still, this type of study is important in judging selenium's overall cancer benefit (or lack thereof).

> "Well-designed and well-conducted RCTs have shown no beneficial effect of selenium supplements in reducing cancer risk (high certainty of evidence)... No clear evidence of an influence of baseline participant selenium status on outcomes has emerged in these studies... Overall, there is no evidence to suggest that increasing selenium intake through diet or supplementation prevents cancer in humans. However, more research is needed to assess whether selenium may modify the risk of cancer in individuals with a specific genetic background or nutritional status, and to investigate possible differential effects of various forms of selenium." – Cochrane Gynaecological, Neuro-oncology and Orphan Cancer Group (2018) [346] Older version PubMed ID#PMC4441528 (2014) [347]

The researchers above did not do any in vitro or in vivo research of their own. They looked at several different studies with differing variables and analyzed them to determine a benefit, or lack thereof. These types of studies are inherently prone to unintended bias as the researchers have to make a lot of subjective decisions on what studies will be included, what variables equal each other (e.g., adults between 100 and 180 lbs may be included in one study, but another study may use participants between 90 and 220 lbs). One study may have asked about a person's drinking habits; another study may not have. The overall conclusion also was based on many different types of cancers and stages, which would tend to obscure benefits that might be seen in preventing specific cancers at stage I or II. This meta-research analysis also conflicts with many other studies on the subject.

The following study looked at non-melanoma skin cancers and selenium.

> "After a total follow-up of 8271 person-years, selenium treatment did not significantly affect the incidence of basal cell or squamous cell skin cancer." – PubMed ID#8971064 (1997) [348]

Recommendations

Selenium's links to cancer prevention appear to be relatively strong. This connection appears to be limited to a higher risk of cancer in a selenium-deficient state. There is no reliable evidence that adding selenium above the body's daily needs helps to further prevent, or treat, cancer.

Several studies have shown selenium's benefits in preventing and treating certain types of cancers: lung, colorectal, breast, melanoma and prostate. The studies showing no benefits were far too broad; they were meta-analysis studies that looked at all forms of cancers and at all stages. Each of those studies used different inclusion criteria, different amounts of selenium and different stages of cancer (preventative to stage IV). This would obscure any benefit that might be found for preventative or stage I or II cancers. Therefore, I think that to *Improve Your Odds*, supplementing selenium, or making sure we get enough through our diets, is something we should be doing.

The body needs proper levels of all minerals to fight cancer, and because many people do not get enough selenium in their diet, I think supplementation may be helpful. The FDA Tolerable Upper Intake Level (UL) for selenium is 400 mcg, and unless more evidence appears that taking higher doses is beneficial for treating or preventing cancer, I think 300 mcg should be the limit that people should supplement. I myself supplement 200 mcg per day. The diet should provide the additional 200 mcg. The best form of selenium to supplement is one derived from yeast, which is what I take.

VITAMINS

Vitamins are organic molecules that are essential micronutrients we require to stay healthy. "Essential" means that our human cells either cannot make them or cannot make enough of them. Because each are essential, one vitamin cannot substitute for another; you must consume enough of each to stay healthy. The amount needed daily is usually relatively small, measured in milligrams, or sometimes micrograms.

Vitamins are not the only essential nutrients to sustain life. Humans also need essential minerals, essential amino acids (from dietary protein) and essential fatty acids (from dietary fats). There are 13 organic molecules that have been classified as "vitamins," and there are many more compounds that are beneficial to human health but not classified as "essential":

1. Thiamine (B1)
2. Riboflavin (B2)
3. Niacin (B3)
4. Pantothenic Acid (B5)
5. Pyridoxine (B6)
6. Biotin (B7)
7. Folate (B9)
8. Cobalamin (B12)
9. Vitamin A
10. Vitamin C
11. Vitamin D
12. Vitamin E
13. Vitamin K

Not all these vitamins will be covered individually, but all are important to general health and the immune system, so it is important to get proper amounts of each of them. Failure to get proper levels will result in a deficiency state that can impact the body's ability to fight cancer cells before they take hold as tumors. Some appear to be more important than others in fighting cancer, and some seem to have some anticancer properties that extend beyond their function as vitamins. Those will be covered in greater detail. Most can be obtained by eating a healthy diet, and that is usually the preferred way of obtaining them.

Updates at - https://improvingyourodds.com

Support at - https://www.facebook.com/groups/cancer.improving.your.odds

VITAMIN AND BETA CAROTENE

Cancers: Most
Body of Evidence: Large
Cost: Low
Recommendation: High (for retinol)

Let's start with the complexities. There are two different types of vitamin A. The first type is retinol; this is called "preformed," and it is only found in animal products such as eggs, meat, poultry and dairy. As the name implies, preformed vitamin A is ready to use "as is." The second kind are carotenoids; these are called "pre-vitamin A." Most people have heard of the carotenoid beta carotene; it is commonly found in carrots, sweet potatoes, dark leafy vegetables (such as spinach), butternut squash, cantaloupe, broccoli and red peppers. Carotenoids need to be converted into retinol by the body before this form of vitamin A can help us, thus why it is known as "pre-vitamin A." This process is inefficient, and several factors can impede this conversion, including genetics, alcohol, intestinal issues, gallbladder issues, low-fat diets or anything that impedes fat absorption.

In this research paper from the *BioMed Research International* journal, several studies were identified showing retinol's ability to treat and prevent various forms of cancer. Studies included in vitro and in vivo research in animals as well as humans. Research indicates up to a 52% reduction in breast cancer risk (in animals with xenografts of human breast cancer cells) with proper vitamin A levels.

> "Epidemiological studies have suggested an inverse correlation between cancer development and dietary consumption of vitamin A. Pharmacological concentrations of vitamin A decrease the incidence of chemically induced experimental tumours. Natural and synthetic retinoids have been demonstrated to inhibit the growth and the development of different types of tumours, including skin, breast, oral cavity, lung, hepatic, gastrointestinal, prostatic, and bladder cancers… Moreover, the addition of RA or synthetic retinoids to human cancer cell lines or human tumour xenografts in nude mice result in growth arrest, apoptosis, or differentiation. It is noteworthy that natural retinoids act as chemotherapeutic agents for the treatment of acute promyelocytic leukemia (APL)… several studies establish an inhibitory role of retinoids in breast cancer. It was reported a 52% reduction in the incidence of mammary cancer in animals treated with retinyl acetate… vitamin A reduces the induction of carcinoma of the stomach by polycyclic hydrocarbons and vitamin A-deficient rats are more susceptible to induction of colon tumours by aflatoxin B than normal animals" – PubMed ID#PMC4387950 (2015) (Open access attribution at the link) [349]

In this study, chemopreventive benefits of retinoic acid were seen against various cancers.

> "The Vitamin A metabolite, retinoic acid, has been shown to have chemo-preventive and therapeutic activity for certain cancers such as head and neck, cervical, neuroblastoma and promyelocytic leukemia. Retinoic acid achieves these activities by inducing differentiation and/or growth arrest." – PubMed ID#15476854 (2004) [350]

Here researchers combined retinol vitamin A with traditional lung cancer therapy and found that retinol greatly improved anti-tumor activity.

> "These results suggest that the combination treatment of SL142 or SL325 (HDAC inhibitors) with retinoic acids (retinol Vitamin A) exerts significant anti-tumor activity and is a promising therapeutic candidate to treat human lung cancer" – PubMed ID#21079797 (2010) [351]

In these studies, new evidence was presented of retinol's ability to treat and prevent several types of cancer, including: breast, skin, lung and hepatoma (liver cancer cells). Vitamin A can help reenable the cancer cells' natural apoptosis function, in which cells that become damaged or cancerous are programmed to die. This is a natural function found in nearly all human cells but that is often turned off in cancer cells. Retinol also helped to prevent metastasis, or the cancer's ability to spread from one location to another.

> "Lung, prostate, breast, ovarian, bladder, oral, and skin cancers have been demonstrated to be suppressed by retinoic acid… low doses and high doses of retinoic acid may respectively cause cell cycle arrest and apoptosis of cancer cells… The biological functions inhibited by retinoic acid include tumor growth, angiogenesis, and metastasis. In addition, retinoic acid has also been found to regulate mitochondrial permeability, death receptors, ubiquitination, and reactive oxygen species, etc… retinoic acid is indeed a potential compound to suppress hepatoma growth and cause hepatoma apoptosis. It's also possible that retinoic acid can work as a helper that cooperates with other treatments and attacks hepatoma." – PubMed ID#PMC4265016 (2014) [352]

> "Retinoids are a class of these compounds that are structurally associated to vitamin A. The retinoids have a wide spectrum of functions. Retinoic acid, which is the active metabolite of retinol, regulates a wide range of biological processes including development, differentiation, proliferation and apoptosis. It suppresses carcinogenesis in tumorigenic animal models for the skin, oral, lung, breast, bladder, ovarian and prostate." – PubMed ID#24239628 (2014) [353]

> "Retinoic acid (RA), a natural metabolite of circulating Vitamin A (retinol) and an irreversible oxidation product of retinol… have been shown to be effective in the prevention of a variety of cancers in experimental animals, and in reversing preneoplastic lesions in humans. The retinoids exhibit a high degree of specificity in cancer chemoprevention… retinoids are anti-tumor promoters" – PubMed ID#12757023 (2003) [354]

"All-trans retinoic acid" (atRA in the study below) is made in the body from vitamin A (retinol) and helps cells to grow.

> "A number of experimental and clinical studies have been performed in the past two decades with retinoids showing that they inhibit or reverse the carcinogenic process in some organs, including hematological malignancy as well as premalignant and malignant lesions in the oral cavity, head and neck, breast, skin and liver… Oral administration of atRA induces differentiation of promyelocytic leukemic cells to mature neutrophils, and leads to a high rates (over 90%) of complete remission." – PubMed ID#15134535 (2004) [355]

There are many research studies of vitamin A (retinol) and its ability to regulate normal gene expression. Many of these studies explore how it regulates gene expression for fighting cancer. It is an important part of our innate immune system; all plants and animals have natural defenses against cancer. Our job is to give the body what it needs to support our innate immune system; without this, we would be missing our primary first defense mechanism against cancer. In today's world we consume a very different diet than our ancestors did, but our innate immune system evolved in our ancient ancestors, not our recent ones. Therefore, we need to make sure our body is receiving similar nutrition to that which existed in ancient times (that does not mean we have to consume the exact same foods, just the same nutrition). One of the components of that diet was higher levels of retinol. Our ancestors ate more fish and preferred organ meats (such as liver) over muscle meat. They also ate foods we would not even consider today (e.g., the organs of small ground animals, birds and fish). These foods were much higher in vitamin A (retinol) than the foods most of us eat today. Though pre-vitamin A from vegetables does have health benefits, research studies show that it is not a substitute for retinol (from animal sources). Therefore, supplementation may be necessary for proper nutrition, chemopreventive properties and chemotherapy uses.

Breast Cancer

There are several synthetic retinoids (vitamin A compounds) being studied for cancer treatment. These are not found naturally in food and are not available over the counter; therefore those will not be discussed here. Often synthetic alternatives are created by drug companies as it is not possible to patent natural compounds and vitamins. The following studies reviewed natural compounds of vitamin A. It should also be pointed out that there are various types and subtypes of breast cancer, and different genetics can affect treatments. What works for one person may not work for another. However, I've found no evidence that the retinol preformed vitamin A has any negative consequences at 25,000 IUs or less per day.

"All-trans retinoic acid and derivatives (retinoids) are promising agents in the management of certain hematologic malignancies and solid tumors, including breast cancer. Retinoids are endowed with anti-proliferative, cyto-differentiating and apoptotic effects… In conclusion, the work of Bosch and colleagues revives interest in retinoids for the treatment and chemoprevention of breast cancer." – PubMed ID#PMC4053099 (2012) [356]

"Retinoids have been reported to inhibit the growth of several breast cancer cell lines in culture and to reduce breast tumor growth in animal models. Furthermore, retinoic acid (RA) can augment the action of other breast cancer cell growth inhibitors both in vitro and in vivo. Clinically, interest has increased in the potential use of retinoids for the prevention and treatment of human breast cancer… A growing body of evidence supports the hypotheses that the RARbeta2 gene is a tumor suppressor gene and the chemopreventive effects of retinoids are due to induction of RARbeta2." – PubMed ID#12452454 (2002) [357]

"We investigated 208 women self-reported as postmenopausal operated on for T(1-2)N(0)M(0) breast cancer who participated in a chemoprevention trial as controls and never received chemotherapy or hormone therapy… At 12 years, patients with low retinol (<2.08 micromol/L, median of distribution) had lower breast cancer survival than those with high retinol (log-rank P = 0.052); the difference was significant for women >or=55 years… CONCLUSIONS: Low plasma retinol strongly predicts poorer prognosis in postmenopausal breast cancer patients." – PubMed ID#19124479 (2009) [358]

"retinoic acid may induce re-differentiation of early transformed breast epithelial cells, suggesting the preventive role retinoic acid plays with respect to breast cancer. Kamal et al. drew attention to the effect of retinoic acid by proteomic analysis in breast cancer cell lines… Retinoic acid was also found to reduce breast cancer growth and lung metastasis" – PubMed ID#PMC4265016 (2014) [359]

Melanoma

The following study shows a clear benefit of retinol supplementation in the prevention of melanoma skin cancer. However, you need to be supplementing 7,500 to 25,000 IU per day to achieve these benefits. Only the preformed retinol form appears to be associated with lower melanoma risk; beta carotene showed no benefit.

> "use of individual retinol supplements at baseline was associated with a decreased risk of melanoma… In this prospective study, we found an inverse association between supplemental intake of retinol and melanoma risk. The risk reduction was statistically significant for current supplemental retinol users… the effect appears to be limited to retinol users who take retinol in doses in excess of that available in a standard multivitamin… Intake of beta-carotene (from supplements, diet or total), was not associated with melanoma risk… Retinoids have powerful effects on cell differentiation and proliferation and inhibits malignant transformation. They have been shown to inhibit the proliferation of human melanoma cell lines and have been shown to inhibit tumor invasion using *in vitro* models. *In vivo*, murine models have shown that retinoids decrease tumor size and improve survival in melanoma" – PubMed ID#PMC3352977 (2012) [360]

The following meta-analysis research study looked at "8 case-control studies and 2 prospective studies comprising 3,328 melanoma cases and 233,295 non-case subjects" and found a significant association of reduced melanoma risk with retinol intake, but no association with total vitamin A or beta carotene. There was a 20% reduction in melanoma risk for those taking higher amounts of retinol.

> "Findings from this meta-analysis suggest that intake of retinol, rather than of total vitamin A or beta-carotene, is significantly associated with reduced risk of melanoma. The subjects with the highest intake of retinol were found to have a 20% (95% CI=8%–31%) reduction in the risk of melanoma, when comparing those with the lowest intake… Our finding of a protective effect of retinol intake on melanoma risk was supported by evidence from experimental and animal studies. Retinol belongs to a class of compounds called retinoids that have been consistently reported to enhance skin repair after ultraviolet light damage" – PubMed ID#PMC4105469 (Open Access attribution at the link) [361]

Here retinoic acid (a metabolite of retinol) was shown to inhibit the growth of human melanoma cells, inhibit invasion (metastasis) and adhesion (cancer cells in the blood need to adhere to normal cells to gain a new foothold). This includes inhibiting highly metastatic melanoma cells.

> "Retinoic acid has been demonstrated to inhibit several biological functions, including tumor growth, angiogenesis and metastasis. Retinoids seem to be

effective in inhibiting proliferation and inducing apoptosis and differentiation…
With regard to the relationship between retinoic acid and melanoma, it has been
demonstrated that retinoic acid are able to inhibit growth of murine and human
melanoma cell lines… vitamin A has been shown to inhibit human melanoma
tumor cell invasion by regulation of EGFR expression which is fundamental for
both growth and invasion. Furthermore, intercellular adhesion molecule gene I
(ICAM-1) is transcriptionally regulated by retinoic acid in melanoma cells [30].
Sengupta et al. found that retinoic acid may also inhibit highly metastatic B16F10
melanoma cells… A recent meta-analysis of randomized controlled trials could
not find a correlation between beta-carotene (a precursor of vitamin A)" –
PubMed ID#PMC4586774 (Open Access attribute at the link) (2015) [362]

In the following study, supplementing with retinol was associated with a significant reduction in melanoma risk when compared with people who did not take retinol supplements. There was no reduction in risk for people who supplemented with carotenoids. This is pretty strong evidence that we should take retinol supplements rather than carotenoids such as beta carotene.

"We examined whether dietary and supplemental vitamin A and carotenoid intake
was associated with melanoma risk among 69,635 men and women who were
participants of the VITamins And Lifestyle (VITAL) cohort study in western
Washington… Baseline use of individual retinol supplements was associated with
a significant reduction in melanoma risk (HR: 0.60; 95% CI: 0.41-0.89). High-
dose (>1,200 µg per day) supplemental retinol was also associated with reduced
melanoma risk (HR: 0.74; 95% CI: 0.55-1.00), as compared with non-users. The
reduction in melanoma risk was stronger in sun-exposed anatomic sites. There
was no association of melanoma risk with dietary or total intake of vitamin A or
carotenoids… Retinol supplementation may have a preventative role in
melanoma among women." – PubMed ID#22377763 (2012) [363]

The following review collected several studies related to retinol and the following cancers: melanoma, hepatoma, lung cancer, breast cancer and prostate cancer. The authors found a common thread where retinol caused cell cycle arrest and apoptosis of cancer cells (meaning it inhibits cancer growth and caused regulated cancer cell death without harming normal cells).

"retinoic acid plays important roles in cell development and differentiation as well
as cancer treatment. Lung, prostate, breast, ovarian, bladder, oral, and skin
cancers have been demonstrated to be suppressed by retinoic acid… Retinoic
acid has been found to have inhibitory effects on growth of murine melanomas

and colony formation of human melanomas… retinoic acid has been proven to cooperate with other effective cancer therapeutic drugs against cancer progression. Retinoic acid becomes a helper to chemo-therapeutic agents, a helper which may decrease both the dosages of these chemo-therapeutic agents required and their side-effects." – PubMed ID#PMC4265016 (2014) (Open Access license, attribute available at the link) [364]

Food Sources

As with many nutrients today, retinol is not easy to obtain in our modern diet. The FDA's recommended Daily Value (DV) is only 5,000 IUs per day, but we really should consume 2 to 4 times this amount from all sources. The following list of foods is meant to show just how hard it is for most people to get even 5,000 IUs of retinol in their diet, unless they consume liver or certain types of fish.

- Beef liver, 3 ounce serving, contains about 26,960 IUs of retinol (540% DV)
- Beef hamburger, 4 ounce serving, contains 0 IUs of retinol, none
- Beef kidney, 3 ounce serving, contains 0 IUs of retinol, again, none
- Chicken breast, 3 ounces, contains 70 IUs of retinol (1% DV)
- Chicken thigh, 3 ounces, contains 125 IUs (2.5% DV)
- Chicken livers, 3 ounce serving, contains 12,078 IUs (243% DV)
- Bluefin tuna, 3 ounce serving, contains 2,142 IUs (43% DV)
- Atlantic cod, 3 ounce serving, contains 40 IUs (1% DV)
- Cod liver oil, 1 tsp, contains 4,500 IUs (90% DV)
- Egg, 2 hard boiled, contains 586 IUs (12% DV)
- Milk, whole, 1 cup, contains 250 IUs (5% DV)
- Butter, 1 tbsp, contains 350 IUs (7% DV)
- Cheddar cheese, 4 ounce serving, contains 566 IUs (11% DV)

As you can see, muscle meat contains very little retinol (or total vitamin A). Oily fish contains far more retinol than non-oily fish. Our ancestors never passed up the chance to consume liver, fish and eggs; these were highly prized foods. Today many people do not like the taste of liver and never consume it. This makes it difficult to get the proper amounts of retinol without supplementing.

Beta Carotene

Cancers: None
Body of Evidence: Moderate
Cost: Low
Recommendation: Avoid supplements

Beta carotene received a lot of press in the 1970s and 1980s as an anticancer nutrient. Some pretty dramatic claims were being made. However, new research has not been nearly as kind to beta carotene, and it has turned out that it may not be nearly as beneficial for cancer as once thought. In fact, in some situations beta carotene supplements may actually increase the chance of cancer. Earlier studies were often done using a retrospective study model, in which people were quizzed about the food they ate. Those who consumed a lot of foods high in beta carotene were assumed to receive any benefit from the beta carotene, when the benefit could have been from eating a diet higher in vegetables, higher in soluble fiber, higher in lycopene, higher in astaxanthin, etc., rather than from the beta carotene in those foods.

Many people do not have the ability to convert beta carotene to retinol (true vitamin A). This is especially true for infants, diabetics, the elderly, people with compromised bile acid production, certain intestinal issues (e.g., SIBO), people who have compromised small intestinal brush borders, people on low-fat diets, etc.

New research shows that smokers should avoid beta carotene supplements, as taking it can increase their risk of lung cancer. It has not been determined if normal amounts found in food can increase this risk as well. (RCT = randomized controlled trial, a study where participants are randomly assigned to either a treatment group or a control group that does not receive the treatment being studied. This is considered the "gold standard" for a research study).

Smokers and Those Exposed to Environmental Pollutants

"The data presented provide convincing evidence of the harmful properties of this compound if given alone to smokers, or to individuals exposed to environmental carcinogens, as a micronutrient supplement. This has now been directly verified in a medium-term cancer transformation bioassay." – PubMed ID#12787812 (2003) [365]

"In subgroup analyses, among smokers and asbestos workers beta carotene significantly increased the risk of all-site cancer (RR 1.08, 95% CI 1.01 to 1.15; two RCTs), lung cancer (RR 1.20, 95% CI 1.07 to 1.34; two RCTs) and stomach cancer (RR 1.54, 95% CI 1.08 to 2.19; one RCT). Beta-carotene at high doses significantly increased the risk of lung cancer (RR 1.16, 95% CI 1.06 to 1.27; six RCTs) and stomach cancer" – PubMed ID#PMH0030452 (2010) [366]

Non-Smokers

In the following meta-analysis of 13 large studies of beta carotene, they found no statistical difference between the groups receiving (or reporting) beta carotene and the control group. There was a significantly higher risk of lung cancer in the group receiving beta carotene (though this may be related to smoking; that wasn't determined in this study).

> "Nine RCTs (13 articles) were included (n=182,323, range 1,621 to 39,876). There was no statistically significant difference between the beta carotene group and the placebo group in the incidence of all-site cancer (eight RCTs) and of stomach (seven RCTs), pancreas (four RCTs), colon-rectum (seven RCTs), prostate (five RCTs), breast (four RCTs) and skin (six RCTs) cancers. The risk of lung cancer was significantly higher in the beta-carotene than the placebo group (RR 1.13, 95% CI 1.04 to 1.24; eight RCTs). There was no statistically significant heterogeneity for any of these analyses." – PubMed ID#PMH0030452 (2010) [367], Full study. [368]

Here beta carotene consumption was significantly associated with higher prostate cancer risk, compared to the control group not receiving beta carotene.

> "Relative prostate cancer mortality was significantly lower among recipients of α-tocopherol than among nonrecipients (RR, 0.84; 95% CI, 0.70–0.99), whereas it was significantly higher among recipients of β-carotene than among nonrecipients (RR, 1.20; 95% CI, 1.01–1.42)... The primary aim of the ATBC Study was to determine whether supplementation with α-tocopherol or β-carotene would reduce the incidence of lung cancer in male smokers. By the end of the intervention period, α-tocopherol had no overall effect, whereas β-carotene increased the incidence by 17%... These temporal effects in both the ATBC Study and CARET suggest that β-carotene in some way accelerated the growth of preclinical tumors" – PubMed ID#PMC3991754 (2014) [369]

> "We conducted a systematic review and dose-response meta-analysis of dietary intake or blood concentrations of carotenoids in relation to PCa (Prostate cancer) risk... Neither dietary β-carotene intake nor its blood levels was associated with reduced PCa risk." – PubMed ID#PMC4570783 (2015) [370]

Much earlier studies, such as this one from 1995, tended to show that beta carotene lowered cancer risk. However, the newer studies above have shown significantly different results.

> "Numerous in vitro expressions have been performed in order to verify the true role played by this agent on cell proliferation and differentiation; until now, findings have been very encouraging, uniformly showing the beta-carotene can

affect carcinogenesis, particularly in early stages, through an antigenotoxic action. Antioxidant functions, immunomodulatory effects and control of intercellular messages via gap junctions are possible action mechanisms of the ability of beta-carotene to block the carcinogenetic process. In vivo animal studies partially confirm the results obtained in vitro showing that beta-carotene is able to reduce the induce cancer development; moreover, the association of the carotenoid with other microelements, such as vitamins E, C and glutathione often appears to be more effective than each agent used alone." – PubMed ID#7647689 (1995) [371]

Recommendation: Consume lots of healthy vegetables; they are good for you for a variety of reasons. But don't count on beta carotene for your vitamin A requirements. See retinol above. There doesn't appear to be a good reason to take beta carotene supplements.

Lycopene

Cancers: Prostate, lung
Body of Evidence: Moderate
Cost: Low
Recommendation: Prostate cancer—high; lung cancer—moderate

Though lycopene is chemically a carotene, it has no vitamin A activity in the body. It does have benefits of its own, but it does not count towards your total vitamin A consumption.

In this 2015 meta-analysis of 21 different studies, lycopene was found to help prevent prostate cancer.

"We summarized the data from 34 eligible studies (10 cohort, 11 nested case-control and 13 case-control studies) and estimated summary Risk Ratios (RRs)... Our meta-analysis indicated that α-carotene and lycopene, but not β-carotene, were inversely associated with the risk of PCa (Prostate cancer)... findings from our study indicate that α-carotene and lycopene, but not β-carotene, are inversely associated with the risk of PCa." – PubMed ID#PMC4570783 (2015) [372]

The following research paper indicates that there is very strong evidence that lycopene inhibits the growth of lung cancer. The study also indicates that lycopene is much more effective from tomatoes, and tomato-based products such as tomato paste, than from pure lycopene supplements. However, if you are trying to fight lung or prostate cancer or these run in your family, you may want to consider taking both a lycopene supplement and consuming tomatoes on an almost daily basis.

> "In vitro studies, despite their relatively artificial nature, demonstrated that lycopene may inhibit the growth of lung cancer cells… various mechanisms have been proposed to explain the inhibitory effects of lycopene, including cell cycle arrest and/or apoptosis induction via a modulation of redox status, a regulation of growth factor signaling, changes in cell growth-related enzymes, an enhancement of gap junction communication, and a prevention of smoke-induced inflammation. In addition, lycopene also inhibited cell invasion, angiogenesis, and metastasis… Lycopene has been reported to deactivate in vitro an array of free radicals, such as hydrogen peroxide, nitrogen dioxide, thyl, and sulphonyl. There are a number of investigations demonstrating in vitro that lycopene is a more potent ROS scavenger than many other dietary carotenoids and other antioxidants, including vitamin E… Many case-control and cohort studies have examined lycopene-rich diets and lung cancer, suggesting an association between lycopene and lung cancer in the protective direction." – PubMed ID#PMC3757421 (2011) (Open Access licensed, attribute at the link) [373]

Most of the studies looking at lycopene involved prostate and lung cancer.

> "the strongest clinical evidence for the benefits of lycopene in cancer are for prostate cancer chemoprevention, the majority of animal studies with lycopene have concerned prostate cancer… There have been relatively few animal studies regarding chemoprevention of other forms of cancer by lycopene." – PubMed ID#PMC3757421 (2011) [374]

In this 2017 research study appearing in the *American Journal of Cancer Research*, it was found that lycopene, administered orally, significantly reduced the metastatic load and significantly reduced the tumor load of ovarian cancer-bearing mice.

> "Lycopene prevention significantly reduced the metastatic load of ovarian cancer-bearing mice, whereas treatment of already established ovarian tumors with lycopene significantly diminished the tumor burden. Lycopene treatment synergistically enhanced anti-tumorigenic effects of paclitaxel and carboplatin… These findings indicate that lycopene interferes with mechanisms involved in the development and progression of ovarian cancer and that its preventive and therapeutic use, combined with chemotherapeutics, reduces the tumor and metastatic burden of ovarian cancer in vivo… Overall, preventive administration of lycopene interfered with tumor metastasis, metastasis-mediating factors and CA125." – PubMed ID#PMC5489781 (2017) [375]

In addition to the metastatic load reduction described in the study above, lycopene was shown to inhibit proliferation and induce apoptosis in prostate cancer cells.

> "Lycopene is a phytochemical that belongs to a group of pigments known as carotenoids. It is red, lipophilic and naturally occurring in many fruits and vegetables, with tomatoes and tomato-based products containing the highest concentrations of bioavailable lycopene. Several epidemiological studies have linked increased lycopene consumption with decreased prostate cancer risk. These findings are supported by in vitro and in vivo experiments showing that lycopene not only enhances the antioxidant response of prostate cells, but that it is even able to inhibit proliferation, induce apoptosis and decrease the metastatic capacity of prostate cancer cells." – PubMed ID#PMC3742263 (2013) [376]

Various studies have shown strong benefits when using lycopene for the treatment and prevention of prostate cancer.

> "Based on the evidence from epidemiologic, animal, and in vitro data and human clinical trials, it is evident that lycopene, a non-provitamin A carotenoid, is a promising agent for prostate cancer chemoprevention. It is also clear that the form of lycopene used (purified versus food sources), dose of lycopene and concomitant use with other carotenoids and antioxidants, duration of exposure, specific target populations, and stage of disease appear to play a major role in determining agonistic or antagonistic effects. Based on our review, there is enough evidence to warrant use of lycopene in phase I and II clinical trials to examine its safety and efficacy as a potential chemopreventive agent for prostate cancer." – PubMed ID#18302908 (2008) [377]

The following paper clearly indicates a significant inverse association between prostate cancer and lycopene consumption. Previous research shows that the consumption of tomato-based products is the best way to get beneficial plasma levels of lycopene.

> "Lycopene, a naturally occurring red carotenoid pigment found in tomatoes, pink grapefruit, watermelon, papaya, guava, and other fruits, has been extensively studied for more than 70 years, with more than 2000 articles published in peer-reviewed journals and 4000 other publications (scientific and otherwise) written on the subject... A significant inverse association between prostate cancer and plasma lycopene concentration [odds ratio (OR) = 0.17, Ptrend = 0.005] was observed between the highest and lowest quintiles of intake... Collectively, these

studies suggest that the consumption of lycopene or lycopene-containing foods reduces the risk for developing prostate cancer… A recent randomized, placebo-controlled, double-blind, crossover trial conducted by Voskuil et al. (2008) determined that tomato-extract supplementation (Lyc-o-Mato®, 30 mg/day lycopene) for two months in premenopausal women with a high breast cancer risk (n = 36) reduced free insulin-like growth factor-I (IGF-I) by 7.0% (p < 0.05). IGF-I is a biomarker associated with increased breast cancer risk in premenopausal women" – PubMed ID#PMC3850026 (2010) [378]

Astaxanthin

Cancers: Oral, bladder, colon, leukemia, hepatocellular, lung, breast
Body of Evidence: Moderate
Cost: Low
Recommendation: High (for oral cancer, bladder carcinogenesis, colon carcinogenesis, leukemia and hepatocellular carcinoma)

Astaxanthin (ATX) is a xanthophyll carotenoid, or keto-carotenoid, widely found in algae, salmon, krill, shrimp, crayfish and other crustaceans. It is what gives salmon meat its red color, as well as shrimp and crayfish their red shell. It has a very low toxicity, even in large amounts, so low that no toxicity symptoms have been identified. Due to the broad number of cancers where ATX has been found beneficial, with no known toxicity, this is a supplement that might be beneficial for anyone with cancer. The following paper contains links to several more astaxanthin research studies and published papers.

"ATX has anti-cancer efficacy in multiple types of cancer, including oral cancer, bladder carcinogenesis, colon carcinogenesis, leukemia and hepatocellular carcinoma. The anti-cancer effects of ATX are reportedly attributed to its effects on the pathological process of cancer cells through a variety of pathways including apoptosis, inflammation and cell junction… these data suggests that ATX could induce mitochondria-mediated apoptosis in cancer cells… Since inflammation affects all stages of cancer, for example, increasing the onset risk, starting the initial genetic mutation, supporting tumor progression and promoting invasion and metastasis, it could be the key target of ATX… by inhibiting invasion factors, ATX may be valuable in preventing cancer cell invasion and metastasis… in human colon cancer cells, ATX also showed anti-cancer effects by inactivation of AKT… the effects of ATX on proliferation, apoptosis, inflammation, invasion and migration has been widely described… A growing number of studies show that ATX emerges as a key player in cancer therapy. It also influences a multitude of molecular and cellular processes." – PubMed ID#PMC4515619 (2015) (Open Access attribution at the link) [379]

Strategy

The research clearly indicates that people need good levels of retinol (the type from animals). There is some evidence that separate benefits are associated with carotenoids (the plant forms). The evidence associated with carotenoids depends on which one you're looking at. The evidence of anticancer effects from beta carotene is on far shakier ground than some of the other carotenoids, with several more recent studies disputing the benefits found in earlier studies.

Remember that the two main forms of vitamin A are not equal: Retinol is by far the preferred version. A retinol supplement of 10,000 to 25,000 IUs per day is recommended (skip the supplement on days you've consumed foods containing 10,000 IUs or more). Over the course of 7 days, you should not consume more than 200,000 IUs in total for the week, from all sources.

Prevention – Consume a minimum of 10,000 IUs of retinol daily from all sources. Your diet should contain plenty of colorful vegetables that are high in carotenoids, as dietary sources are the best for carotenoids. To obtain more lycopene, consume fresh tomatoes and tomato-based products, such as tomato paste, on regular basis.

Complementary treatment – Consume 25,000 IUs of retinol daily from all sources. If you are not a smoker, you can also take a 2,000 to 2,500 IU (retinol equivalent) supplement of "mixed carotenoids" (e.g., "carotenoid complex"). This will likely contain beta carotene, lutein, zeaxanthin, lycopene, astaxanthin and alpha carotene. Additional amounts of lycopene and astaxanthin are recommend if you have one of the cancers they benefit; these two carotenoids have no vitamin A (retinol) activity, so they do not count towards the weekly limit. Continue to consume a healthy diet that contains natural sources of retinol, lycopene and other carotenoids.

VITAMIN B

"B" vitamins are an area that I will not cover in detail. Suffice it to say that we need proper levels of each B vitamin, and there is a fairly wide margin for error. This means we can consume 2, 4, or even for some, 10 times (or more) of the DV with no ill effects. In fact, some of the B vitamins are sold in strengths up to 10,000% the recommended Daily Value. This is not necessary and might even be detrimental to health. One large study (n = 77,118) found that people taking high doses of vitamin B6 or B12 were at greater risk of lung cancer.

> "use of vitamin B6 and B12 from individual supplement sources, but not from multivitamins, was associated with a 30% to 40% increase in lung cancer risk among men. When the 10-year average supplement dose was evaluated, there was an almost two-fold increase in lung cancer risk among men in the highest categories of vitamin B6 (> 20 mg/d; hazard ratio, 1.82; 95% CI, 1.25 to 2.65) and B12 (> 55µg/d; hazard ratio, 1.98; 95% CI, 1.32 to 2.97) compared with nonusers." – PubMed ID#28829668 (2017) [380]

Eating a healthy diet full of bioavailable vitamins, as described in Chapter 4, is very important. If done properly most people will not need to supplement B vitamins. There are exceptions; for example, some people with gut issues may not absorb vitamin B12 as well as others. If you do supplement B vitamins, I recommend that they are naturally sourced when possible and kept at reasonable levels. There is definitely a bell curve, but it is a very wide bell, where too little is bad for you and way too much is also bad for you. Luckily, with most B vitamins there is a lot of room for error.

A deficiency of any of the B vitamins can lead to a weakened immune system, and this can lead to an inhibited ability to fight and prevent cancer. However, more is not always better, especially when it comes from supplements. There is also no evidence that you can treat any cancer with mega-doses of B vitamins.

Recommendation

- Consume a diet high in vegetables, including colorful ones.
- Use an online nutrition tracking website or app to make sure you are getting enough B vitamins. Examples include MyFitnessPal.com and Cronometer.com; both of these have phone apps.
- Have your B12 levels (along with red blood cell markers) checked to make sure you are getting enough B12 and that it is working the way it should.
- Aim for at least the RDA/DV of each of the B vitamins. If obtained only from food, you don't need to worry if you go over this number. You can use the chart on this website to find out the RDA for each vitamin. [381]

Folate (Vitamin B9)

AKA: Vitamin B9, folic acid, folinic acid

Folate, often called folic acid, is an essential water-soluble B vitamin (B9). It is found in dark leafy green vegetables, asparagus, beets, Brussels sprouts, eggs and legumes. "Folate" is the natural form of vitamin B9; folinic acid is a form that the body easily converts to folate. "Folic acid" (note the spelling difference) is a synthetic form of folate and is used in many supplements and to fortify some foods (more on this later). It can sometimes be difficult to get folate from the diet as bioavailability can vary from 10% to 98% depending on many factors, including the pH of the intestines, digestive enzyme status, alcohol use and antinutrients in the diet. Some people also have genetic issues on the MTHFR gene that can greatly affect how these people utilize folate.

Folate has many health benefits. Studies have shown the benefits of proper folate levels include: reduced risk of heart disease, anti-aging properties, brain health benefits, positive mood and less depression, promotion of fetal development and prevention of neural tube defects, and promotion of liver health.

A deficiency of folate has been associated with the development of several cancers, including: pancreatic, cervical, prostate and colon cancer. In at least one study they found that the spleen produced fewer NK (natural killer) cells if there was a deficiency of folate. NK cells are a type of lymphocyte (a white blood cell), and they play a major role in defense against cancer cells. You certainly want to make sure you are not deficient.

Several studies have shown that a folate deficiency increases the risk of developing several different cancers. Proper levels of folate are very important to good health, but I would like to point out that, once again, no benefits have been shown in taking more than the recommended Daily Value, nor will consuming large amounts treat an existing cancer. See the recommendations at the end of this section. The following study excerpts show the importance of proper folate levels.

Beneficial Findings

> "Naturally occurring folates are water soluble, labile compounds that rapidly lose activity in foods over periods of days or weeks, consequently it is estimated that half or even three-quarters of initial folate activity may be lost between harvest and consumption… The major putative relationship between cancer and folate status relates to the role of folate in providing precursors for DNA repair and synthesis… The cancer protection potential of folates has been demonstrated by large-scale epidemiological and nutritional studies indicating that decreased folate

status increases the risk of developing certain cancers. These data indicate that folic acid deficiency affects the stability of cellular DNA at the chromosomal and molecular levels... Folate supplementation, particularity localized to areas of elevated demand, is thus proposed as a strategy to enhance genomic integrity and prevent the development of cancer." – PubMed ID#PMC3795437 (2012) [382]

Suboptimal folate status in humans is widespread." – PubMed ID#20544289 (2011) [383]

"Folate is proposed as a cancer prevention target for its role in providing precursors for DNA repair and replication... The cancer prevention potential of folate has been demonstrated by large-scale epidemiological and nutritional studies indicating that decreased folate status increases the risk of developing certain cancers." – PubMed ID#PMC3795437 (2012) [384]

"Folate deficiency has been implicated in the development of several cancers, including cancer of the colorectum, breast, ovary, pancreas, brain, lung and cervix... people who habitually consume the highest level of folate, or with the highest blood folate concentrations, have a significantly reduced risk of developing colon polyps or cancer." – PubMed ID#20544289 (2011) [385]

"folic acid is crucial for normal DNA synthesis and repair. Folate deficiency may cause an imbalance in DNA precursors, uracil misincorporation into DNA, and chromosome breakage... It also assesses the evidence from cellular, animal and human studies that folic acid can modulate DNA by such mechanisms." – PubMed ID#10746348 (1999) [386]

"evidence suggests that folate may also play a role in cancer prevention. Two recently published large, prospective epidemiologic studies suggest that maintaining adequate levels of serum folate or moderately increasing folate intakes from dietary sources and vitamin supplements can significantly reduce the risk of pancreatic and breast cancer, respectively. This protective effect of folate appears to be operative in subjects at risk for developing these cancers, namely, male smokers for pancreatic cancer and women regularly consuming a moderate amount of alcohol for breast cancer." – PubMed ID#10575908 (1999) [387]

"Adequate folate intake appears to help sustain normal patterns of DNA methylation and minimize DNA damage... inadequate folate availability impairs DNA synthesis in rapidly dividing tissues such as the epithelium of the gastrointestinal tract… Therefore, adequate folate status is crucial for accurate DNA synthesis and cell division." – PubMed ID#PMC2790187 (2009) [388]

Harmful Findings

There is a difference between natural folate and folic acid supplements. In most people, moderate supplementation of folic acid allows the body to convert it to folate in the body. However, in other people the synthetic folic acid form does not convert properly to the natural folate form. In those people, folic acid supplementation can inhibit the utilization of dietary folate (from vegetables), and thus it should be avoided. Because it is difficult to know who can convert folic acid to folate and who can't, I recommend taking methyl folate 5-MTHF or folinic acid if taking supplements. These forms convert to folate much more easily and do not block the natural form. The difference between the forms makes it difficult to evaluate in vivo human studies, as the outcome of the study can vary from person to person based on their DNA.

> "There is no evidence that folic acid is effective in the chemoprevention of colorectal adenomas or colorectal cancer for any population." – PubMed ID#20085565 (2010) [389]

Here the development of breast cancer was increased by 20% in women taking folic acid supplements. However, this might have been due to some of the women having genetics that prevent them from converting folic acid to folate, in which case they would essentially have been contributing to a folate deficiency by taking folic acid supplements. The study did not control for that variable, so in my humble opinion, this seems likely. Simply by taking another form of folate, this could have been avoided.

> "In this study, the risk of developing breast cancer was significantly increased by 20% in women reporting supplemental folic acid intake > or = 400 microg/d compared with those reporting no supplemental intake… food folate intake was not significantly related to breast cancer risk" – PubMed ID#17063929 (2006) [390]

The following study appeared in a 2014 edition of the journal *PLoS One*; it looked at 14 prospective studies that reported data on 677,858 individuals.

> "daily folate intake of 200–320 µg was associated with a lower breast cancer risk; however, the breast cancer risk increased significantly with a daily folate intake >400 µg… folate intake had little or no effect on the risk of breast cancer; moreover, a dose-response meta-analysis suggested a J-shaped association between folate intake and breast cancer." – PubMed ID#PMC4059748 (2014) [391]

This paper looked at "folic acid," the synthetic form of folate. It shows that folic acid can block natural forms of folate, especially in people with impaired MTHFR genes.

> Folic acid "inhibits methylenetetrahydrofolate reductase (MTHFR) by which high concentrations of folic acid could inhibit the formation of 5-methyl tetrahydrofolate... concerns about excess intake of the pharmaceutical form of folate, folic acid... long-term supplementation with high doses of folic acid might also affect intestinal and renal folate uptake processes by down-regulating folate carriers" – PubMed ID#PMC2790187 (2009) [392]

There is a pretty good chance that "folic acid" is what caused the increased levels of cancer in the studies above. This is due to "food intake" of folate not being associated with a higher risk of cancer, regardless of the level consumed.

Recommendations

Several studies indicate that the supplementation of over 400 mcg of folate can increase the odds of getting cancer, especially breast cancers, and therefore it is best that most people get their folate through diet. If you do supplement, do not take more than 400 mcg of methyl folate 5-MTHF or folinic acid per day; these forms convert easily to folate and do not block natural folate found in food. Note, it is recommended that you do not supplement "folic acid" unless other forms are not available. You may also want to avoid processed foods that have been "enriched" with folic acid.

Studies showing anticancer benefits of folate are comparing deficiency states with a normal folate status. People with a deficiency of folate are more likely to get certain cancers. Therefore, it is important to eat a healthy diet that includes the foods listed below.

The adult RDA for folate is 400 mcg/day, and the tolerable upper intake level (UL) of folic acid is 1,000 mcg (or 1 mg). However, I recommend never supplementing more than 400 mcg of any form of folate. Do not supplement folic acid, and avoid supplements that contain it. Consume a diet high in natural folate. Foods high in natural folate include:

- Liver (organic grassfed is best)
- Garbanzo beans (chickpeas)
- Lentils, peas and non-waxy beans
- Spinach
- Beets
- Brussels sprouts
- Broccoli
- Dark green leafy vegetables
- Asparagus
- Rice

VITAMIN C

AKA: Ascorbic acid, sodium ascorbate, calcium ascorbate, potassium ascorbate, ascorbyl palmitate, ascorbyl stearate

When reading health articles on the internet, you are bound to find almost nothing bad about vitamin C. You're also likely to find plenty of opinions (even links to very old research) touting the benefits of high-dose vitamin C for cancer. However, the studies regarding high-dose vitamin C and cancer are decidedly mixed. Early studies showed that it helped retard cancer growth; but most of these studies have been found to be flawed, usually due to lack of randomized controls or because they were purely observational. More recent studies using high-dose (e.g., 10 grams or more) intravenous vitamin C (intravenous administration of vitamin C has been found to produce plasma levels 25 to 70 times higher than oral doses) have shown just the opposite effect. These very high doses of vitamin C increase angiogenesis (new blood vessel supplies to cancer tumors, which is a very bad thing), reduce cancer cell apoptosis (also very bad) and increase metastasis (basically the spreading of cancer from one location to another. This is as bad as it gets). Research now considers intravenous vitamin C (and other very high dose methods) to be very dangerous, except possibly in very limited situations.

Ascorbic acid - The medical and scientific communities (around the world) recognize no difference in "ascorbic acid" and "whole vitamin C"—they are one and the same. Ascorbic acid can be extracted from natural foods or produced through a bacterial process (much like what happens when bacteria ferments cabbage and increases its vitamin C content). Other cofactors that may, or may not, be found in foods containing vitamin C are not part of the vitamin C molecule (vitamin C is ascorbic acid). Some in the alternative health community seem to have a different (non-scientific) opinion about this. Yet, when they quote studies citing the benefits of vitamin C, those studies used ascorbic acid.

Beneficial Findings

"The results suggest that doses of vitamin C induce oxidative stress in cancer cells… results indicated that treatment of malignant lymphocytic cell lines with vitamin C (0.25–1 mM) for 24 h led to a marked dose-dependent decrease of cell proliferation… A similar result was obtained with cells containing over 90% of blasts from patients with AML. In these cell lines, induction of apoptosis by vitamin C demonstrated a dose-dependent effect. In addition, vitamin C weakly induced apoptosis in ovarian cell lines, including SK-OV-3, OVCAR-3 and 2774. For many of the cancer cell lines, ascorbate concentrations caused a 50% decrease in cell survival… vitamin C dramatically increased intracellular GSH oxidation and reactive oxygen species (ROS) levels within 3 h in a concentration-dependent manner… No side effects were reported for most patients, while 59 were reported to have lethargy or fatigue out of 11,233 patients that received intravenous vitamin C" – PubMed ID#PMC3798917 (2013) (Open Access license attribution can be found at the link)

Ascorbic acid (in vitro) kills 86% of melanoma cells in 24 hours and 43% of neuroblastoma cells. How ascorbic acid works in vivo (in the body), especially if taken orally, was not determined by this study. Vitamin C, though an antioxidant, quickly oxidizes in the body; this oxidized form will harm our efforts to fight cancer.

"ascorbate causes cell death of approximately 86% of B-mel cells within 24 h. SK-N-BE(2) neuroblastoma cells are more resistant, 32% and 43% cell death for peroxide and ascorbate, respectively. In all cases, cell death causes hypodiploic DNA staining, evaluated by flow cytometry. Both cell lines can efficiently metabolise ascorbate due to significant levels of NADH-dependent semidehydroascorbate reductase and glutathione-dependent dehydroascorbate reductase. The cell death observed suggests a pro-oxidant, rather than anti-oxidant, role for ascorbic acid at physiological concentrations under these experimental conditions." – PubMed ID#7576946 (1995)

"The redox-active form of vitamin C, ascorbate, shows therapeutic efficacy in tumor cells. These antitumor effects of ascorbate are mainly based on its extracellular action and, in addition to the induction of apoptosis, also include an anti-proliferative effect by inducing cell cycle arrest. Furthermore, ascorbate treatment specifically enhances the cytostatic potency of certain chemotherapeutics, which implicates therapeutic benefit during tumor treatment." – PubMed ID#PMC3082037 (2010) [393]

Harmful Findings

There are several studies that show that high-dose vitamin C can kill various cancer cell lines in vitro. However, things get much more complicated in vivo. For one thing, the overall immune system becomes very important. Vitamin C has been shown to be cytotoxic to several cancer cells; however, we need to be cautious with nutrients that show high antioxidant potential, as some of these have been shown to prevent cancer drugs, and our immune system, from utilizing high levels of ROS against cancer cells (see Vitamin E for a more complete discussion on this topic). High levels of ROS in the tumor microenvironment put huge stress on cancer tumors and can help kill them. It has frequently been suggested that vitamin C may abrogate the effects of chemotherapy drugs (as these can introduce ROS in cancer tumors). The following research, which was published in the *Journal of Cancer Research*, supports this theory.

> "Vitamin C is an antioxidant vitamin that has been hypothesized to antagonize the effects of reactive oxygen species-generating antineoplastic drugs… vitamin C caused a dose-dependent attenuation of cytotoxicity… **Vitamin C treatment led to a dose-dependent decrease in apoptosis in cells** treated with the antineoplastic agents… administered prior to mechanistically dissimilar antineoplastic agents antagonizes therapeutic efficacy in a model of human hematopoietic cancers by preserving mitochondrial membrane... These results support the hypothesis that vitamin C supplementation during cancer treatment may detrimentally affect therapeutic response." – PubMed ID#PMC3695824 (2008) [394]

This tends to indicate that vitamin C use should be restricted during any cytotoxic treatment, especially chemotherapy and probably radiation therapy. This is not limited to chemotherapy, as ROS also can exist around tumors due to our immune response. You certainly do not want to decrease apoptosis in cells you are trying to kill.

Angiogenesis is the formation of new blood supplies to tumors; without this, cancer tumors cannot grow. Tumors release substances that force the body to make new blood vessels. Tumor cells release various pro-angiogenic factors, including angiogenin, vascular endothelial growth factor (VEGF), fibroblast growth factor (FGF) and transforming growth factor-β (TGF-β). There are many cancer treatment drugs that target these factors in order to inhibit tumor growth. We do not want to increase angiogenesis, and high-dose vitamin C does this.

> "restriction of the availability of ascorbic acid would suppress tumor growth, perhaps through diminishing angiogenesis. Ascorbic acid plays an essential role in angiogenesis as a cofactor for prolyl hydroxylase in catalyzing hydroxyproline synthesis… Tumor growth and metastasis are dependent on angiogenesis… investigators found that animals given high doses of ascorbic acid showed accelerated tumor growth… Tumors have been found to have an unusual metabolism of ascorbic acid, actively concentrating ascorbic acid relative to surrounding normal fluids and tissues… **ascorbic acid, in addition to supporting angiogenic activities, may also promote tumor cell survival and protect against oxidative stress**." – PubMed ID#PMC1804324 (2007)

Vitamin C is known to increase interleukin 1 (IL-1) and TNFα (TNF-alpha). Though an integral part of the immune system, these two compounds are also known to stimulate cancerous tumor growth. Some tumors are known to produce IL-1 and/or induce neighboring healthy cells to produce it for them. The following three studies show the negative consequences of raising IL-1 and TNFα.

"Ten subjects in each group received daily vitamin C (1 g ascorbic acid), vitamin E... or vitamins C and E for 28 days... interleukin 1 (IL-1), interleukin 6 (IL-6), and tumor necrosis factor alpha (TNF-alpha) in the culture supernates were assayed by enzyme-linked immunosorbent assay methods. Production of **IL-1 beta and TNF-alpha in the group supplemented with vitamins C and E was significantly higher**" – PubMed ID#8942423 (1996)

"Solid tumors in which IL-1 has been shown to be up regulated include breast, colon, lung, head and neck cancers, and melanomas, and patients with IL-1 producing tumors have generally bad prognoses... **IL-1 exhibits autocrine behavior by stimulating the tumor cell itself to invade and proliferate**... IL-1 induces expression of metastatic genes such as matrix metalloproteinases (MMP) and stimulates nearby cells to produce angiogenic proteins and growth factors such as VEGF, IL-8, IL-6, TNFα, and tumor growth factor beta (TGFβ)... Recent studies have determined the necessity of IL-1 in tumor growth, metastasis, and angiogenesis" – PubMed ID#PMC1660548 (2006)

"As a pro-inflammatory cytokine, TNF is secreted by inflammatory cells, which may be involved in inflammation-associated carcinogenesis... TNF could be an endogenous tumor promoter, because **TNF stimulates cancer cells' growth, proliferation, invasion and metastasis, and tumor angiogenesis**... its anticancer property is mainly through inducing cancer cell death, a process that could be used for cancer therapy. On the other hand, TNF stimulates proliferation, survival, migration, and angiogenesis in most cancer cells that are resistant to TNF-induced cytotoxicity, resulting in tumor promotion. Thus, TNF is a double-edged sword that could be either pro- or anti-tumorigenic." – PubMed ID#PMC2631033 (2009)

In this meta-analysis of 696 research studies, papers and case studies, they concluded that vitamin C does not improve cancer survival, nor does it enhance the benefits of chemotherapy or reduce its toxicity.

"Conclusion: There is no high-quality evidence to suggest that ascorbate supplementation in cancer patients either enhances the antitumor effects of chemotherapy or reduces its toxicity... No RCTs [random control trials] reported any statistically significant improvements in overall or progression-free survival or reduced toxicity with ascorbate relative to control arm." – PubMed ID#25601965 (2015) [395]

Recommendations

There is mounting evidence that high-dose vitamin C (especially intravenous) can worsen many, if not most, cancers. Therefore, this is not something that I can recommend, and I will not take it myself. Though there may be some very specific uses for certain cancers, this will need to be extensively studied and doses determined in order to prevent doing more harm than good. Only then can it be used safely. The evidence is clear that the misapplication of high-dose vitamin C can not only worsen cancer, but also can defeat the benefits of other cancer treatments.

Therefore, my recommendation is to supplement no more than about 250 mg of oral vitamin C daily, and to avoid intravenous treatments unless given by a licensed oncologist. I know this goes against a lot of what you'll read online, but I can find little evidence that more than 250 mg is needed, and too much can be counterproductive. I would avoid intravenous use of vitamin C supplements until more research is done showing the circumstances under which it is appropriate. Unless new evidence to the contrary comes out, I would not worry about normal dietary consumption of vitamin C in fruits and vegetables. Because of their other cancer-fighting benefits, I recommend consuming lemon, lime, avocados and vegetables as your food source of vitamin C (in normal dietary amounts).

There are some studies that show fruit, and especially citrus such as lemons, limes and oranges, does have beneficial effects against cancer. However, these results do not seem to be related to their vitamin C content.

> "Pooled results from observational studies showed an inverse association between citrus fruits intake and the risk of breast cancer." – PubMed ID#PMC3625773 (2013)

Low-Sugar Sources of Vitamin C

- 1 lemon or lime, about 45 mg of vitamin C, 2.1 grams of sugar
- Avocado, ½ an avocado, about 10 mg of vitamin C, 0.6 grams of sugar
- Broccoli, ½ cup boiled, 51 mg of vitamin C, 1 gram of sugar
- Sweet potato, 1 cup cooked and cubed, 16 mg of vitamin C, 16 grams of sugar
- Cabbage, 1 cup boiled and drained, 56 mg of vitamin C, 4 grams of sugar
- Cauliflower, 100 grams/1 cup, 46 mg of vitamin C, 2.4 grams of sugar
- Tomato, 1 medium raw, 28 mg of vitamin C, 6.1 grams of sugar
- Tomato juice, 1 cup, 45 mg of vitamin C, 8.5 grams of sugar

VITAMIN D

AKA: Vitamin D2 (ergocalciferol and calciferol), vitamin D3 (cholecalciferol)

Cancers: Most
Body of Evidence: Large
Cost: Low
Recommendation: High

The first observation of an inverse correlation between sunlight exposure and overall cancer incidence and mortality in North America was published almost 80 years ago. Since then several observational studies have confirmed those results; the more sunlight an area receives, the lower its overall incidence of cancer. Vitamin D has been shown to be preventative, and beneficial in treating, several forms of cancer. This is even more fascinating when one considers that researchers don't seem to want to use doses of vitamin D that our body is accustomed to. When evaluating research studies of the benefit of vitamin D, one must take into account that most studies used almost insignificant amounts of vitamin D. When our skin is exposed to UV-B from the sun, it is capable of producing 10,000 to 25,000 IUs of vitamin D per day (up to 50,000 IUs if we're getting a sunburn inducing level of sun, which, of course, we don't want), in addition to a few hundred IUs of vitamin D that we receive from our diet. When you consider that research studies usually use between 200 and 3,333 IUs of vitamin D, and that many people receive very little daily vitamin D due to our modern lifestyle, the amounts used in these studies are insufficient to show optimal benefits. When studies do show benefits, even with the relatively small doses used, it makes me wonder how much better the results may have been if the dosage were closer to what the human body actually needs per day (probably between 7,500 and 10,000 IUs total on average, not including what it needs to store up for the winter).

The Endocrine Society has defined vitamin D deficiency as a blood test of 25(OH)D below 20 ng/mL (50 nmol/L), and vitamin D insufficiency as a measurement of 25(OH)D of 21–29 ng/mL (52.5–72.5 nmol/L). No major organization has stuck its neck out to define the "optimal" vitamin D level; there is a lot of debate as to what the optimal vitamin D levels are. The following 2014 study looked at 32 research studies conducted between 1966 and 2013 that looked at "serum 25-hydroxyvitamin D in association with all-cause mortality combined." What it found was the lowest "all cause" mortality was achieved (lowest rate of death from any cause) when people had vitamin D levels starting at 45 ng/mL. The lowest rate of mortality stayed the same up to 70 ng/ml and beyond.

> "This study confirmed an inverse association between serum 25(OH)D concentrations and age-adjusted all-cause mortality rates. Overall, individuals whose 25(OH)D concentrations were in the lowest quantile (0–9 ng/mL) had nearly twice the age-adjusted death rate as those in the highest quantile (> 35 ng/mL)." – PubMed ID#PMC4103214 (2014) [396]

Research studies also fail to consider the important cofactors for either proper vitamin D utilization or proper utilization of calcium (calcium levels increase with higher levels of vitamin D intake, as vitamin D helps with absorption from the small intestine). For instance, studies are now showing vitamin K2 (which is not the same as regular vitamin K) is needed by the body to properly utilize calcium (vitamin K2 is discussed in detail later in this chapter). Vitamin K2 helps the body remodel (repair and rejuvenate) its bones and teeth; without this, the calcium circulates in the blood much longer than it should and often ends up collecting in tissue (such as blood vessels). Vitamin K2 is primarily found in the fat of grass-fed animals. The bacteria in their guts convert regular vitamin K into vitamin K2. They then store it in their body fat for future use. Dairy from grass-fed animals is therefore high in vitamin K2. Certain fermented foods (foods that would have a high level of vitamin K if not fermented, such as cabbage (sauerkraut) and the fermented soy product natto) also contain high levels of vitamin K2, this too is due to a bacterial process. Because vitamin D increases calcium levels, calcium and vitamin K2 are very important topics to consider when discussing vitamin D (and will be discussed again later).

> "more than 50% of the world's population is at risk for vitamin D deficiency. This deficiency is in part due to the inadequate fortification of foods with vitamin D and the misconception that a healthy diet contains an adequate amount of vitamin D. Vitamin D deficiency causes growth retardation and rickets in children and will precipitate and exacerbate osteopenia, osteoporosis and increase risk of fracture in adults. The vitamin D deficiency has been associated pandemic with other serious consequences including increased risk of common cancers, autoimmune diseases, infectious diseases and cardiovascular disease." – PubMed ID#18348443 (2008) [397]

As you can see from the following research, vitamin D is a critical piece of the cancer-fighting/prevention puzzle. There are now over 100 observational studies (in vivo) of vitamin D and its relation to cancer risk. There are hundreds of additional in vitro studies. There is simply an overwhelming amount of evidence that maintaining proper vitamin D levels is a key component in preventing and treating cancers. It may not cure your cancer on its own, but it is certainly a piece of the puzzle and necessary for "*Improving Your Odds*."

> "These findings provide strong evidence that vitamin D status plays an important role in controlling the outcome of cancer. Support for the UVB-vitamin D-cancer theory is now scientifically strong enough to warrant use of vitamin D in cancer prevention, and as a component of treatment." – PubMed ID#19269856 (2009) [398]

> "vitamin D has shown that its active form not only regulates calcium and phosphate metabolism but also has significant antimitotic and cell differentiation effects. It can inhibit proliferation, angiogenesis and metastatic potential in cancer tissue. Insufficient vitamin D plasma levels are found in 20-60% of cancer

---

patients at diagnosis… vitamin D deficiency is associated with higher aggressivity of tumor and shorter survival of patients." – PubMed ID#25882019 (2015) [399]

"The correlation between decreased morbidity and mortality of cancer and exposure to sunlight is known. The many biological functions of vitamin D that contribute to cancer prevention have only recently begun to be appreciated. Once activated 1,25-dihydroxyvitamin D [1,25(OH)2D3] functions as a potent inhibitor of normal and cancer cellular proliferation. Vitamin D deficiency in mice led to a 60% increase in colon tumor growth, compared to vitamin D-sufficient mice." – PubMed ID#16886659 (2006) [400]

"1,25(OH)2D3 (blood levels of vitamin D) was one of the most potent hormones for inhibiting both normal and cancer cell proliferation… men who had metastatic prostate cancer and received 2000 IU/d vitamin D had as much as a 50% reduction in prostate-specific antigen levels… mice that were injected with mouse colon cancer cells (MC-26) and were vitamin D sufficient had a 40% decrease in the growth of their tumors compared with mice that were treated in an identical manner but were vitamin D deficient… women who ingested 1400 to 1500 mg/d calcium and 1100 IU/d vitamin D3 for 4 yr reduced their risk for developing cancer by 60%… A wide variety of other tumor cell lines including leukemia; melanoma; and lung, breast, and prostate cancer cells have been shown to respond to the antiproliferative and prodifferentiating activity of 1,25(OH)2D3" – PubMed ID#PMC4571149 (2008) [401]

The following research shows several ways that vitamin D can help prevent and treat various cancers. It also points out the various immune system benefits of vitamin D, especially those with benefits to fighting cancer. One of the critical improvements is the enhancement of apoptosis activity against various types of cancer cells.

"evidence suggest that vitamin D or its metabolites have a direct inhibitory action on the development and progression of various cancers. Some population-based studies show that low serum 25 hydroxyvitamin D (25OH D) levels are associated with increased risk of cancers of the colon, breast, and prostate as well as other cancers. Studies in animals have shown that severe vitamin D deficiency or deletion of the vitamin D receptor (VDR) gene increase cancer risk. In addition there are a number of studies that show a reduction in cancer (tumor incidence or tumor size) in animals injected with chemical analogs of the vitamin D" – PubMed ID#PMC4572477 (2015) [402]

As shown in this study, the higher the levels of vitamin D, the lower the risk of contracting most forms of cancer, including, but not limited to, breast, colorectal, leukemia, lymphoma, melanoma and prostate. These are very different forms of cancer. Studies have also shown a lower risk of recurrence and mortality, as well as overall improved outcomes, in patients with higher levels of vitamin D.

> "Vitamin D has now been convincingly shown both in vitro and in preclinical animal models to alter the differentiation, proliferation, and apoptosis of cancer cells… Epidemiologic and observational data relating circulating 25(OH)D levels and cancer risk suggest an inverse relationship for most cancers including breast, colorectal, leukemia and lymphoma, and prostate… previous epidemiologic studies have demonstrated inverse relationships between circulating 25(OH)D levels and breast cancer development, recurrence risk, and mortality… patients in the highest quintile having a 40% decreased risk (of colorectal cancer development) when compared with those in the lowest quintile… A recent prospective cohort study of 390 patients with newly diagnosed chronic lymphocytic leukemia evaluated the relationship between 25(OH)D levels and both overall survival (OS) and time-to-treatment (TTT)… comparison of the highest 25(OH)D quartile to the lowest quartile revealed a 57% reduction (OR 0.43; 95% CI 0.24–0.76) in lethal prostate cancer risk" – PubMed ID#PMC3899831 (2013) [403]

Here it was shown that vitamin D promoted apoptosis in cancer cells. This is the natural programmed death of cells that have become cancerous, damaged or just old (allowing them to be replaced by new, healthy cells). The apoptosis process is usually defective or turned off in cancer cells. Reenabling this process is vital to preventing and treating all forms of cancer.

> "1,25(OH)$_2$ D treatment promoted apoptosis in the undifferentiated gastric cancer cell line… a number of studies have found that transcripts for genes encoding proteins that control apoptosis are regulated by 1,25(OH)2 D treatment… these transcript level changes suggest that 1,25(OH)2 D induces apoptosis by transcriptionally activating or repressing various genes… Taken together, it is possible that 1,25(OH)2 D directly regulates the expression of a variety of genes whose protein products are involved in DNA damage repair and programmed cell death, thereby offering protection against carcinogenesis… Conclusion: There is now a large amount of population-based evidence showing that higher vitamin D status can protect against a variety of cancers." – PubMed ID#PMC4572477 (2012) [404]

Several studies have now shown that people in more northern climates are at a higher risk of being diagnosed with several types of cancer. This is due to receiving less UV-B light—UV-B is what our skin uses to manufacture vitamin D.

> "The negative association of the latitude where people live and the incidence of non cutaneous cancer in that population in North America have been demonstrated in many studies for many types of cancer. Since the intensity of UVB exposure decreases with increasing latitude, and UVB exposure provides the mechanism for vitamin D production in the skin, the hypothesis that increased vitamin D provides protection against the development of cancer has been proposed…. animal studies have been quite consistent in their demonstration that vitamin D and/or its active metabolite 1,25 dihydroxyvitamin D (1,25(OH)2D) can prevent the development and/or treat a variety of cancers in a variety of animal models. Furthermore, 1,25(OH)2D has been shown to impact a number of cellular mechanisms that would be expected to underlie its anticancer effects." – PubMed ID#24402695 (2014) [405]

Vitamin D has been shown to exert several beneficial effects against cancer, showing that its benefits are not an accidental occurrence, but a very important part of our innate and adaptive immune system.

> "There is increasing evidence that Vitamin D (Vit D) and its metabolites… exert antiproliferative, pro-differentiating, and immune modulatory effects on tumor cells in vitro and may also delay tumor growth in vivo… Experimental and clinical observations suggest that Vit D and its analogues may be effective in preventing the malignant transformation and/or the progression of various types of human tumors including breast cancer, prostate cancer, colorectal cancer, and some hematological malignances. These findings suggest the possibility of the clinical use of these molecules as novel potential chemopreventive and anticancer agents." – PubMed ID#25856702 (2015) [406]

The body uses vitamin D (again, a pro-hormone) in several ways to combat cancer cells. These are outlined in the following research paper.

> "Experimental observations suggest that the chemopreventive effects of Vit D appear to be mainly due to its modulating activity on important biological functions such as cell proliferation, cell differentiation, growth factors gene expression, signal transduction, and apoptosis… recent clinical observations showed a significant inverse association between 1,25(OH)2D3 serum concentration and risk of breast cancer… Vit D was associated with a 50% decrease in risk of colorectal tumor" -- doi: 10.3109/13880209.2014.988274 [407]

In this 8-year study, the risk of getting colon cancer decreased 3-fold in people with vitamin D blood levels greater than 20 ng/ml. It also points out that people living at higher latitudes (further from the equator) have lower vitamin D levels and higher cancer risk and mortality.

> "an eight-year prospective case-control study of adults living in Washington County and reported that the risk of getting colon cancer decreased three-fold in people with a serum 25(OH)D > 20 ng/ml. These results together suggested that living at higher latitudes meant less exposure to vitamin D producing sunlight and therefore the connection with the first association with latitude and cancer mortality could be linked to an inverse relationship with cancer mortality and vitamin D status… A meta-analysis of studies reporting cancer incidence rates for more than 100 countries including Australia, China, Japan, Spain among others revealed an inverse relationship with solar UVB exposure for 15 types of cancer including bladder, breast, cervical, colon, endometrial, esophageal, gastric, lung, ovarian, pancreatic, rectal, renal and vulvar cancer as well as Hodgkin's and non-Hodgkin's lymphoma… a quantitative meta-analysis on the optimal status for colorectal cancer prevention showed that a 25(OH)D level of 34 ng/ml was associated with a 50% reduced risk of developing colorectal cancer." – PubMed ID#PMC3897598 (2013) (Open Access license, attribute at the link) [408]

In this 2017 meta-study, the authors found an inverse relationship between vitamin D blood levels and 20 different types of cancer (so the higher the blood levels of vitamin D, the lower the risk of coming down with one of these cancers).

> "Many reports showed an inverse association between serum vitamin D concentration and incidence of several cancers, including breast, colorectal, kidney, lung, and pancreatic. About 20 different cancers have incidence rates inversely related to solar UV-B doses and serum vitamin D concentration… circulating vitamin D levels (levels ≥45 ng/mL) may protect against breast cancer… The meta-analysis conducted by Chen et al11 revealed that women with the highest quantile of circulating 25(OH)D was associated with a 45% (odds ratio [OR] = 0.55, 95% confidence interval [CI] = 0.38-0.80) decrease in breast cancer risk when compared with those women with the lowest quantile of blood 25(OH)D." – PubMed ID#PMC5802611 (2017) (Creative Common Open Access attribute at the link) [409]

Another meta-research study from 2017 found the same results as the research above.

"A vast amount of preclinical and epidemiologic studies have focused on the impact vitamin D has on disease progression and mortality of cancer. High circulating levels of vitamin D are associated with a reduced risk of developing certain cancer types (breast, colorectal, gastric, hematological, head and neck, kidney, lung, ovarian, pancreatic liver, prostate and skin cancer). It has been demonstrated that vitamin D inhibits proliferation and induces differentiation of carcinoma cells in vitro and in vivo." – PubMed ID#PMC5713297 (2017) [410]

"A Review of the Evidence Supporting the Vitamin D-Cancer Prevention Hypothesis in 2017… three clinical trials do support the hypothesis. In general, the totality of the evidence, as evaluated using Hill's criteria for causality in a biological system, supports the vitamin D-cancer prevention hypothesis." – PubMed ID#29374749 (2018) [411]

"Several lines of population-based studies revealed an inverse correlation between serum 25-hydroxyvitamin D (25(OH)D) levels and high risk of colon, breast, prostate, gastric, and other cancers. Moreover, there are strong evidences from several cell culture and animal studies to support the antitumorigenic effects of vitamin D… several epidemiological, clinical, preclinical, and in vitro experimental data strongly suggest that the activation of vitamin D signaling could be a promising strategy for prevention, as well as treatment of many types of cancer." – PubMed ID#PMC5938036 (2018) [412]

Melanoma

Some people are genetically more likely than others to get melanomas from too much sun exposure. So, there is a delicate dance between getting enough vitamin D from the sun, but not so much that one raises the risk of melanoma. See the Strategy sub-section for more information on this. It is obvious, however, that we need to keep our vitamin D levels above 35 ng/ml to help avoid melanoma.

"An association between deficient levels of vitamin D3 and several types of malignant neoplasms, notably colon, breast and skin cancer, has already been shown… Some studies suggest that normal levels of vitamin D3 at the time of diagnosis are associated to a better prognosis in patients with melanoma… vitamin D may reduce cancer risk through several biologic pathways. In particular, in vitro studies indicate that 1,25(OH)D may inhibit cell growth in human melanoma cell lines [9]. High circulating vitamin D concentration has been found to be associated with reduced melanoma progression and improved survival… In 2011 Vinceti et al. have examined the association between vitamin D and melanoma risk through a population-based case-control study. They described an inverse association between dietary intake of vitamin D and melanoma risk, in particular among males and older subjects. A similar inverse association has also been described by a US-hospital-based case-control study" – PubMed ID#PMC4586774 (Open Access attribution at the link) (2015) [413]

The following study looked at 252 metastatic melanoma patients who had vitamin D (25(OH)D3) levels recorded within one year after diagnosis. There was a clear association between low vitamin D levels (below 20 ng/ml) and significantly worse outcomes (HR 4.68, or in plain English, about 368% worse!). This study confirms the results of several other studies that show a clear association between low vitamin D levels and poor prognosis with several forms of cancer, especially metastasizing melanoma. This study also shows significant benefits to raising vitamin D levels after being diagnosed with melanoma.

"A worse melanoma prognosis was associated with vitamin D deficiency (P=0.012), higher stage (P<0.001), ulceration (P=0.001), and higher mitotic rate (P=0.001) (HR 1.93, 95% CI 1.15-3.22). In patients with stage IV metastatic melanoma, vitamin D deficiency was associated with significantly worse melanoma-specific mortality (adjusted HR 2.06, 95% CI 1.10-3.87). Patients with metastatic melanoma who were initially vitamin D deficient and subsequently had a decrease or ≤20 ng/mL increase in their 25(OH)D3 concentration had significantly worse outcomes (HR 4.68, 95% CI 1.05-20.88) compared to non-deficient patients who had a >20 ng/mL increase. Our results suggest that initial vitamin D deficiency and insufficient repletion is associated with a worse prognosis in patients with metastatic melanoma… metastatic melanoma patients with vitamin D deficiency who are unable to raise their 25(OH)D3 levels have a worse prognosis compared to those who are vitamin D replete initially or are vitamin D deficient, but are able to markedly (>20 ng/mL) increase their 25(OH)D3 levels." – PubMed ID#PMC5351676 (2017) [414]

Open Access attribution - Timerman, Dmitriy et al. "Vitamin D deficiency is associated with a worse prognosis in metastatic melanoma." Oncotarget vol. 8,4 (2017): 6873-6882. doi:10.18632/oncotarget.14316

"Median serum 25(OH)D concentrations were significantly lower (p = 0.004) in melanoma patients (median = 13.6 ng/ml) as compared to controls (median = 15.6 ng/ml). Primary tumors of patients with low serum 25(OH)D concentrations

---

(<10 ng/ml) had significantly (p=0.006) greater Breslow thickness (median: 1.9 mm) as compared to patients with higher levels (>20 ng/ml; median: 1.00 mm). Patients with 25(OH)D serum concentrations in the lowest quartile had inferior overall survival (median: 80 months) comparing with the highest quartile (median: 195 months; p=0.049)." – PubMed ID#25437008 (2014) [415]

"This inhibitory effect of the hormone on melanoma cell proliferation was dose-related and represents the first demonstration of a 1,25-(OH)2D3 mediated action on tumor cells." – PubMed ID#6257495 (1981) [416]

Colorectal

There are many studies showing an inverse relationship between vitamin D levels and colorectal cancer risk. The lower the levels of vitamin D in the blood (25(OH)D), the higher the risk of contracting colorectal cancer. In addition to the studies below, there are several studies earlier in this section that mention colorectal cancer (those studies mentioned other cancers as well).

"In this cohort of healthy women, we found a significant inverse association between prediagnostic 25(OH)D levels and risk of incident colorectal cancer, and a borderline significant inverse association between prediagnostic 25(OH)D levels and colorectal cancer-related mortality. These results support a possible association between plasma 25(OH)D and risk of colorectal cancer in women." – PubMed ID#25813525 [417] (2015) (Full Study) [418]

"A wealth of scientific evidence supports a role for vitamin D in decreasing colorectal cancer incidence, and possibly mortality. This reduction in risk is related to inhibition of cellular proliferation and stimulation of differentiation." – PubMed ID#21309673 [419]

The following research took an in-depth look at scientific studies of vitamin D and colon cancer. What the researchers found was a substantial amount of evidence showing the clear benefit of vitamin D to cancer prevention and treatment. The research included in vitro and in vivo studies.

"Since Garland et al. proposed vitamin D for colon cancer prevention 25 years ago, functional studies on vitamin D or its analogs have provided supportive evidence for its anti-tumour effect in colorectal cancer. Evidence from both in vitro and in vivo experiments suggests that anti-proliferation, pro-differentiation, pro-apoptosis, anti-angiogenesis, immune modulation, and microRNA regulation are involved in the anti-tumour effect of vitamin D. Recent studies also explore the local expression and impact of vitamin D metabolizing enzymes and VDR, which may lead to discovery of predictive biomarkers for vitamin D treatment response." – PubMed ID#PMC4890569 (2016) [420]

Breast and Ovarian Cancer

"Several studies suggested that living at higher geographical latitudes increased the risk of developing and dying of colon, prostate, breast and other cancers. People exposed to sunlight were noted to less likely develop cancer. Several studies evaluated circulating levels of 25(OH)D and its possible association with cancer. Case-control studies and laboratory tests have consistently demonstrated that vitamin D plays an important role in the prevention of breast cancer. Vitamin D supplementation is a much needed, low cost, effective, and safe intervention strategy for breast cancer prevention that should be implemented. It has been shown that vitamin D levels are lower in ovarian cancer patients. Low 25(OH) D concentration associated with lower overall survival rate might suggest for the important role of severe deficiency in more aggressive course of ovarian cancer." – PubMed ID#23700865 (2013) [421]

This study of breast cancer risk and progression in African-Americans and Hispanics showed that low levels of vitamin D were a clear indicator of a higher risk of breast cancer and a poor survival rate. A blood level "below 26 ng/mL predicts a decrease in disease-free survival."

"A total of 237 African-American (Cases = 119, Control = 118) and 423 Hispanic women (Cases = 124, Control = 299)… The results showed that 69.2% of African-Americans and 37.8% of Hispanics had 25(OH)D3 levels below 20 ng/mL. The 25(OH)D3 level below 20 ng/mL was significantly associated with breast cancer in both African-Americans (OR = 2.5, 95% CI = 1.3–4.8) and Hispanics (OR = 1.9, 95% CI = 1.1–3.0). However, the predicted probabilities of breast cancer in African-Americans were significantly higher than in Hispanics ($p < 0.001$). The 25(OH)D3 below 20 ng/mL was significantly associated with triple negative breast cancer (TNBC) in African-Americans (OR = 5.4, p = 0.02, 95% CI = 1.4–15), but not in Hispanics in our cohort of participants. Levels of 25(OH)D3 below 26 ng/mL predicts a decrease in disease-free survival" – PubMed ID#PMC5664083 (2017) [422]

"For breast cancer–controlled studies, case-control studies consistently find an inverse correlation between 25(OH)D and breast cancer risk.15,16 Bilinski et al15 showed that 25(OH)D concentration below 75 nmol/L at diagnosis was associated with a significantly higher risk of breast cancer… Other studies have found similar reduction in the risk for breast cancer… The prevalence of vitamin D deficiency in breast cancer population has ranged from 23% to 95.6%… women in the fourth quartile of serum 25(OH)D level had 3 times lower risk of developing breast cancer compared with those in the first quartile… Similar results were reported by Shaukat et al who studied 42 newly diagnosed breast cancer cases and 52 controls. They found that serum vitamin D levels were significantly lower in cases (85.7%) compared with controls (55.8%). The unadjusted and adjusted ORs for breast cancer in cases and controls showed a statistically significantly increased risk of breast cancer… women with 25(OH)D concentration more than 20 ng/mL had 67% lower risk of any invasive cancer compared with serum 25(OH)D less than 20 ng/mL… Low levels of vitamin D were recorded among patients with breast cancer compared with healthy controls. Moreover, low vitamin D levels were common at breast cancer diagnosis and were associated with a poor prognosis; about 94% women with vitamin D level less than 20 ng/mL develop metastases and 73% die of the advanced disease… This review shows that most of the vitamin D studies support the inverse association between vitamin D level and breast cancer risk, and retrospective and prospective epidemiologic studies revealed that vitamin D deficiency is associated with increased breast cancer risk." – PubMed ID#PMC5802611 (2017) (Creative Commons license, attribute at the link) [423]

Atoum M, Alzoughool F. Vitamin D and Breast Cancer: Latest Evidence and Future Steps. Breast Cancer (Auckl). 2017;11:1178223417749816. Published 2017 Dec 20. doi:10.1177/1178223417749816

Recent research studies clearly show that lower blood vitamin D levels are associated with increased ovarian cancer risk and lower survival rates.

"The odds ratio for epithelial ovarian cancer risk (10,065 cases) estimated by combining the individual SNP associations using inverse variance weighting was 1.27 (95% confidence interval: 1.06 to 1.51) per 20 nmol/L decrease in 25(OH)D concentration. The estimated odds ratio for high-grade serous epithelial ovarian cancer (4121 cases) was 1.54 (1.19, 2.01)… In conclusion, we demonstrate an association between low 25(OH)D concentration and risk of ovarian cancer in women of European ancestry, with our MR approach providing estimates which are unaffected by the confounding or biases present in observational studies. Whilst our results cannot guarantee causality, placed in the context of other epidemiological studies, they provide additional evidence supportive of a causal link between vitamin D and risk of ovarian cancer." – PubMed ID#PMC5100621 (2016) [424]

"Both vitamin D and its receptor have a protective role in gynecological cancers. Low levels of vitamin D are found in ovarian, cervical and vulvar cancer. As a response to cancer, the expression of the vitamin D receptor is upregulated in endometrial, ovarian, cervical and vulvar cancer… Ecological studies have demonstrated a lower incidence of ovarian cancer in southern countries, indicating a positive correlation between factors which inhibit vitamin D synthesis (e.g., latitude, sun exposure) and ovarian cancer risk… Vitamin D and its receptor have been shown to suppress epithelial ovarian cancer invasion into the omentum… this paper indicates a key role of vitamin D and its receptor in gynecological cancers." – PubMed ID#PMC5713297 (2017) [425]

The following study looked at putting patients on a high-calcium, low-lactose diet and increasing their sun exposure. This study found that this combination lowered the risk of ovarian cancer. However, it did not show which of these three variables, or which combination of two variables, were responsible for the lower ovarian cancer risk.

"Our findings suggest that a high-calcium, low-lactose diet, and sun exposure in summer months may reduce the risk of ovarian cancer in African-American women." – PubMed ID#27632371 (2016) [426]

Strategy

Vitamin D has been shown in a vast number of studies to benefit a wide variety of cancers, diseases and health conditions. Obtaining enough of this vitamin is highly recommended.

It is best to have your vitamin D levels tested, and if your levels are under 40 ng/ml, you should work to get them up between 40-60 ng/ml. This will require supplementing more than what the body normally uses per day (or getting more mid-day sun). The recommendations below assume that your blood levels are already at or above 40 ng/ml. Few people in northern climates have this level unless they routinely take vitamin D supplements or work or play outdoors during the mid-day sun, and their levels generally drop below that by the end of the winter months.

If you are a cancer patient, it is usually not a problem to get insurance to pay for vitamin D testing (if ordered by your oncologist). If you are wanting to prevent cancer, you may need a good reason to get your doctor to order it, such as: getting very little sun, working in an office all day, sun avoidance, or frequent colds and flus. If you have to pay for it yourself, you can get a vitamin D test for $60 to $100 online (you'll have to go to a local lab to get blood drawn); a good company to use is DirectLabs.com. [427] Their vitamin D test is $59, and that includes the price of the blood draw.

Prevention: Supplement 5,000 IUs of vitamin D daily; if your levels are already normal, you can skip supplementing on days that you've received more than 15 minutes of strong sun over most of your body, or 45 minutes for arm, legs and face exposure. Shoot for blood levels in the 40-60 ng/ml range and adjust your supplementation appropriately. See the recommendations below regarding the need to take vitamin K2 as well.

Complementary/Adjuvant Treatment: Shoot for blood levels of around 60 ng/ml. Discuss your supplementation with your oncologist. Levels up to 100 ng/ml have been shown to be safe, but no additional benefits have been found above 60 ng/ml.

Non-Skin Cancers: Obtain mid-day sun over most of your body for 15 to 45 minutes per day. This varies by person, skin color (people with darker skin need more time) and sun strength (time of the year, time of day, latitude). Start with 10 minutes, and add 5 minutes per day until you notice it causing a very slight pink skin color (for Caucasians) an hour or so after getting out of the sun. This is your maximum exposure. As your skin tans, you will be able to add more sun. Avoid getting more sun exposure (especially if you are fair skinned), even if you seem to tolerate it well. The UV-B wavelength is what makes vitamin D in the skin; UV-B is filtered by the atmosphere in the morning and evening, so mid-day sun is best. UV-B is also blocked by glass and even thin clothing.

Supplement 5,000 IUs per day in the spring, autumn and winter; depending on how far north you live, you may need more than that. If during the summer you are unable to get at least 15 minutes of mid-day sun, supplement 5,000 IUs of vitamin D on those days. Taking a high-quality cod liver oil once per day can provide another source of natural vitamin D (be sure to get one with a lemon or orange flavor added. This really helps with the taste. Read the label to see how much vitamin D it provides you).

Skin Cancers: Follow your doctor's directions for sun exposure; ask if 15 minutes is allowable. The amount of time will greatly depend on the time of year, where you live, skin color, amount of haze, etc. The goal if you have skin cancer is to get just enough sun that any pink you get doesn't last more than a couple hours. You do not want to overdo it, even if you don't burn easily. Expose as much skin as circumstances allow; this allows you to make more vitamin D in less sun exposure time. Supplement 5,000 IUs of vitamin D3 per day on days you cannot get sun. As mentioned above, take a high-quality cod liver oil.

See recommendations below regarding the need for taking vitamin K2 as well.

> "Biochemical vitamin D toxicity consists of 25(OH)D >200 ng/ml, hypercalcemia and a suppressed PTH level with no clinical symptoms, but none of the participants had that either. Because most labs identify the normal range

for 25(OH)D at 30-100 ng/ml, some physicians believe any 25(OH)D above 100 ng/ml is toxicity. It is not" – <u>Vitamin D Research Council</u> [428]

Magnesium

The mineral magnesium is required for the body to properly utilize vitamin D (and vice versa—vitamin D is also needed for the body to properly utilize magnesium). You need to make sure you are getting enough magnesium, especially once you start to supplement more vitamin D or start getting more sun. Few people get enough magnesium from their diet, so a supplement may be necessary. I recommend a liquid "ionic" (or nano particle) magnesium as they are the easiest to absorb and can be mixed into any liquid without affecting the flavor of the drink. Try to obtain at least 400 mg of magnesium per day from all sources (food and supplements). The FDA recommends not supplementing more than 350 mg/day. I do not recommend taking the following forms of magnesium, as they aren't absorbed by the gut very well and thus can cause diarrhea: carbonate, chloride, gluconate, sulfate and oxide. Whole books have been written about magnesium (e.g., *The Magnesium Miracle* by Carolyn Dean); for this conversation it is just important to know that you need to get enough magnesium if you are getting plenty of vitamin D.

Recommendation: Eat foods high in magnesium, such as: spinach, Swiss chard, dark chocolate, avocado, pumpkin seeds, almonds, kefir and black beans. Take a magnesium supplement in the range of 200 to 350 mg per day.

Vitamin K2

Vitamin K2 is not the same as "vitamin K," or K1. Vitamin K2 is needed for the proper utilization of calcium. Since increasing vitamin D levels can also increase calcium levels, one needs to make sure they are consuming enough K2. Without proper K2 levels, calcium is not properly utilized for bone remodeling, and it stays in the bloodstream longer than it should. This can lead to cardiovascular disease. K2 is found in <u>grass-fed</u> meat, butter and dairy. If the cow was not fed green grass, it won't have much K2 in its fat stores, and thus we won't obtain much K2 from it. Some K2 is also available from certain fermented foods, such as live cultured sauerkraut, miso and a fermented soy product called natto. K2 supplements can often be found combined with vitamin D3, and this is the way I advise obtaining it. There is no known toxicity level for vitamin K2, so don't worry about taking a K2 supplement and obtaining more from food.

Much like magnesium, whole books have been written about vitamin K2 (e.g., *Vitamin K2 and the Calcium Paradox: How a Little-Known Vitamin Could Save Your Life* by Kate Rheaume-Bleue), and for good reason—K2 can be very beneficial for cardiovascular disease, osteoporosis, etc.

"This study shows that high dietary menaquinone (VK2) intake, but probably not phylloquinone (VK1), is associated with reduced coronary calcification. Adequate menaquinone intakes could therefore be important to prevent cardiovascular disease." – PubMed ID#18722618 (2009) [429]

Recommendation: Make sure you are supplementing between 50 and 1,000 mcg per day of K2. This is a wide range, but research shows that even 50 mcg helps prevent arterial wall calcification and supports healthy bone density. I would also try to consume grass-fed beef and butter on a regular basis. Also see the Vitamin K2 section later in this chapter, as this important vitamin has anticancer benefits of its own.

VITAMIN E

AKA: α-Tocopherol, topopherol and tocotrienols

Vitamin E (along with vitamin C) is one of the rare natural supplements that may be able to prevent cancers from forming but can also hinder the ability to fight tumors once they've formed.

Vitamin E from food sources is safe (see recommendations in the Strategy section) and may even be useful in preventing and treating certain cancers. Low-dose mixed tocopherol vitamin E supplements may also be safe. However, vitamin E supplements should not be used along with anticoagulants like warfarin without consulting your doctor. Supplementing with high-dose vitamin E (above 400 IU per day) long-term has been shown to be associated with increased risk of all-cause mortality and increased risk of certain cancers.

Vitamin E is a strong antioxidant, and thus it can help prevent cellular DNA and mitochondria damage from free radicals. This is thought to be how normal cells first become cancerous. Reactive oxygen species (ROS) are a natural byproduct of normal cell metabolism and are detoxified by the body. In the early stages of development, cancer cells utilize moderate levels of ROS as part of their development process. Thus, if antioxidants can help prevent oxidative stress and reduce ROS levels, it may help prevent those cells from becoming cancerous.

Once a tumor has formed, cancer cells start to produce high levels of ROS, which, if left unchecked, can inhibit tumor growth and induce apoptosis (cancer cell death). Cancer depends on its ability to regulate ROS levels and efficiently detoxify high levels. Most chemotherapy and radiotherapy treatments kill cancer cells by increasing ROS stress on cancer cells at a much higher rate than normal cells, to levels that the tumor cannot detoxify. If we take high levels of certain antioxidants, it will help reduce ROS stress on cancer cells, helping them to grow, and this can impede apoptosis. Since apoptosis is nature's way of causing defective cells (such as cancer cells) to die, impeding this process is not something we want!

More vitamin E than what people would normally consume in their diet may do more harm than good, and mega-doses most certainly will (especially alpha-Tocopherol). For many years the alternative medicine crowd has encouraged the use of very high levels of antioxidant vitamins, such as vitamins E and C. Current science shows us that this is not always a good idea, especially if someone has cancer (even small undetected tumor cells).

There is also evidence emerging that the most common form of vitamin E, α-Tocopherol (αT), may be the least effective form for fighting cancer. Some of the less common (and, in the past, less studied) forms seem to have far more benefit, with natural, mixed-tocopherol forms being far superior. In fact, some studies have shown that supplementing 400 IU of alpha-Tocopherol per day (the most common dosage in supplements) may raise the risk of being diagnosed with certain cancers (most likely due to small, undetected cancers benefiting from high alpha-Tocopherol supplements). These other forms of vitamin E are also much better at reducing inflammation and seem to target cancer cells, inducing apoptosis, preventing epigenetic changes in normal cells, and having general antiproliferation effects, as shown here.

> "Natural Forms of Vitamin E as Effective Agents for Cancer Prevention and Therapy… accumulating mechanistic and preclinical animal studies show that other forms of vitamin E, such as γ-tocopherol (γT), δ-tocopherol (δT), γ-tocotrienol (γTE), and δ-tocotrienol (δTE), have far superior cancer-preventive activities than does αT. These vitamin E forms are much stronger than αT in inhibiting multiple cancer-promoting pathways… The existing evidence strongly indicates that these lesser-known vitamin E forms are effective agents for cancer prevention or as adjuvants for improving prevention, therapy, and control of cancer." – PubMed ID#PMC5683003 (2017) [430]

> "recent results in animal models have shown the cancer preventive activity of γ- and δ-tocopherols as well as a naturally occurring mixture of tocopherols, and the lack of cancer preventive activity by α-tocopherol. On the basis of these results as well as information from the literature, we suggest that vitamin E, as ingested in the diet or in supplements that are rich in γ- and δ-tocopherols, is cancer preventive; whereas supplementation with high doses of α-tocopherol is not." – PubMed ID#PMC3502042 (2012) [431]

The following paper links to various vitamin E research studies showing the benefits and limitations of vitamin E in cancer therapy.

> "The therapeutic potential of vitamin E isoforms in cancer therapy has been widely studied and thoroughly reviewed. Vitamin E members could be beneficial against a variety of cancer types, including breast, prostate, and colon through various possible mechanisms, including stimulation of wild-type p53 tumor suppressor gene, down-regulation of mutant p53 proteins, activation of heat shock proteins (HSPs), and possession an anti-angiogenic effect mediated by the blockage of transforming growth factor (TGF)" – PubMed ID#PMC4365088 (2015) [432]

Some studies have shown no anticancer benefits to taking 400 IU vitamin E (alpha-Tocopherol) supplements. The following study followed over 1,000 patients for an average of 7 years; half were taking 400 IU of alpha-Tocopherol, and half were not. I think the lack of benefits was due to only using alpha-Tocopherol (rather than a full-spectrum vitamin E with the other 7 forms) and to using too much—400 IU. The following study appeared in appeared in *JAMA* (*Journal of the American Medical Association*).

> "A randomized, double-blind, placebo-controlled international trial (the initial
> Heart Outcomes Prevention Evaluation [HOPE] trial... Among all HOPE
> patients, there were no significant differences in the primary analysis: for cancer
> incidence, there were 552 patients (11.6%) in the vitamin E group vs 586 (12.3%)
> in the placebo group... among patients enrolled at the centers participating in the
> HOPE-TOO trial, there were no differences in cancer incidence, cancer deaths,
> and major cardiovascular events, but higher rates of heart failure and
> hospitalizations for heart failure." – PubMed ID#15769967 (2005) [433]

There is definitely a "Goldilocks Zone" for vitamin E, especially alpha-Tocopherol. Too little is associated with increased cancer risk, and too much is associated with poor cancer outcomes and increased heart disease.

Breast Cancer

There have been some studies showing that women with very low vitamin E intake have a much higher risk of breast cancer (up to 50% higher risk). However, vitamin supplementation with alpha-Tocopherol acetate supplements (by far the most common vitamin E supplement) fail to reduce breast cancer incidence for most women. Research is showing that by far the best sources of vitamin E are food sources.

In fact, in a recent (2016) study, alpha-Tocopherol acetate was shown to accelerate breast cancer cell growth while reducing ROS level and p53 expression in vitro (gleaned from the full study). Though this study is preliminary, and only in vitro, you may wish to consider not taking vitamin E supplements if you have breast cancer or a history of breast cancer. Natural vitamin E from food sources would be a much better alternative.

> "Vitamin E supplement in the chow significantly accelerated breast cancer cell
> growth in vivo. ROS level and p53 expression were decreased in tumor tissues.
> Water-solvable vitamin E Trolox significantly promoted MCF7 cell proliferation
> in vitro, while reducing intracellular ROS level and p53 expression. p53
> knowdown by p53-siRNA transfection inMCF7 cells significantly reduced p53
> expression and increased MCF7 cell proliferation." – PubMed ID#27383327 [434]
> Full Study [435] (2016)

Again, apoptosis means "programmed cell death." This is a process whereby cells destroy themselves if they become damaged beyond repair, as in cancer cells. However, cancer normally turns off this function. Anything that can turn it back on without damaging normal cells is a

---

good thing. This paper links to studies that show that vitamin E can do this (in vitro) with several cancer cell lines, including breast cancer.

> "some in vitro studies have reported that vitamin E succinate may trigger apoptosis in several cell lines, including breast, prostate, intestine and liver cancer… it has been demonstrated that vitamin E succinate may promote breast tumor dormancy" – PubMed ID#PMC4586774 (2015) [436]

Though too much alpha-Tocopherol can possibly increase cancer metastasis and proliferation, too little has been shown to increase breast cancer risk (see recommendations below in the Strategy section). The following is from a meta-study that did a meta-analysis of 40 different studies.

> "Severe α-tocopherol deficiency could increase breast cancer risk. The association between plasma vitamin C and breast cancer was only significant in case-control studies." – PubMed ID#25316441 (2015) [437]

Melanoma

The following study looked at vitamin E with melanoma in mice (in vitro and in vivo). They found that vitamin E inhibited cancer growth by promoting apoptosis. I took a look at the full study, and they were just using d-alpha-Tocopherol ("d" is the natural form). This seems to conflict with other studies (such as those outlined in the paper below) that show that vitamin E can worsen metastasis. The amount seems to be important; mega-dose levels have been shown to make many cancers worse, but several studies using lower amounts show that it can be used to treat existing cancers (as well as help prevent cancers from forming). My take on this is that the jury is still out. Personally, I've decided to go with a low-dose mixed tocopherol and tocotrienols supplement as described in the Strategy section below, as well as increased consumption of vitamin E-rich vegetables. The following study is out of the Department of Surgery at Southern Illinois University School of Medicine in Springfield, Illinois. The first quote is from the online abstract available at PubMed, and the second quote is from the full study.

> "Vitamin E inhibits melanoma growth in mice - This is the first report of the antimelanoma effect of VES (vitamin E succinate) in vivo. The mechanism of the antimelanoma effect of VES in vivo involves the promotion of tumor cell apoptosis" – PubMed ID#11812968 (2002) [438]

> "Tumors in the control groups grew rapidly, reaching an average volume of 2350 ± 798μL by day 15 after the inoculation of B16F10 melanoma cells. In contrast, the inhibition of tumor growth on mice that were administered VES intraperitoneally was profound, with tumor volume remaining at an

average of 367 ± 136µL... Several other in vitro studies have shown that VES triggers apoptosis in many cell lines, including breast, prostate, intestine, liver, tongue, and heart." -- doi:10.1067/msy.2002.119191

Below is some of the evidence showing that vitamin E supplementation (and other strong antioxidants) can actually worsen established cancers (especially malignant melanoma). This is because the immune system uses oxidation to attack cancer cells. This is not a new idea; it has been shown in several studies, but this concept has been slow to gain support in the alternative medicine community. Since chemo and radiation therapy trigger oxidative ROS damage in cancer cells, you probably should not be taking high-dose vitamin E (or high-dose vitamin C) while receiving these treatments. Check with your oncologist to be sure. NAC (mentioned in the first study) is also an over-the-counter nutritional supplement; from analyzing the full study, it is apparent that NAC should be avoided in people with preexisting cancers.

"we describe the effects of two widespread antioxidants, N-acetylcysteine (NAC) and vitamin E, on malignant melanoma progression... using a transgenic mouse model and a panel of human cell lines... The results show that dietary antioxidant supplementation increases metastasis in malignant melanoma, and that this is dependent on new glutathione synthesis and activated RHOA. The data also indicates that mitochondria-targeted antioxidants do not inhibit cancer progression...dietary vitamin E markedly increased the number of lymph metastases but not primary tumors in mice, which was in agreement with our previous in vitro observations. These results suggest that cancer patients and people with high risk of developing cancer should avoid the use of antioxidant supplements." -- University of Gothenburg (2018) [439]

"Treatment with NAC or vitamin E also spurred the growth of human lung-cancer cells grown in culture. In both mouse models and human cells, the antioxidants seemed to protect cancer cells by reducing the amount of DNA damage." – Nature.com (2014) [440]

"supplementation of antioxidants does not result in the presumed health benefit, but paradoxically a high intake of antioxidants is associated with increased mortality. More than 68 randomized control trials were analyzed for the effects of β-carotene, vitamin A and vitamin E on mortality. All these compounds, given in a relatively high dose as a single compound or in different combinations, had no beneficial effects." -- doi.org/10.1016/j.redox.2014.12.017 (2015) [441]

"Natural antioxidants like vitamin C, vitamin E, carotenoids, and polyphenols like flavonoids, are at present generally considered to be beneficial components from fruit and vegetables… at higher doses or under certain conditions antioxidant-type functional food ingredients may exert toxic pro-oxidant activities." -- doi.org/10.1016/S1382-6689(02)00003-0 (2002) [442]

Strategy

This is one of those vitamins that I recommend obtaining mostly from food sources; this is the best way of getting mixed tocopherols and tocotrienols. Juicing vegetables is also a good way to obtain natural vitamin E. As you can see from the food list below, getting just the RDA from food may be somewhat difficult for some people; thus, the importance of eating 3 balanced meals per day, with vegetables at each meal. Empty-calorie meals are a lost opportunity to obtain good nutrition.

Supplements – Standard alpha-Tocopherol supplements have been shown to speed tumor growth in several studies and should be avoided. There are some mixed tocopherol and tocotrienol supplements on the market; just make sure they haven't added large amounts of alpha-Tocopherol in order to boost the IU number (under 50 IU is OK). Look for a bottle that lists all 8 of the tocopherol and tocotrienols and the amount of each. The book's website should list a brand that meets these requirements. Because of the recent research regarding high doses of vitamin E possibly worsening many cancers, I recommend not taking mega-doses—no more than 50 IU of alpha-Tocopherol, and under 400 IU total of mixed tocopherol / tocotrienols (about 268 mg). The FDA's RDA for adults is 15 mg or 22.4 IU.

Foods High in Vitamin E

- Turnip greens (1 cup cooked, 14% DV) (dandelion and Swiss chard are also good)
- Spinach (1 cup cooked, 17% DV)
- Avocado (1 cup cubed, 16% DV) (avocado oil is an even better source)
- Eggs (2 large chicken eggs, 6% DV)
- Butternut squash (1 cup cooked, 13% DV)
- Tomatoes (1 cup cooked, 7% DV), tomato sauce (1 cup, 17% DV)
- Hamburger meat (3 oz serving, 2% DV)
- Cod (1 fillet, 231 g, 7% DV)
- Salmon (1/2 fillet 198 g, 12% DV)
- Almonds (1 oz, 38% DV), hazelnuts (1 oz, 20% DV)
- Sunflower seeds (1/4 cup, 60% DV; 1 oz per day will give you 37% DV)
- Wheat germ oil (1 Tbsp, 101% DV)
- Flaxseed oil (1 Tbsp, 12% DV)

Vitamin K

AKA: Vitamin K1, phylloquinone

Many studies, and especially older ones, do not differentiate between vitamin K (or K1, phylloquinone) and vitamin K2 (menaquinone). Though they are related, there is a big difference between the two, and one cannot substitute for the other. Many nutritionists still do not understand the differences. Vitamin K can be found in high amounts in most green vegetables, especially green leafy vegetables. Vitamin K2 (discussed in the next section) is usually made from vitamin K by bacteria in the gut of an animal. Most of the anticancer benefits are found in vitamin K2, but there are other benefits to regular vitamin K as well. Due to the ease of availability and the other health benefits of vegetables, I recommend getting vitamin K from food sources.

The following study is one of the few to show that vitamin K1 can prevent cancer (half of the cancers in the placebo group were breast cancers, and the other half were other cancers).

> "Higher mean serum vitamin K levels over the duration of the study correlated with lower cancer incidence ($p < 0.05$)... We also detected a lower incidence of cancers in the vitamin K–supplemented group... half of the cases were breast cancers (one in the vitamin K group and six in the placebo group)... Recent data suggest that the K vitamins may have anticancer effects. In conclusion, vitamin K1 supplementation at a daily dose of 5 mg does not protect against age-related decreases in BMD, but may reduce the incidence of fractures and cancers" – PubMed ID#PMC2566998 (2008) [443]

Increasing vitamin K1 (phylloquinone) was associated with a significantly lower risk of cancer and all-cause mortality. However, the study muddies things when talking about cancer, as it includes dietary changes of both phylloquinone and menaquinone (vitamin K2). The following study looked at "dietary intake" changes, with those consuming foods high in vitamin K having better health outcomes. However, these foods also have many other health benefits, making it very difficult to determine if the health benefit came from increased vitamin K intake or from the other benefits associated with increased vegetable intake.

> "Energy-adjusted baseline dietary phylloquinone intake was inversely associated with a significantly reduced risk of cancer and all-cause mortality after controlling for potential confounders (HR: 0.54; 95% CI: 0.30, 0.96; and HR: 0.64; 95% CI: 0.45, 0.90, respectively). In longitudinal assessments, individuals who increased their intake of phylloquinone or menaquinone during follow-up had a lower risk of cancer (HR: 0.64; 95% CI: 0.43, 0.95; and HR: 0.41; 95% CI: 0.26, 0.64, respectively) and all-cause mortality (HR: 0.57; 95% CI: 0.44, 0.73; and HR: 0.55;

> 95% CI: 0.42, 0.73, respectively) than individuals who decreased or did not change their intake… An increase in dietary intake of vitamin K is associated with a reduced risk of cardiovascular, cancer, or all-cause mortality in a Mediterranean population at high cardiovascular disease risk." – PubMed ID#24647393 (2014) [444]

However, most studies found little benefit to increasing K1 (phylloquinone) intake, anticancer benefits were mostly seen with vitamin K2 (menaquinone).

> Cancer risk reduction with increasing intake of menaquinones [K2] was more pronounced in men than in women, mainly driven by significant inverse associations with prostate (P for trend = 0.03) and lung (P for trend = 0.002) cancer. We found no association with phylloquinone [K1] intake. – PubMed ID#20335553 (2010) [445]

Most of the research shows little improvement in cancer risk by increasing vitamin K1 intake. I think this is due to using K1 in isolation. Vitamin K1 is found in green plant matter. When we consume it, the bacteria in our gut are supposed to convert the K1 to the more beneficial K2. In part because this requires soluble fiber to help feed these bacteria, this fiber is not found in vitamin K1 supplements. This process of conversion is what happens in a strong, healthy microbiome, such as that of our ancestors. Today, few people consume enough vegetables, or the variety, that our ancestors consumed. We also take medications (such as antacids and antibiotics) that reduce the microbial diversity of our gut. So, we have largely lost the ability to convert vitamin K1 to K2 and must rely on obtaining vitamin K2 from the food we eat (primarily from cheese, grass-fed beef, butter made from grass-fed dairy, and fermented vegetables). We have probably been slowly losing this ability since the start of agriculture, some 10,000 years ago.

The foods that contain vitamin K1 are still very healthy for us (in other ways) and we should still consume them. If we consume a wide variety of green vegetables and get our guts in good working order, we can probably start making some vitamin K2 again. So, my recommendation is to consume a healthy diet full of green leafy vegetables, and not to take a vitamin K1 supplement. The next section will cover vitamin K2, where I will recommend taking a supplement.

Recommendations

I'm working under the assumption that a vitamin K1 deficiency is not a good thing and may increase the risk of some cancers. If one is not deficient, adding more vitamin K1 may have no anticancer benefits. However, since vitamin K1 is very easy to get in the diet, and the food sources of K1 have other anticancer benefits, my recommendation is to eat more of those foods. You will receive more vitamin K1, but the benefits will most likely come from the other nutritional benefits of these foods.

Foods high in vitamin K1:

- Green leafy vegetables, including but not limited to: kale, turnip greens, collards, Swiss chard, spinach, mustard greens, parsley, romaine lettuce

- Many vegetables, including: broccoli, Brussels sprouts, cauliflower, cabbage (including sauerkraut and kimchi)

- Fish, meat, liver, eggs

❖ VITAMIN K2

AKA: Menaquinone

Cancers: Most
Body of Evidence: Large
Cost: Low
Recommendation: High

Vitamin K2 (menaquinone), though sharing similarities to Vitamin K, is very different biologically. However, you may still find a lot of ambiguous references to "vitamin K" that do not specify which one they're talking about, especially in older research. Because most of the benefits are found in K2, it is important to know which one is being discussed. Bacteria in the guts of animals convert K1 into K2; this happens to a much lesser degree in humans as well. It is thought that the human gut once had a much better ability to convert K1 to K2, but after generations of more modern living and altered diet, we have largely lost this ability. Another reason we may have lost this ability is that we became more efficient hunters and started eating animals that had already made this conversion for us. Large amounts of K2 can be found in the fat of animals that consume green grass, such as bison, cows, deer, sheep, etc. When we consume the organs, milk or adipose (fat) of these grass-fed animals, we get a good dose of K2 as well.

Here vitamin K2 was shown to work in conjunction with chemotherapy agents. K2 has a very wide margin of safety, and no toxicity level has been identified for it.

> "Consistent with the results of clinical studies, data from animal studies indicated that VK2 treatment significantly inhibited tumor growth, without any evident side effects… VK2 can inhibit the proliferation of cancer cells by inducing the cell-cycle arrest of cancer cells, in which inhibition of nuclear factor-κB (NF-κB) activity has a crucial role. NF-κB is a regulatory factor that can be simulated by cytokines to participate in the immune and inflammatory reaction… the induction of the cell-cycle arrest and apoptosis has a crucial role in the antitumor mechanism of VK2… In addition to PKC, protein kinase A (PKA), which can lead to cell-cycle arrest at the G1 and G2-M phase, is another type of kinase

involved in the mechanism of VK2 against tumor cells… In several cases, the combination of VK2 with other chemotherapy agents can produce stronger effects than the use of either alone." – PubMed ID#PMC5958717 (2018) [446]

The following study shows that vitamin K2 can substantially reduce prostate cancer growth and reduce tumor size through apoptosis). The study also references several past studies of vitamin K2 and its benefits in treating other cancer types. Note the 80% decreased risk in developing hepatocellular carcinoma!

"In recent years, several studies have shown that vitamin k2 (VK2) has anticancer activity in a variety of cancer cells… Our investigations show that VK2 is able to suppress viability of androgen-dependent and androgen-independent prostate cancer cells via caspase-3 and -8 dependent apoptosis… In recent years, various reports have shown that VK2 has antioncogenic effects in various cancer cell lines, including leukemia, lung cancer, ovarian cancer, and hepatocellular cancer. Although the exact mechanisms by which VK2 exert its antitumor effect are still unclear, processes such as cell cycle arrest, apoptosis and induction of differentiation appear to contribute to the therapeutic effects of VK2… a randomized trial of 43 women with viral hepatitis treated with high dose VK2 showed an 80% decreased risk of developing hepatocellular carcinoma… These studies thus suggest that the intake of VK2 may be beneficial in preventing the progression of prostate cancer. Moreover, VK2 is also shown to enhance the chemotherapeutic efficacy of conventional anticancer drug Sorafenib in hepatocellular carcinoma… there are no known side effects associated with ingestion of high doses of VK2… Our results show that VK2 treatment at concentrations from 50 to 100 µM concentration significantly inhibited the secretion of PSA… Our results of this study show that VK2 is able to suppress viability of androgen-dependent and androgen-independent prostate cancer cell lines in a dose dependent manner. We also show here that the reduced proliferation induced by VK2 is the result of caspase-3 and -8 dependent apoptosis. Thus, our study reiterates the apoptotic potential of VK2 against prostate cancer cells as has been previously reported for other cancer types… The anti-proliferative effect of VK2 was confirmed in vivo, where tumor growth was substantially reduced following treatment with VK2" – PubMed ID#PMC3767046 (2013) (Open Access license, attribute at the link) [447]

Samykutty A, Shetty AV, Dakshinamoorthy G, et al. Vitamin k2, a naturally occurring menaquinone, exerts therapeutic effects on both hormone-dependent and hormone-independent prostate cancer cells. *Evid Based Complement Alternat Med.* 2013;2013:287358. doi:10.1155/2013/287358

Though the following study points out some of the ways vitamin K2 treats and prevents breast cancer, K2's range of action is much broader than just breast cancer.

> "A significant dose-dependent, growth inhibitory effect was found when cells were treated at these concentrations. These effects were seen in both adhesion and proliferation phases and show a dramatic reduction in cell growth. Additional analysis of MDA-MB-231 cells treated with VK2 (100 µmol/L) in combination with a low-glucose nutrient media showed a further decrease in adhesion and viability. This is the first study of its kind showing the real-time effects of VK derivatives on breast cancer cells and suggests that dietary factors may be an important consideration for patients." – PubMed ID#26082424 (2015) [448]

Though "anticancer" is mentioned in this research, it is important to note the other benefits as well, such as anticalcification, bone forming and insulin sensitizing. The first two are from K2's ability to help calcium work properly in the body. Without K2, calcium circulates in the blood, eventually calcifying arteries; with K2, the calcium does what it is supposed to do, remodeling bones and teeth. The ability to sensitize cells to insulin can help diabetes, metabolic syndrome and even cancer. Diabetes doubles the risk of pancreas, liver and endometrial cancers, and it increases the risk of colorectal, breast and bladder cancer by 20% to 50%. This could be because cancer cells love sugar, and if our cells are not utilizing sugar (and insulin) properly, then more sugar is available to cancer cells.

> "Research has shown that vitamin K is an anticalcification, anticancer, bone-forming and insulin-sensitising molecule… Vitamin K2 has been shown to inhibit the growth of human cancer cell lines, including hepatoma lines, as well as to treat myelodysplastic syndrome." – PubMed ID#PMC4600246 (2015) [449]

Once again, a natural treatment, vitamin K2, can induce apoptosis (natural self-destruction of cancer cells) without harming normal cells in any way. A healthy body with a healthy immune system is normally able to deal with cancer as it develops. Apoptosis is one of the main ways it goes about doing this. Restoring this natural ability to fight cancer is of utmost importance.

> "We originally reported that vitamin K2 (VK2) analogs, including menaquinone 4 (MK4) but not vitamin K1, effectively induce apoptosis in various types of primary cultured leukemia cells and leukemia cell lines in vitro. It has also been reported by others that VK2 showed the differentiation-inducing activity in leukemia cell lines… These data suggest that VK2 also shows the differentiation inducing effects on leukemia cells which are resistant against VK2-inducing apoptosis. The dichotomous nature of VK2 against leukemia cells appears to

---

have clinical benefits for the treatment of patients with leukemias and myelodysplastic syndromes." – PubMed ID#11455981 (2001) [450]

This study from 1999 also showed vitamin K2's ability to induce apoptosis in cancer cells—in this study, specifically leukemia cells. Vitamin K2 seems to have cancer-fighting benefits across a wide array of cancers. This is not so much because vitamin K2 fights cancer, as because it gives our cells and immune system one of the raw ingredients that it uses to fight cancer. Vitamin K2 is not killing the cancer cell directly; it is restoring a natural function of the cancer cell, which is to self-destruct (through apoptosis) because it is no longer a healthy human cell.

"We have previously reported that vitamin K2 (VK2) has a potent apoptosis inducing activity toward various types of primary cultured leukemia cells including acute myelogenous leukemia arising from myelodysplastic syndromes (MDS). As previously reported for cultured primary leukemia cells, exposure to VK2, but not to VK1, resulted in induction of apoptosis of MDS-KZ cells in a dose-dependent manner… VK2-induced inhibition of cell growth, suggesting that caspase-3 is, at least in part, involved in VK2-induced apoptosis." – PubMed ID#10482991 (1999) [451]

The following review looked at vitamin K and prostate cancer. Here it shows a broad-spectrum benefit against several cancers, as well as inducing apoptosis to help slow cancer development and progression.

"recent studies reveal that VK inhibits the growth of cancer cells through other mechanisms, including apoptosis, cell cycle arrest, autophagy, and modulation of various transcription factors such as Myc and Fos. In the present review, we focus on the anticancer effect of dietary VK and its analogs on prostate cancer… In this review, we have summarized the recent progress of VK in various cancers especially PCa. Collective data from different studies indicate that VK is a potential anticancer compound. In particular, the following observations make VK a unique therapeutic agent for treatment of various cancers: (a) It exhibits a broad-spectrum of toxicity toward a wide range of human cancer cells of different origins; (b) It induces apoptosis by interfering with multiple mechanisms that are considered central to cancer development and progression; (c) It can inhibit multiple signaling pathways which are frequently deregulated in human cancers and associated with drug resistance." – PubMed ID#PMC5593683 (2017) [452]

"Vitamin K2 (menaquinone-4: VK2) induces apoptosis and differentiation in leukemia cells. We recently reported that VK2 also induces apoptosis in lung cancer cell lines. In the present study, we focused on the in vitro combined effects of imatinib mesylate plus VK2 on SCLC cell lines such as LU-139, LU-130, NCI-H69 and NCI-H128." – PubMed ID#15586222 (2005) [453]

Other Vitamin K2 Benefits

The following manuscript was published in *Open Heart Journal*, part of the *British Medical Journal*. Here they cover many of the additional benefits of vitamin K2 supplementation. These are very significant improvements in health risks. The improvement in insulin sensitivity can also significantly reduce cancer risk.

"A recent meta-analysis has shown that vitamin K2 (45 mg/day) significantly reduces hip (77% reduction), vertebral (60% reduction) and all non-vertebral fractures (81% reduction)."

"Vitamin K administration has been shown to significantly delay the progression of CAC (coronary artery calcification) and, in addition, it has also been shown to significantly delay the deterioration of arterial elasticity… Cross-sectional and cohort data have shown a lower risk of coronary heart disease (CHD), CHD mortality, all-cause mortality and severe aortic calcifications with higher vitamin K2 (menaquinone) intake. This was not shown with vitamin K1 intake"

"Warfarin has been shown to cause severe arterial calcifications in the aorta and the carotid arteries of rats. However, when high-dose therapy with vitamins K1 or K2 (100 µg/g of chow) was given, the progression of calcifications ceased and there was also a 37% reduction in prior calcifications induced by warfarin. Moreover, high-dose vitamin K1 or vitamin K2 restored arterial distensibility back to that seen in control rats.38 Thus, animal data indicate that vitamin K (K1 or K2) may be able to reverse arterial calcifications and at the same time improve arterial compliance."

Insulin sensitivity - "In a 3-year randomised, double-blind, controlled trial of 355 patients, vitamin K significantly improved insulin sensitivity in men with diabetes. Vitamin K is involved in pancreatic β-cell proliferation, insulin sensitivity, production of adiponectin and increased glucose tolerance, all of which may have contributed to these results." – PubMed ID#PMC4600246 (2015) [454]

Open Access citation - DiNicolantonio, James J et al. "The health benefits of vitamin K." *Open heart* vol. 2,1 e000300. 6 Oct. 2015, doi:10.1136/openhrt-2015-000300

Vitamin K2 can help prevent vascular calcification and osteoporosis, two very good reasons why everyone should take a vitamin K2 supplement. Vitamin K2 helps the body utilize calcium to remodel bones and teeth (bones and teeth are not static; they need constant maintenance by the body, and this requires calcium). Without vitamin K2, the calcium continues to circulate in the blood, which can lead to vascular calcification.

> "Vitamin K2 deficiency has recently been recognized as a protagonist in the development of vascular calcification and osteoporosis. Data reported so far are promising and, dietary supplementation seems a useful tool to contrast these diseases." – PubMed ID# 24089220 (2013) [455]

Several studies have shown significant benefits to those with type 2 diabetes. Because high blood glucose levels have been linked to higher cancer rates, reducing glucose levels can only help in fighting cancer.

> "In recent years, evidence from prospective observational studies and clinical trials has shown T2DM (type 2 diabetes mellitus) risk reduction with vitamin K2 supplementation. We thus did an overview of currently available studies to assess the effect of vitamin K2 supplementation on insulin sensitivity, glycaemic control and reviewed the underlying mechanisms. We proposed that vitamin K2 improved insulin sensitivity through involvement of vitamin K-dependent-protein osteocalcin, anti-inflammatory properties, and lipid-lowering effects. Vitamin K2 had a better effect than vitamin K1 on T2DM." – PubMed ID#29196151 (2018) [456]

> "Vit K2 administration could improve glycemic status in type 2 diabetic rats by induction of OC gene expression. Osteocalcin could increase β-cell proliferation, energy expenditure, and adiponectin expression. Different concentrations of Vit K2 were required to affect glucose metabolism and insulin sensitivity." – PubMed ID#29429532 (2018) [457]

Strategy

Vitamin K2 is one of the safest supplements one can take to help treat and prevent cancer, as well as help prevent heart disease. No overdose, or maximum tolerable level, has been identified for it. Taking vitamin K2 along with a vitamin D capsule each day is a very easy and inexpensive step everyone should take.

High-fat dairy from grass-fed animals (whole milk, cream, butter), high-fat meat/organs from grass-fed animals, true fermented vegetables, natto and miso are all very good natural sources of vitamin K2. There are good reasons to consume these anyway, and K2 is yet another very good reason.

If you consume green leafy vegetables on a regular basis, you will get all of the vitamin K1 that you need. Normally there is no need to supplement vitamin K1. However, if you don't consume these foods, taking a supplement with both vitamin K1 and K2 is a good idea. Remember, one does not substitute for the other.

Most people taking both a good amount of vitamin D3 and a vitamin K2 supplement will not need to supplement additional calcium. Eat a healthy diet that includes green leafy vegetables and hard cheeses (to avoid lactose), and this will meet the calcium needs of most people. Often, people develop osteoporosis due to not obtaining enough vitamin D3 and vitamin K2.

My recommendation is to take at least 80 mcg of vitamin K2 menaquinone-7 (MK-7) (and/or 1,000 mcg of menaquinone-4 (MK-4)). There is no drawback to taking more, and from my review of the literature, taking up to 250 mcg of MK-7 per day may show additional benefit. There are some differences between MK-7 and MK-4; I personally take a supplement that has both. If you must choose one form, MK-7 is the form you want to take. MK-7 is far more bioavailable (so you can take less), and it lasts longer in the body. In addition to MK-7, adding some MK-4 may slightly *Improve Your Odds*, but the research on that is limited.

> *Because of my melanoma, I don't get as much sun as I used to. This makes it difficult to keep my vitamin D levels up. Since there is no harm in getting plenty of vitamin K2, I use both a D3/K2 capsule and liquid drops (sublingual). Fermented vegetables, such as sauerkraut and kefir, are also high in K2, and I usually consume at least one serving of those 3 to 4 times per week.*

FOODS AND FOOD FRACTIONS

In addition to the diet information in Chapter 4, some foods should be consumed to supplement the diet. Many people eat foods simply because they are what they grew up with, or because that is what tastes good to them. However, in order to prevent and treat cancer, we must feed the immune system what it needs. Usually this means the type of foods our ancient ancestors would have consumed. Though these may not be the exact foods our ancestors would have consumed (they ate a much more diverse diet than we do), they are similar and contain many of the same, or related, compounds.

The foods listed in this section have known cancer-fighting properties.

❖ ASPARAGUS

AKA: *Asparagus officinalis*

I'm not going to spend a lot of time on this topic as there isn't a lot of research available, and no human in vitro studies, but there seems to be something to asparagus for fighting cancer, so it deserves a mention. Asparagus is high in folate (natural folic acid), potassium, vitamin C, vitamin B6 (pyridoxine), vitamin B1 (thiamine), vitamin K1 and fiber. It has a lot of antioxidants and has been shown to be anti-inflammatory. One reason for this is that it is also high in glutathione. Some sources say it has been used medically for over 2,000 years.

There is no doubt that asparagus is a healthy vegetable. Regarding cancer, asparagus also contains unique polysaccharides and saponins that have shown anticancer/antiproliferation properties against several diverse cancers.

> "Asparagus polysaccharide has been clinically adopted to treat various cancers including breast cancer, leukemia, and lung cancer... Asparanin A, a steroidal saponin isolated from A. officinalis, has displayed antiproliferative activities against many cancers, such as esophageal cancer, gastric cancer, lung cancer and leukemia" – PubMed ID#PMC4808884 (2016) (Open Access attribution available at the link) [458]

> "asparagus saponins (HTSAP), mainly protodioscin and HTSAP-10 have higher cytotoxic activity than HTSAP-1, HTSAP-6, and HTSAP-8. This study links the potential anticancer effect of asparagus to specific saponins and unveils the triguero Huétor-Tájar asparagus as a nutraceutical particularly in colon cancer therapies." – PubMed ID#30156381 (2018) [459]

"asparagus polysaccharide potentiated the effects of mitomycin both in vitro and in vivo. Mechanistic studies revealed that deproteinized asparagus polysaccharide might exert its activity through an apoptosis-associated pathway by modulating the expression of Bax, Bcl-2, and caspase-3. In conclusion, deproteinized asparagus polysaccharide exhibited significant anticancer activity against hepatocellular carcinoma cells and could sensitize the tumoricidal effects of mitomycin, indicating that it is a potential therapeutic agent (or chemosensitizer) for liver cancer therapy." – PubMed ID#24310501 (2014) [460]

Recommendation – Certainly try to include asparagus in your diet, along with a wide variety of other vegetables.

❖ BILBERRY/BLUEBERRY EXTRACTS

Berries contain many bioactive compounds that have shown benefits against various cancers. These compounds include a diverse range of phytochemicals (e.g., flavonols, phenolic acids, tannins, anthocyanins and anthocyanidins), all of which have shown anticancer properties in various research studies.

Some the most exciting studies are for the compounds anthocyanin and anthocyanidin (these two compounds are related, so I will usually just refer to them as "anthocyanins"). Bilberry, blueberry and hibiscus extracts are all high in these compounds. While reading this research, just keep in mind that the benefits of these bilberries and blueberries are broader than just these compounds; they are very strong antioxidants and are high in potassium and vitamin C. If you're looking for a tasty superfood, you need look no further. But for maximum treatment benefits, I recommend also adding a powdered berry extract.

The following study looked at two blueberry extracts (anthocyanins and anthocyanidins) and found that they were generally as effective against (B16-F10) melanoma cells as doxorubicin (a chemotherapy drug), with far less toxicity towards normal cells. Furthermore, they found that the blueberry extracts could induce apoptosis in the melanoma cells (through the upregulation of caspase-3 and p53 levels).

"studies found that anthocyanins and their aglycones selectively inhibited the growth of cancers, but exerted little or no effect on the growth of normal cells… blueberry anthocyanidins and anthocyanins exerted a strong cytotoxicity on B16-F10 (melanoma) cells… Yi and co-workers reported that blueberry anthocyanins induced apoptosis in HT-29 (colorectal cancer cells) and Caco-2 cells (colorectal cancer cells), and resulted in a two- to seven-fold increase in DNA fragmentation.

Faria et al. demonstrated that blueberry anthocyanin extracts significantly reduced the proliferation of two breast cancer cell lines (MDA-MB-231 and MCF7) and exhibited obvious anti-invasive potential in both cell lines… the anthocyanin-rich fraction of blueberries was found to inhibit proliferation, stimulate apoptosis, and increase lactate dehydrogenase leakage activity in B16-F10 melanoma murine cells. In another study, mulberry anthocyanin extract was proven to prevent atherosclerosis and inhibit melanoma metastasis… Faria et al. demonstrated that blueberry anthocyanin extracts significantly reduced the proliferation of two breast cancer cell lines (MDA-MB-231 and MCF7) and exhibited obvious anti-invasive potential in both cell lines… these results reveal that both anthocyanin and anthocyanidin extracts exhibited strong inhibitory effects against B16-F10 cells in a dose-dependent manner, and low or no cytotoxicity to L929 cells (non-cancerous cells used as a baseline)" – PubMed ID#PMC5492086 (2017) [461]

Open Access Citation - Wang E, Liu Y, Xu C, Liu J. Antiproliferative and proapoptotic activities of anthocyanin and anthocyanidin extracts from blueberry fruits on B16-F10 melanoma cells. Food Nutr Res. 2017;61(1):1325308. Published 2017 Jun 19. doi:10.1080/16546628.2017.1325308

This study found that of the 10 edible berries they looked at, the bilberry extract was the most effective at inhibiting cancer growth in human leukemia and colorectal cancer cells. This is due to having the highest concentration of phytochemicals, especially anthocyanins. Because of this, bilberry extract will likely be the best choice for all forms of cancer, followed by blueberries.

"Induction of apoptosis in cancer cells by Bilberry (Vaccinium myrtillus) and the anthocyanins… Among ethanol extracts of 10 edible berries, bilberry extract was found to be the most effective at inhibiting the growth of HL60 human leukemia cells and HCT116 human colon carcinoma cells… bilberry contained the largest amounts of phenolic compounds, including anthocyanins, and showed the greatest 1,1-diphenyl-2-picrylhydrazyl (DPPH) radical scavenging activity. Pure delphinidin and malvidin, like the glycosides isolated from the bilberry extract, induced apoptosis in HL60 cells. These results indicate that the bilberry extract and the anthocyanins, bearing delphinidin or malvidin as the aglycon, inhibit the growth of HL60 cells through the induction of apoptosis. – PubMed ID#12502387 (2003) [462]

Anthocyanin was shown to be effective against two different breast cancer cell lines. They both inhibited proliferation of the cancer and acted as anti-invasive factors (preventing cancer cells from invading normal cells).

"An anthocyanin extract from blueberry (extract I) and an anthocyanin-pyruvic acid adduct extract (extract II) were tested on two breast cancer cell lines (MDA-

MB-231 and MCF7)… Both extracts (250 µg/mL) demonstrated significant antiinvasive potential in both cell lines. Furthermore, they did not demonstrate any capacity for chemotaxis. In conclusion, blueberry anthocyanins and the respective anthocyanin-pyruvic acid adducts demonstrated anticancer properties by inhibiting cancer cell proliferation and by acting as cell antiinvasive factors and chemoinhibitors." – PubMed ID#20564502 (2010) [463]

The following research study looked at how various fruits and vegetables affected the relative risk of developing estrogen receptor (ER)-negative breast cancer. What they found was a clear association for lower ER breast cancer rates from blueberry, peach, strawberries and winter squash consumption. The relative risk reduction for blueberries was exceptionally high.

"During 24 years of follow-up, we documented 792 cases of ER− post menopausal breast cancer. Intakes of total fruits plus vegetables and total vegetables were only marginally associated with lower risk of ER− breast cancer (table 2). On the other hand, there was no association with total fruits intake. When we explored the associations with individual fruits and vegetables, we noted a RR of 0.82 for an increment of 2 servings/week of berries. When we separately examined strawberries and blueberries, the two berries item in our FFQ, the RR for every 2 servings/week for strawberries was 0.80, and for blueberries was 0.67." – PubMed ID#PMC3641647 (2013) [464]

Again, anthocyanin is one of the active ingredients in bilberry, blueberry and (to a lesser extent) hibiscus extracts. ARF below stands for "anthocyanin rich fractions." ARF-T was simply one of the distributers.

"The anthocyanin rich-fraction… was shown to have the highest anthocyanin content and antioxidant activity, and inhibited B16-F10 melanoma murine cells proliferation at concentrations higher than 500 µg/ml. In addition, ARF-T stimulated apoptosis and increased total LDH activity in metastatic B16-F10 melanoma murine cells. These results indicate that the anthocyanins from blueberry cultivar could be used as a chemopreventive or adjuvant treatment for metastasis control." – PubMed ID#23890760 (2013) [465]

Another study showing that anthocyanins from blueberries and bilberries both prevented proliferation and triggered apoptosis. Reenabled apoptosis in cancer cells is a very important part of stopping cancer growth and treating existing tumors.

"Antiproliferative and proapoptotic activities of anthocyanin and anthocyanidin extracts from blueberry fruits on B16-F10 melanoma cells… Anthocyanins have been proven to affect multiple cancer-associated processes in different cancer cell lines. However, relatively few studies have investigated the effects of blueberry anthocyanins on metastatic melanoma. Thus, this study focuses on evaluating the chemopreventive potential of blueberry anthocyanins and their aglycones (anthocyanidins) in B16-F10 melanoma cells… These data suggest that both anthocyanin and anthocyanidin extracts inhibit the proliferation and trigger the apoptosis of B16-F10 cells" – PubMed ID#28680383 (2017) [466]

Recommendations

I'm impressed by the quantity and quality of the research on this. Even though a lot of the research has been on melanoma (which is the type of cancer I had), there is enough research on several types of cancer to lead me to believe that these berries should show benefits against many types of cancer and could be an important part of any prevention protocol. I personally use a powdered bilberry extract and take about 1 tsp per day (1/2 tsp, twice per day). It mixes well into my chaga/mushroom tea base.

I recommend taking a concentrated extract so as to get the most benefit. However, it always helps to consume the whole food as well. Often there are cofactors in the whole food that might be missing in the supplement or extract.

Foods high in anthocyanin:

- Blueberries
- Bilberries
- Blackberries
- Hibiscus
- Black rice
- Black raspberries
- Red cabbage

❖ BUTYRATE

Butyrate is a short-chain fatty acid (SCFA) that is normally produced in our colon by certain beneficial bacteria. When the gut is working correctly, we probably make enough of this to meet our needs and help prevent cancer, especially colorectal cancer (CRC).

However, most people do not have the strong microbiome (basically, our gut bacteria) that our ancestors had. We eat a poor diet, don't consume enough soluble fiber, don't eat enough vegetables (especially dark green leafy vegetables), drink alcohol, eat too much sugar, are prescribed antibiotics/steroids/antacids, drink chlorinated water, have caesarian section births (so we're born with a weaker intestinal microbiome), etc., etc., etc. All of this adds up to the fact that for many or most of us, our guts simply do not produce as much butyrate as our bodies need.

Colorectal cancer is probably the most studied cancer for butyrate benefits, as butyrate feeds the epithelial cells of the colon. In the following study it was shown the butyrate decreases cancer cell proliferation, helps the immune system "see" cancer cells better, and induces apoptosis in colorectal cancer cells. It can also help decrease proliferation of CRC.

> "Colorectal cancer is characterized by an increase in the utilization of glucose and a diminishment in the oxidation of butyrate, which is a short chain fatty acid. In colorectal cancer cells, butyrate inhibits histone deacetylases to increase the expression of genes that slow the cell cycle and induce apoptosis. Understanding the mechanisms that contribute to the metabolic shift away from butyrate oxidation in cancer cells is important in in understanding the beneficial effects of the molecule toward colorectal cancer. Here, we demonstrate that butyrate decreased its own oxidation in cancerous colonocytes… At physiologically relevant doses, butyrate decreases cell proliferation, increases cell differentiation and induces apoptosis in colorectal cancer cells… butyrate has been shown to decrease proliferation in cancerous colonocytes and increase proliferation in non-cancerous colonocytes" – PubMed ID#PMC6007476 (2018) (Open Access attribution available at the link) [467]
>
> "Colorectal cancer (CRC) is one of the most common solid tumors worldwide. A diet rich in dietary fiber is associated with a reduction in its risk. Butyrate (BT) is one of the main end products of anaerobic bacterial fermentation of dietary fiber in the human colon. This short-chain fatty acid is an important metabolic substrate in normal colonic epithelial cells and has important homeostatic functions at this level, including the ability to prevent/inhibit carcinogenesis" – PubMed ID#24160296 (2013) [468]
>
> "A diet rich in fiber is associated with a low risk of developing colorectal cancer. The fermentation of the dietary fiber by intestinal microflora results in production of butyrate, which plays a plurifunctional role on the colonocytes, and it has also been reported as a chemopreventive agent" – PubMed ID#26224132 (2015) [469]

Breast Cancer

"NaBu induced a dose and time-dependent cell toxicity in breast cancer cells which was related to the cell cycle arrest and induction of apoptosis… Moreover, sodium butyrate induced both intrinsic and extrinsic pathway of apoptosis in human pancreatic cancer cell lines… The results of the current study also our previous study [20] have revealed that sodium butyrate deceased the rate of viable breast cancer cells in a dose and time dependent manner… The data presented herein demonstrated that sodium butyrate manipulates breast cancer cell growth and mediates induction of apoptosis through activation of caspase 3 and 8, enhancement of intracellular ROS level, depletion of mitochondrial membrane potential ($\Delta\psi$m) and induction of cell cycle arrest. Also, our results revealed no significant differences on the effect of sodium butyrate on the aforementioned assays in normal breast cells (MCF10A)." – PubMed ID#PMC5669027 (2017) [470]

Pancreatic Cancer

"Pancreatic cancer is characterised by a highly malignant phenotype with a marked resistance to conventional therapies and to apoptotic activators. Here, we demonstrate that sodium butyrate (NaBt), an inhibitor of histone deacetylases, sensitises human pancreatic cancer cell lines to both mitochondria- and Fas-mediated apoptosis." – PubMed ID#16109447 (2005) [471]

Melanoma

"Conclusion: Sodium butyrate could effectively inhibit B16 melanoma growth through suppressing tumor associated macrophage proliferation and reduce relevant pro-tumor macrophage factors expression… NaB (Sodium Butyrate) could induce apoptosis in A375 melanoma cell line by up-regulating p53 protein [5]… B16 melanoma growth was suppressed in vitro and vivo by NaB" – PubMed ID#PMC4443161 (2015) [472]

It has been known for some time that butyrate produced in the colon gets absorbed into the systemic environment (e.g., the bloodstream), where it can have many beneficial effects. For butyrate to show in vivo benefits for melanoma, it is obvious that it is making it into the bloodstream. The following study proves this.

In this study from 1992, it was shown that butyrate levels would significantly increase within 15 to 45 minutes of the synthetic carbohydrate lactulose being injected in the colon (during surgery).

The beneficial bacteria in the gut were consuming the lactulose (which is not the same as the dairy sugar "lactose") and producing butyrate. The butyrate would then be absorbed into the blood.

> "The major end products of fermentation, short chain fatty acids (acetate, propionate, butyrate) were measured in portal and peripheral venous blood after the caecal instillation of lactulose at surgery in patients undergoing elective cholecystectomy. Blood samples for short chain fatty acid measurement were taken before and at 15 minute intervals... After lactulose there was a rapid rise in portal short chain fatty acids with peak concentrations being reached in 15 to 45 minutes." – PubMed ID#PMC1379496 (1992) [473]

Recommendation

The best way to obtain butyrate, especially for cancer prevention, is through a healthy diet containing lots of vegetables high in soluble fiber. This feeds our beneficial bacteria and allows them to create butyrate (and other beneficial SCFAs). High-fat dairy foods from grass-fed cows are also high in butyrate. Most Westerners no longer consume enough of these foods. See Chapter 3 for ideas about how to restore the microbiome of the gut.

There are butyrate supplements, and these can be very beneficial for increasing blood levels of butyrate. However, they should be unnecessary in the prevention of cancer if you consume a healthy diet (as described in this book). If you already have cancer, they can be useful to raise blood levels of butyrate. Right now, the level of evidence is not very high for most cancers; the only cancers I think have enough evidence that butyrate may help treatment are colon cancer and perhaps breast cancer.

There are many reasons to consume more vegetables, and those high in soluble fiber are also usually high in nutrients needed for a healthy immune system. The recommendation here is to eat more, and a greater variety, of vegetables, especially green leafy vegetables. Foods high in beta-glucans are also a good way to feed the microbiome (and thus make more butyrate), and oatmeal and mushrooms are very high in beta-glucans.

❖ CRUCIFEROUS VEGETABLES

Cruciferous vegetables (CVs) such as broccoli, Brussels sprouts, cabbage and cauliflower contain a range of benefits. When they say "eat your vegetables," this is a great place to start! This is one food that has strong evidence of reducing one's cancer risk.

There are many research studies showing CVs can benefit:

- High blood pressure
- Heart disease
- Kidney disease
- Diabetes
- Neurodegenerative disease
- Atherosclerotic vascular disease
- And, of course, cancer!

Eating just 3 to 5 servings of cruciferous vegetables per week can result in a 50% to 60% reduction in cancer risk! These results are even better than when looking at "all fruits and vegetables" (which saw a 20% to 50% reduction—but that diet would also have included some cruciferous vegetables) and "green leafy vegetables." (Brassica = cruciferous vegetables)

> "eating 3–5 servings of crucifers a week (the highest US intake group), are often associated with a 50%, or even 60% decrease in (cancer) risk compared to those who eat fewer than one serving of crucifers per week" – PubMed ID#18327874 (2008, from the full study) [474]

> "The consumption of both alliaceous and cruciferous vegetables have been associated with health benefits, including a reduced risk of developing various cancers including breast, prostate, lung, pancreatic and gastrointestinal (Herr & Buchler, 2010)… For cruciferous vegetables, these health benefits are associated with the consumption of glucosinolates, the sulphur-rich compounds that accumulate in cruciferous vegetables, and their metabolic derivatives" – PubMed ID#PMC5460521 (2017) [475]

> "The results of 7 cohort studies and 87 case-control studies on the association between brassica consumption and cancer risk are summarized. The cohort studies showed inverse associations between the consumption of cabbage, cauliflower, and broccoli and risk of lung cancer; between the consumption of brassicas and risk of stomach cancer; between broccoli consumption and risk of all cancers taken together; and between brassica consumption and the occurrence of second primary cancers." -- PubMed ID#8877066 (1996) [476]

The following study compared lung cancer risk of smokers who consumed high levels of "fruits and vegetables" to those who just consumed higher levels of cruciferous vegetables. There was no detectable risk benefit for the fruits and vegetables, but there was a 30% to 47% decrease in risk for those who consumed high levels of cruciferous vegetables. There is obviously something to this!

> "Inverse linear trends were observed between intake of fruits, total vegetables, and cruciferous vegetables and risk of lung cancer (ORs ranged from 0.53-0.70, with P for trend < 0.05)… Our findings indicate that cruciferous vegetables may play a preventive role in lung cancers that are smoking-related, rather than the more general effect of other vegetables and fruits that may be overshadowed by the strong effect of smoking." – PubMed ID#PMC2874783 (2010) [477]

One of the most beneficial compounds in cruciferous vegetables is sulforaphane (SFN). SFN is an organic sulfur compound created when glucoraphanin (found in CVs) comes into contact with the enzyme myrosinase, also found in CVs. The SFN is created when the cruciferous vegetables are chewed, mashed, etc.

Broccoli sprouts contain 10 to 100 times the amount of glucoraphanin than mature plants, making them an excellent source of sulforaphane (SFN). Glucoraphanin is one of the glucosinolates mentioned in the following study. Glucoraphanin is converted to sulforaphane as described above.

> "Epidemiological evidence strongly suggests that consumption of dietary phytochemicals found in vegetables and fruit can decrease cancer incidence. Among the various vegetables, broccoli and other cruciferous species appear most closely associated with reduced cancer risk in organs such as the colorectum, lung, prostate and breast. The protecting effects against cancer risk have been attributed… their comparatively high amounts of glucosinolates, which differentiate them from other vegetables. Glucosinolates, a class of sulphur-containing glycosides, present at substantial amounts in cruciferous vegetables, and their breakdown products such as the isothiocyanates, are believed to be responsible for their health benefits." – PubMed ID#23679237 (2013) [478]

This research shows that a consuming sulforaphane-containing foods (such as broccoli sprouts) can affect the epigenetic expression of genes passed on to a child in the womb. This can greatly reduce the risk of the child developing breast cancer later in life, while helping the mother prevent cancer in herself as well! Amazing!

> "Bioactive dietary components such as sulforaphane (SFN), an isothiocyanate from cruciferous vegetables including broccoli sprouts (BSp), cabbage, and kale, has been shown to reduce the risk of developing many common cancers through regulation of epigenetic mechanisms… These results suggest that a temporal exposure to epigenetic-modulating dietary components such as cruciferous vegetables could be a key factor for maximizing chemopreventive effects on

human breast cancer… The elucidation of the efficacy of early, in utero, chemoprevention of breast cancer using epigenetic dietary intervention is the most novel aspect of this investigation. Our study provides important implications for the efficient use of BSp during pregnancy and postnatal early life on prevention of breast cancer in later life, and potential epigenetic mechanisms may be involved in this process." – Cancer Prevention Research [479]

Of course, inhibiting metastasis is one of the most important attributes we can look for in an anticancer treatment. Rarely does the original tumor cause death; it is usually metastasis to a vital organ. Apoptosis (where cells are programmed to die if they become defective, such as in cancer cells) is also very important. SFN has shown both of these abilities.

"SFN inhibits the metastasis of B16F-10 melanoma cells in both in vivo and in vitro models… SFN-induced apoptosis was associated with the activation of caspases 3 and 9, Bax, and p53 and the downregulation of Bcl-2, caspase-8, Bid, and NF-kB. Caspase-3 is a most likely candidate to mediate SFN-induced apoptosis" – PubMed ID#21649489 (2011) [480]

The following research appeared in the *Asian Pacific Journal of Cancer Prevention*. The study found that SFN induces apoptosis in breast cancer cells, while reducing inflammation. When taken along with the chemotherapy drug gemcitabine, it showed even greater benefits and minimized the toxicity to normal cells.

"Sulforaphane inhibits growth of human breast cancer cells and augments the therapeutic index of the chemotherapeutic drug, gemcitabine… Notably, SFN was found to significantly downregulate the expression of Bcl-2, an anti-apoptotic gene, and COX-2, a gene involved in inflammation, in a time-dependent manner. These results indicate that SFN induces apoptosis and anti-inflammatory effects on MCF-7 cells via downregulation of Bcl-2 and COX-2 respectively. The combination of SFN and gemcitabine may potentiate the efficacy of gemcitabine and minimize the toxicity to normal cells… SFN may be a potent anti-cancer agent for breast cancer treatment." – PubMed ID#24289589 (2013) [481]

"SFN has several benefits and may be an effective therapy for the reduction of tumor size as well as for combating multiple pathways of cancer… Various studies reveal SFN to be an effective inhibitor of HDACs and an inducer of apoptosis through multiple pathways in different cancer types as well as a repressor of human telomerase reverse transcriptase (hTERT) gene and its protein product in breast cancer cells… There is more than just one mechanism by which CVs negatively impact cancer progression. Indoles, another derivative of glucosinolates, are found in abundance in CVs, and indole-3-carbinol (I3C) is showing promising evidence as a cancer preventive therapeutic." – PubMed ID#PMC4354933 (2015) [482]

"Amongst a number of related variants of isothiocyanates, sulforaphane (SFN) has surfaced as a particularly potent chemopreventive agent based on its ability to target multiple mechanisms within the cell to control carcinogenesis. Anti-inflammatory, pro-apoptotic and modulation of histones are some of the more important and known mechanisms by which SFN exerts chemoprevention. The effect of SFN on cancer stem cells is another area of interest that has been explored in recent years and may contribute to its chemopreventive properties." – PubMed ID#28735362 (2018) [483]

"Sulforaphane (SFN) is a phytochemical converted from cruciferous plants… Due to its extensive sources, hypotoxicity, and diverse biological functions, SFN has been intensively investigated in many cancers. For example, SFN inhibits the phase I enzymes but induces the phase II enzymes, promotes the apoptosis and cell cycle arrest, and inhibits the metastasis and angiogenesis. In addition, SFN has been demonstrated to target multiple pathways involved in cancer cells in combination with other anticancer compounds. For example, SFN potentiates the efficacy of imatinib and sorafenib against chronic myeloid leukemia cells and pancreatic cancer cells, respectively; in addition, SFN also acts synergistically with human tumor necrosis factor-related apoptosis ligand in advanced prostate cancer cells" – PubMed ID#PMC5099878 (2016) [484]

Recommendation

Don't just "eat your vegetables." If your goal is to "*Improve Your Odds*" against cancer, make sure you consume your cruciferous vegetables, including: broccoli, Brussels sprouts, cabbage, cauliflower, bok choy, kale, collard greens, Napa cabbage, mustard seeds, daikon and radish. You will get the most benefit from consuming sprouts of these vegetables. The sprouts contain 10 to 100 times the amount of glucoraphanin (which converts to sulforaphane (SFN)), which is what research shows has most of the cancer fighting abilities. These vegetables are also very high in vitamins, minerals and other phytonutrients.

Cooking these vegetables can destroy the myrosinase enzyme. Without myrosinase, glucoraphanin cannot create sulforaphane (the active, cancer-fighting compound). Researchers have found that steam cooking for fewer than 5 minutes will preserve myrosinase. Another good way to cook it is "sous vide" (where the food is sealed in a vacuum bag and then cooked in water). Boiling or microwaving for even less than a minute destroyed the majority of the myrosinase. If you want to eat well cooked cruciferous vegetables and still get your sulforaphane, consume a raw food high in myrosinase along with the cooked vegetable. Adding ground mustard seed, wasabi, arugula, daikon or broccoli sprouts or consuming with raw cabbage (such as in coleslaw) are excellent ways to restore the needed myrosinase. Mustard seed seems to be an especially good choice as it contains a more resilient isoform of myrosinase. [485] I make a coleslaw with raw daikon sprouts, a few small pieces of broccoli florets and a bit of ground mustard seed. It is yummy and provides all the raw ingredients needed for a good dose of sulforaphane.

The research on this is strong: Sulforaphane is clearly beneficial in preventing and treating cancer. So, it is worth it to include cruciferous vegetables in your diet and to consume them correctly.

You can purchase broccoli sprout supplements (in capsule and powder forms). Just make sure to purchase those made from the "sprouts"; if it just says "broccoli powder," it is made from the mature plant. Mature plant supplements are OK, but not nearly as good as those made from the sprouts.

There is a common misconception that raw cruciferous vegetables can be goitrogens (interfere with thyroid hormones). However, research shows that one would have to consume a very large amount of raw CVs in order for this to be an issue, and it will likely only affect people who are iodine-deficient. So, consuming a serving or two of cruciferous vegetables every day is perfectly fine.

I recommend consuming all these vegetables whenever possible, especially the sprouts. If you don't think you can consume one at least once per day for treatment (3 times per week for prevention), you may want to use a supplement as well. After researching this, I've added a broccoli sprout supplement to what I take, just to cover my bases.

Note: If CVs give you gas, you can take a supplement containing alpha-galactosidase (such as Beano), a digestive enzyme that helps break down complex sugars found in legumes (beans, peas and lentils) and cruciferous vegetables such as cauliflower, broccoli and cabbage.

❖ FLAXSEED

Flaxseed is often considered a "superfood" due to its many health benefits. It is very nutritious, containing high amounts of protein and omega-3 (ALA) fats, a good amount of soluble fiber and a variety of vitamins and minerals. Flaxseed also contains high levels of "ligands"; ligands are "phytoestrogens," a plant estrogen that can help us balance and utilize our own estrogens better (in both men and women). Some cancers are estrogen sensitive. Flaxseed is credited with helping lower cholesterol, lowering blood pressure, improving bowel movements, controlling blood sugar levels, controlling hunger, and yes, preventing and fighting certain cancers. Of note, flaxseed oil does not contain lignans and lacks the antioxidant properties of ground flaxseed, so stick to ground flaxseed as described at the end of this section.

In this study, mice were injected with breast cancer tumor cells. Half of the mice were fed their normal mouse chow diet; the other half had 10% of their diet substituted with flaxseed. In the group with the flaxseed, they found that tumor growth was inhibited by 45%. Though this may not translate directly to humans, the research is very significant.

"In animal studies with mice injected with breast tumor cells, feeding them with flaxseed caused a decrease in tumor incidence, number, and size… Their experimental study was conducted in mice to which tumors were administered, along with the introduction in their diet of a mixture of lignan. The result was a decrease in the tumor load due to the presence of flaxseed and lignan SDG in the mice diet… While the cancer was progressing, the mice were on a regular diet for 8 weeks after cancer cells' injection. One group was fed with 10% of flaxseed, while the other group kept the same kind of diet. The rate of the tumor growth was reduced by 45% due to flaxseeds" – PubMed ID#PMC5808339 (2018) [486]

Here the research study looked at breast cancer metastasis. Mice were injected with human breast cancer cells (MDA-MB-435) into the mammary fat area. After the cancer was established (at week 8), the mice were divided into two groups, the control group ("BD" below) and the group that was fed 10% of their diet as flaxseed ("FS" group). The mice that were fed flaxseed experienced a very significant reduction in metastasis to the lungs and lymph nodes: "Metastatic lung tumor number was reduced by 82%"!

"Dietary flaxseed inhibits human breast cancer growth and metastasis… Lung metastasis incidence was 55.6% in the BD group and 22.2% in the FS group, while the lymph node metastasis incidence was 88.9% in the BD group and 33.3% in the FS group. Mean tumor number (tumor load) of total and lymph node metastasis was significantly lower in the FS than in the BD group. Metastatic lung tumor number was reduced by 82%, and a significantly lower tumor trend was observed in the FS group." – PubMed ID#12588699 (2002) [487]

The phenols and lignans in flaxseeds have been shown in various studies to prevent cancer and help stop the spread of established cancers.

"Flaxseeds contain a good amount of phenolic compounds. These phenolic compounds are well known for anticancer and anti-oxidative properties… Flaxseed lignans play an important role in preventing various types of cancer specially the hormone sensitive ones… Epidemiological studies indicate that phytoestrogens rich diets reduce the risk of various hormone dependent cancers, heart diseases and… Anticancer activity of lignans is attributed to its ability to scavenge hydroxyl free radicals (Prasad 1997; Hu et al. 2007; Sok et al. 2009).

SECO, SDG also play an important role in reduction of hypercholesterolemia, atherosclerosis, hypertension and diabetes (Prasad 2000, 2004)… Lignans, enterodiol and enterolactone are believed to be partly responsible for growth inhibition of human prostate cancer" – PubMed ID#PMC4375225 (2014) [488]

The anticancer benefits of flaxseed extend beyond estrogen-sensitive cancers, such as breast cancers, to other cancers, even melanoma. Here groups of mice with melanoma were fed flaxseed as a percentage of their diet. Those fed the most (10%) had a 63% lower number of tumors than mice in the control group.

"The present study investigated the effect of dietary supplementation of flaxseed, the richest source of lignans, on experimental metastasis of B16BL6 murine melanoma cells in C57BL/6 mice… The median number of tumors in mice fed the 2.5, 5 and 10% flaxseed-supplemented diets was 32, 54 and 63% lower than that of the controls, respectively. The addition of flaxseed to the diet also caused a dose-dependent decrease in the tumor cross-sectional area and the tumor volume. These results provide the first experimental evidence that flaxseed reduces metastasis and inhibits the growth of the metastatic secondary tumors in animals." – PubMed ID#9500208 (1998) [489]

Once again, the following research shows that flaxseed in the diet led to a significant reduction in (mouse) melanoma metastasis to the lungs: 22% in the group fed SDG (flaxseed contains a large amount of SDG) versus 59% in the control group.

"Flaxseed is the richest source of providing lignan precursor such as secoisolariciresinol diglucoside (SDG)… It is proposed that the anticancer activity of SDG is associated with the inhibition of enzymes involved in carcinogenesis… Similar, the anti carcinogenic effect of SDG molecule has been observed in pulmonary metastasis, mammary gland and breast cancer metastasis. The studies showed that the supplementation of SDG in mice diet resulted in reduction of volume, area and numbers of tumors significantly as compared to control mice group. The two week supplementation of SDG in mice diet led to 22% more pulmonary metastasis tumors in melanoma cells than average tumors as compared to control group having 59% more tumors than average" – PubMed ID#PMC4517353 (2015) [490]

The amount of evidence for flaxseed (and its lignans) continues to grow.

Recommendations

As you can see from the above, it is well worth including flaxseed in your diet. The lignans work differently than most of the other anticancer food compounds, so the effects can work synergistically. But even by itself, the 30% to 65% reduction in tumors found in some of these studies is an outstanding improvement. I would try to consume a small amount daily.

Like most things discussed in this book, obtaining the full benefits of flaxseed requires a little knowledge and/or effort. To start with, if you just eat whole flaxseeds, they will mostly just pass through you; flaxseeds have a tough outer shell that won't digest in the human gut. Secondly, raw flaxseeds contain anti-nutrients; these are substances found in many grains and seeds and are intended by nature to help the seeds pass through the animal, so that the seeds can be spread by the animal rather than digested (with a pile of dung to help them grow). These anti-nutrients also interfere with our digestive enzymes and prevent nutrition in the other food we're eating from being absorbed!

However, there is a simple solution to these problems. Purchase sprouted flaxseeds. Sprouting bursts the hull (so that we can absorb the nutrition within), and the germination process neutralizes the antinutrients, increases the nutrition of the seeds and extends their shelf life. So, what is the drawback? Price: Sprouted flaxseed is about 2 to 3 times the cost of unsprouted. I would argue that it is well worth the price difference, especially if you are planning to consume the seed uncooked (as cooking can help reduce the anti-nutrients, but you will still need to grind the unsprouted seeds before cooking). In my opinion, nothing is more expensive than something that doesn't work. You can also germinate the seeds yourself. Simply search the internet for "how to germinate flaxseeds," and you will find instructions and videos.

Flaxseed lignans are available in capsule supplements. However, supplements do not capture all of the benefits of flaxseed, and they are much more expensive. This is one area where I think it is better to consume the whole food. I purchase sprouted seeds as I use them in what I call "sludge." I use 1 tsp of sprouted seeds in a drink that contains larch tree fiber, mushroom powders, liquid mineral drops, 1 drop of cinnamon oil, etc. You can also sprinkle it over salads or casseroles, mix it in salad dressings, soups or stews, sprinkle it over yogurt, etc. I find it very easy to use ground flaxseed as it has a very mild, savory flavor, much like mild toasted nuts.

> *Search Google for "how to cook with flaxseeds" and "how to eat flaxseeds daily," and you'll find plenty of ideas.*

❖ KEFIR

Kefir is a thick liquid, a yogurt-like, probiotic drink that is naturally carbonated. It has a slightly tart flavor, somewhat like buttermilk, but not as sour. Kefir has been consumed in basically the same form for thousands of years. Kefir is believed to have originated in the Caucasus mountain region, in what is now part of the Russian Federation. It was originally a nutritious dairy drink made in a leather bag and carried by horsemen, where it continued to ferment in the saddlebags. The fermentation process preserved the milk so that it could be carried for days or weeks while remaining wholesome. A benefit quickly noticed was that this process also allowed lactose-intolerant adults the ability to consume milk (in the form of kefir) without the nasty side effects; the bacteria in the kefir consume the lactose. Human adults have been mostly lactose intolerant (malabsorbing lactose in the small intestine) for hundreds of thousands of years. Kefir's beneficial cultures produce antibacterial compounds that not only help keep the milk safe to drink, but also help control undesirable bacteria and yeast growth in the gut. All the while, kefir remains a very nutritious drink, high in bioavailable forms of calcium, B vitamins, folic acid and amino acids.

"Anticancer properties of kefir have been linked to the presence of a number of bioactive components including peptides, polysaccharides, and sphingolipids which have significant roles in several signaling pathways and regulation of some cellular processes including cell proliferation, apoptosis and transformation."

Breast Cancer - In-vitro "After 6 days of cell with kefir products… the final kefir product (K4) showed significant dose-dependent suppressive effects on malignant cells proliferation with no inhibitory effects on normal cells."

In-vivo "The result of this study showed that 2 days cyclical administration of both products diminished tumor growth"

Colon Cancer - "Khoury, et al. also reported that kefir significantly reduced proliferation of human colorectal adenocarcinoma cells in a time-and dose-dependent manner"

Sarcoma - "One week after tumor inoculation, with oral administration of 5mL/kg/day of different treatments for 30 days, tumor growth was inhibited 64.8% and 70.9%"… Shiomi, et al.21 studied the effect of a water-soluble polysaccharide (KGF-C) isolated from isolated from kefir grain on the two types of sarcoma tumor cells inoculated in male mice. Oral administration of KGF-C, compared to the controls, inhibited the growth of both tumor cells which was measured by the difference between tumor weight in the intervention and control groups. Also, in vitro direct cytotoxicity of KGF-C on tumor cells was investigated. There was no or little direct cytotoxicity against the tumor cell based on the ratio of the dead cells to the total cells…

> In conclusion, evidence suggests a beneficial effect on cancer prevention and treatment." – Archives of Iranian Medicine, Vol 18, No. 12, December 2015 (Creative Commons CC BY 4.0 license, further attribution available at the link) [491]

In this study they found that a 2-day cyclic feeding worked best (compared to consuming kefir every day). Kefir was diluted 1:100 in sterile water and was used to replace the water mice received for 2 consecutive days per week. This goes to show that we do not need to consume kefir on a daily basis to receive benefit from it.

> "Administration of kefir and a kefir cell-free fraction (KF) to mice injected with breast tumor cells… administration of both products delayed tumor growth and increased the number of IgA(+) cells in the mammary gland. Changes in the balance between CD4+ and CD8+ cells in the mammary gland were observed in mice from the group fed KF cyclically for 2 d, such that the number of CD4+ cells increased when the number of CD8+ cells remained constant. Mice that received 2-d cyclic administration of KF showed significant increases in the number of apoptotic cells and decreases in Bcl-2(+) cells in the mammary gland, compared with the tumor control group… Immunostimulation by fermented milks as a means of keeping the host immune system in a permanent state of readiness has been shown to successfully prevent different cancers" – PubMed ID#17369232 (2007) [492]

The following study, published in the *Integrative Cancer Therapies* journal, found that kefir both significantly reduced 4T1 breast cancer tumors as well as substantially increased the immune system's anticancer T cells (500% to 700%). As described in Chapter 2, T cells are very important for fighting and preventing cancer (with or without immunotherapy). This study used "water kefir." From other research I've seen, dairy kefir probably works even better as it has a higher percentage of immunomodulating peptides.

> "kefir can aid in alleviating lactose intolerance, inflammation, and high total cholesterol as well as exhibiting immunomodulation properties. It has also been reported that kefir has the ability to induce cytotoxicity and reduce cancer growth in vivo…. A significant reduction in tumor size and weight (0.9132 ± 0.219 g) and a substantial increase in helper T cells (5-fold) and cytotoxic T cells (7-fold) were observed in the kefir water–treated group. Proinflammatory and proangiogenic markers were significantly reduced in the kefir water–treated group. Conclusions. Kefir water inhibited tumor proliferation in vitro and in vivo mainly through cancer cell apoptosis, immunomodulation by stimulating T helper cells and cytotoxic T cells, and anti-inflammatory, antimetastatic, and

antiangiogenesis effects… The percentage of migrating cells was reduced by 88.03% ± 1.44% when treated with 12.5 mg/mL kefir water. The same pattern can be observed in the invasion assay, where the invaded cells were reduced in number when exposed to higher concentration of kefir water, with 72.83% ± 4.01% of cell invasion being suppressed at 12.5 mg/mL." – PubMed ID#PMC5739168 (2016) (Creative Commons / Open Access license attributions available at the link) [493]

The following study looked at the effects of using kefir on leukemia cells. They found that it exhibited antiproliferation qualities (that is, it helped prevent the cancer from spreading) and was proapoptotic (it caused cancer cells to resume programmatically dying as they should, i.e., apoptosis).

"The results obtained in this study indicate that kefir exhibits an antiproliferative and proapoptotic effect in HTLV-1-negative malignant T-lymphocytes… This is also consistent with the previously reported antitumor effect of kefir on many types of cancer, such as slowing down Sarcoma 180 growth in mice by introducing kefir both orally and intraperitonially, inhibition of pulmonary metastasis in Lewis lung carcinoma by orally administered polysaccharide fraction from kefir grains, reduction of proliferation and apoptosis induction in Sarcoma 180 in vitro, as well as the regression of human mammary cancer demonstrated by Kubow et al… Kefir reduces proliferation and induces apoptosis of leukemic cells without exhibiting any significant necrotic effect on normal cells." – PubMed ID#PMC3064404 (2011) [494]

Stimulating, or modulating, T cell lymphocytes is extremely important. See Chapter 2 for more information.

"In recent years, reports have shown that dietary probiotics such as kefir have a great potential for cancer prevention and treatment… Kefir is fermented milk with Caucasian and Tibet origin, made from the incubation of kefir grains with raw milk or water… some of the bioactive compounds of kefir such as polysaccharides and peptides have great potential for inhibition of proliferation and induction of apoptosis in tumor cells. Many studies revealed that kefir acts on different cancers such as colorectal cancer, malignant T lymphocytes, breast cancer and lung carcinoma." – PubMed ID#28956261 (2017 – Medical Oncology) [495]

"Kefir is a unique cultured product that contains beneficial probiotics… (it) exhibits numerous beneficial qualities such as anti-inflammatory, immunomodulation, and anticancer effects… inhibited tumor proliferation in vitro and in vivo mainly through cancer cell apoptosis, immunomodulation by stimulating T helper cells and cytotoxic T cells, and anti-inflammatory, antimetastatic, and antiangiogenesis effects… The percentage of migrating cells was reduced by 88.03% ± 1.44% when treated with 12.5 mg/mL kefir water." – PubMed ID#PMC5739168 (2016 – Integrative Cancer Therapies) [496]

Fermented foods have been called "the poor man's dish and the rich man's medicine." They contain a large amount of beneficial bacteria, usually far more in one serving than your average probiotic pill.

When reading research studies, one needs to pay close attention to whether they are discussing fermented foods with no live cultures (such as alcohol, cheese and chocolate) versus those with live cultures (kefir, kimchi, certain sauerkrauts). Those without live cultures have been shown to have no added benefits, whereas those with live cultures do have added health benefits.

Recommendations

Kefir has many health benefits. Besides the direct anticancer effects shown above, it also helps to strengthen the immune system, heal the gut and restore the gut's microbiome (another huge benefit to the immune system). Kefir is usually lactose-free (as the fermentation process has consumed the lactose), and even the sometimes-problematic casein proteins have been predigested (meaning people who have issues digesting milk protein may be able to drink it in comfort). Due to the many benefits it provides, I recommend consuming it. Since one of the studies above showed that it had the most benefit when not consumed daily, I recommend drinking 4 to 6 ounces, 3 to 4 days per week.

Kefir is now available in most grocery stores, and I recommend the whole-fat, unsweetened varieties (sometimes called "Greek" style). If made from grass-fed milk, you will also be receiving a good amount of vitamin K2 (another cancer fighter). Another option is to make your own. It is very easy to do once you purchase the kefir "grains" used to make it. These grains contain a symbiotic culture of bacteria and yeast (SCOBY), and this is the traditional way to make kefir (store-bought kefir simply uses a bacteria starter culture). You can find instructions and purchasing options on *The Gut Health Protocol*'s website at this link. [497]

❖ LARCH TREE ARABINOGALACTAN FIBER

Arabinogalactan fiber, usually made from the larch tree plant, is a biopolymer composed of arabinose and galactose monosaccharides (simple sugars). In nutrition it is classified as a soluble fiber (soluble fiber dissolves in water or absorbs it; insoluble fiber does neither).

I first came across larch tree arabinogalactan fiber (LTAF) in researching intestinal health for *The Gut Health Protocol* (my first book, available on Amazon). This fiber has unique properties in feeding good bacteria in the colon, not contributing to bacterial overgrowth in the small intestine, and helping to control certain pathogenic bacteria in the intestine.

When LTAF feeds beneficial bacteria in the colon, it helps the bacteria produce the short-chain fatty acid (SCFA) butyrate (discussed earlier in this chapter). Butyrate gets absorbed into the bloodstream, where it circulates to the site of cancer cells. Butyrate has been shown to be effective in fighting many cancers (again, more information on butyrate can be found earlier in this chapter). Arabinogalactan has also shown strong immune system benefits that directly affect our ability to prevent and fight cancer. Here it was shown to benefit both breast cancer and pancreatic cancers.

> "sodium butyrate deceased the rate of viable breast cancer cells in a dose and time dependent manner… Our results showed that the cytotoxic effect of sodium butyrate was related to the induction of apoptosis in both cell lines… Natoni et all, have shown that sodium butyrate can also sensitize human pancreatic cancer cell lines to both intrinsic and extrinsic pathway of apoptosis… sodium butyrate exerts its anti tumorgenic effect via pharmalogical silencing of oncogene Bim1 in tongue cancer… The data presented herein demonstrated that sodium butyrate manipulates breast cancer cell growth and mediates induction of apoptosis through activation of caspase 3 and 8, enhancement of intracellular ROS level, depletion of mitochondrial membrane potential ($\Delta\psi$m) and induction of cell cycle arrest." – PubMed ID#PMC5669027 (2017) [498]

LTAF has been shown in several studies to improve the immune system. The following study looked at general immune system markers, such as NK cells (NK stands for "natural killer"—that's just how powerful they are). NK cells are a very important aspect of the immune system's ability to fight cancer.

> "Studies done in vivo report that the number of mouse spleen NK cells more than double compared to control after 14 days exposure to intra-peritoneally injected larch arabinogalactan… Grieshop et al.'s in vivo study on dogs, demonstrating that oral administration of larch arabinogalactan (at doses of 0.55 g/day or 1.65 g/day for 10 days) increases the number of circulating white blood cell counts… Larch arabinogalactan seems to positively influence NK cells, macrophage activities and pro-inflammatory cytokine production." – DOI: 10.1186/s12986-016-0086-x (2016) [499]

The following is only one of hundreds of studies on the benefits of strengthening and directing the immune system against cancer.

"Cancer immunotherapy seeks to strengthen and direct the patient's natural immune mechanisms against malignant cells, with the aim of targeting the disease while minimizing effects to surrounding healthy tissue (1). Preliminary data display the potential of immunotherapy, specifically natural killer (NK) cell-based immunotherapy, for targeting the quiescent cancer stem cell (CSC) population" – PubMed ID#PMC5585139 [500]

In this study appearing in the journal *Biomedicine and Pharmacotherapy*, they looked at the effect of a combination of larch tree arabinogalactan and curcumin (discussed in the next section under Turmeric and Curcumin) on the growth of breast cancer. The full study showed that the combination of arabinogalactan and curcumin could reduce breast cancer cell growth by up to 70% in vitro, in a dose-dependent manner. Each was able to reduce breast cancer cell growth independently, but there were clear benefits to using both.

"Combination of arabinogalactan (AG) and curcumin (Cur) significantly decreased cell growth in human breast cancer cells without any significant effect on normal cell growth. This combination could increase cell population in sub-G1 phase, which was indicative of apoptosis… Our findings suggest that the combination of AG and Cur is of great potential to induce apoptosis in breast cancer cells in vitro and in vivo." – PubMed ID#28152473 (2017) [501]

As indicated in Chapter 2 on Immunotherapy, increasing the number of Bifidobacteria throughout the colon is extremely important for a good immune response to cancer. Larch tree fiber feeds Bifidobacteria.

"Evidence also indicates human consumption of larch arabinogalactan has a significant effect on enhancing beneficial gut microflora, specifically increasing anaerobes such as Bifidobacteria and Lactobacillus. Larch arabinogalactan has several interesting properties which appear to make it an ideal adjunctive supplement to consider in cancer protocols. Experimental studies have indicated larch arabinogalactan can stimulate natural killer (NK) cell cytotoxicity, enhance other functional aspects of the immune system, and inhibit the metastasis of tumor cells to the liver." – PubMed ID#10231609 (1999) [502]

"These three studies performed in healthy adults suggest that larch arabinogalactan might influence TNF-α secretion and modulate the proportion of immune cells proportions" – PubMed ID#PMC4828828 "arabinogalactan, a highly purified polysaccharide… was effective in activating macrophages to cytotoxicity against tumor cells and micro-organisms (Leishmania enriettii). Furthermore, this polysaccharide induced macrophages to produce tumor necrosis factor (TNF-alpha), interleukin-1 (IL-1), and interferon-beta 2." – PubMed ID#2785214 (1989) [503]

In the following study, arabinogalactan was obtained from rice hull polysaccharides (RHPS). The end result should be the same or similar to the results from larch tree arabinogalactan, as both are highly refined into arabinogalactans.

"TNF-related apoptosis-inducing ligand, perforin, and granzyme B of NK-92MI cells and induced the secretion of IFN-γ and TNF-α. In the in vivo experiment, colon cancer CT26-bearing mice were used to investigate the effects of RHPS in cytotoxicity and anticancer. The results revealed that RHPS inhibited cancer weight and volume in CT26-bearing mice and significantly upregulated splenic cytotoxicity and NK-cell population." – PubMed ID#30471400 (2019) [504]

When trying to fight or prevent cancer, one of the most important assets is a strong adaptive immune system. You want the immune system to be able to build a strong response once it has identified the cancer threat. Here, the benefits of arabinogalactan on the immune system were shown against K562 leukemia cells using various immuno-markers.

"Arabinogalactan-mediated enhancement of NK cytotoxicity was not initiated directly but was found to be governed by the cytokine network. Generally, arabinogalactan pretreatment induced an increased release of interferon gamma (IFN gamma), tumor necrosis factor alpha, interleukin-1 beta (IL-1 beta) and IL-6" – PubMed ID#8439987 (1993) [505]

"Experimental studies have indicated larch arabinogalactan can stimulate natural killer (NK) cell cytotoxicity, enhance other functional aspects of the immune system, and inhibit the metastasis of tumor cells to the liver. The immune-enhancing properties also suggest an array of clinical uses, both in preventive medicine, due to its ability to build a more responsive immune system, and in clinical medicine, as a therapeutic agent in conditions associated with lowered immune function, decreased NK activity, or chronic viral infection." – PubMed ID#10231609 (1999) [506]

Recommendation

Larch tree arabinogalactan is a natural soluble fiber. It can be mixed into a drink, much like most soluble fiber powdered supplements. It can also be mixed in with food (such as a casserole) when cooking. The benefits extend well beyond those of cancer prevention and treatment; it feeds the beneficial bacteria of the gut. The beneficial bacteria provide many benefits to us, not least of which is the production of short-chain fatty acids, such as butyrate. Butyrate, produced by beneficial bacteria consuming fiber such as larch tree, has been shown to decrease inflammation of the brain (and thus, most likely, reduce the likelihood of Alzheimer's and Parkinson's, though the research is still being done on this).

As the studies above show, larch tree fiber has strong anticancer properties. This is in no small part due to increasing Bifidobacteria and the effects this has on the immune system (see Chapter 2). General benefits to gut health (such as increased butyrate production and increased microbial diversity) also help our ability to fight cancer.

I highly recommend taking this fiber on a daily basis. The fiber can be easily mixed in with water or your favorite drink; it has very little flavor, especially when mixed with something that does (even a tea). There is also no grit. It is healthy for anyone, whether they have cancer or not.

Consume 1 tsp, 2 to 3 times per day, mixed in with your favorite (non-alcoholic) beverage. To avoid gas and bloating, start with ½ tsp once per day, and work up to the full amount over 3 weeks.

❖ L-ARGININE

The following study shows the benefits of L-arginine supplementation in the treatment of breast cancer.

> "L-Arg (L-Arginine) is involved in many biological activities, including the activation of T cells. In breast cancer patients, L-Arg is depleted by nitric oxide synthase 2 (NOS2) and arginase 1 (ARG-1) produced by myeloid-derived suppressor cells (MDSCs)… L-Arg treatment inhibited tumor growth and prolonged the survival time of 4 T1 TB mice. The frequency of MDSCs was significantly suppressed in L-Arg treated TB mice. In contrast, the numbers and function of macrophages, CD4+ T cells, and CD8+ T cells were significantly enhanced. The IFN-γ, TNF-α, NO levels in splenocytes supernatant, as well as iNOS, IFN-γ, Granzyme B mRNA levels in splenocytes and tumor blocks were significantly increased… L-Arg supplementation significantly inhibited tumor growth and prolonged the survival time of 4 T1 TB mice, which was associated

with the reduction of MDSCs, and enhanced innate and adaptive immune responses." – PubMed ID#PMC4888479 (2016) (Open Access article, the full study and attribution can be found on PubMed) [507]

"We have studied the effect of dietary supplementation with L-arginine (30 gm/day for 3 days) on host defenses in patients with breast cancer… Dietary supplementation with L-arginine in patients with breast cancer significantly enhances host defenses and therefore may have a role in adjuvant treatment." – PubMed ID#8310409 (1994) [508]

"The amino acid L-arginine can significantly enhance natural killer (NK) and lymphokine-activated killer (LAK) cell cytotoxicity in patients with locally advanced breast cancer. In this study, the effect of L-arginine supplementation on natural cytotoxicity was determined in patients with breast cancer receiving CHOP chemotherapy… L-Arginine was able to repeatedly stimulate NK and LAK cell cytotoxicity in patients who were receiving CHOP chemotherapy" – PubMed ID#8076711 (1994) [509]

On the other hand:

"This study demonstrates that, in contrast to animal studies, L-arginine stimulates human tumours in vivo. This represents the first direct evidence that a single amino acid can modulate the behaviour of a human cancer." – PubMed ID#1315652 (1992) [510]

Special Note

L-arginine is an amino acid that is a healthy part of any diet. However, some cancer cells lack an enzyme (ASS) to convert citrulline to arginine. These cancers must rely on external sources of arginine to survive.

There is some indication that adding extra L-arginine to the diet may be contraindicated for those with certain types of cancers, such as melanoma, hepatocellular carcinoma, pancreatic cancer, prostate cancer and mesothelioma. These may lack ASS expression in the tumor lesions; therefore, those with these types of cancers should not take extra L-arginine without consulting their oncologist (see PubMed ID#PMC3534294 [511]). Arginine avoidance is not a good preventative strategy for someone without cancer.

Currently there is no evidence that dietary restriction of foods containing L-arginine is helpful (again, unless recommended by your oncologist). There are drugs currently undergoing research that block the ability of these cancer cells to utilize L-arginine, without harming normal cells. One of these is ADI-PEG 20 [512] by Polaris Pharmaceuticals, Inc.

This does not apply to most breast cancers; adding L-arginine may be able to help doctors treat breast cancer (see studies above).

Usage

This amino acid can be found in several food sources (such as turkey, pork loin, chicken, dairy and chickpeas). When obtained through food, it can compete with other amino acids for uptake in the body. Taking L-arginine as a powdered supplement between meals helps it to be more readily taken up by the body. It can be mixed into a low-sugar smoothie or water. I would recommend not exceeding the directions on the bottle unless advised by your healthcare professional.

This is one supplement that I do not recommend unless advised by your oncologist. Whether it is beneficial or harmful greatly depends on your specific type/subtype of cancer.

❖ MODIFIED CITRUS PECTIN

AKA: MCP

Modified citrus pectin (MCP) has been shown in research studies to help with persistent diarrhea, hypercholesterolemia and several types of cancer. The cancer benefits span several different types, including, but certainly not limited to: prostate, melanoma, colon, breast, multiple myeloma, hemangiosarcoma and liver. There are dozens of studies, most in vitro and some in vivo. In vivo research has shown oral intake to induce apoptosis and inhibit metastasis in melanoma cells. Angelan, a pectin-derived polysaccharide found in MCP, enhances the immune function of macrophages, B lymphocytes and natural killer (NK) cells. Studies on oral intake have also shown that MCP inhibits the growth and metastasis of colon and liver cancers in xenograft in vivo studies with mice (xenograft is where human cancers are grafted into mice, where they behave very much like they would in humans).

> "Heat-Modified Citrus Pectin Induces Apoptosis-Like Cell Death and Autophagy in HepG2 and A549 Cancer Cells… In vivo, it has been shown that angelan, a pectin-derived polysaccharide, could prevent melanoma cell growth and metastasis, and angelan was also reported to be an immunomodulator that enhances the immune function of B cells, macrophages and natural killer cells [8]. Oral intake of soluble pectin fragments inhibits the growth and metastasis of transplanted tumors in mice [9,10], and it has been shown that modified citrus pectin inhibits the growth of colon cancer and liver metastasis… Modified Citrus Pectin induced apoptosis in mouse androgen-dependent and -independent prostate cancer cells" – PubMed ID#PMC4368604 (2015) [513]

The following study found that MCP has strong benefits in fighting prostate cancer. It also works well as an adjuvant treatment alongside chemotherapy and immunotherapy drugs. Excess galectin-3 in the body can promote chronic inflammation, which is known to promote, or worsen, certain cancers. Galectin-3 can also be responsible for uncontrolled abnormal cell growth and cancer metastasis; MCP can help prevent this by naturally blocking galectin-3.

> "Due to its anti-adhesive, apoptosis-promoting, and apoptosis-inducing properties, it appears that MCP is capable of targeting multiple critical rate-limiting steps involved in cancer metastasis (Fig. 3). In addition, by inhibiting Gal-3 anti-apoptotic function and enhancing apoptosis induced by cytotoxic drugs, it holds the potential to increase dramatically the efficiency of a conventional chemotherapy." – PubMed ID#PMC2782490 (2008) [514]

Modified citrus pectin (MCP) is a known galectin-3 inhibitor. Inhibiting galectin-3 has been shown to help prevent metastasis and can help treat many forms of cancer. Here MCP was given orally to mice that had (xenografted) urinary bladder cancer (UBC). MCP was shown to have "remarkable inhibitory effects."

> "oral administration of MCP to the T24 xenograft-bearing nude mice inhibited the tumor growth significantly… overexpression of galectin-3 was associated with high tumor grade with lymph node metastasis, poor overall survival in UBC patients. Considering the remarkable inhibitory effects of MCP on UBC cell proliferation and survival in vitro and in vivo mainly through galectin-3, which is upregulated in UBCs, MCP may become an attractive agent, as a natural dietary fiber, for prevention and therapy of UBCs." – PubMed ID#29769742 (2018) [515]

The following research showed that MCP made prostate cancer (PCa) more sensitive to ionizing radiation (IR). Once again it was due to MCP being a natural galectin-3 inhibitor. There is evidence that galectin-3 inhibitors can interfere with metastasis, improve apoptosis and inhibit several forms of cancer.

Galectin-3 is a lectin protein produced by humans; it has various functions within the body. Galectin-3 is also upregulated by tumor cells; it physically blocks our immune system's CD4 and CD8 T cells from killing tumor cells (see Chapter 2 for an explanation of just how important this is).

> "Our findings demonstrated that MCP (Modified Citrus Pectin) sensitized PCa cells to IR by downregulating anti-apoptotic Gal-3, modulating DNA repair pathways, and increasing ROS production. For the first time the correlation between MCP, radiotherapy, and Gal-3 for prostatic cancer treatment was found. In addition, MCP reduced the metastatic properties of PCa cells. These findings provide MCP as a radiosensitizing agent to enhance IR cytotoxicity, overcome radioresistance, and reduce clinical IR dose." – PubMed ID#30043669 (2018) [516]

MCP is shown to block the negative effects of galectin-3. High levels of galectin-3 have been shown to promote metastasis and inhibit apoptosis. MCP reverses this. Here MCP shows a strong ability to block the galectin-3 protein and help "inhibit the growth and metastasis" of many types of cancer cells.

"The number of liver metastases in high MCP concentration group was significantly less than that in low and middle MCP concentration groups… galectin-3 protein on the surface of cancer cells would be almost completely blocked by MCP molecules… The results of our study show that MCP could effetely inhibit the growth and metastasis of implanted colon cancer in mouse spleen. The number of liver metastases and tumor volume in high MCP concentration group were significantly less and smaller than those in control group, indicating that MCP can inhibit the growth and metastasis of colon cancer in a dose-dependent manner, which is consistent with the reported data." – PubMed ID#PMC2778124 (2008) [517]

"Galectin-3 is expressed in many tumors and possibly plays an important role in tumor progression and metastasis… However, the intensity of the galectin-3 expression in tumors depends on the type of tumor, its invasiveness, and metastatic potential. For example, increased expression of galectin-3 is observed in colon, head and neck, gastric, endometrial, thyroid, liver, bladder cancers, and breast carcinomas… anti-apoptotic functions of cytoplasmic galectin-3 has been consistently shown in many types of cancer cells, including breast, prostate, thyroid, bladder, colorectal, pancreatic, gastric, myeloid leukemia, neuroblastoma, and some B-cell lymphoma… MCP was shown to inhibit in vitro tumor cell adhesion to endothelium138 and homotypic aggregation as well as in vivo formation of metastatic deposits of human breast and prostate carcinoma cells in lungs and bones" – PubMed ID#PMC4662425 (2015) [518]

Creative Commons attribution - Ahmed H, AlSadek DM. Galectin-3 as a Potential Target to Prevent Cancer Metastasis. Clin Med Insights Oncol. 2015;9:113–121. Published 2015 Nov 25. doi:10.4137/CMO.S29462

Excess galectin-3 has been found to be associated with many cancers, including melanoma. Blocking galectin-3 can significantly interfere with cancer growth and metastasis.

"Galectin-3 Contributes to Melanoma Growth and Metastasis via Regulation of NFAT1 and Autotaxin… In cancers, increased expression of galectin-3 has been correlated with the progression of glioma, melanoma, thyroid, pancreatic, and breast cancer… Silencing galectin-3 reduced NFAT1 protein expression which resulted in decreased autotaxin expression and activity. Reexpression of autotaxin in galectin-3 silenced melanoma cells rescues angiogenesis, tumor growth and metastasis in vivo… mice fed with Modified Citrus Pectin, a carbohydrate binding inhibitor of galectin-3, significantly reduced spontaneous metastasis of MDA-MB-431 breast cancer cells" – PubMed ID#PMC3500452 (2012) [519]

Here is another method whereby MCP inhibits tumor growth, prevents metastasis and promotes normal apoptosis (where abnormal cells, such as cancer, are programmed to destroy themselves).

"LCP (low-molecular-weight citrus pectin) effectively inhibits the growth and metastasis of gastrointestinal cancer cells, and does so in part by down-regulating Bcl-xL and Cyclin B to promote apoptosis, and suppress EMT. Thus, LCP alone or in combination with other treatments has a high potential as a novel therapeutic strategy to improve the clinical therapy of gastrointestinal cancer." – PubMed ID#PMC4870717 (2016) [520]

Recent studies have also shown benefits of using galectin-3 blockers along with immunotherapy. Although adjuvant research to date has been limited to pharmaceuticals, there is no reason to believe that modified citrus pectin wouldn't be beneficial as well.

Recommendations

This is one of those natural supplements that works across a wide range of cancers and has little to no downside. I would certainly consider adding modified citrus pectin to your diet. I've added this to my permanent regime of supplements as it has many health benefits beyond those of treating and preventing cancer.

Take 5 grams (usually one scoop of powder) per day for prevention and 10 grams per day for adjuvant cancer treatment, or as directed by your oncologist. I take this along with larch tree fiber and other powders mixed in with chaga tea. It can be mixed with regular tea, water, almond milk, etc.

Some people may experience a little gas or bloating when starting out. If this happens to you, simply cut back to ¼ the daily dose and work up to the full dose over 2 weeks. Usually this gas indicates you haven't been getting enough soluble fiber in your diet, or that you have a bacterial dysbiosis (too much of the wrong kind of bacteria). Normally your gut will adjust to MCP in 7 to 14 days.

❖ OMEGA-3 FATTY ACIDS

Cancers: Most
Body of Evidence: Large
Cost: Low
Recommendation: High

Omega-3 polyunsaturated fatty acids (PUFA), such as those found in fish and seafood, have a great deal of evidence showing that they can induce apoptosis in cancer cells and in vivo (in the body) tumors. It is selectively cytotoxic towards cancer cells, with little to no toxicity towards normal human cells.

The broad category "PUFA" is the type of fat found in "vegetable" oils, nuts, fish, seafood and grain-fed meat. PUFA in the human diet is made up mostly of omega-3, omega-6 and omega-9 fatty acids. Omega-3 and -6 are "essential" fats, meaning that our body cannot make them and must obtain them from our diet. In today's world most people have no trouble getting enough omega-6. Our ancestors consumed a diet with a ratio of fatty acids of approximately 1:1 omega-6 to omega-3 fatty acids. Today that ratio is closer to 20:1 (perhaps even higher) due to the high consumption of vegetable oils and the fact that much of the meat we eat comes from animals that consumed a diet high in omega-6 fats (this gets passed down to us).

> "while the intake of omega-6 fatty acid increased and the omega-3 fatty acid decreased, resulting in a large increase in the omega-6/omega-3 ratio from 1:1 during evolution to 20:1 today or even higher." – PubMed ID#PMC4808858 (2016) [521]

We are consuming too little beneficial omega-3 today, and far too much omega-6; such consumption has been found to be pro-inflammatory and thus can lead to cancer, impaired immune function, heart disease and other degenerative diseases.

> "Overconsumption of ω-6 PUFAs, and an increased proportion of ω-6:ω-3 PUFA ratio observed in general in Western diets, leads to the activation of pathogenesis mechanisms for a wide range of pathologies, including cardiovascular diseases, metabolic or immune pathologies, and cancer" – PubMed ID#PMC5776638 (2018) [522]

For these reasons, it is important that we both increase our intake of omega-3 fatty acids, especially those from fish (see below), and reduce omega-6 levels.

The important components of omega-3 are EPA and DHA. These components are generally only found in omega-3 obtained from seafood. When you see canola oil advertised as being "high in omega-3," this is alpha-linolenic acid (ALA). Canola oil/ALA contains no beneficial EPA or DHA. They will claim that ALA converts to EPA/DHA in the body; however, less than 5% of ALA gets converted to EPA, and less than 0.5% (one-half of one percent) of ALA gets converted to DHA. This assumes that the omega-3/ALA in canola oil is used uncooked, and that it hasn't already gone rancid in the bottle (a problem with all liquid PUFA "vegetable" oils). Do not rely on ALA sources to obtain EPA/DHA. The only reliable sources are fish, seafood and fish oil supplements. I find this to be a problem for people consuming a vegan diet. See the Strategy section below for how to consume a diet higher in omega-3s.

Omega-6 fatty acids are found in nearly all "vegetable" liquid oils. Some of the worst oil sources are sunflower, corn, sesame, soybean, cottonseed, peanut, canola and chicken fat. "Vegetable oil" is often a mixture of two or more of these oils. These oils should be avoided when practical. A small amount of sesame oil can be used for flavoring, but it is best to add it after cooking. For the best fats to use for cooking, see the Strategy section below.

Vegetable oils can go rancid very quickly, as PUFAs are simply very delicate. They also do not hold up well under high heat and light exposure, and thus are best consumed in their natural, fresh state—not from a bottle (which can vary in age and storage conditions). Again, researchers believe that humans in ancient times consumed a diet with an omega-6-to-omega-3 ratio of approximately 1:1; with today's diet ratio being approximately 20:1, very few people need to supplement omega-6. When too much omega-6 is consumed, it is inflammatory in the body, and excessive/chronic inflammation may lead to cancer. In fact, this is one of the primary causes of systemic inflammation in the body. Too much omega-6 can have negative consequences throughout the body. The following research shows just how important it is to improve our omega-6-to-omega-3 ratio.

"Excessive amounts of omega-6 polyunsaturated fatty acids (PUFA) and a very high omega-6/omega-3 ratio, as is found in today's Western diets, promote the pathogenesis of many diseases, including cardiovascular disease, cancer, and inflammatory and autoimmune diseases, whereas increased levels of omega-3 PUFA (a low omega-6/omega-3 ratio) exert suppressive effects. In the secondary prevention of cardiovascular disease, a ratio of 4/1 was associated with a 70% decrease in total mortality. A ratio of 2.5/1 reduced rectal cell proliferation in patients with colorectal cancer, whereas a ratio of 4/1 with the same amount of omega-3 PUFA had no effect. The lower omega-6/omega-3 ratio in women with breast cancer was associated with decreased risk. A ratio of 2-3/1 suppressed inflammation in patients with rheumatoid arthritis, and a ratio of 5/1 had a beneficial effect on patients with asthma, whereas a ratio of 10/1 had adverse consequences." – PubMed ID#12442909 (2002) [523]

"in contrast to traditional therapies, n-3 PUFAs appear to cause selective cytotoxicity towards cancer cells with little or no toxicity on normal cells... n-3 polyunsaturated fatty acids (PUFAs), eicosapentaenoic acid (EPA) and docosahexaenoic acid (DHA), can exert anti-neoplastic activity by inducing apoptotic cell death in human cancer cells either alone or in combination with conventional therapies… Several studies have demonstrated that n-3 PUFAs, EPA and DHA have inhibitory effects on tumor growth by inducing cancer cell death via apoptosis, either alone or in combination with conventional anticancer therapies… the mechanisms are still not completely understood… it appears to be selective, in that n-3 PUFAs cause cytotoxicity against cancer cells with little or no toxicity on normal cells… *n*-3 PUFAs, EPA and DHA can induce apoptosis in tumor cells *in vitro* and *in vivo*, in a dose- and time-dependent manner. They induce apoptosis *in vitro,* in tumor cell lines derived from a wide range of solid tumors including colorectal carcinoma, esophageal and gastric cancers, hepatocellular carcinoma, pancreatic cancer, cholangiocarcinoma, breast, ovarian, prostate and bladder cancers, neuroblastoma and glioma, lung cancer, squamous cell carcinoma (SCC) and melanoma" – PubMed ID#PMC4773771 (2016 – Open Access attribution available at the link) [524]

Seafood is the best source of omega-3 fatty acids. Though some seafood can be high in mercury, there are plenty of very low-mercury sources.

Low-mercury choices for obtaining omega-3 include:

- Atlantic mackerel – 2,270 mg omega-3 per 3-ounce serving. Avoid king and Spanish mackerel as these have higher mercury content.
- Salmon – Contains 700 to 1,800 mg of omega-3 per 3-ounce serving. The exact amount depends on the type of salmon. The fattier the better.
- Anchovies – 1,750 mg omega-3 per 3-ounce serving
- Herring – 1,200 mg of omega-3 per 3-ounce serving
- Sardines – 830 mg of omega-3 per 3-ounce serving
- Rainbow trout – 830 mg of omega-3 per 3-ounce serving
- Oysters – 370 to 585 mg omega-3 per 3-ounce serving, with Pacific oysters being the highest in omega-3
- Catfish – 391 mg omega-3 per 3-ounce serving. Not recommended for routine consumption as most catfish are farm raised and grain fed. This results in more omega-6 (745 mg) than omega-3. Wild-caught catfish are most likely much lower in omega-6.
- Shrimp – 450 mg omega-3 per 3-ounce serving, low omega-6
- Atlantic cod – 166 mg omega-3 per 3-ounce serving
- Lobster – 73 mg omega-3 per 3-ounce serving, moderate mercury risk for kids 0 to 5 years old

See http://seafood.edf.org [525] for additional information.

> "The omega-3 fatty acid intakes recommended for healthy individuals are not likely to be effective in chronic inflammatory conditions, given the level of omega-6 fatty acids in our diets [15,23,25,28]. If the ratio of EPA + DHA to AA in blood or tissue is the key factor, an intake of ~2 to 3 g/day combined EPA and DHA, or at least 2% of calories, is likely to be needed to result in a tissue level ratio of EPA + DHA to AA that approaches or exceeds unity. Doses generally exceeding 2 g/day combined EPA + DHA are needed to reduce prostaglandin E2 levels and doses of 3 to 3.5 g/day combined EPA + DHA are most often used in the treatment of hypertriglyceridemia or inflammatory disorders such as rheumatoid arthritis. No tolerable upper limit has been set for EPA and DHA, although the US Food and Drug Administration recognizes doses of up to 3 g/day as safe and the European Safety Union up to 5 g/day as safe." – PubMed ID#PMC4418048 (full Open Access paper) [526]

Strategy

Increase your omega-3 consumption from fish, reduce your omega-6 consumption, and in the process, improve your omega-6-to-omega-3 ratio.

- Ditch the vegetable oil. You can cook with refined coconut oil, avocado oil and ghee. For low-heat cooking, butter and olive oil can be used. Do not use any hydrogenated fats. Animal fats, such as real lard (not hydrogenated versions) and beef tallow, can be good choices if grass fed and organic, but if they are grain fed, their fat will contain high levels of omega-6. Chicken fat is very high in omega-6 and is not recommended for cooking. Simply reducing omega-6 levels will have a positive impact on omega-6-to-omega-3 ratios, and thus has benefits even without increasing omega-3 levels. Nearly all commercial mayonnaise is made from soybean oil and is thus high in omega-6. However, it is very easy to make your own using olive oil or avocado oil, and it tastes much better (see the following recipe [527]).

- Take a high-quality fish oil supplement daily. The goal here is freshness, the highest EPA/DHA levels and ultra-low mercury levels. Most companies include things like soy oil or glycerin (glycerol), in capsules, so I use a liquid form without these added ingredients. Be sure to find one that is quality tested for mercury levels. Supplements that have been steam or molecularly distilled have the lowest mercury levels. Once you receive your bottle of fish oil, stick it in the refrigerator, especially after opening.

- Consume more fish and seafood. See the listing above for those with the lowest mercury content and the highest omega-3 content.

- For cancer prevention, strive for 2 grams of EPA/DHA per day, from all sources. For adjuvant cancer treatment, discuss with your doctors whether you can take up to 4 grams per day.

> *I myself take a liquid fish oil supplement (Carlson). During treatment I took 2 tsp, twice per day, for a total dose of 5.2 grams of EPA/DHA per day. Now that I'm in complete remission, I have cut back to 1 tsp, once per day. I also try to eat more fish.*

❖ Soy (Genistein)

Soy presents a mixed bag of good and bad attributes. Remember that plants have incorporated various chemicals into their biology for their own purposes, not for ours. We simply adapted to consume and utilize plants, and their unique chemical properties, for our own good. Soy is not edible in its natural raw form; it must be properly prepared and cooked, or fermented, before it can be consumed. In their raw form, soybeans contain trypsin inhibitors that make them toxic to humans and many animals. Because of this, humans haven't fully adapted to consume soy; even cooked, many people are allergic to soy or have issues with some of its compounds (such as oxalates).

Soy contains phytoestrogens, which are plant-based estrogens. The research is mixed as to whether these estrogens can interfere with testosterone and affect the balance of other hormones. Soy also contains phytates and oxalates, commonly called antinutrients, which can bind (tie up) minerals such as calcium, zinc and iron, making them unavailable to us. A person with "leaky gut" (a common intestinal malady where small protein molecules can pass through the intestinal wall) can be functionally allergic to soy (where soy can cause symptoms without anaphylaxis).

Fermented soy products do not have most of these issues. Well-cooked soy products are also less likely to cause problems (e.g., cooking mostly neutralizes phytates), and not everyone will have problems with processed soy products. Tofu (probably the most commonly consumed soy product in Asia) is well cooked and well processed when you purchase it. Though it is not fermented, it is unlikely to cause issues from antinutrients. Fermented soy products such as natto, miso, tempeh and soy sauce are usually fine if a person is not allergic to soy. Supplements containing genistein isolated from soy are also OK—again, if a person is not allergic to soy. Be cautioned that most soy products today are made from GMO (genetically modified) soybeans; if you can find GMO-free or organic soy products, they are worth the added cost.

"Present in soy, genistein prevents any cancer cells that persist after surgery from invading new organs and spreading (Vantyghem SA et al 2005). This potential to arrest the spread of cancer is linked to genistein's ability to reduce production of the growth factor VEGF, a prerequisite for cancer spread and invasion (Ravindranath MH et al 2004)." – Life Extension [528]

"This review compares and contrasts literature in terms of the anti-cancer and cancer-promoting effects of soy isoflavones and estrogen in humans and animal models. In conclusion, current human and animal data provide evidence for several anticancer properties of soy and/or its isoflavones. Although the specific quantities and constituents responsible for the observed anti-cancer effects have not been elucidated, it appears that soy isoflavones do not function as an estrogen, but rather exhibit anti-estrogenic properties." – PubMed ID#23919747 (2013 metadata review) [529]

"studies show that among Asian women higher soy consumption is associated with an approximate 30% reduction in risk of developing breast cancer… Despite the interest in the role of soy in reducing breast cancer risk concerns have arisen that soy foods, because they contain isoflavones, may increase the likelihood of high-risk women developing breast cancer and worsen the prognosis of breast cancer patients. However, extensive clinical and epidemiologic data show these concerns to be unfounded. Clinical trials consistently show that isoflavone intake does not adversely affect markers of breast cancer risk, including mammographic density and cell proliferation. Furthermore, prospective epidemiologic studies involving over 11,000 women from the USA and China show that postdiagnosis soy intake statistically significantly reduces recurrence and improves survival." – PubMed ID#27161216 (2016, full study available at the link) [530]

"it has been shown that genistein inhibits the activation of NF-kappa B and Akt signaling pathways, both of which are known to maintain a homeostatic balance between cell survival and apoptosis. Genistein is commonly known as phytoestrogen, which targets estrogen- and androgen-mediated signaling pathways in the processes of carcinogenesis. Furthermore, genistein has been found to have antioxidant property, and shown to be a potent inhibitor of angiogenesis and metastasis. Taken together, both in vivo and in vitro studies have clearly shown that genistein, one of the major soy isoflavones, is a promising reagent for cancer chemoprevention and/or treatment." – PubMed ID#14628433 (2003) [531]

Strategy

If you have had breast cancer, or are simply wanting to *Improve Your Odds* of avoiding breast cancer, adding processed soy products, such as tofu, miso, etc., to your diet is a good idea. They can easily be incorporated into any diet. Try adding small squares of firm tofu to any broth-based soup or frying it alongside breakfast eggs (rather than potatoes). There are thousands of recipes online. A quick search for "tofu recipes" will turn up many; I found a "Tofu and Mushroom Stir-Fry" that looks very good.

Taking a genistein supplement is also an option.

❖ SWEET POTATOES

The sweet potato is a starchy vegetable (or tuber) that grows underground as a root. They have historically been a staple food for indigenous populations across the globe and have been cultivated for at least 10,000 years (probably much longer). Though the United States grows over 1 million tons of sweet potatoes each year, China grows over 80 million tons, and Africa, 14 million tons! China and countries in Africa also have much lower cancer rates than those in Western countries (yes, probably for many reasons).

Sweet potatoes are known to be packed with nutrition and fiber, and they contain vitamin B5, B6, thiamin, niacin, riboflavin, vitamin C, vitamin E, as well as beta carotene (a pre-vitamin A discussed earlier). Beyond these obvious benefits, sweet potatoes contain unique polysaccharides (complex sugars) that have medicinal properties (much like mushrooms do). They also contain "anthocyanins," a water-soluble pigment and a type of flavonoid with very powerful antioxidant properties.

Recent research of the ubiquitous sweet potato has been focused on proteins called sporamins, which have anticancer properties. Sporamin is the most common protein found in the sweet potato, comprising over 80% of its protein.

> "Proteins isolated from sweet potato can be separated into sporamin A (31 kDa) and sporamin B (22 kDa)… Previous studies have identified the sweet potato protein (SPP) as a type of Kunitz-type trypsin inhibitor (KTI) with potential therapeutic effects in a variety of cancer models. For instance, Huang et al reported that KTI purified from sweet potato inhibited proliferation and induced apoptosis of NB4 promyelocytic leukemia cells. Additionally, Yao et al showed that SPP inhibited proliferation and induced apoptosis of human tongue carcinoma… KTIs isolated from other sources… have been shown to exert antiproliferative, anti-invasion and antimetastatic activities in a variety of

malignant cells, animal models and cancer patients" – PubMed ID#PMC3671082 (2013) [532]

"Sporamin, a Kunitz-type trypsin inhibitor (TI) from sweet potato tuberous roots, has demonstrated anti-tumor activity through poorly defined mechanisms… Sporamin significantly inhibited the cell viability and proliferation activity and induced apoptosis in PANC-1 and BxPC-3 cells. Consistently, in sporamin-treated PANC-1 and BxPC-3 cells, the anti-apoptotic proteins Bcl-2 and Bcl-XL were downregulated and the pro-apoptotic protein Bax was upregulated. Moreover, nuclear factor kappa B activation and I$\varkappa$Bα phosphorylation were inhibited, and total I$\varkappa$Bα expression was increased" – PubMed ID#28714369 (2017) [533]

"We investigated the effects of sporamin, the major soluble protein with a kunitz-type trypsin inhibitory activity in the root tuber of the sweet potato, on cell proliferation, apoptosis, Akt/GSK-3 signaling and its related genes to provide more insights in the mechanism behind the inhibitory effects of sporamin in a human tongue cancer line Tca8113. In this study, sporamin inhibited cell proliferation and induced apoptosis in Tca8113 cells in a concentration-dependent and time-dependent manner." – PubMed ID#20408878 (2011) [534]

"Sporamin suppresses growth of human esophageal squamous cell carcinoma cells (ESCC) by inhibition of NF□$\varkappa$B via an AKT□independent pathway… In conclusion, sporamin may suppress the growth of human ESCC cells via NF□$\varkappa$B□dependent and AKT□independent mechanisms and may act as a promising natural therapeutic agent for the treatment of human ESCC." – PubMed ID#29039512 (2017) [535]

The "purple-fleshed" sweet potato is the one consumed almost daily by people in Okinawa, which has one of the longest life expectancies in the world and very low rates of cancer.

"Purple-fleshed sweet potato (PFSP) (Ipomoea batatas L. Lam) has been known to possess high amount of anthocyanins which contribute to its antioxidant activity… exhibited anti-inflammatory activities by suppressing the production of NO and proinflammatory cytokines, such as NF-$\varkappa\beta$, TNF-α, and IL-6, in LPS-induced macrophage cells. Anticancer activities of these extracts were displayed through their ability to inhibit the growth of cancer cell lines, such as MCF-7 (breast cancer), SNU-1 (gastric cancer), and WiDr (colon adenocarcinoma), in concentration- and time-dependent manner. Further studies also revealed that SP

> extracts could induce apoptosis in MCF-7 and SNU-1 cancer cells through extrinsic and intrinsic pathway" – PubMed ID#26509161 (2015) [536]

> "Ipomoea batatas (L.) Lam, also known as sweet potato, is an extremely versatile and delicious vegetable that possesses high nutritional value. It is also a valuable medicinal plant having anti-cancer, antidiabetic, and anti-inflammatory activities. Sweet potato is now considered a valuable source of unique natural products, including some that can be used in the development of medicines against various diseases and in making industrial products." – PubMed ID#24921903 (2014) [537]

Sweet potato proteins (sporamins, or SPP below) have been shown to decrease proliferation and metastasis with several different cancers; this has been shown both in vitro and in vivo (with human cancers xenografted into mice or rats). The following study looked at the effect of sporamins on colorectal and lung cancers (ip = intraperitoneal, an injection into the body cavity; ig = intragastric, infusion via a stomach tube). The exciting part here is that "significant" benefits were seen in vivo even if the proteins were consumed orally. This means benefits should be seen when consuming sweet potatoes as a normal part of your diet.

> "Notably, ig and ip administration of SPP induced a significant decrease in spontaneous pulmonary metastatic nodule formation in C57 BL/6 mice (21.0 ± 12.3 and 27.3 ± 12.7 nodules/lung vs 42.5 ± 4.5 nodules/lung in controls, respectively, P < 0.05) after 25 d treatment. Moreover, the average weight of primary tumor nodules in the hind leg of mice decreased from 8.2 ± 1.3 g/mice in the control to 6.1 ± 1.4 g/mice in the ip group (P = 0.035)... SPP exerts significant antiproliferative and antimetastatic effects on human colorectal cancer cell lines, both in vitro and in vivo." – PubMed ID#PMC3671082 (2013) [538]

Anthocyanins are found in many fruits and vegetables, including: eggplant, purple corn, red cabbage, purple cauliflower, bilberries, blueberries, raspberries and the purple Okinawan sweet potato. Anthocyanins have been found to have anticancer properties against several kinds of cancer, including (but not limited to): breast, skin (melanoma), leukemia, colon, liver, fibrosarcoma, lung, pancreatic and prostate cancers, in both in vitro and in vivo studies. They work through various mechanisms, including inducing apoptosis in cancer cells, inhibiting angiogenesis (the creation of new blood vessels to tumors) and inhibiting metastasis. Though I don't think pure anthocyanin supplements are available (at least not over the counter), you can get bilberry extracts that are very high in anthocyanins; these are usually sold for eye health.

> "Anthocyanins are a class of water□soluble flavonoids, which show a range of pharmacological effects, such as prevention of cardiovascular disease, obesity

control and antitumour activity. Their potential antitumour effects are reported to be based on a wide variety of biological activities including antioxidant; anti☐ inflammation; anti☐mutagenesis; induction of differentiation; inhibiting proliferation by modulating signal transduction pathways, inducing cell cycle arrest and stimulating apoptosis or autophagy of cancer cells; anti☐invasion; anti☐metastasis; reversing drug resistance of cancer cells and increasing their sensitivity to chemotherapy." – PubMed ID#PMC5429338 (2017) [539]

Recommendations

Though sweet potatoes have some obvious beneficial nutritional properties, they are also high in carbohydrates and sugar; 1 cup of cooked and cubed sweet potato, about 200 grams, contains approximately 41 total grams of carbohydrates, of which 6.5 grams are fiber and 13 grams are sugar. If you are on a low-sugar or ketogenic diet (as discussed in Chapter 4), you will need to restrict how much sweet potato you consume, but even a little can be beneficial. If you are on a low-sugar diet, you can consume up to ½ cup per day (1 medium sweet potato, defined as approximately 5" long by 2" in diameter). It will have about 17 grams of net carbohydrates. Depending on other carbohydrates you've consumed that day, you can still remain in ketosis (most people can remain in ketosis while consuming up to 50 grams of carbohydrates per day, and more if you exercise).

It is a good idea to consume a little sweet potato on a regular basis, especially purple sweet potatoes when you can find them. We need a variety of vegetables each day, but only a small amount of each is necessary. For that reason, soups, stews and stir-fries make an excellent way to consume this variety. Soups and stews also keep well and can even be frozen. Your soup or stew can be thought of as your tasty nutritional cancer supplement, as it should contain a variety of cancer-fighting vegetables (I even add soluble fiber powders to mine). You can make it in quantity and then consume 1 to 3 cups per day (you can eat more if it is relatively low-carb) as a side to whatever else you are eating.

Try to consume a minimum of ½ cup of sweet potato, 3 times per week.

❖ TAURINE

Taurine is an amino acid with benefits throughout the body. Concentrations of taurine are naturally found in the brain, heart, spinal cord, muscles and other organs. Though taurine is not considered "essential" (as the body can make small amounts of it), dietary consumption of taurine is needed for optimal health, and therefore it is often referred to as "conditionally essential." It was first identified in the bile of the ox (*Bos taurus*), thus its name. Taurine, as an amino acid, is a building block of proteins and can be found in seafood, beef, lamb, dark chicken/turkey meat and eggs; smaller amounts can be found in seaweed. One of the primary jobs of taurine (or glycine) is to conjugate with bile acid to form bile salts; without it, bile cannot solubilize fats (and fat-soluble vitamins) in the gut, which facilitates their digestion and absorption.

Even though it isn't difficult to obtain taurine in the diet, many studies have shown benefits to supplementation. Taurine has been shown to naturally lower cholesterol, improve the action of insulin (benefiting diabetics), treat gallbladder disease, reduce blood pressure and treat heart disease, and it has cytoprotective properties (protecting cells from harmful substances). It has been proposed as adjuvant therapy for several other diseases and conditions.

Taurine has been shown in several studies to have anti-tumor effects (in many different types of cancer) by reducing proliferation, increasing apoptosis and controlling inflammation. It has also shown benefits in adjuvant therapy alongside chemotherapy drugs.

> "In this study, we found that taurine inhibits the proliferation of murine melanoma B16F10 cells via apoptosis. Taurine can block melanoma cell proliferation and induce apoptosis through a mitochondrial pathway." -- DOI 10.1007/978-3-319-15126-7 (2015) [540]

PUMA and BAX, mentioned below, are pro-apoptotic, meaning that they encourage apoptosis. Taurine was found to upregulate compounds in tumors. This study looked at lung cancer cells, but the effect has been seen in several diverse cancers (such as colorectal and breast cancers).

> "Expression of PUMA and Bax were upregulated in the xenograft tumors following taurine treatment, whereas Bcl-2 was downregulated. In addition, the inhibitory effect of taurine and exogenous PUMA on tumor growth was significantly higher than that of a single treatment of taurine or exogenous PUMA. It can therefore be concluded that taurine can inhibit cell proliferation of the human lung cancer A549 cell line and the growth of the xenograft tumors, whereas PUMA serves an important role in taurine-induced growth suppression… serum level of taurine was found to be significantly lower in patients with breast cancer than in patients in the high-risk breast cancer group or the healthy control group… it was also demonstrated that taurine could induce apoptosis and suppress proliferation in colorectal and breast cancer cells… PUMA serves a critical role in the action of taurine against lung cancer… The combined use of taurine and the chemotherapeutic agent cisplatin enhanced the antitumor effect" – PubMed ID#PMC5840730 (2018 – Open Access attribution at the link) [541]

Taurine was studied here for its ability to induce apoptosis in breast cancer cells. They found that taurine increased "p53 upregulated modulator of apoptosis" (PUMA), also known as Bcl-2-

binding component 3 (BBC3). PUMA is a pro-apoptotic protein that induces apoptosis in cancer cells.

> "In the study, Tau (Taurine) inhibited growth and induced apoptosis of the two cell lines in a concentration- and time-dependent manner. Notably, the inhibitory effect of Tau on p53-/- cancer cells was clearly significant compared to the p53+/+ cancer cells. Further studies showed that Tau promoted apoptosis in human breast cancer cells and inhibited the growth of tumor in nude mice by inducing the expression of PUMA, which further up- and downregulated the expression of Bax and Bcl-2 protein, giving rise to increased activation of caspase-3. Collectively, these results indicate that Tau is a potent candidate for the chemotherapy of breast cancer through increasing the PUMA expression independent of p53 status." – PubMed ID#25395275 (2015) [542]

> "In B16F10 mouse melanoma cells, Tau functions by upregulating superoxide dismutase genes, glutathione peroxidase and catalase, while inhibiting cell growth by decreasing the concentration of reactive oxygen species in a dose-dependent manner. In addition, following treatment with Tau for liver fibrosis, the levels of hydrogen peroxide lipids, transforming growth factor-β and hydroxyproline in the blood and liver are significantly reduced, and liver damage and fibrosis are decreased… application of Tau with curcumin promotes immunity in an organism… the effect of Tau on the apoptosis of human cervical carcinoma cells has been demonstrated to be time- and dose-dependent" – PubMed ID#PMC4486811 (2015) [543]

Recommendation

Research studies used a typical therapeutic dosage of taurine of 2 grams taken 3 times daily (in addition to a normal diet). When I was treating my cancer, I was supplementing 3 grams twice per day as it fit into my schedule better; I also consumed a low-carb diet that is high in foods that contain taurine (now that I am cancer-free, I rely on diet to obtain enough taurine). Some studies have used up to 12 grams of taurine per day with no ill effects. The most common side effect of using high doses of taurine is intestinal discomfort. If this occurs, cut back on the amount you're taking.

Amino acids somewhat compete with each other in the body, and therefore when treating cancer, it is best to take taurine supplements and not rely solely on dietary sources. Some have speculated that it might be best to take taurine between meals (to avoid its competing with other amino acids); however, this has not been shown in research. I take it mixed in with my "sludge" drink that contains several different powder and liquid supplements, including larch tree fiber and mushroom powders. Because this is rather filling, I do usually drink it between meals.

❖ NUTS

Everyone knows that nuts are a healthy part of our diet. They have always been consumed by humans, even in very ancient times, in much the same form as today. No wonder our bodies have learned to utilize their goodness.

The following meta research study looked at 36 different observation studies, with a total of over 36,000 patients. This study only looked at "development" of these cancers, not treating them once they are developed. It also looked at mortality rates and found that nut consumption reduced total mortality (during the study period) in a "dose-response" manner. That means the more you consume, the better the results, and nuts decreased mortality from cancer and heart disease.

> "Observational studies suggest nut consumption is inversely associated with the incidence of cardiovascular disease and cancer... After summarizing all of the available evidence, nut intake was found to be associated with a decreased risk of developing colorectal cancer, endometrial cancer, and pancreatic cancer." – PubMed #18296370 (2008) [544]

The Nurses' Health Study is one of the largest studies of chronic health issues ever conducted (and is still ongoing as of 2019), with over 121,700 participants. There have been many smaller studies conducted from the data it has gathered. In this study, they found that nut consumption decreased mortality from cancer and heart disease in a "dose-response manner." In other words, people who consumed more nuts had better outcomes.

> "A large cohort study using data from the Nurses' Health Study and the Health Professionals Follow-up Study found that nut consumption could decrease total mortality in a dose–response manner. Moreover, nut consumption was associated with decreased mortality from cancer and heart disease... practical recommendation for individuals interested in making better food choices to reduce the risk of cancer and heart disease is to consume nuts 4–5 times per week, to aim for a serving size of 1–1.5 ounces... Overall, nut consumption was significantly associated with a reduced risk of developing cancer (RR 0.85, 95%CI 0.76–0.95; I2 66.5%)." – PubMed ID#PMC4560032 (2015) [545]

This meta-analysis looked at 29 different studies on the health benefits of nuts. This also showed an association with reduced risk of cancer.

"Higher nut intake is associated with reduced risk of cardiovascular disease, total cancer and all-cause mortality, and mortality from respiratory disease, diabetes, and infections." – PubMed #PMC5137221 (2016) [546]

"During 3,038,853 person-years of follow-up, 16,200 women and 11,229 men died. Nut consumption was inversely associated with total mortality among both women and men… Significant inverse associations were also observed between nut consumption and deaths due to cancer, heart disease, and respiratory disease." – PubMed ID#9786231 (2013) [547]

The average durations of the studies mentioned below were 30 years in the Nurses' Health Study and 24 years for the Health Professionals Follow-up Study. During this period, the combined risk of dying over the 24- to 30-year period was 20% lower for those who consumed 1 ounce of nuts (they examined those who consumed nuts less than once per week, once per week, 2 to 4 times per week, 5 to 6 times per week, and 7 or more times per week). Though this study found similar benefits for both peanuts and tree nuts, other studies found greater benefits for tree nuts, especially pecans and walnuts. Regardless, 20% is a huge improvement.

"Data from two large prospective studies – the Nurses' Health Study (NHS, 76,464 women) and the Health Professionals Follow-up Study (HPFS, 42,498 men) were analyzed to determine the association between nut consumption and subsequent total and cause-specific mortality… A total of 27,429 deaths (16,200 women and 11,229 men) occurred over 3,038,853 person-years of follow-up. There was a significant, dose-dependent inverse relationship between nut consumption and total mortality in both the studies. The pooled multivariate hazard ratios for death among participants who ate nuts were 0.93, 0.89, 0.87, 0.85 and 0.80 for those who consumed nuts less than once per week, once per week, two to four times per week, five or six times per week, and seven or more times per week, respectively" – PubMed ID#PMC4121755 (2014) [548]

The following study on walnuts and breast cancer was released while this book was being written. Though there have been several in vitro studies and a number of xenograft in vivo (mouse) studies, this is one of the first in vivo studies on humans. What they found was a clear benefit to gene expression that would improve breast cancer survival, including slowed proliferation and increased apoptosis. This study verifies previous animal studies and may give further weight to studies that involved other cancers.

"Consumption of walnuts has slowed breast cancer growth and/or reduced the risk of mammary cancer in mice. The benefit against cancer was associated with altered expression of genes for cancer growth and survival. We hypothesized that walnut consumption would alter gene expression in pathologically confirmed breast cancers of women in a direction that would be expected to decrease breast

> cancer growth and survival, as was seen in mice… women in the walnut group began to consume 2 oz of walnuts per day until follow-up surgery… RNA sequencing expression profiling revealed that expression of 456 identified genes was significantly changed in the tumor due to walnut consumption. Ingenuity Pathway Analysis showed activation of pathways that promote apoptosis and cell adhesion, and inhibition of pathways that promote cell proliferation and migration. These results support the hypothesis that, in humans, walnut consumption could suppress growth and survival of breast cancers." – PubMed ID#30979659 (2019) [549]

These are some very large, well run studies, and all of them showed much lower cancer rates, better outcomes from cancer, and longer life expectancy in those consuming the most nuts. Nuts, especially walnuts and pecans, have been shown to have many health benefits besides cancer prevention. Here are just a few examples: Type II diabetes, [550] cardiovascular disease, [551] coronary heart disease, [552] and stomach and pancreatic cancers. [553] Most of these studies were epidemiological studies looking at people's cancer risk based on past nut consumption; no one was forced to eat nuts. Therefore, the research did not look at any risks from overconsumption; everything has a bell curve (where too little is unhealthy, and too much is also unhealthy). Nut consumption seems to be more forgiving than many foods and food fractions, but you still should not overdo it.

Recommendation

When *Improving Your Odds*, eating healthy—and specifically, eating foods found to help prevent cancer—can't hurt. With the last study above (from 2019), it is clear that at least walnuts can also help treat certain cancers. I myself try to eat 1 to 2 ounces of pecans or walnuts per day, and I will always consume an ounce or so of other nuts when offered or available.

HERBALS/BOTANICALS

If you are on any medications or have other health issues, be sure to look up any herbal/botanical that you plan to take, in order to find any contraindications. One of the best ways to do this is on the Memorial Sloan Kettering Herbs and Dietary Supplements website. [554] It is not uncommon for dietary supplements to interfere with certain medications. Even though the herbal might otherwise be very healthy, you don't want to interfere with any medications you might be taking.

Many herbals have a variety of bioactive properties, and some of these may interfere with any other treatment you might be on. Though the link above is a good first check for contraindications, it is always best to discuss with your oncologist any herbs or botanicals you plan to supplement. In many cases, moderation is best, and this is an example of how "more is not always better."

In a study appearing in the medical journal *JAMA Oncology*, [555] they found that relying on supplements instead of traditional allopathic treatment while suffering from breast, colorectal, lung and prostate cancer can double the risk of dying from these cancers over the study period. The study also looked at whether the use of supplements along with allopathic treatment shortened survival times, and they found that it did not. They did not look at whether choosing to do both complementary medicine and allopathic treatments extended people's lives (strange that they wouldn't look at this). They also did look at specific complementary treatments—and there are a lot of people doing a lot of things that do not help them or make their condition worse (thus the point of this book, which is a science-based approach).

The point here is that you should not give up your allopathic treatments in favor of herbal treatment.

Updates at - https://improvingyourodds.com/

Support at - https://www.facebook.com/groups/cancer.improving.your.odds

ALOE VERA

Aloe vera is known for many health benefits and has been used medicinally for centuries. Most people are familiar with some of its external uses, such as soothing sunburn, cuts and burns. It is also often used in skin and beauty products. Even in ancient times, aloe vera was used internally for constipation, stomach ailments and as a general tonic for the nervous system.

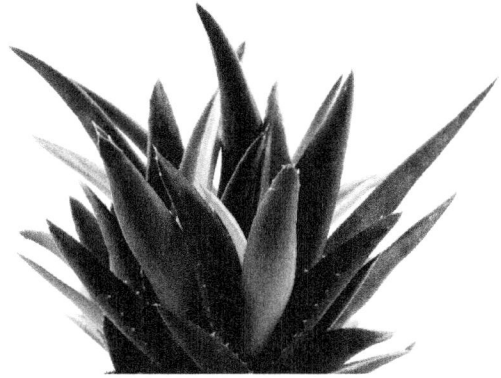

In recent history there has been increased interest in using aloe vera in preventing and fighting cancer. The main interest is the polysaccharides, known as glyconutrients, glycans (special complex sugars with medicinal benefits) and glycoproteins, found in the plant. It is also high in beneficial phytochemicals.

Only the gel of aloe vera should be used internally, not the sap/latex or the rest of the leaves. If you grow your own aloe, do not use the yellow ooze from the skin; you only want to use the clear gel within.

> "Many of the anti-cancer agents currently used have an origin in natural sources including plants. Aloe vera is one such plant being studied extensively for its diverse health benefits, including cancer prevention... In this study, the cytotoxic potential of Aloe vera crude extract (ACE) alone or in combination with cisplatin in human breast (MCF-7) and cervical (HeLa) cancer cells was studied... Exposure of cells to ACE resulted in considerable loss of cell viability in a dose- and time-dependent fashion, which was found to be mediated by through the apoptotic pathway... ACE did not have any significant cytotoxicity towards normal cells, thus placing it in the category of safe chemopreventive agent. Further, the effects were correlated with the downregulation of cyclin D1, CYP 1A1, CYP 1A2 and increased expression of bax and p21 in MCF-7 and HeLa cells." – PubMed ID#25854386 (2015)[556] (Open Access attribution available at Asian Pacific Journal of Cancer Prevention [557])

An aloe vera and honey combination were tested in vivo with tumor-bearing rats. They found that this mixture decreased the size of tumors (as judged by the relative weight of the tumors between the two groups of rats). They also found that it reduced cancer cell proliferation and increased apoptosis.

> "tumour-bearing rats that received a gavage with a 670 µL/kg dose of Aloe vera
> and honey solution daily, and the CW group - tumour-bearing rats which received
> only a 0.9% NaCl solution. The effect of Aloe vera and honey against tumour
> growth was observed through a decrease in relative weight (%) and Ki67-LI in
> tumours from the WA group compared with those from the CW group. The
> Bax/Bcl-2 ratio increased in tumours from the WA group at all tested timepoints.
> These data suggest Aloe vera and honey can modulate tumour growth by
> reducing cell proliferation and increasing apoptosis susceptibility." – PubMed
> ID#20839215 (2011) [558]

Aloe extract has shown antiproliferation activity in many cancer cell lines (meaning that it slows
the growth and spread of cancer). Here it was tested on colon cancer cells, and researchers found
that it is also apoptosis-promoting.

> "Aloe emodin (AE), a natural anthraquinone, is reported to have antiproliferative
> activity in various cancer cell lines. In this study, we analyzed the molecular
> mechanisms involved in the growth-inhibitory activity of this hydro-
> xyanthraquinone in colon cancer cell… This is the first study indicating that the
> AE induces apoptosis specifically through the activation of caspase-6." – PubMed
> ID#22343391 (2012) [559]

The following study investigated the use of aloe vera (topical gel and oral extract) on stage 2 skin
carcinogenesis in Swiss albino mice. Group I below is the control group. The cancer was reduced
the most in Group III, the group taking oral aloe vera; tumor development decreased by 60% in
this group.

> "The animals were randomly divided into 4 groups and treated as follows: Group
> I, DMBA + croton oil only (controls); Group II, DMBA + croton oil + topical
> aloe vera gel; Group III, DMBA + croton oil + oral aloe vera extract; Group I V,
> DMBA + croton oil + topical aloe vera gel + oral aloe vera extract. Results
> showed that body weight was significantly increased from 78.6% in the control
> group (Group I) to 92.5%, 87.5%, and 90.0% in Groups II, III, and I V,
> respectively. A 100% incidence of tumor development was noted in Group I,
> which was decreased to 50%, 60%, and 40% in Groups II, III, and I V,
> respectively. Also in Groups II, III, and IV, the cumulative number of papillomas
> was reduced significantly from 36 to 12, 15, and 11; tumor yield from 3.6 to 1.2,
> 1.5, and 1.1; and tumor burden from 3.6 to 2.4, 2.50, and 2.75, respectively, after
> treatment with aloe vera." – PubMed ID#20932247 (2010) [560]

In vivo testing (using human cancers transplanted to mice) found clear cancer-preventative
benefits with all cancers tested.

> "In vivo, active principles exhibited significant prolongation of the life span of tumor-transplanted animals... A. vera active principles exhibited significant inhibition on Ehrlich ascite carcinoma cell (EACC) number, when compared to positive control group... active principles showed a significant concentration-dependent cytotoxicity against acute myeloid leukemia (AML) and acute lymphocytes leukemia (ALL) cancerous cells. Furthermore, in MTT cell viability test, aloe-emodin was found to be active against two human colon cancer cell lines (i.e. DLD-1 and HT2), with IC(50)... Our data suggest that the tested A. vera compounds may exert their chemo-preventive effect through modulating antioxidant and detoxification enzyme activity levels, as they are one of the indicators of tumorigenesis... The results... clearly indicate that tested active principles exhibited a significant dose-dependent inhibitory effect on all cancer cell lines examined, with varying effect on the different cell lines." – PubMed ID#19941474 (2010) [561]

Aloesin is one of the active ingredients in aloe vera. It has been shown to inhibit tumor growth and metastasis in ovarian cancer.

> "It was found that aloesin inhibited cell viability and cell clonality in a dose-dependent manner. It arrests the cell cycle at the S-phase and induced apoptosis in SKOV3 cells. In an in vivo experiment, it was observed that aloesin inhibited tumor growth. Moreover, it inhibited migration and invasion of cancer in SKOV3 cells... In summary, the present study identified aloesin as a novel therapeutic compound to inhibit tumor growth and metastasis in ovarian cancer." – PubMed ID#PMC5494088 (2017) [562]

Aloe vera extracts have been shown to improve apoptosis in this study with skin cancer. The nice thing here is that they found that a standard water extract was just as effective as a methanol extract, meaning that you can just use fresh aloe vera with no special processing.

> "The well documented immunostimulant effect of the plant leaf extracts (Im et al. 2010; Srivastava et al. 2014) as well as their antioxidant activity (Ozsoy et al. 2009) could also have had an influence on the selective cytotoxic effectiveness... The benefits of A. vera extracts and aloe derivatives on skin as well as their demonstrated anticancer properties, makes the plant a good target for studies on skin related diseases and skin cancer. We have demonstrated in the present study the cytotoxic effect of A. vera extracts and AE and their apototic/necrotic mechanisms, on a skin cancer cell type. No difference was observed between the

cytotoxic effects of aqueous and methanolic extracts as well extracts obtained from fresh or dried leaves. A. vera gel and AE are thus potential targets for anticancer drug research." -- DOI: 10.5152/IstanbulJPharm.2017.0013 (2017) [563]

The external use of aloe vera can be helpful in treating radiotherapy (radiation therapy)-induced dermatitis (skin inflammation—that is, itchy rash and/or swollen, reddened skin).

"Patients were given a lotion of Aloe vera to use on one half of the irradiated area, with no medication to be used on the other half. The grade of dermatitis in each half was recorded weekly until 4 weeks after the end of radiotherapy… The findings in our trial demonstrate a protective effect of Aloe vera lotion against radiation-induced dermatitis. The effect was more evident in patients undergoing radiotherapy with larger treatment fields and higher doses of radiation." – PubMed ID#PMC3728063 (2013) [564]

Recommendation

This is another supplement that can't hurt. Purchase good aloe vera sold for oral consumption or grow your own. It is important to use the gel, and not the rind, nor liquid from the rind. Once opened, the bottle needs to be refrigerated.

When first starting aloe vera, some people report mild intestinal discomfort and perhaps light diarrhea. If that is the case, start slowly, perhaps 1 tsp per day, and work up to the full amount over 2 to 4 weeks. This is most often seen in people with a weak microbiome (little in the way of beneficial gut bacteria). Aloe vera is a pretty good prebiotic (beneficial bacteria food) and can help build up the microbiome.

You can find instructions for extracting the gel from fresh aloe vera leaves on WikiHow, and be sure to read the comments at the end, as they can help address some questions you might have. [565]

California has listed "non-decolorized" aloe vera as being known to cause cancer or toxicity (under CA Proposition 65). Always purchase from a reputable brand to ensure safety and quality.

> *I was consuming 2 Tbsp per day of the gel for 6 months; I stopped taking it as I was taking other medicinal polysaccharides (e.g., mushrooms and beta-glucans) and I wanted to scale back on the number of supplements once my cancer tumors were under control (NED). I took this one by spoon, not mixing it with anything. However, many people mix it into a smoothie.*

ARTEMISININ

Artemisinin, an extract of the sweet wormwood (*Artemisia annua*) plant, has a fascinating history in China, one that would nearly have been lost if it hadn't been for the Vietnam War! During the Vietnam War, Ho Chi Minh, the Communist leader of North Vietnam (which was at war with South Vietnam), was losing a large number of troops to drug-resistant malaria. In 1967, Ho turned to his ally, China, for help. Because China also had a malaria problem in its southern provinces, it decided to help. They set up a secret research project to test thousands of ancient Chinese herbs and herbal recipes against malaria. At first, they weren't successful. Then they found one effective compound in an ancient recipe called "Emergency Prescriptions Kept Up One's Sleeve." It was a recipe for an artemisinin, and the recipe was over 1,600 years old! It described artemisinin as working against "intermittent fevers," something malaria is known for. Their first round of testing on mice was unsuccessful. But when they went back to the recipe, they found that it said the artemisinin should be "steeped in cold water"—the scientists had boiled it. The hot water must have damaged the active ingredients. Further testing showed that the cold-water extract was 100% effective in mice and monkeys against malaria. Their work in isolating and describing artemisinin led to further research that ended up in a malaria drug that has saved the lives of millions of people. The Chinese scientist Tu YouYou won the Nobel Prize in Medicine on 5 October 2015 for this work; she was the first woman in China to win the Nobel Prize.

Now science is finding new uses for this ancient wormwood extract, and artemisinin has been found in many studies to selectively kill cancer cells! Cancer cells are well known for their ability to rapidly divide, doing so much faster than most normal cells. Many chemotherapy drugs take advantage of this trait. Iron is required for cell division, and many cancer types accumulate iron for that very purpose. Most cancers have a large number of iron-attracting receptors on their cell surface compared to normal cells. Artemisinin binds to iron and is carried to the cancer cells. It has been shown that artemisinin selectively kills cancer cells; some in vitro studies have shown that artemisinin kills nearly 100% of cancer cells within 24 hours when these cancer cells are "pre-loaded" with iron. As of yet, this discovery has not worked its way into a medically approved cancer treatment—again, because artemisinin is a natural product (available in health food stores) and there is no profit incentive (drug companies are looking at ways to produce a patentable synthetic form).

> "(recently) studies have been carried out to assess the potential of artemisinin and its derivatives to inhibit the growth and proliferation of cancer cells. It has been shown that they selectively kill tumor cells. This specificity is due to certain tumor cell characteristics, such as increased metabolism, elevated concentration of iron and transferrin, and susceptibility to Reactive Oxygen Species (ROS)... clinical trials and studies have demonstrated the drug's efficacy to selectively eliminate cancer cells both in vitro and in vivo, synergistic activity when combined with

> regular chemotherapeutic regimes and minimal toxicity." – PubMed
> ID#PMC5872176 (2018 – Open access attribute at the link) [566]

> "In the present investigation, we analyzed the inhibitory effects of artemisinin on
> migratory ability of melanoma cell lines (A375P and A375M, low and medium
> metastatic properties, respectively). We demonstrate that artemisinin induces cell
> growth arrest in A375M, and affects A375P cells viability with cytotoxic and
> growth inhibitory effects" – PubMed ID#18956140 (2009) [567]

Here artemisinin was investigated in vivo. When human cancer cells are implanted in animals for research, it is called a "xenograft"; xenograft cancer cells work much the same way in the animal as they would in humans. Artemisinin leads to "rapid induction of apoptosis in cancer cells," leading to the death of those cells without harm to normal cells.

> "Artemisinin is a chemical compound extracted from the wormwood plant,
> Artemisia annua L. It has been shown to selectively kill cancer cells in vitro and
> retard the growth of implanted fibrosarcoma tumors in rats. In the present
> research, we investigated its mechanism of cytotoxicity to cancer cells… DHA
> (dihydroArtemisinin) treatment significantly decreased cell counts and increased
> the proportion of apoptosis in cancer cells compared to controls (chi2=4.5, df=1,
> p<0.035)… This rapid induction of apoptosis in cancer cells after treatment with
> DHA indicates that artemisinin and its analogs may be inexpensive and effective
> cancer agents." – PubMed ID#15330172 (2004) [568]

The following study looked at using artemisinin and iron against 5637 (bladder cancer) and 4T1 (breast cancer) cell lines. The artemisinin/iron combination causes excess free radical damage in cancer cells, while not harming normal cells. [569] I do not recommend adding iron supplements unless under the care of a healthcare practitioner.

> "Anticancer properties of artemisinin and its derivatives have been shown in
> many experiments… In four groups treated with different doses of artemisinin
> and iron, dose-dependent changes were observed. These changes included
> apoptosis and necrosis with dominance of apoptosis." – PubMed ID#25579554
> (2014) [570]

Recommendations

I recommend taking no more than 200 mg twice per day unless working with a medical practitioner. Pregnant and nursing women should consult their physician.

> *I take 150 to 200 mg artemisinin per day (depending on the brand, that is one capsule). The brand that I take is refined to 98% purity (whereas the sweet wormwood plant contains 0.3-0.5% artemisinin). Look for something similar. Now that I'm NED, I will stop taking this in a couple of months.*

❖ ASHWAGANDHA

AKA: *Withania somnifera,* **Indian winter cherry, Indian ginseng, winter cherry,** *Physalis alkekengi* **(Chinese lantern)**

Ashwagandha is known as an "adaptogen," or something that can help us deal with stress (physical, emotional and environmental). It is also known for lowering blood sugar levels, reducing cortisol, improving immune system function, boosting testosterone in men, boosting brain function and helping to fight anxiety and depression. This seems like a lot for one humble herb. But there is actually quite a bit of research on it, including its ability to fight cancer, and that is what this section will focus on.

> "Withaferin A (WA), a major bioactive component of the Indian herb Withania somnifera, induces cell death (apoptosis/necrosis) in multiple types of tumor cells, but the molecular mechanism underlying this cytotoxicity remains elusive."
> – PubMed ID#26230090 (2015) [571]

Because ashwagandha acts as an immunomodulator, it should be helpful in fighting most cancers. If your immune system is aware of the cancer, ashwagandha should be able to help by improving the immune response.

> "W. somnifera significantly altered the level of leucocytes, lymphocytes, neutrophils, immune complexes and immunoglobulins (Ig) A, G and M. The azoxymethane induced colon cancer and immune dysfunction was better controlled by W. somnifera. These results suggested that the immunomodulatory effects of W. somnifera could be useful in the treatment of colon cancer." – PubMed ID#20840055 (2010) [572]

This shows that ashwagandha can help mitigate some of the side effects of cancer.

Updates at - https://improvingyourodds.com

Support at - https://www.facebook.com/groups/cancer.improving.your.odds

"Over, based on the data providing a correlation Withania somnifera along with paclitaxel provide stabilization of membrane bound enzyme profiles and decreased lipid peroxidation against benzo(a)pyrene induced lung cancer in mice." – PubMed ID#17003952 (2006) [573]

Breast Cancers

Ashwagandha seems to be able to help breast cancers in several different ways.

"Effect of Withania somnifera root extract on spontaneous estrogen receptor-negative mammary cancer in MMTV/Neu mice… These results indicate that the root extract reduced the number of mammary carcinomas that developed and reduced the rate of cell division in the carcinomas." – PubMed ID#25368231 (2014) [574]

Withaferin A (WA below) is a constitute of ashwagandha. Here it was found to significantly reduce the mean area of invasive breast cancer.

"WA administration resulted in a statistically significant decrease in macroscopic mammary tumor size, microscopic mammary tumor area, and the incidence of pulmonary metastasis. For example, the mean area of invasive cancer was lower by 95.14% in the WA treatment group compared with the control group… Mammary cancer prevention by WA treatment was associated with increased apoptosis, inhibition of complex III activity, and reduced levels of glycolysis intermediates. Proteomics confirmed downregulation of many glycolysis-related proteins in the tumor of WA-treated mice compared with control, including M2-type pyruvate kinase, phospho glycerate kinase, and fructose-bisphosphate aldolase A isoform 2." – PubMed ID#23821767 (2013) [575]

"Withaferin A inhibits in vivo growth of breast cancer cells accelerated by Notch2 knockdown… Notch2 functions as a tumor growth suppressor in TNBC and WA offers a novel therapeutic strategy for restoring this function." – PubMed ID#PMC4867258 (2016) [576]

"Withaferin A-mediated apoptosis in breast cancer cells is associated with alterations in mitochondrial dynamics… Withaferin A (WA), a steroidal lactone derived from a medicinal plant (Withania somnifera), inhibits cancer development in transgenic and chemically-induced rodent models of breast cancer" – PubMed ID#30685490 (2019) [577]

Immune System/Stress Response

The immune system has a <u>huge</u> effect on cancer; it is our first and best line of defense. After chemotherapy and radiation, there are always viable cancer cells left; some are free-floating metastasizing cells in the blood and lymphatic system. It is the immune system, if properly functioning, that will clean up what is left and help prevent a recurrence. Chronic stress, or an improper response to stress, can have a huge negative effect on the immune system.

> "The biologically active constituents of Ashwagandha leaves include alkaloids, steroidal lactones and saponins that have been proposed to possess anti-stress, anti-oxidant, analgesic, immunomodulatory, adaptogenic and immunostimulant properties. Some studies have also reported anticancer, neuroregeneration and cholinergic activities in Ashwagandha extracts" – PubMed ID#PMC3214041 (2011) [578]

> "it may therefore be concluded that there were distinct modulation in the immune response exhibited by the three chemotypes of Withania somnifera and NMITLI 101R appeared to possess a better immunostimulatory activity than the other chemotypes at lower doses." PubMed ID#22182427 (2012) [579]

> "The treatment group that was given the high-concentration full-spectrum Ashwagandha root extract exhibited a significant reduction ($P<0.0001$) in scores on all the stress-assessment scales on Day 60, relative to the placebo group. The serum cortisol levels were substantially reduced ($P=0.0006$) in the Ashwagandha group, relative to the placebo group. The adverse effects were mild in nature and were comparable in both the groups. No serious adverse events were reported… The findings of this study suggest that a high-concentration full-spectrum Ashwagandha root extract safely and effectively improves an individual's resistance toward stress and thereby improves self-assessed quality of life." – PubMed ID#PMC3573577 (2012) [580]

> "Sixty-two abstracts were screened; five human trials met inclusion criteria… Conclusions: All five studies concluded that WS intervention resulted in greater score improvements (significantly in most cases) than placebo in outcomes on anxiety or stress scales." – PubMed ID#PMC4270108 (2014) [581]

Recommendations

Ashwagandha can be helpful in improving the immune system and the immune response to cancer. It can be especially helpful if you are dealing with a lot of stress and tend to get sick easily, or more frequently than those around you. As ashwagandha improves the immune response, adding it to your daily regimen can only help, especially if you are on immunotherapy.

❖ ASTRAGALUS ROOT

AKA: Bei qi, huang qi, hwanggi, milk vetch, ogi

Astragalus is a Chinese flowering plant that is used in traditional Chinese medicine (TCM). The roots contain medicinal polysaccharides believed to have some anticancer properties. There are over 2,000 species of astragalus, some poisonous, but the ones used in common supplements are safe (just don't identify or use plants on your own unless you really know what you're doing).

There are very few in vivo studies of astragalus root for the treatment of cancer. I've included it here as it is commonly used in complementary medicine. The following study used xenografts of colorectal cancer (CRC) tumors into mice. At the end of the study, the results did show an approximately 30% reduction in tumor size when compared to the controls.

> "In the present study, we have demonstrated that AM can effectively reduce the tumor growth in nude mice without significantly altering the mouse body weight… our preliminary results show that crude extract of AM inhibits growth of CRC in vivo without apparent toxicity and side effect." – PubMed ID#PMC4689484 (2016) [582]

There is some limited evidence that astragalus may help halt proliferation of certain gastric cancers. This evidence was obtained from small-scale in vitro and in vivo (mouse xenograft) studies. There have been no well done in vivo human studies to date.

> "We found that AE inhibited proliferation but caused apoptosis in human gastric cancer cells. Furthermore, the tumor growth and volume were reduced by AE administration in nude mice implanted with gastric cancer cells… Overall, AE enhances apoptosis in gastric cancer cells in vitro and in vivo, which is associated with decreased activation of IL-6/Stat3 signals." – PubMed ID#27731799 (2016) [583]

In this meta-analysis on 19 non-small cell lung cancer studies, astragalus root was not found to have any benefits and did not extend the lives of patients.

"The positive results described from the 19 studies of low quality are of questionable significance. No well-designed, randomized placebo-controlled trial with objective outcome measures has been conducted. Most of the trials were of very low methodological quality and the interpretation of any positive findings for the efficacy of the included AGI (Astragalus injection) for treating NSCLC (nonsmall cell lung cancer) patients should be made with caution. Based on this systematic review, there is no strong evidence to support the objective effectiveness and safety of AGI" – PubMed ID#PMC6426520 (2019) [584]

Recommendation

Unless you have gastric or colorectal cancer, this is not a supplement I would recommend. There is more high-quality research showing no benefits than there is research showing any benefit. Those showing benefit are mostly in vitro. The limited benefits also do not seem to be systemic (throughout the body), but instead limited to the gastrointestinal tract.

❖ BERBERINE

Cancers: Gastric, liver, colorectal, mostly due its anti-inflammatory and anti-tumor activities

Used in Chinese medicine for over 5,000 years, berberine has, in recent years, been studied for a variety of uses. It has been used in both Ayurvedic and Chinese medicine. These uses include inflammation, diabetes, arrhythmia, metabolic syndrome and cancer. It also has some antibiotic, or antiseptic, qualities. Berberine is found in several different plants, including: *Berberis vulgaris* (barberry), *Hydrastis canadensis* (goldenseal), *Mahonia aquifolium* (Oregon grape) and *Berberis aristata* (tree turmeric or chutro). It has a strong yellow color, much like turmeric, and it has been used as a wool dye, especially in India and China.

Berberine has been studied for its effects on many different types of cancer, including (but not limited to): breast, liver, bladder, brain, cervical, chondrosarcoma, endometrial, esophageal, gastric, leukemia, lung, multiple myeloma, melanoma, ovarian, prostate and pancreatic. Because of its strong abilities to control inflammation, it is also being studied for conjunctive therapy alongside traditional chemotherapy and radiotherapy cancer treatments.

This study evaluated berberine for its anti-tumor effect on ovarian cancer cells. They found that berberine inhibited cancer cell proliferation and induced apoptosis. It also has beneficial effects on breast, liver and colorectal cancer.

"Berberine exhibits antitumor effects in human ovarian cancer cells... Berberine possesses antitumor effect via inhibition of cell proliferation and induction of apoptosis in ovarian cancer cells. Berberine could synergistically enhance the cell killing effect of other antitumor agents... has been demonstrated to have effects on the expression proteins involved in apoptosis, autophagy, cell cycle progression and invasion... BBR has been shown to have minimal effects on "normal cells" but has anti-proliferative effects on cancer cells (e.g., breast, liver, CRC cells)" – PubMed ID#25544381 (2015) [585]

The following study looked at using berberine to improve cancer cell sensitivity chemotherapy. They found that it was able to increase cancer cell sensitivity to chemotherapy, including cells that were resistant to chemotherapy. It also was shown to have antiproliferation and apoptosis effects.

"low-dose berberine can enhance DOX sensitivity in drug-resistance breast cancer cells through AMPK-HIF-1α-P-gp pathway. On the other hand, high-dose berberine alone directly induces apoptosis through the AMPK-p53 pathway with the independence of HIF-1α expression. Taken together, our findings demonstrate that berberine sensitizes drug-resistant breast cancer to DOX chemotherapy and directly induces apoptosis through the dose-orchestrated AMPK signaling pathway in vitro and in vivo. Berberine appears to be a promising chemosensitizer and chemotherapeutic drug for breast cancer treatment." – PubMed ID#PMC5535724 (2017) [586]

Inflammation may be indicated in the development of up to 15% of all tumors; it is also found in nearly all developed tumors, as the cancer will cause inflammation. Being able to control this inflammation, without interfering with the body's ability to fight the tumors, is very important. Berberine is also able to fight cancer through other mechanisms.

"Epidemiological studies have indicated that the occurrence and development of up to 15% of tumors are related to infections and that chronic inflammation can especially increase the risk of cancer... chronic inflammation is thought to be particularly harmful and related to cell carcinogenesis. carcinogenic mechanisms caused by chronic inflammation are complicated and include genetic mutation induction, angiogenesis promotion and cell proliferation... anti-inflammatory activity of berberine was detected by the reduction of proinflammatory cytokines such as TNF-α, IL-13, IL-6, IL-8 and IFN-γ... anti-tumor activity of berberine mainly includes inhibiting the growth of tumor cells, promoting tumor cell apoptosis, inducing the differentiation of tumor cells and inhibiting the expression and metastasis of tumor cells. – DOI:10.1038/aps.2016.125 (2017 – Open Access attribution at the link) [587]

> "Berberine exerted anti-cancer effect in various cancer cell lines, and was also implied in the treatment of metabolic related diseases… Our result showed that berberine regulated the reprogramming metabolism through three aspects simultaneously, including mitochondrial oxidative phosphorylation, glycolysis and macromolecular synthesis." – PubMed ID#25212656 (2015) [588]

In an in vivo mouse model of human metastatic melanoma cancer, the following study found that berberine could "significantly" inhibit metastasis (migration and invasion) to the lungs.

> "Administration of berberine resulted in significant suppression of B16F-10 melanoma induced tumor nodule formation and enhanced the survival of tumor-bearing mice. Berberine treatment also decreased various biochemical parameters associated with lung metastasi" – PubMed ID# (2012) [589]

The following paper shows the various ways that berberine inhibits cancer growth. These effects have been noted in several studies and several different cancer lines.

> "Berberine is also able to inhibit the growth of various types of cancer cells, promote the apoptosis of tumor cells, induce the differentiation of tumor cells, and suppress the metastasis of tumor cells… Overall, these effects of berberine may lead to cell cycle arrest, induce cell death via apoptosis and activate autophagy… Berberine is able to inhibit the proliferation and induce the apoptosis of gastric cancer cells… berberine (10 μg/mL) can cause G0/G1 cell arrest and cell apoptosis… Previous studies have confirmed the anti-tumor effects of berberine on the human hepatocellular carcinoma (HCC) cell line by inhibiting proliferation and inducing apoptosis in HCC cells… As a natural compound with both anti-inflammatory and anti-tumor activities, berberine shows great potency in cancer treatment." – PubMed ID#PMC5309756 (2017, Open Access attribution available at the link) [590]

Berberine also has the ability to control high blood sugar levels, perhaps as well as the prescription drug metformin. This may have anticancer benefits in its own right. Metformin is also being investigated for its anti-tumor benefits. (PubMed ID#PMC5839379 [591])

Strategy

Though berberine does show anti-tumor activity against several cancers, it is also a "broad-spectrum" antibacterial. This means that it may have a negative impact on the human microbiome (or beneficial gut bacteria). For this reason, I do not advise taking it to prevent cancer. However, adding it to your treatment regimen for established tumors might be worth the risk. The antibacterial properties are not as strong as those of antibiotics, and for most people, these effects are most likely temporary, lasting as long as the treatment. These risks may be partially mitigated by following the steps in Chapter 3 on Gut Health.

❖ BITTER MELON

AKA: *Momordica charantia*

Bitter melon is a member of the *Cucurbitaceae* family, related to gourds, squash and cucumbers. As the name denotes, it has a somewhat bitter flavor. Bitter melon is commonly used in Asian dishes where both the flesh of the melon and its leaves are used in cooking. Extracts are also available in pill form.

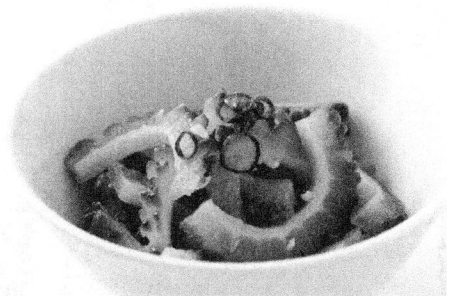

The bitter melon has been used medicinally for centuries and is commonly used to treat diabetes and other blood sugar-related conditions. It has also been used for treating asthma, herpes (EBV) and cancer. Recent research has shown that it indeed has beneficial properties for these conditions. More recent research has begun looking at fractions from bitter melon for possible anticancer drugs. Several studies have found that bitter melon contains multiple fractions that show positive benefits in the treatment and prevention of several different cancers. The research below will outline some of these.

"In a melanoma model, the mice which received fruit and leaf extracts of Momordica at the doses of 500 and 1000 mg/kg body weight for 30 days showed increase in life span of animals and tumour volume was significantly reduced as compared to control values… a single application of Momordica extracts at doses of 500, 1000 and 1500 mg/kg body weight, 24 hours prior the i.p. administration of cyclophosphamide, significantly prevented micronucleus formation and chromosomal aberrations in a dose dependent manner in bone marrow cells of mice. The present study demonstrate chemopreventive potential of Momordica fruit and leaf extracts on DMBA induced skin tumorigenesis, melanoma tumour and cytogenicity." – PubMed ID#20843118 (2010) [592]

"In mice given free access to extract of Bitter Melon (0.5%) or Ginger (0.125%) in drinking water, the development of mammary tumors was significantly inhibited. Furthermore, the former inhibited uterine adenomyosis with a common pathological background to mammary tumors and the latter inhibited mammary tumor growth. While the mechanism of the effects of these natural products remains to be clarified, there were no adverse effects of chronic treatment with these agent" – PubMed ID#12230008 (2002) [593]

Special polysaccharides (biologically active, usually non-digestible sugars) from certain plants and fungi are showing a lot of promise in cancer treatment research; mushroom polysaccharides were discussed earlier in this chapter. As we see here, it is the polysaccharides in bitter melon that are showing the most promise. Bitter melon has shown "strong anticancer activity against various tumors," inducing apoptosis and inhibiting metastasis "without noticeable toxicity."

"Polysaccharides are among the important bioactive components of M. charantia. It has been shown that polysaccharides from M. charantia fruits possess various bioactivities, such as antioxidant, antidiabetic, immune enhancing, neuroprotective, antitumor and antimicrobial… M. charantia extracts and its monomer components have shown strong anticancer activity against various tumors such as lymphoid leukemia, lymphoma, choriocarcinoma, melanoma, breast cancer, skin cancer and prostate cancer… M. charantia juice activated AMPKs in human pancreatic carcinoma cells, decreased cell viability in all four pancreatic carcinoma cell lines (BxPC-3, MiaPaCa-2, AsPC-1 and Capan-2 cells), exerted strong apoptosis-inducing activity and significantly inhibited MiaPaCa-2 tumor xenograft growth without noticeable toxicity… M. charantia can depress cancer cells proliferation in experimental settings; its antitumor activities may be partially attributed to MAP30, α-MMC, β-MMC and other medicinal proteins. In summary, bioactive components of M. charantia act as anti-tumor agents mainly through inhibiting tumor cell proliferation, inducing tumor cell apoptosis, influencing energy metabolism, depressing tumor cell metastasis and enhancing the relevant tumor suppressor gene activity" – PubMed ID#PMC5751158 (2017) (Open Access attribution available at the link) [594]

In the below study, bitter melon is described as having "significant anti-cancer efficacy" against various diverse cancers. It also shows "significant" "inhibition of EBV-EA" (Epstein-Barr virus, or human herpes virus). EBV inhibition is correlated to anti-tumor activity. In other words, what inhibits EBV usually inhibits cancer, even though we may not always know why (this also does not mean EBV causes or promotes a specific cancer).

"bitter melon extract or its isolated constituents have shown significant anticancer efficacy against lymphoid leukemia, lymphoma, and breast, skin, prostate, colon, bladder and pancreatic cancers... In these preliminary experiments, all eighteen compounds displayed their potential against 12-O-tetradecanoylphorbol-13-acetate (TPA)-induced activation of Epstein-Barr virus early antigen (EBV-EA). These results are significant as inhibition of EBV-EA induction is recognized to be correlated with anti-tumor promoting activities in cancer chemoprevention studies... showed significant cyto-toxic effects (in MTT assay) against MCF-7 (breast cancer), HepG2 (hepatocellular cancer), HEp-2 (laryngeal cancer), and WiDr (colon cancer) cells" – PubMed ID#PMC5067200 (2016) [595]

Conclusions

Besides the direct anticancer benefits of bitter melon, it also has very powerful blood sugar modulating properties. High blood sugar has a strong correlation with various cancers; therefore, it only makes sense to include a natural food that has both anticancer benefits and blood sugar regulation. The anticancer evidence for bitter melon is not as strong as it is for some of the other foods and supplements. However, the cost of bitter melon supplements is not very high, and therefore, supplementing with it is something you may wish to consider.

Recommendations

Bitter melon can be consumed in food dishes—there are many recipes online—or it can be consumed as a supplement in capsule form. Capsules are certainly more convenient. I take a bitter melon supplement that contains 5% bitter principles, 500 mg, once or twice per day.

❖ BLACK SEED EXTRACT

AKA: *Nigella sativa,* **black cumin seed**

The following paper reviewed numerous research studies on *Nigella sativa* showing benefits in fighting various cancers, including but not limited to: breast, colon, liver, lymphoma, carcinoma, sarcoma, pancreatic, leukemia, melanoma, lung, prostate and cervical cancers. It can inhibit these cancers through various mechanisms, including improving apoptosis, downregulating expression of anti-apoptotic genes, helping to prevent metastasis, and even some cytotoxic abilities.

"This review focuses on analyzing experimental findings related to the ability of N. sativa to exert anti-proliferative, pro-apoptotic, anti-oxidant, cytotoxic, anti-mutagenic, anti-metastatic, and NK cytotoxic activity enhancing effects against various primary cancer cells and cancer cell lines. Moreover, we underline the molecular mechanisms of action and the signal transduction pathways implicated in the suppression of tumorigenesis by N. sativa… an effective therapeutic potential of N. sativa to suppress tumor development, reduce tumor incidence, and ameliorate carcinogenesis… findings reported in the last two decades strongly suggest that N. sativa fractions could serve, alone or in combination with known chemotherapeutic drugs, as effective agents to control tumor initiation, growth, and metastasis, and hence, treatment of a wide range of cancers." – PubMed ID#PMC5052360 (2016) [596]

The following paper reviews the benefits of N. *sativa* oil against several different cancers (in vitro and in vivo) and found that it has some ability to protect cells from radiation therapy.

"N. sativa may be a beneficial agent in protection against ionizing radiation-related tissue injury… N. sativa were found to be effective in vitro in inactivating MCF-7 breast cancer cells… TQ, the major constituent of N. sativa oil extract, induced apoptosis and inhibited proliferation in PDA (pancreatic ductal adenocarcinoma) cells… TQ (from N. sativa) blocked angiogenesis in vitro and in vivo, prevented tumor angiogenesis in a xenograft human prostate cancer (PC3) model in mouse, and inhibited human prostate tumor growth at low dosage with almost no chemotoxic side effects" – PubMed ID#PMC3252704 (2011) [597]

The following research makes a very good case for the use of N. *sativa* as an adjuvant treatment to conventional cancer therapies. It outlines dozens of research studies, in vivo and in vitro, that show the benefits of using it alongside radiotherapy, chemotherapy and immunotherapy. Several different types of cancer are covered.

"Thymoquinone (TQ), the main bioactive component of Nigella sativa, has been found to exhibit anticancer effects in numerous preclinical studies. Due to its multitargeting nature, TQ interferes in a wide range of tumorigenic processes and counteracts carcinogenesis, malignant growth, invasion, migration, and angiogenesis. Moreover, TQ can specifically sensitize tumor cells toward conventional cancer treatments (e.g., radiotherapy, chemotherapy, and immunotherapy) and simultaneously minimize therapy-associated toxic effects in normal cells… In addition to its cell death and tumor growth inhibitory activities, TQ is found to interfere with other tumorigenic processes including angiogenesis, invasion, and metastasis… TQ also displayed promising results both in vitro and in vivo in an orthotopic model of pancreatic cancer… the prevention of radiation-induced metastatic progression of breast cancer cells by TQ through restoration of TGF-β… A significant attenuation has been reported in breast, gastric, and colon cancer xenografts after intra peritoneal administration of TQ… TQ treatment also showed promising results in doxorubicin-resistant human breast cancer cells" – PubMed ID#PMC5466966 (2017) (Open Access citation available at the link) [598]

"thymoquinone exerts its inhibitory effect on migration of human and mouse melanoma cells by inhibition of NLRP3 inflammasome. Thus, our results indicate that thymoquinone can be a potential immunotherapeutic agent not only as an adjuvant therapy for melanoma, but also, in the control and prevention of metastatic melanoma." – PubMed ID#23583630 (2013) [599]

Recommendations

Research shows that black seed extract (*N. sativa*) offers many benefits in prevention and treatment of cancer. It's also well suited as an adjuvant treatment to conventional therapies.

Therapeutic doses are in the range of 1.5 to 2 grams (1,500 to 2,000 mg) per day. This should be taken in 2 to 3 divided doses, preferably with a meal. Because black seed has some antibacterial properties, be sure to take measures to improve your microbiome, beneficial bacteria diversity and Bifidobacteria (see Chapters 2 and 3).

❖ BOSWELLIA SERRATA

AKA: Indian frankincense, Salai, Salai Guggul, Gajabhakshya, olibanum

Boswellia serrata, better known as frankincense, originates in India, Africa and the Middle East. It has long been used to make incense and perfumes and is mentioned by name 17 times in the Bible (the word meaning incense is used 113 times, and it is assumed that many of those references are also to frankincense). Frankincense was one of the gifts given to the newborn Jesus. Frankincense was also used medicinally at that time and was used medicinally in China at least back to 500 BCE. Evidence shows that it was traded in the Middle East and North Africa at least 5,000 years ago. Frankincense is made from the resin of trees of the genus *Boswellia*, including *B. serrata*, *B. sacra*, *B. frereana*, *B. carterii* and *B. thurifera*.

Here *Boswellia* is shown to mediate cancer cell death in 3 different breast cancer cell lines, without harming normal cells.

"Boswellia sacra essential oil-mediated cell viability and death were studied in established human breast cancer cell lines (T47D, MCF7, MDA-MB-231) and an immortalized normal human breast cell line (MCF10-2A)… All three human breast cancer cell lines were sensitive to essential oil treatment with reduced cell viability and elevated cell death… Boswellia sacra essential oil prepared from hydrodistillation has tumor cell-specific cytotoxicity in multiple cancer cell types. Consistent with anti-proliferative, pro-apoptotic, and anti-invasive activities in cultured breast cancer cells, Boswellia sacra essential oil is shown to induce tumor cell cytotoxicity in a drug resistant and metastasized breast cancer" – PubMed ID#PMC3258268 (2011) (Open Access citation available at the link) [600]

"Boswellia sacra essential oil Fraction IV exhibited anti-proliferative and pro-apoptotic activities against pancreatic tumors in the heterotopic xenograft mouse model… All fractions of frankincense essential oil from Boswellia sacra are capable of suppressing viability and inducing apoptosis of a panel of human pancreatic cancer cell lines… Although chemical component(s) responsible for tumor cell cytotoxicity remains undefined, crude essential oil prepared from hydrodistillation of Boswellia sacra gum resins might be a useful alternative therapeutic agent for treating patients with pancreatic adenocarcinoma, an aggressive cancer with poor prognosis." – PubMed ID#23237355 (2012) [601]

In the following study, a 39-year-old woman with stage I breast cancer, with no metastasis or lymph node involvement, went to her doctor complaining of headaches and nausea. A computer tomography (CT, or CAT) scan was done of her head. It found multiple metastasized tumors, several large tumors and many small ones scattered throughout the brain. Several of these tumors were severe and inoperable. That is when doctors decided to try *B. serrata* (an oxidoreductase plant lipoxygenases, or LOX, inhibitor). *Boswellia* had been used for years in brain tumor patients in Germany, along with radiation therapy. After just 10 weeks of therapy, she underwent another CT scan, and it showed a complete disappearance of the tumors! She was continued on 800 mg of *B. serrata* 3 times per day as maintenance. As of the publication of the research 4 years later, she showed no further signs of brain tumors. Normally the prognosis after being diagnosed with multiple brain metastasis is a 3- to 5-month life expectancy. The LOX inhibitor attributes of *B. serrata* have shown treatment benefits in meningeoma and glioblastoma brain cancers, as well as prostate cancer, pancreatic cancer, breast cancer and some forms of melanoma.

"Boswellia serrata, a lipoxygenase inhibitor was applied for this inhibition. Multiple brain metastases were successfully reversed using this method in a breast cancer patient who had not shown improvement after standard therapy. The results suggest a potential new area of therapy for breast cancer patients with brain metastases that may be useful as an adjuvant to our standard therapy." – PubMed ID#17001517 (2007) [602]

The following study looked at melanoma in a mouse model and found that administering a LOX inhibitor (such as *B. serrata*) was able to inhibit melanoma.

"These results give new insights to the mechanisms through which inflammation may contribute to tumor progression and suggest that LOX has an important role in tumor progression associated with an inflammatory state in the presence of apoptosis, which may be a consideration for apoptosis-inducing treatments, such as chemotherapy and radiotherapy." – PubMed ID#19737966 (2009) [603]

The following research looked at using *B. serrata* in conjunction with DOX (a chemotherapy drug) to treat hepatocellular carcinoma (HCC). HCC is the most common type of primary liver cancer in adults and the most common cause of death in people with cirrhosis. Caspases are crucial mediators of programmed cell death (apoptosis); caspase-3 is a frequently activated death protease.

"Recent studies on brain tumors, leukemic, and colon cancer cells indicate that boswellic acids from B. serrata may have antiproliferative effects. DOX is one of the most commonly used anticancer agents against HCC; however, it is associated with severe toxicities to vital organs… B. serrata extract containing boswellic acids in combination with DOX was effective in a synergistic manner in inhibition of tumor growth of HCC in vitro and also protected against toxicity in vivo. Our results indicate that the anticancer activity of B. serrata alone and in combination with DOX was mediated via activation of caspase cascade and induction of apoptosis… Induction of caspase-3 has been demonstrated following boswellic acid treatment in colon cancer, lukemic cells, and prostate cancer cells. Induction of apoptosis and expression of cleaved caspase 3 was significantly induced in vitro" – PubMed ID#PMC4142179 (2014) [604]

The following paper looked at the research showing efficacy in fighting various cancers, including: prostate, colorectal, glioma, leukemia, bladder, pancreatic, multiple myeloma, neuroblastoma and cervical cancer.

"The anti-cancer potential of boswellic acid is well evidenced by several in vitro, in vivo, and clinical studies in different cancers that implicate its inhibitory actions against different hallmarks of cancer such as survival, proliferation, angiogenesis, invasion, and metastasis… BA, especially AKBA, ß-boswellic acid, and acetyl-ß-boswellic acid have been shown to exert marked cytotoxicity on malignant glioma cells even at lower micromolar concentrations, primarily through

apoptosis induction, and it is independent of free radical formation. --
doi:10.1016/j.canlet.2016.04.017 (2016) [605]

In this report they describe the cancer preventative effects of oral *B. serrata* administration alone in a case of high-grade invasive papillary UCC (urothelial carcinoma, a type of urinary cancer) during 2-year follow-up.

"The use of Boswellia-derived products in the management of cancer has been well document in other published studies… Boswellia species have been demonstrated to have anticarcinogenic activity in chemically induced mouse skin cancer models, as well as antiproliferative and pro-apoptotic activities against rat astrocytoma cell lines and in human leukemia cell lines. Clinically, extracts from the resins have been shown to reduce the peritumoral edema in glioblastoma patients and reverse multiple brain metastases in a breast cancer patient…The patient reported the absence of any adverse effect from daily oral administration of BSGRH… a daily dose of 3 mL of BSGRH seems to have a cancer preventive effect as the patient is free of UCC in his urinary bladder in the last 14 months after the last recurrence as per cystoscopic surveillance." – PubMed ID#PMC5739138 (2017) (Open Access license attribution at the link) [606]

Boswellia was shown below to inhibit human cancer cells through a variety of mechanisms, including: inhibiting proliferation, blocking new blood vessels to tumors, inhibiting migration and inducing apoptosis (programmed cell death, which is normally turned off in cancer cells). As with many natural cancer treatments, *Boswellia* is likely to show these benefits across a wide variety of cancers. Due to funding limits, it has only been studied against a few cancers.

"Boswellia specious, has been used in traditional and modern medicine for treating various diseases with very minimal side effects. In the current study, we investigated the anti-cancer activity of methanolic extract of Boswellia serrata (B. serrata) on HT-29 human colon cancer cells… Boswellia specious, has been used in traditional and modern medicine for treating various diseases with very minimal side effects. In the current study, we investigated the anti-cancer activity of methanolic extract of Boswellia serrata (B. serrata) on HT-29 human colon cancer cells… Our findings suggest that B. serrata extract inhibits proliferation, angiogenesis and migration and induces apoptosis in HT-29 cells by inhibiting of mPGES-1 and decreasing the PGE2 level and its downstream targets." – PubMed ID#28549801 (2017) [607]

The following study appeared in the medical journal *Cancer Genomics Proteomics* and looked at using *Boswellia serrata* extract (BSE) to treat triple-negative breast cancer (TNBC). TNBC is a difficult cancer to treat as it does not respond to hormone receptor-based chemotherapies. This study did not look at other cancers. (ER = endoplasmic reticulum, UPR = unfolded protein response; these two pathways are closely tied to activated programmed cell death (APCD).)

> "The anti-cancer effects of the historically used frankincense sap (BSE) appear to involve major impact on the ER/UPR response, concomitant to effecting multiple targets counter to the growth, proliferation and metastasis of TNBC cancer cells." – PubMed ID#29109091 (2017) [608]

Commercial frankincense (*B. serrata*) essential oil was used to determine its effect on bladder cancer cells, compared to normal bladder cells. The study found that *B. serrata* oil suppressed bladder cancer cell viability but had no effect on normal bladder cells.

> "Frankincense oil-induced cell viability was investigated in human bladder cancer J82 cells and immortalized normal bladder urothelial UROtsa cells… frankincense oil suppressed cell viability in bladder transitional carcinoma J82 cells but not in UROtsa cells. Comprehensive gene expression analysis confirmed that frankincense oil activates genes that are responsible for cell cycle arrest, cell growth suppression, and apoptosis in J82 cells… Frankincense oil appears to distinguish cancerous from normal bladder cells and suppress cancer cell viability." – PubMed ID#PMC2664784 (2009) [609]

> "We found that AKBA alone suppressed the proliferation and metastasis of human CRC. This correlated with the downregulation of various biomarkers linked to inflammation, cell proliferation, cell survival, invasion, and angiogenesis… We found that AKBA at 50 mg/kg significantly inhibited CRC growth in an orthotopic mouse model, but when the dose was increased to 200 mg/kg, it further enhanced the antitumor effects… More than 70% of tumor growth was inhibited by 200 mg/kg AKBA, and this level of inhibition was also seen in dose-dependent manner. The animals tolerated AKBA very well" – PubMed ID#PMC3246525 (2011) [610]

Strategy

Some reports indicate that frankincense oil does not contain the *Boswellia* acids (triterpenoids) of the *B. serrata* sap. Though the essential oil does contain some anticancer benefits, the *Boswellia* acids seem to show the most benefits. Therefore, I would recommend taking a capsule supplement that contains at least 50% *Boswellia* acids (the one I took contains 65%).

The study above used 800 mg, 3 times per day as maintenance. It does not mention the treatment dose, nor does it mention the amount of *Boswellia* acids it contained. I personally took 500 mg twice per day; my supplement contains 65% *Boswellia* acids. I've seen recommendations of up to 2,600 mg per day, but again, these did not mention the percentage of *Boswellia* acids. There just have not been enough human studies to come up with an accurate optimal dosage.

B. serrata has an excellent safety record; however, no recommended Tolerable Upper Intake Level (UL) has been set or proposed. Experiments with mice have tested it up to 500 mg/kg of body weight with no adverse effects (this equates to 25 grams (25,000 mg) for a 50 kg/110 lb person). Therefore, taking considerably less than that should be considered safe.

To err on the safe side, from what I'm seeing I would not exceed 2,400 mg/day of 65% *Boswellia* acids unless instructed to do so by a healthcare provider. I personally do not take this for maintenance, although a dose of up to 500 mg twice per day seems like a reasonable maintenance dose.

CANNABIS CBD OIL / MARIJUANA

AKA: Cannabidiol oil, cannabis, marijuana

Cancers: Unknown
Body of Evidence: Weak
Cost: Moderate
Recommendation: Low

The popularity of medical marijuana and CBD (cannabidiol) oil is soaring. It is hard to find a disease or condition that advocates aren't claiming can be cured or improved by cannabis. Though there are certainly some medical benefits to cannabis, few of the claims have been studied with anywhere near the rigor of prescription drugs, over-the-counter medications or even most vitamins and nutrients. We all know the reasons for this; marijuana is illegal at the federal level in the US and most Western countries (at least at publication). That and the political environment make research and funding very difficult. But simply because politics has prevented proper research does not mean cannabis can cure every disease, nor does it mean that it doesn't. However, this book is based on natural solutions that have scientific evidence of efficacy, so that is where the focus in this section will remain.

Your body produces its own cannabinoids, known as "endocannabinoids" ("endo" for internal), which perform various functions within the body. Some cells in the body contain cannabinoid receptors, of which there are two types, CB1 and CB2. The cannabinoid THC can attach to either of these. Brain cells contain cannabinoid receptors, and this is the reason we get "high" when smoking marijuana. Another function of cannabinoid receptors is in the regulation of the inflammation process. When the inflammation gets out of hand, endocannabinoids (and thus cannabis cannabinoids) can signal cells to stop sounding the inflammation siren, and thus break the inflammation cycle. This is why cannabis is often used to calm inflammation. There is a lot of research being done on cannabinoids and inflammation, especially for topical skin applications.

Because our bodies utilize endocannabinoids for a wide range of functions (and many more yet to be discovered), there is great interest in investigating cannabis cannabinoids for medical applications. Cannabinoids aren't only familiar to our body; they are essential. Therefore, it only makes sense that exocannabinoids (cannabinoids originating outside the body, e.g., THC from marijuana) would have great potential for treating certain medical conditions. As stated earlier, this research is still in its infancy, and simply because our cells are familiar with cannabinoids doesn't mean that cannabis can cure cancer or whatever else ails you (our cells are very familiar with sodium too, and that doesn't mean it cures cancer).

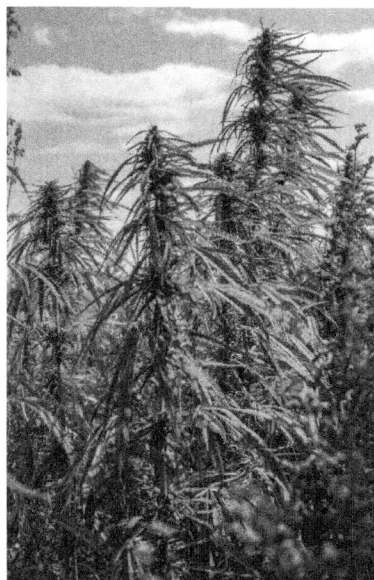

What I found while researching this topic is that there is some evidence that the various forms of cannabis may benefit prevention and treatment of <u>some</u> cancers, in some situations. But I also found that these same forms of cannabis can impede the immune system and, in some cases, may make other cancers worse. If the thought of adding CBD oil or medical marijuana scares or confuses you, this section may not help calm those feelings, as even the experts admit there is much to be learned. If you are bound and determined to use cannabis products, including non-THC varieties of CBD oil, I recommend you read this entire section before making up your mind. I also recommend that you consult with your oncologist first, as **certain types of cancers have been shown to be worsened by cannabis. There are also studies showing that cannabis products can interfere with some immunotherapy drugs.** Cannabinoids are complex biochemicals, and as such, usage for disease treatment can also be complicated.

First, let me see if I can cover some more of the basics. CBD (cannabidiol) oil is made from the *Cannabis sativa* plant. CBD is one of the cannabinoids found in cannabis. Most CBD products on the market do not contain THC (the psychoactive chemical that makes people high) and are therefore legal in many states (if it contains THC, it should be labeled as such and will only be legally sold in states where it is allowed). When purchasing CBD oil, be sure it states that it is "CBD" oil, and not just "hemp oil." CBD is derived from the leaves and stalks of the hemp plant. It contains 3% to 4% cannabinoids, the active chemicals that may have some health promoting and disease fighting properties (including perhaps fighting some cancers). You will find that CBD oil is a lot more expensive than hemp oil.

Products labeled as "hemp oil" are made from the seeds and contain only trace amounts of cannabinoids. Both are made from the same "hemp" plant; yes, it is confusing. Hemp oil may have some nutritional benefits, but it is not the form used for medicinal purposes. Some people may try to convince you that hemp oil has helped them; if true, this is most likely due to it being high in alpha-linolenic acid (ALA). ALA is an omega-3 precursor to EPA/DHAs, and thus can help reduce inflammation. There really is nothing special about ALA; in fact, it is a rather poor source of EPA/DHA (what the body really needs). If this is what you are looking for, I recommend that you purchase a good fish oil supplement to obtain even more beneficial omega-3s (fish oil contains much more beneficial forms of omega-3s than ALA from hemp oil, and no conversion from ALA to EPA/DHA is necessary).

Marijuana is a high-THC version of the hemp plant. It is usually smoked but can also be made into food and other products. THC is one of the 113 cannabinoids identified in cannabis (cannabidiol, or CBD, being one of the other primary cannabinoids), and it is the principal psychoactive constituent of cannabis. THC is what gets people "high." High-THC products, including marijuana, are still illegal in most countries and most of the states in the USA. THC has been found to have some health benefits of its own, but at this time it is not known if THC is needed to get the full medicinal benefits of cannabis. In short, THC is a cannabinoid that can get people high, but most of the other cannabinoids do not get people high.

Currently, the evidence for the use of CBD (cannabidiol) oil for cancer prevention and treatment is rather weak (yes, possibly due to a lack of research). Most studies that have been done are in vitro (in the test tube) or small in vivo studies involving rats or mice. At the time of this writing, there has only been one very small study of cannabinoids on humans and cancer. This study was on nine terminal patients with recurrent glioblastoma who were resistant to standard therapy. The THC was injected directly into the tumors (and thus the patients didn't exhibit any psychoactive effects). In this study, 2 of the 9 patients achieved some benefits, but THC did not eradicate their cancer. Glioblastoma is a very aggressive cancer with no known cure, and all of the patients in this study died from their cancer. Therefore, this was not a very helpful study to determine the benefits, or lack of benefits, of cannabis.

When considering anecdotal accounts about hemp or CBD oil, we must always consider the placebo effect. It is real, and it is frequently seen in research studies that do not use rigorous controls, such as double-blind controls. People think a substance is helping them, and therefore, they feel better and they report benefits (and may even have some benefits due to lowered stress from the perceived benefits). In addition, some of the research papers I found have declared "conflicts of interest" (e.g., researchers being paid by companies selling medical marijuana or papers written by the "executive director" of a Canadian nonprofit formed to promote cannabis products). For the sake of scientific rigor, I will not be including these papers.

Much of the research on cannabis has focused on nausea, appetite and pain relief, rather than chemotherapy or immunomodulating benefits. None of this means that CBD doesn't help treat or prevent cancer, but there simply isn't good evidence, currently, that it does. However, there is pretty good evidence that it helps in treating nausea, appetite suppression and pain.

Beneficial Findings

What follows is a sampling of the research that is currently available on cannabis derivatives and cancer. This is by no means inclusive of all the research that is available. I tried to include abstracts of the most unique part of each paper or research study, without being duplicative (even cautionary warnings have been excluded here). Some of these papers may include a lot more interesting information, but due to copyright restrictions, I am limited in how much can be quoted. I recommend that if a study interests you, you read the rest of the abstract or full text from the included link. If the paper is not available in full (e.g., it is only available behind a "paywall"), then you may be able to get it from a university library or your doctor.

The following paper has declared conflicts of interest.

> "Aside from symptom management, an increasing body of in vitro and animal-model studies supports a possible direct anticancer effect of cannabinoids by way of a number of different mechanisms involving apoptosis, angiogenesis, and inhibition of metastasis. Despite an absence of clinical trials, abundant anecdotal reports that describe patients having remarkable responses to cannabis as an anticancer agent, especially when taken as a high-potency orally ingested concentrate, are circulating. Human studies should be conducted to address

critical questions related to the foregoing effects." – PubMed ID#PMC4791148 (2016 – Declared conflicts of interest) [611]

Here they looked at cannabinoids that exclude the psychoactive THC compound. The study found that the cannabinoids could inhibit angiogenesis (formation of the new blood vessels required for cancer growth).

> "local administration of a nonpsychoactive cannabinoid to mice inhibits angiogenesis of malignant gliomas as determined by immunohistochemical analyses and vascular permeability assays. In vitro and in vivo experiments show that at least two mechanisms may be involved in this cannabinoid action: the direct inhibition of vascular endothelial cell migration and survival as well as the decrease of the expression of proangiogenic factors" – PubMed ID#12514108 (2003) [612]

Pharmaceutical companies are looking to create drugs that inhibit the VEGF pathway. VEGF is a signaling protein produced by cells that stimulates the formation of blood vessels. Without these new blood vessels, tumors would be unable to grow. Research shows that cannabinoids can selectively do this, in vitro and in mice, for glioma cancer cells. Glioma is a type of brain and spinal cord cancer.

> "vascular endothelial growth factor (VEGF) pathway plays a critical role in tumor angiogenesis… cannabinoids depressed the VEGF pathway by decreasing the production of VEGF and the activation of VEGF receptor (VEGFR)-2, the most prominent VEGF receptor, in cultured glioma cells and in mouse gliomas." – PubMed ID#15313899 (2004) [613]

In this study from 2010, THC, the active ingredient in cannabis, was shown both in vitro and in vivo (in mice) to be active against glioblastoma cells (a form of brain cancer). They also tested cannabidiol (CBD, another cannabis derivative) and THC together and found they worked even better together.

> "The cannabinoid 1 (CB(1)) and cannabinoid 2 (CB(2)) receptor agonist Delta(9)-tetrahydrocannabinol (THC) has been shown to be a broad-range inhibitor of cancer in culture and in vivo, and is currently being used in a clinical trial for the treatment of glioblastoma. The treatment of glioblastoma cells with both compounds led to significant modulations of the cell cycle and induction of reactive oxygen species and apoptosis as well as specific modulations of extracellular signal-regulated kinase and caspase activities. These specific changes

were not observed with either compound individually, indicating that the signal transduction pathways affected by the combination treatment were unique… Our results suggest that the addition of cannabidiol to Delta(9)-THC may improve the overall effectiveness of Delta(9)-THC in the treatment of glioblastoma in cancer patients." – PubMed ID#20053780 (2010) [614]

In this 2018 study out of Radiation Oncology unit of Brigham and Women's Hospital and Harvard Medical School, both in Boston, Massachusetts, the authors found that the addition of CBD to radiotherapy (RT) or smart radiotherapy biomaterials (SRBs) significantly reduced in vivo (mouse model) tumors for both lung and pancreas cancers. CBD treatment was found to be even more beneficial than the radiation therapy, but the two used together showed the most benefit. In the lung cancer group, 60% of the mice in the combined CBD+SRB group were still alive at the end of the study (40 days), while none of the mice in the control, CBD or SRB groups were alive. In the pancreatic tumor study, after 20 days, 50% of the control group were alive, whereas 80% of the CBD group and 100% of the combined CBD+SRB group were alive.

"Pancreatic cancer is one of the deadliest cancers, with a dismal 5-year survival rate of less than 5%. Meanwhile lung cancer is amongst the top killers… study results showing synergistic outcomes when using CBDs in combination with RT are in consonance with previous work… Clonogenic assay results are shown in Figures Figures2A,B2A,B demonstrating substantially enhanced tumor cell killing when using CBDs with RT. Significant synergy is observed in the study arm combining 2 μg of CBD with RT at 4 Gy. Such synergy may allow for greater effective tumor cell killing while reducing the dose of RT. Remarkably, 5 μg of CBD was found to achieve greater tumor cell killing than 4 Gy of RT. This supports findings in previous studies that CBDs can induce apoptosis, with potential mechanism being the generation of highly potent reactive oxygen species (9). This effect combined with DNA damage by RT could account for the observed synergistic outcomes." – PubMed ID#PMC5928848 (2018) [615]

The following paper is out of the Poznań University of Life Sciences in Poznań, Poland, and it discusses the ability of cannabinoids to inhibit tumor proliferation, metastasis and angiogenesis (the tumor's ability to form new blood vessels). It also discusses the ability of CBDs to activate apoptosis in tumors without affecting healthy cells. It concludes by pointing out that cannabinoids' benefits still must overcome their immunosuppressive characteristics, which can make them a poor choice for some cancers and patients.

"About 100 phytocannabinoids have been described, of which Δ9 □ tetrahydrocannabinol (THC) is main psychoactive compound. Action of THC in human organism relies on mimicking endogenous agonists of CB receptors— endocannabinoids. It is responsible for euphoria and has analgesic, antiemetic, and anti□inflammatory properties, however, its psychoactivity strongly limits medical potential. Another phytocannabinoid which gains medical attention is cannabidiol (CBD)… Many cannabinoids… have shown ability to inhibit proliferation, metastasis, and angiogenesis in a variety of models of cancer… the main effect of cannabinoids in a tumor is the inhibition of cancer cells' proliferation and induction of cancer cell death by apoptosis. It has been shown that CB1 and CB2 receptor agonists stimulate apoptotic cell death in glioma cells… It has been shown that cannabinoids induce process of autophagy in cancer cell lines such as glioma, melanoma, hepatic, and pancreatic cancer. Moreover, some additional mechanisms have been demonstrated to contribute to the process of an induction of cell death by cannabinoids in certain cell lines… Viability of noncancerous cells seems to remain unchanged or sometimes even elevated by cannabinoids… Cannabinoids show antitumor activity in cell lines and in animal models of cancer, but we still do not have data concerning their efficacy and safety from well☐prepared clinical trials. Moreover, antitumor effects of cannabinoids have to overcome their known immunosuppressive effects which can be potentially protumorigenic." – PubMed ID#PMC5852356

Creative Commons attribution - Śledziński, Paweł et al. "The current state and future perspectives of cannabinoids in cancer biology." Cancer medicine vol. 7,3 (): 765-775. doi:10.1002/cam4.1312 (2018 - Full Open Access attribution at the link) [616]

Anandamides, also known as N-arachidonoylethanolamine or AEA, are a class of bioactive lipids known as fatty acid amides. Anandamide plays an important role in the regulation of appetite, pleasure and our reward system; AEA is produced by humans in the cell membranes and tissues of the body. Anandamide is known as the "bliss molecule" for its effects on the brain; THC (the active ingredient in cannabis that gets a person high) and anandamides have a very similar chemical structure. Researchers believe that theobromine, found in chocolate, helps increase anandamides in the brain. The following study shows that THC can inhibit the growth of cancer cells due to its strong similarity to anandamide (that truly would be "bliss"!).

"It has been shown that anandamide, potently and selectively, inhibited proliferation of human breast cancer cells… have shown antitumor activities of five natural cannabinoids, cannabidiol, cannabigerol, cannabichromene, cannabidiol acid, and $\Delta(9)$-tetrahydrocannabinol (THC), and suggested that cannabidiol was the most potent inhibitor of breast cancer cell growth. Both cannabidiol and the cannabidiol-rich extract also inhibited the growth of MDA-MB-231 breast carcinoma cells in athymic nude mice." – PubMed ID#18199524 (2008) (Excerpt from the full study) [617]

Cannabinoids have been found to inhibit cancer cells through various mechanisms: angiogenesis (inhibiting new blood vessel growth to tumors), cell migration (their ability to move from one location to another), metastasis (the development of new tumors at distance from the original tumor) and carcinogenesis (inhibiting normal cells from becoming cancerous). They are also shown to calm cancer-induced inflammation.

> "Intriguingly, antitumour effects mediated by cannabinoids are not confined to inhibition of cancer cell proliferation; cannabinoids also reduce angiogenesis, cell migration and metastasis, inhibit carcinogenesis and attenuate inflammatory processes." – PubMed ID#19589225 (2009) [618]

There is a lot of interest in researching CBD and THC cannabinoids for glioblastoma, a very aggressive form of brain cancer. This is due to its large number of CB2 cannabinoid receptors. Currently, this form of cancer is almost always fatal within 2 years (if treated conventionally, and within weeks if not treated). CBD and THC are being considered for adjuvant therapy to perhaps improve the success of conventional therapies. If someone you know has glioblastoma, this might be something they should discuss with their oncologist. Do not expect an oncologist to bring up this topic, or anything that is not an FDA-approved medication or treatment, unless it is part of an approved trial. This is something the patient would have to do on their own, but you will need to make sure that CBD/THC do not interfere with the oncologist's other treatment and that the oncologist is aware this is being done.

Note here where it states, "low doses of cannabinoids may enhance proliferation, whereas high doses of cannabinoids usually induce growth arrest or apoptosis." This is that "Goldilocks Zone" I've mentioned, where too little and too much are counterproductive; however, it is very difficult to determine what is "just right."

> "cannabinoids induce growth arrest or apoptosis in a number of transformed neural and non-neural cells in culture. In addition, cannabinoid administration induces regression of malignant gliomas in rodents by a mechanism that may involve sustained ceramide generation and extracellular signal-regulated kinase activation. In contrast, most of the experimental evidence indicates that cannabinoids may protect normal neurons from toxic insults, such as glutamatergic overstimulation, ischaemia, and oxidative damage. Regarding immune cells, low doses of cannabinoids may enhance proliferation, whereas high doses of cannabinoids usually induce growth arrest or apoptosis." – PubMed ID#12182964 (2002) [619]

Here CBD was found to inhibit the migration of glioma cells in vitro (in the test tube) in a rather wide range of concentrations. However, translating this in vitro range (where the concentration is applied directly to the cancer cells) to a human in vivo (in the body) concentration (when taken orally, intravenously or smoked) will be very difficult and require many trials. Keep in mind that getting the concentration wrong can worsen the patient's prognosis.

"The present study shows, for the first time, that CBD can inhibit the migration of U87 human glioma cells in vitro… we found that CBD caused concentration-related inhibition of glioma cell migration in a range of concentrations starting from 0.01 up to 9 μM… In conclusion, the present study demonstrates, for the first time, that CBD can inhibit the migration of tumoral cells… data further support the use of cannabinoids as antimetastatic drugs as previously demonstrated for met-fluoro-anandamide on rat thyroid cancer cell... This antimigratory property, together with the known antiproliferative and apoptotic features of CBD, strengthen the evidence for its use as a potential antitumoral agent." – PubMed ID#PMC1576089 (2005) [620]

This research shows the probable mechanism whereby THC induces apoptosis in glioma cells.

"delta9-Tetrahydrocannabinol (THC), the major active component of marijuana, induced apoptosis in C6.9 glioma cells… THC stimulated sphingomyelin hydrolysis in C6.9 glioma cells. THC and N-acetylsphingosine, a cell-permeable ceramide analog, induced apoptosis… Results thus show that THC-induced apoptosis in glioma C6.9 cells may rely on a CB1 receptor-independent stimulation of sphingomyelin breakdown." – PubMed ID#9771884 (1998) [621]

In this 2009 study out of Complutense University in Madrid, Spain, they showed that the cannabinoid THC promotes autophagic death in human and mouse cancer cells. This promoted the apoptotic death of cancer cells. Various cell lines were investigated, including glioblastoma.

"In this study we show that cannabinoids, a new family of potential antitumoral agents, induce autophagy of cancer cells and that this process mediates the cell death–promoting activity of these compounds. Several observations strongly support this idea: (a) THC induced autophagy and cell death in different types of cancer cells but not in nontransformed astrocytes, which are resistant to cannabinoid killing action, (b) pharmacological or genetic inhibition of autophagy prevented THC-induced cell death, (c) autophagy-deficient tumors were resistant to THC growth-inhibiting action, and (d) THC administration activated the autophagic cell death pathway in 3 different models of tumor xenografts as well as in 2 human tumor samples." – PubMed ID#PMC2673842 (2009) [622]

Activation of CB2 receptors by cannabinoids can impede the VEGF signaling protein that triggers vascular growth to support tumors' growth.

> "The abundant expression and distribution of CB2 receptors in glioblastoma and particularly endothelial cells of glioblastoma indicate that impaired tumor growth in presence of CB may be associated with CB2 activation. Selective CB2 agonists might become important targets attenuating vascular endothelial growth factor (VEGF) signalling and thereby diminishing neoangiogenesis and glioblastoma growth." – PubMed ID#19480992 (2009) [623]

The following paper outlines the large amount of research that was available in 2003 for using THC to treat various cancers.

> "The antitumour effects Delta9-THC and its analogues were first identified in the 1970s. Antineoplastic activities were reported in Lewis lung adenoma cells, L1210 leukaemia cells and HeLa S3 cells. As detained below, numerous investigations have since identified antiproliferative, apoptotic, antiangiogenic, and antimestastatic properties of cannabinoids… Rather than inducing apoptosis, the endocannabinoid AEA arrested the proliferation of human breast cancer cells by halting progression through the cell cycle at the G1/S transition… Clearly, cannabinoid receptor systems provide a therapeutic target for tumour intervention, including cancers such as malignant astrocytomas, gliomas, breast, thyroid, prostate, non-melanoma skin cancers, and lymphoblastic disease." – PubMed ID#14640910 (from the full study DOI: 10.1517/14728222.7.6.749) (2003) [624]

The following research investigated the use of Met-F-AEA (a stable anandamide, a brain chemical that binds to the cannabinoid CB1 receptors, much like THC does). This study may, or may not, apply to THC and other cannabis-derived cannabinoids.

> "Stimulation of cannabinoid CB1 receptors by 2-methyl-arachidonyl-2'-fluoro-ethylamide (Met-F-AEA) inhibits the growth of a rat thyroid cancer cell-derived tumor in athymic mice by inhibiting the activity of the oncogene product p21ras… Our findings indicate that CB1 receptor agonists might be used therapeutically to retard tumor growth in vivo by inhibiting at once tumor growth, angiogenesis, and metastasis." – PubMed ID#12958205 (2003) [625]

In this study, which used xenografted, metastasizing lung cancer tumors in mice, they found that injections of THC reduced tumor weight by around 50%.

> "Δ-9 Tetrahydrocannabinol inhibits growth and metastasis of lung cancer... THC (5mg/kg body wt.) was administered once daily through intraperitoneal injections for 21 days. The mice were analyzed for tumor growth and lung metastasis. A significant reduction (~50%) in tumor weight and volume were observed in THC treated animals compared to the vehicle treated animals. THC treated animals also showed a significant (~60%) reduction in macroscopic lesions on the lung surface" – AACR (2007) [626]

These studies, taken together, tend to indicate whole CBD oil, as well as marijuana, would be more beneficial than fractionated CBD oil (one without THC) due to the greater variety of cannabinoids.

Harmful Findings

Though there is a growing body of evidence showing the promise of using cannabinoids for cancer, there is also research showing it can make some cancers worse (especially breast cancers). The last sentence here says it best.

> "Here, we demonstrate that anandamide, Delta(9)-tetrahydrocannabinol (THC), HU-210, and Win55,212-2 promote mitogenic kinase signaling in cancer cells. Treatment of the glioblastoma cell line U373-MG and the lung carcinoma cell line NCI-H292 with nanomolar concentrations of THC led to accelerated cell proliferation... **concentrations of THC comparable with those detected in the serum of patients after THC administration accelerate proliferation of cancer cells instead of apoptosis and thereby contribute to cancer progression in patients.**" – PubMed ID#15026328 (2004) [627]

The study below indicates that breast cancer cell lines are resistant to Delta-9-THC (the psychoactive component of cannabis that also has anticancer properties). However, they only looked at THC's ability to induce apoptosis (the natural process of cells killing themselves if they become defective). Other studies (cited above) show that THC inhibits cancer through several means: "Rather than inducing apoptosis, the endocannabinoid AEA arrested the proliferation of human breast cancer cells by halting progression through the cell cycle at the G1/S transition" (see PubMed ID# 14640910 above).

> "We demonstrated that the human breast cancer cell lines MCF-7 and MDA-MB-231 and the mouse mammary carcinoma 4T1 express low to undetectable levels of cannabinoid receptors, CB1 and CB2, and that these cells are resistant to Delta9-THC-induced cytotoxicity. Furthermore, exposure of mice to Delta9-

> THC led to significantly elevated 4T1 tumor growth and metastasis due to
> inhibition of the specific antitumor immune response in vivo… Such findings
> suggest that marijuana exposure either recreationally or medicinally may increase
> the susceptibility to and/or incidence of breast cancer as well as other cancers
> that do not express cannabinoid receptors and are resistant to Delta9-THC-
> induced apoptosis." – PubMed ID#15749859 (2005) [628]

Several studies have indicated that low levels of cannabinoids (such as THC) may accelerate the
growth of breast cancer tumors. The solution in each of these studies was to increase the dosage.
The problem is that these studies have been done in vitro and in mice. The proper dose for
humans, for each cancer, still needs to be determined (and too much is also a problem—it's that
"Goldilocks Zone"). This problem appears to be limited to cancer cells that do not have the CB1
and CB2 cannabinoid receptors. Again, if you wish to consume cannabis products, you should
work with your oncologist to see if your particular cancer can benefit from THC or if it will be
exacerbated.

In the following mouse study, they administered the equivalent of 340 mg to a human (figuring
a 150 lb/68 kg person) four times per week (1,360 mg/week). When you consider that the
average "joint" weighs 0.3 grams and delivers approximately 12 mg of THC (based on a relatively
strong 11% THC cannabis variety), a person would need to smoke 113 joints per week to obtain
the same dosage as what was used in this study. I've met some potheads in my day, but I've never
met one who could smoke this much marijuana. In the full study, they note other research
showing that marijuana suppresses the immune system (not what you want, especially when on
immunotherapy).

> "intermittent administration of THC (5 mg/kg, four times/wk i.p. for 4 wk) led
> to accelerated growth of tumor implants compared with treatment with diluent
> alone… Our findings suggest the THC promotes tumor growth by inhibiting
> antitumor immunity by a CB2 receptor-mediated, cytokine-dependent pathway….
> The THC-mediated modulation of immune reactivity has previously been studied
> in infectious disease models (17). Newton and associates (16) injected mice with
> THC before infecting them with a sublethal dose of an opportunistic lung
> infection, Legionella pneumophila. While control mice developed cell-mediated
> immune responses and became immune to repeated infection, mice pretreated
> with THC failed to react and died when rechallenged." – PubMed ID#10861074
> (2000) [629], Full Study [630]

Most of the following research paper outlines the anti-tumor effects of cannabinoids; however,
it also shows some of the risks with this type of treatment.

> "a few studies have shown that, under certain conditions, cannabinoid treatment
> can stimulate cancer cell proliferation in vitro and interfere with the tumour-
> suppressor role of the immune system… various studies have associated the

expression levels of cannabinoid receptors, endocannabinoids, or endocannabinoid-metabolizing enzymes with tumour aggressiveness, which suggests that the endocannabinoid system might be overactivated in cancer and hence pro-tumourigenic" – PubMed ID#PMC4791144 (2016) [631]

The following showed that THC enhanced both breast cancer growth and metastasis. Whenever the immune system is suppressed, this can have a negative impact on the body's ability to fight cancer.

"McKallip et al. have earlier shown that Δ(9)-tetrahydrocannabinol enhanced breast cancer growth and metastasis specifically in cells expressing low levels of cannabinoid receptors by suppressing the antitumor immune response, suggesting that cannabinoid exposure may increase the incidence of breast cancer as well as other cancers that do not express cannabinoid receptors." – PubMed ID#18199524 (2008) (Excerpt from the full study) [632]

Though I find the research above to be credible, there is much more work that needs to be done on humans to determine dosing. Because of the ethical questions of treating patients with something that might make their conditions worse, this will be delicate and time-consuming research. The optimal dose may vary from person to person, and it may be influenced by weight, age, genetics, general health, immune health, other drugs/treatments, etc. It will also vary from cancer to cancer. It seems likely that cannabis, and especially THC, has a benefit (for some cancers, and especially for those with cannabinoid receptors) at moderate doses, but it is immunosuppressing at lower and higher doses. What is considered "moderate" still needs to be determined.

Symptom Relief

Here the research is a lot clearer. A 2018 prospective research study published in the March 2018 edition of *European Journal of Internal Medicine* analyzed data from 2,970 people living with cancer. The most frequent types of cancer were: breast (20.7%), lung (13.6%), pancreatic (8.1%) and colorectal (7.9%), with over 51% of these patients having stage 4 cancer. The patients were treated with medical cannabis between 2015 and 2017. The researcher's conclusions were that cannabis is "well tolerated, effective and safe" for people with cancer who have sleep problems, pain, weakness, nausea and lack of appetite.

"The main symptoms requiring therapy were: sleep problems (78.4%), pain (77.7%, median intensity 8/10), weakness (72.7%), nausea (64.6%) and lack of appetite (48.9%). After six months of follow up, 902 patients (24.9%) died and 682 (18.8%) stopped the treatment. Of the remaining, 1211 (60.6%) responded;

95.9% reported an improvement in their condition, 45 patients (3.7%) reported no change and four patients (0.3%) reported deterioration in their medical condition… Cannabis as a palliative treatment for cancer patients seems to be well tolerated, effective and safe option to help patients cope with the malignancy related symptoms." – PubMed ID#29482741 (2018) [633]

"since 2007, the Israeli Ministry of Health has been providing authorizations for medical cannabis use. Nowadays there are >30,000 patients in Israel taking cannabis, especially for the palliation of cancer symptoms… Bar-Lev Schleider et al. provide a valuable epidemiological insight into ~3000 of those cancer patients who had been prescribed cannabis for managing their malignancy-associated symptoms… 95.9% of patients reported an (either significant or moderate) improvement in their condition. Likewise, only 18.8% of patients reported good/very good quality of life before treatment initiation, whereas 69.5% did so after the 6-month cannabis regime. Regarding overall safety, cannabis was generally well tolerated, and most side effects reported, such as dizziness, dry mouth, and somnolence, could be considered as mild, especially in the context of an advanced cancer patient population." – PubMed ID#PMC5961457 (2018) [634]

However, there is also recent research showing cannabinoids having little to no benefit for improving appetite, nausea/vomiting, greater than 30% pain improvement, or sleep problems in cancer patients.

"We provide a systematic review and meta☐analysis on the efficacy, tolerability, and safety of cannabinoids in palliative medicine… In cancer patients, there were no significant differences between cannabinoids and placebo for improving caloric intake… appetite… nausea/vomiting… >30% decrease in pain… or sleep problems" – PubMed ID#PMC5879974 (2018) [635]

Yet again, there is conflicting evidence about the usage of cannabinoids. My goal here is not to convince you one way or the other, but to present the evidence. If I were faced with the question to try it or not, I would consider the following:

- Are conventional treatments not working well enough? Or do they have too many side effects?
- Are cannabinoids safe to take for my type of cancer?
- I'm not taking immunotherapy
- Is my oncologist OK with my taking them along with my other treatments?
- Can I obtain them where I live?

If the answer to all these questions is "Yes," then I would probably give it a try.

> *I personally have genetic issues that prevent me from taking opioid-based painkillers, and my gastrointestinal tract can't handle NSAIDs. Right now, that leaves me Tylenol and cannabis for pain relief. Someday I may have to make this decision myself.*

Recommendation

There is a lot of buzz right now surrounding medical marijuana and CBD oil. Low-THC CBD oil is legal in many states, but unlike what you may have heard, it is <u>not</u> legal in all 50 states. In fact, low-THC CBD oil is not even legal at the federal level (yes, that means it is technically illegal everywhere in the US—at least when this went to press). Although the DEA has stated that small personal amounts are not an <u>enforcement priority</u>, [636] it is still possible to get in trouble (and the DEA can change its mind again at any time). CBD oil should also not be sent through the US mail, or any other common carrier, across state lines. You should <u>never</u> take it on a trip to another country, even to those where it is legal, as you can be searched leaving the US and when you come back in.

Judging from the research above, it is obvious that there is a lot of potential for using cannabis extracts medicinally to treat some forms of cancer. However, I'm afraid this topic is much more complex than other botanicals and nutrients covered in this book, and a clear recommendation cannot be given. Cannabis is a complex plant. Even when looking at just the THC fraction, there is a lot of conflicting research; for some cancers (and cancer subtypes), a little THC may worsen the cancer, a moderate amount of THC <u>may</u> help treat it, and taking a little too much is also problematic, again worsening the cancer. THC is also a psychoactive drug; people really shouldn't stay stoned all the time. The "Goldilocks Zone" (the "just right" level) has yet to be determined and will most certainly vary depending on the person and cancer type.

Other constituents of cannabis, especially terpenes (e.g., myrcene, α-pinene and β-caryophyllene), have received very little attention and research. It is quite possible that some of these substances may provide positive or negative effects as well. When smoking marijuana, you are inhaling much more than just cannabinoids (such as THC).

Cannabinoids, CBD oil and marijuana do not seem to have enough positive research, at this time, to recommend them for anti-cancer treatments or prevention, simply based on the science. I think the research shows that certain cannabinoids might be useful under very specific circumstances for certain types of cancer, especially in conjunction with more traditional treatments. However, these substances do not appear to be suitable for self-administration for the treatment or prevention of cancer. The research showing immunosuppressing effects simply cannot be ignored.

If you do partake in either marijuana or non-THC cannabinoids, I recommend moderation. Though science has not determined the goalposts of that "Goldilocks Zone", there seems to be one. Overconsumption (or underconsumption) could be very detrimental.

> "The most studied and established roles for cannabinoid therapies include pain, chemotherapy-induced nausea and vomiting, and anorexia. Moreover, given their breadth of activity, cannabinoids could be used to concurrently optimize the management of multiple symptoms, thereby reducing overall polypharmacy." – PubMed ID#PMC5176373 (2016) (Current Oncology) [637]

Stress can be a big factor in immune system health. If marijuana calms you, and it is legal in your state, then it may have benefits in that regard. If it is illegal in your state, the added risk and worry (not to mention paranoia) of consuming illegal marijuana will probably negate any stress relief benefits.

Cannabis products have been used for years for nausea, appetite and pain treatment benefits. Several studies have shown them to have benefits in those regards. However, recent research is calling even this into question. Using cannabinoids for this purpose may be something to consider if other options don't work for you. However, this should be done under supervision of your oncologist to ensure that cannabinoids won't make your particular cancer worse. If I were diagnosed as terminal and I agreed with this prognosis, I would not hesitate to consider marijuana for pain relief, nausea or even appetite enhancement. Even if it turned out to be a placebo effect, who cares? I personally have a genetic issue that precludes the use of opioids, and NSAIDs (including aspirin) affect my stomach and cause tinnitus, so I'm running out of options. Many of you may also not want to take opioids if you can avoid it, as they can be quite addictive.

If all of this has left you more confused about cannabis than before you read it, you are not alone. The topic is very complex, and as with most natural alternatives, research money is scarce unless it may lead to a patentable drug or strengthen the government's stance against legalization. After reading around 100 studies and research papers on the topic, I myself am left unsure as to whether cannabis will *Improve Your Odds* with cancer or not; there is a very large *it depends* associated with that question.

Check in at the book's website for any updates on this very important and rapidly changing topic.

CHRYSIN

AKA: Propolis

Chrysin is the biologically active component of honey, and the only component that shows cancer fighting properties. Because of honey's very high sugar content, it is recommended that chrysin be used to obtain the anticancer benefits, rather than consuming honey. Chrysin is a type of flavonoid, a flavone. Flavones and other flavonoids are commonly found in foods, especially spices and red/yellow/purple vegetables.

Chrysin has shown benefits with a wide range of cancers; this is a good sign that it may help with most cancers. The following study indicates that chrysin showed significant benefits treating melanoma cancers transferred to mice (xenografts), as compared to the control group.

> "The results showed that chrysin inhibited cancer cell growth at a dose-dependent manner by inducing apoptosis and cell cycle arrest at G2/M phase. Moreover, chrysin suppressed melanoma tumor growth at an average of 60% (after 14 days of treatment) and 71% (after 21 days of treatment) compared to the tumor-bearing group. Furthermore, chrysin treatment increased the cytotoxic activity of NK, CTL and macrophages. The findings showed that chrysin antitumor action on the murine melanoma model was very promising, suggesting that chrysin could be a potentially good candidate for future use in alternative anti-melanoma treatments." – PubMed ID#29352974 (2018) [638]

The full study discussed in the abstract below looked at chrysin in two melanoma lines. They found that chrysin inhibited cellular growth by 40% to 50% in one cell line. In the other cell line, it was classified as "cytotoxic," with a metabolic activity reduction of over 90% in only 24 hours. They found significant cancer inhibition in all levels of chrysin tested, but with a clear dose-dependent pattern. For the techies out there, chrysin blocked the cell cycle of melanoma cells in the G0/G1 phase and induced hyperploid progression; this led to apoptosis and cancer cell death. There were no negative effects on normal cells.

> "results suggest that the anti-proliferative effects of honey are due mainly to the presence of chrysin. Chrysin may therefore be considered a potential candidate for both cancer prevention and treatment." – PubMed ID#20811719 (2010) [639]

> "Chrysin at 30–100 µM levels selectively reduced the viability of melanoma cells without affecting the viability of scleral fibroblasts and RPE cells. Chrysin increased mitochondrial permeability, the levels of cytosol cytochrome c, and caspase-9 and −3 activities, but not capase-8 activity in uveal melanoma cells. The

results of the present study indicate that chrysin induces apoptosis of human uveal melanoma cells via the mitochondrial signaling pathway and suggest that chrysin may be a promising agent in the treatment of uveal melanoma." – PubMed ID#PMC5228444 (2016) [640]

The following looked at chrysin in colon cancer. What I found interesting was the oral dosing. Significant benefits were found at dosing of 10 mg / kg. For a 180 lb (82 kg) adult, that would equate to 820 mg.

"chrysin accomplishes anti-cancer effect on colon cancer cells via induction of the apoptosis and attenuation of the sall4 the expression… the oral administration of chrysin at 8 and 10 mg.kg-1 has led to a significant regression in the tumors' volume as compared to the control group… The pro apoptotic effect of chrysin has been reported in breast carcinoma, cervical cancer, leukemia, lung cancer (NSCLC), and colon cancer in vitro… chrysin possess moderate cytotoxic effect on CT26 cells in a concentration dependent manner." – PubMed ID#PMC5492241 (2016) [641]

Recommendations

Due to the strong results seen in a variety of cancers, this is a supplement that I recommend taking. Chrysin is relatively inexpensive and has few to no side effects.

Because it has shown very strong benefits with human melanoma, it is a supplement that I take 500 mg of, twice per day. This is the dose I recommend if you currently have cancer—up to 1,000 mg twice per day, unless working with a healthcare professional. For prevention, 500 mg once per day is commonly recommended.

❖ CINNAMON EXTRACTS

AKA: *Cinnamomum zeylanicum,* Ceylon

Cancers: Most
Body of Evidence: Large
Cost: Low
Recommendation: High

Cinnamon has been in common use for thousands of years. It was used by the Egyptians over 4,000 years ago and was even mentioned in the Old Testament. It spread quickly to Europe, where its consumption became a status symbol among the upper elite due to its high cost at the time.

Cinnamon extracts, such as the essential oil, seem to be one of those rare substances that have a great number of benefits and very few drawbacks. Besides being a very popular spice, it has many medicinal uses, including potent anticancer benefits (both prevention and treatment).

> "prevention and treatment of serious illnesses, such as diabetes, cardiovascular diseases, Alzheimer's disease, and cancer. Cinnamon is known to have antioxidant, antibacterial, anti-inflammatory, and other therapeutic properties."— PubMed ID#PMC4488098 (2015) [642]

The essential oil of cinnamon has several studies showing its ability to treat cancer tumors and improve the cancer fighting abilities of the immune system. Many of the studies are on human cancer cells; the studies on mice are both in vivo and in vitro. It is becoming common to take human cancer cells and xenograft them to mice. This allows researchers to study human cancers in a biological system without the costs, difficulties and risks of human trials. This type of research has proven to be very similar to human in vivo studies.

> "we have demonstrated the potent anti-tumor efficacy of cinnamon extract and have elucidated its underlying mechanism using a mouse melanoma model system. Cinnamon extract significantly reduced tumor progression by down-regulating the tumor-associated growth factors such as EGF, VEGF-a, TGF-b, Cox-2, HIF-1, and neovascularization, while increasing the cytolytic activity of CD8+ T cells… long term treatment of cinnamon extract (more than 48 h) could induce active cell death and growth inhibition in several cancer lines such as melanoma, breast cancer, colorectal cancer, and hepatoma cell lines" – PubMed ID#19203831 (from the full study doi:10.1016/j.canlet.2009.01.015) (2009) [643]

This same team went on to publish an additional study that showed additional pathways where cinnamon extracts could be used to treat tumors. This research shows that cinnamon extracts can be a "potent anti-tumor" agent that shows promise across a range of different cancers. Increasing apoptosis in cancer cells is extremely valuable. Apoptosis is the cell's natural ability to detect damage to itself (including cancer) and self-destruct. This is one of the functions that cancer turns off. Turning this back on, and enhancing its action, has the potential to cure cancer.

> "Our study suggests that anti-tumor effect of cinnamon extracts is directly linked with enhanced pro-apoptotic activity and inhibition of NFκB and AP1 activities and their target genes *in vitro* and *in vivo* mouse melanoma model. Hence, further elucidation of active components of cinnamon extract could lead to development of potent anti-tumor agent or complementary and alternative medicine for the treatment of diverse cancers." – PubMed ID#PMC2920880 (2010) [644]

Solid tumors need a good blood supply to grow. Without being able to add new blood vessels, they would not be able to grow beyond a few millimeters in size. Tumors can initiate the process of creating new blood vessels (angiogenesis) by giving off chemical signals (such as VEGF) that stimulate angiogenesis. They can also stimulate nearby healthy cells to produce angiogenesis signals. Being able to stop tumors from initiating angiogenesis is a very important treatment method.

> "Although many anti-angiogenesis agents are available for cancer treatment, their side effects limit their application for cancer prevention... Previously, we demonstrated an extract from cinnamon, as well as its main component, procyanidins, was a potent inhibitor of angiogenesis through suppressing VEGF receptor kinase activity on endothelial cells... CE and another main component, cinnamaldehyde, effectively inhibited cancer cell VEGF expression through suppression of HIF-1a gene expression and protein synthesis. Thus, components of cinnamon have dual effects on angiogenesis and tumor cell growth—while cinnamaldehyde prevents the expression of VEGF by cancer cells, procyanidins inhibit the action of VEGF kinase activity on endothelial cells. As a result, CE potently inhibited angiogenesis and tumor growth in mice. – PubMed ID#27253180 (Extracts from the full study doi: 10.1002/mc.22506) [645]

> "Cinnamon extract inhibits VEGF-induced endothelial cell proliferation, migration, and tube formation in vitro, sprouts formation from aortic ring ex vivo, and tumor-induced blood vessel formation in vivo... Taken together, this study revealed novel activity in cinnamon and identified a natural inhibitor of VEGF signaling that could potentially be useful in cancer prevention and/or treatment." – PubMed ID#PMC2901047 (2010) [646]

VEGF is being studied extensively by pharmaceutical companies looking for new cancer-fighting drugs. VEGF is one of the important factors in tumor growth, as cancer cells utilize this natural function to build new blood vessels (angiogenesis) to feed tumor growth. Being able to block abnormal angiogenesis is yet another important benefit of cinnamon oil (cinnamaldehyde).

> "Angiogenesis, the formation of new vessels from preexisting vasculature, is an important mechanism used by tumors to promote growth and metastasis... Vascular endothelial growth factor (VEGF) is one of the most critical and specific angiogenesis factors regulating normal physiological and tumor angiogenesis... in the presence of CE, the number of migratory cells was significantly reduced in response to VEGF, in a concentration-dependent manner... Compared with controls, CE treatment led to a significant reduction in (tumor) blood vessel density indicated by reduced expression of CD31. These data indicated that CE is an angiogenesis inhibitor in vivo... As a natural

inhibitor of VEGFR2, CE has the potential to be routine diet-based strategy for cancer prevention or treatment." – PubMed ID#PMC3105590 (2010) [647]

A few of these studies use ground cinnamon, but the concentration of cinnamaldehyde is what is important. This is the reason most research studies use the essential oil of cinnamon (most often zeylanicum or Ceylon cinnamon bark); it has a high concentration of this active ingredient.

"β-Caryophyllene (BCP) is a sesquiterpene found in various plants… BCP exhibited cytotoxic activity against BT-20 human breast cancer cells, HeLa human cervical cancer cells, HTB140 human melanoma cells and B16F10s... these results indicate that increasing the intake of spices such as cloves, oregano, cinnamon and black pepper would help to prevent melanoma growth and metastasis." -- Carcinogenesis, Volume 36, Issue 9, 1 September 2015 [648]

"In vitro and in vivo system, cinnamon treatment strongly inhibited the expression of pro-angiogenic factors and master regulators of tumor progression not only in melanoma cell lines but also in experimental melanoma model. In addition, cinnamon treatment increased the anti-tumor activities of CD8(+) T cells by increasing the levels of cytolytic molecules and their cytotoxic activity." – PubMed ID#19203831 (2009) [649]

Many of the studies looked at very specific cancers. However, the findings are often applicable to other forms of cancer as well.

"Cinnamon alters the growth kinetics of SiHa cells in a dose-dependent manner. Cells treated with ACE-c exhibited reduced number of colonies compared to the control cells. The treated cells exhibited reduced migration potential that could be explained due to downregulation of MMP-2 expression. Interestingly, the expression of Her-2 oncoprotein was significantly reduced in the presence of ACE-c. Cinnamon extract induced apoptosis in the cervical cancer cells through increase in intracellular calcium signaling as well as loss of mitochondrial membrane potential. Conclusion: Cinnamon could be used as a potent chemopreventive drug in cervical cancer… cinnamon reduced the migration of cancer cells in a significant manner, further strengthening its potential use as an anti-cancer drug in cervical cancer." – PubMed ID#PMC2893107 (2010) [650]

Reactive oxygen species (ROS) are found in nearly all forms of cancer; they are very important to cancer development. However, research has shown that there is a delicate balance of ROS and that cancer cells also generate antioxidant proteins to help keep ROS in balance (allowing the tumor growth to continue). Disrupting this process is one of the goals of cancer treatment research.

> "Cinnamaldehyde induces apoptosis by ROS-mediated mitochondrial permeability transition in human promyelocytic leukemia HL-60 cells... our data indicate that cinnamaldehyde induces the ROS-mediated mitochondrial permeability transition and resultant cytochrome c release. This is the first report on the mechanism of the anticancer effect of cinnamaldehyde." – PubMed ID#12860272 (2003) [651]

The word "apoptosis" refers to a cell's built-in programming to die. This can be a process of renewal that kills cells as they get older, or a clean-up process that kills cells that are genetically defective or damaged. Cinnamaldehyde "induces" (or restores) the cancer cells' apoptosis—their ability to kill themselves. Apoptosis would have normally happened shortly after a normal cell became damaged or cancerous. Apoptosis is often turned off in established cancer cells, which is one of the things that makes cancer so dangerous. Cinnamaldehyde can help restore that natural ability.

> "Cinnamaldehyde (CA) is a bioactive compound... that has been identified as an antiproliferative substance with pro-apoptotic effects on various cancer cell lines... Compared with the control group, the proliferation inhibition rate of the human colorectal cancer cells following treatment with CA increased in a dose- and time-dependent manner. The invasion and adhesion abilities of the cells were significantly inhibited... In conclusion, CA has the potential to be developed as a new antitumor drug. The mechanisms of action involve the regulation of expression of genes involved in apoptosis, invasion and adhesion via inhibition of the PI3K/Akt signaling pathway." – PubMed ID#26677144 (2016) [652]

The following study looked at human colorectal cancer cells and found that cinnamaldehyde (CA) significantly inhibited CRC by interfering with cancer invasion and adhesion cells. Cell adhesion molecules play a significant role in cancer progression and metastasis; blocking them is an important step in preventing the spread of cancer. In most cancers, it usually isn't the original tumor that kills; it is the spread (metastasis to organs). CA was also able to reactivate apoptosis in cancer cells, causing them to die as a damaged cell should.

> "CA inhibits CRC cell proliferation in vitro... the inhibition rates of the cells were significantly higher compared with the control group at the same time points (p<0.01), and the inhibition by CA was exhibited in an approximate dose- and time-dependent manner... The invasion and adhesion abilities of the cells were significantly inhibited... CA also elevated the apoptotic rate... CA has attracted a great deal of research interest for its anticancer properties. It has been

used to inhibit the growth and induce the apoptosis of cancer cells as a natural bioactive substance in several studies. Its potential in the development of an effective anticancer and chemopreventive agent has been a focus in previous studies" – PubMed ID#26677144 (doi: 10.3892/or.2015.4493) [653]

Cinnamaldehyde is the active ingredient in cinnamon that has received the most research; it also contains eugenol and polyphenols, all of which have been found to have anticancer properties. Cinnamon attacks cancer in several different ways and has been shown to be very safe for human cells.

"Cinnamon extract strongly inhibited tumor cell proliferation in vitro and induced active cell death of tumor cells by up-regulating pro-apoptotic molecules while inhibiting NFkappaB and AP1 activity and their target genes such as Bcl-2, BcL-xL and survivin. Oral administration of cinnamon extract in melanoma transplantation model significantly inhibited tumor growth with the same mechanism of action observed in vitro… Our study suggests that anti-tumor effect of cinnamon extracts is directly linked with enhanced pro-apoptotic activity and inhibition of NFkappaB and AP1 activities and their target genes in vitro and in vivo mouse melanoma model. Hence, further elucidation of active components of cinnamon extract could lead to development of potent anti-tumor agent or complementary and alternative medicine for the treatment of diverse cancers." – PubMed ID#20653974 (2010) [654]

Though studies have used both *Cinnamomum cassia* and *Cinnamomum zeylanicum, cassia* is much higher in a chemical called "coumarins," which can be toxic at high doses. No more than 5 grams of *cassia* oil should be taken per day (based on a 50 kg body weight). This is approximately 100 drops of cinnamon oil (one drop weighs approximately 50 mg), far more than anyone needs to take (more is <u>not</u> better). *C. zeylanicum* (Ceylon) would have an even better safety margin (many times better). Research studies on humans have used up to 6 grams per day without ill effects. *C. zeylanicum* is also the essential oil used in most studies.

The following is a study using cinnamon oil in the treatment of diabetes.

"A meta-analysis by Allen *et al.* done for 10 randomized controlled trials including 543 patients has established that cinnamon, when taken in a dose of 120 mg/day to 6 g/day for approximately 4 months leads to a statistical decrease in levels of fasting plasma glucose along with an improvement in the lipid profile." – PubMed ID#PMC4466762 (2015) [655]

The following is from a well-respected book by healthcare professionals about using essential oils.

> "We agree with the Commission E Monographs daily oral maximum of 200mg for the (cinnamon essential) oil." -- Essential Oil Safety - E-Book: A Guide for Health Care Professionals

These safety concerns were most likely due to the high levels of coumarin in *cassia* cinnamon. *C. zeylanicum* contains far less coumarin and has a much higher margin of safety.

Strategy

The studies above are just a small sampling of those showing the benefits of using cinnamon oil to fight cancer and tumors. This is one supplement that I take and will continue to take. Besides its strong cancer-fighting and preventative properties, it also has several general health benefits.

For the reasons stated above, you should limit your daily intake of cinnamon oil to no more than 4 drops of *C. zeylanicum* (AKA: *Cinnamomum verum*, Ceylon) essential oil per day unless instructed otherwise by a healthcare professional who can monitor your treatment. I personally take 1 to 2 drops per day; higher amounts can reduce the diversity of the gut's microbiome. Up to 4 can be taken if you are trying to get rid of unwanted bacteria in your gut (cinnamon oil is very selective in the bad bacteria that it kills). This is well within the margin of safety, and again, more is not necessarily better. After three years of NED (no evidence of disease), I may drop this to a maintenance dose of 1 drop every 2 to 3 days.

Be sure to only use *C. zeylanicum* (Ceylon) bark, steam distilled essential oil, 100% pure (you want nothing added to it!). See this book's website for recommendations. When taking the oil, it should be diluted in a carrier oil, such as MCT oil (what I use); coconut, olive and avocado oils and ghee (clarified butter) are also OK. This combination can be mixed in warm tea, water, cocoa or coffee; I personally use a coffee frother to make sure everything is well combined. You should make sure you consume at least 4 ounces of liquid for every drop consumed. This can have a mild *bite*, but it isn't too bad. You can reduce this by adding ½ to 1 tsp of larch tree fiber to the mix (which you should be taking anyway), and then froth or blend well. This fiber allows the oil and water to mix (emulsify) and reduces the "bite" of the cinnamon.

When reporting this to your doctor, you can report taking 50 mg of cinnamon oil per day per drop (e.g., if you are taking two drops per day, report that you are taking 100 mg of cinnamon oil). Some oncologists want to know about everything that you eat and supplement. However, they don't always know if something will interfere with the treatment they've prescribed you, so they may ask you to stop all supplements. They tend to take the easy way out and have people stop taking everything, just in case. Personally, I would make them earn their pay and have them show you a study or advisory that cinnamon oil (or other supplements mentioned in this book) is contradicted before stopping it.

❖ Essiac Tea

Essiac tea is a mixture of four herbs: *Arctium lappa* (burdock), *Rumex acetosella* (sheep sorrel), *Ulmus rubra* (slippery elm) and *Rheum officinale* (Chinese rhubarb). Other mixtures are reported to contain burdock root, Indian rhubarb, sheep sorrel, inner bark of slippery elm, watercress, blessed thistle, red clover and kelp. Reportedly, Essiac tea was created by the Ojibwa tribe of Canada. As you can see, there is no standardized formula for Essiac tea, which makes judging its effectiveness difficult as the formula can change from study to study.

In recent years, Essiac tea has been widely discussed as a homeopathic treatment for cancer. Some studies do show that it is a strong antioxidant and is DNA-protective. As discussed in other areas of this book, strong antioxidant properties are not always a good thing when treating existing cancers. The research done with Essiac tea has not been promising, with some research showing that it can actually make some cancers worse. There are some anecdotal reports of people getting better after consuming it daily; however, people do sometimes beat cancer with no intervention (medical, nutritional or herbal). Anecdotal evidence of this sort is very unreliable, especially when weighed against studies showing no benefit (and appearing in alternative medicine journals, no less).

The following in vitro study that appeared in the *Journal of Alternative and Complementary Medicine* found mixed results. At low doses, Essiac tea appeared to boost important T cell levels, but at higher doses it inhibited T cells. Because translating in vitro dosing to human in vivo dosing is difficult, it isn't clear what the proper in vivo dose should be. It is also possible the dose might be different for people with an impaired, or weakened, immune system.

> "We found in vitro evidence of decreased proliferation of both noncancerous transformed (CHO) and cancerous prostate cell line (LNCaP) when Essiac was present in the culture media. A dose response for inhibition was demonstrated by a linear regression performed on the data for both the CHO and LNCaP cells... **At low doses of Essiac, augmentation of proliferation of these T cells was demonstrated, but at higher doses Essiac was inhibitory to T-cell proliferation.**" – PubMed ID#15353028 (2004) [656]

In this in vivo (in the body) study appearing in the journal *Nutrition and Cancer*, they found that no toxicity was noted in mice. However, they also found that Essiac tea had no effect on tumor size or proliferation of cancer cells.

> "Toxicity in nude mice was tested, and efficacy in inhibiting PC-3 xenograft growth. No toxicity or tumour size difference was observed dosing up to 240 mg/kg QD, over 28 days, excepting the positive control group treated with paclitaxel. Ki-67 and PCNA expression was analyzed in treated tumors, but no

difference in expression of either marker was observed. These evaluations suggest **Essiac has no marked antiproliferative effect on the models tested.**" – PubMed ID#17640165 (2007) [657]

Recommendation

Until more research is available, my advice would be to avoid this one. If consumed in low amounts, it might be harmless, but that level has not been clarified. There are many other natural supplements here (without registered trademarks) that have plenty of evidence as to their efficacy.

If you can handle green tea (see that section and the notes on COMT), that would be a much better choice. However, I would consume that in moderation as well.

❖ FUCOIDAN

Cancers: Possibly all
Body of Evidence: Moderate
Cost: Low
Recommendation: High

Fucoidan is a complex sulfated polysaccharide found in several species of brown seaweed, such as kombu and bladderwrack. Kombu is found in Japanese, Korean and Chinese cuisine, often in soups. Wakame, another brown seaweed that contains fucoidan, is one of the main ingredients in miso soup. Evidence that these seaweeds have been consumed in Asian cultures goes back over fifteen thousand years, and they have probably been consumed much longer than that.

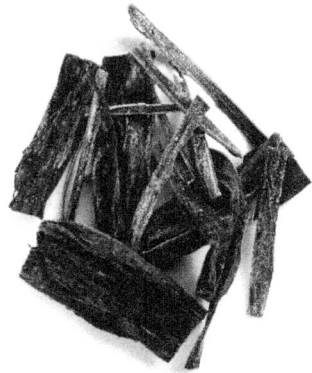

Kombu (as well as other brown seaweeds) and the fucoidan extract have been shown in various studies to be an immunomodulatory, to prevent and treat cancers, and to reduce inflammation. They are also anti-arthritic, radioprotective (they benefit people on radiation therapy), reduce osteoarthritis symptoms, inhibit the influenza virus, display potent antiviral activity against all forms of herpes, help prevent some of the cellular damage caused by Alzheimer's disease, help protect cells from radiation and chemotherapy damage, and can help lower blood pressure.

The following paper looked at the current research available for fucoidan and concluded that fucoidan contains strong anticancer activity. It also has immunomodulating benefits and possesses protective effects against the development of chemotherapy and radiation side effects.

"Fucoidan, a natural component of brown seaweed, has anti-cancer activity against various cancer types by targeting key apoptotic molecules. It also has beneficial effects as it can protect against toxicity associated with chemotherapeutic agents and radiation. Thus the synergistic effect of fucoidan with current anti-cancer agents is of considerable interest. This review discusses the mechanisms by which fucoidan retards tumor development, eradicates tumor cells and synergizes with anti-cancer chemotherapeutic agents… The anti-cancer property of fucoidan has been demonstrated in vivo and in vitro in different types of cancers" (continued below)

Fucoidan has multiple anticancer mechanisms as well as immunomodulator effects. It is also protective against both radiation and chemotherapy side effects. Fucoidan itself rarely causes any side effects and is beneficial for general health. This makes it an excellent adjuvant therapy that can be used in conjunction with almost any other therapy and most any type of cancer (but always check with your oncologist).

"Fucoidan mediates its activity through various mechanisms such as induction of cell cycle arrest, apoptosis and immune system activation. Additional activities of fucoidan have been reported that may be linked to the observed anti-cancer properties and these include induction of inflammation through immune system, oxidative stress and stem cell mobilization… A number of in vitro and in vivo studies have indicated that fucoidan contains strong anti-cancer bioactivity. Since fucoidan also possesses immunomodulatory effects, it is postulated that it may have protective effects against development of side effects when it is co-administered with chemotherapeutic agents and radiation." – PubMed ID#PMC4413214 (2015) (Open Access attribution at the link) [658]

Fucoidan stimulates the immune system's ability to produce NK (natural killer) cells, one of our primary cancer fighting tools. It also impedes overactive cell division (one of the hallmarks of cancer).

"The survival of mice was prolonged when Mekabu fucoidan was administered for 4 days before tumor cell inoculation, compared with non-treated mice. Fucoidan significantly enhanced the cytolytic activity of NK cells and increased the amount of IFN-gamma produced by T cells up to about 2-fold compared with non-treated mice. The anti-tumor effect of Mekabu fucoidan appears to be mediated by IFN-gamma-activated NK cells." – PubMed ID#12929574 (2003) [659]

Fucoidan has the ability to restore apoptosis in cancer cells. It can also inhibit the proliferation of cancer. In this study of breast cancer cells, it was found that apoptotic death was caused by several mechanisms, while not affecting normal cells.

> "Fucoidan is an active component of seaweed that has been shown to inhibit proliferation and induce apoptotic cell death in several tumor cells… In the present report, we investigated the effect of fucoidan on the induction of apoptosis in human breast cancer MCF-7 cells. Our data demonstrated that fucoidan reduced the viable cell number of MCF-7 cells in a dose- and time-dependent manner. In contrast, fucoidan did not affect the viable cell number of normal human mammary epithelial cells." – PubMed ID#19754176 (2009) [660]

Here it was shown that fucoidan induces apoptosis of human T cell leukemia virus type 1-infected T cell lines and primary adult T cell leukemia cells.

> "Fucoidan significantly inhibited the growth of peripheral blood mononuclear cells of ATL patients… Fucoidan induced apoptosis of HTLV-1-infected T-cell lines… Further analysis showed that fucoidan inactivated NF-kappaB and activator protein-1 and inhibited NF-kappaB-inducible chemokine, C-C chemokine ligand 5 (regulated on activation, normal T expressed and secreted) production, and homotypic cell-cell adhesion of HTLV-1-infected T-cell lines. In vivo use of fucoidan resulted in partial inhibition of growth of tumors of an HTLV-1-infected T-cell line transplanted subcutaneously in severe combined immune deficient mice." – PubMed ID#16201850 (2005) [661]

In this study out of Fukuoka University in Japan, they looked at fucoidan's ability to suppress sarcoma, Lewis lung carcinoma and B16 melanomas. They found that another action of fucoidan is the prevention of tumor-induced angiogenesis (tumor-induced formation of new blood vessels meant to feed the tumor). This is in addition to the anti-tumor actions shown above, such as cell cycle arrest, apoptosis and immune system activation.

> "Fucoidan, a sulfated polysaccharide extracted from brown seaweed… shows an inhibitory action on the progression and metastasis of malignant tumors… The inhibitory action of fucoidan was also observed in the growth of Lewis lung carcinoma and B16 melanoma in mice. These results indicate that the antitumor action of fucoidan is due, at least in part, to its anti-angiogenic potency and that increasing the number of sulfate groups in the fucoidan molecule contributes to the effectiveness of its anti-angiogenic and antitumor activities." – PubMed ID#12504793 (2003) [662]

In addition to the anti-tumor and antimetastatic (inhibiting metastasis) activity, fucoidan also potentiated the toxic effect of cyclophosphamide (a chemotherapy drug).

"Antitumor and antimetastatic activities of fucoidan, a sulfated polysaccharide isolated from Fucus evanescens (brown alga in Okhotsk sea), was studied in C57Bl/6 mice with transplanted Lewis lung adenocarcinoma. Fucoidan after single and repeated administration in a dose of 10 mg/kg produced moderate antitumor and antimetastatic effects" – PubMed ID#18239813 (2007) [663]

Cancer has developed ways of turning off apoptosis, allowing the cancer to grow uncontrolled. Whenever we can support apoptosis, or turn it back on again, that is a very good thing.

"Fucoidan (FE) is a potent inducer of apoptosis in various cancer cell lines… Several studies have shown that fucoidan induces extrinsic or intrinsic apoptotic signaling in different cancer cell types via alteration of expression or activities of mitochondria-associated proteins, cell cycle regulatory proteins, proteases, and transcription factors… Two cervical cancer patients (a 49-year-old female and a 24-year-old female), a renal cancer patient (81-year-old male), and a liver cancer patient (74-year-old female) also experienced improvement in their symptoms after receiving fucoidan extract orally at 30–40 mg/kg/day… In conclusion, our study demonstrates that FE inhibits growth of the MCF-7, MDA-MB-231, HeLa, and HT1080 cell lines. We present evidence that FE induces a caspase-independent mitochondria-mediated apoptotic pathway in MCF-7 cells." – doi.org/10.1371/journal.pone.0027441 (2011) (Open Access attribution available at the link) [664]

"the present data suggest that fucoidan induces apoptotic and autophagic cell death, and both apoptotic and autophagic mechanisms contribute to the fucoidan☐induced AGS cell death." – doi.org/10.1111/j.1750-3841.2011.02099.x (2011) [665]

Additional research can be found in PubMed ID#PMC6266495 (2018). [666]

Adjuvant Treatment

Adjuvant treatment is a treatment given in conjunction with another, primary, treatment to either improve its effectiveness, decrease recurrence or reduce side effects.

"Results showed that fucoidan regulated the occurrence of fatigue during chemotherapy. Chemotherapy with fucoidan was continued for a longer period than chemotherapy without fucoidan. Additionally, the survival of patients with fucoidan treatment was longer than that of patients without fucoidan, although the difference was not significant. Thus, fucoidan may enable the continuous administration of chemotherapeutic drugs for patients with unresectable advanced or recurrent colorectal cancer, and as a result, the prognosis of such patients is prolonged." – PubMed ID#22866084 (2011) [667]

Chemotherapy and radiation therapy can lead to inflammation, sometimes severe. This inflammation has many negative consequences, from reduced quality of life (QOL) to increased tumor proliferation, angiogenesis and metastasis. [668] Fucoidan has been shown to help reduce this excess inflammation and thus improve most of the associated side effects.

"Conventional anticancer therapies still cause difficulties with selective eradication and accompanying side effects that reduce patients' quality of life (QOL). Fucoidan is extracted from seaweeds and has already exhibited broad bioactivities, including anticancer and anti-inflammatory properties… The main proinflammatory cytokines, including interleukin-1β (IL-1β), IL-6, and tumor necrosis factor-α (TNF-α) were significantly reduced after 2 weeks of fucoidan ingestion. QOL scores, including fatigue, stayed almost stable without significant changes during the study period. The univariate and multivariate analyses revealed that the responsiveness of IL-1β was a significant independent prognostic factor." – PubMed ID#28627320 (2018) [669]

In a study (dual blind randomized control trial) of 54 patients with colorectal cancer, half of the patients received 4 grams of fucoidan powder in addition to chemotherapy. This resulted in a DCR (disease control rate) of 92%, compared to 69% in the placebo control group.

"54 patients were enrolled, of whom 28 were included in the study group and 26 in the control group. The primary endpoint was the disease control rate (DCR), and secondary endpoints included the overall response rate (ORR), progression-free survival (PFS), overall survival (OS), adverse effects (AEs), and quality of life (QOL). Results: The DCRs were 92.8% and 69.2% in the study and control groups" – PubMed ID#PMC5408268 (2017) [670]

I should point out that fucoidan may not be appropriate for all forms of cancer. A 2017 study of uveal melanoma (ocular melanoma of the eye) cell lines (in vitro) found that fucoidan may not be protective against this type of cancer. Currently, they do not know if this finding applies only to uveal melanoma, or to some other cancers as well. They also do not know if these results will be replicated with in vivo studies, nor have the results been confirmed by other research.

I have two types of melanoma; neither are ocular, so I do take this supplement as I think it has a lot of potential.

Recommendations

Most studies used between 500 mg and 4,000 mg of fucoidan per day. I recommend taking 500 mg of fucoidan twice per day unless advised by a treatment professional to take more (or less). Fucoidan is also a prebiotic (it feeds beneficial bacteria in the gut), so if you develop gas or bloating, scale back to one capsule per day until your gut adjusts to it, and then try twice per day again (you may have to repeat this a few times until your gut adjusts to the fiber). A healthy microbiome is also known to strengthen the immune system and help it fight cancer.

Consuming brown seaweed in food is also fine and probably has even more benefits, with some yet to be identified. The taste can be a little fishlike, but if you use it in moderation (e.g., ½ tsp per serving to start), you can obtain the benefits without imparting a strong flavor. I enjoy making and consuming miso soup. Miso is a great probiotic; the fermented soy contains genistein (discussed earlier), and it contains brown seaweed (for fucoidan). Miso is also easy to make; just be sure you have a food thermometer, as you do not want to add the miso to the wakame broth until the temperature has fallen below 120°F (49°C), in order to maintain the probiotic benefits. You'll find plenty of recipes online, but they don't all mention this point.

Note: If you are on anticoagulants such as warfarin and heparin, you should discuss taking this with your doctor, as fucoidan is also an anticoagulant. Your doctor may need to reduce the dosage of your prescription medications. The fucoidan extract contains iodine (though less than seaweed), so if you have Hashimoto's, you should discuss with your doctor whether you should take it.

Fucoidan is relatively inexpensive, fights cancer by various mechanisms, and benefits gut health (and thus the immune system). Certainly, it is worth including in any protocol.

GARLIC

AKA: *Allium sativum*

Cancers: Liver, stomach, colon, prostate, bladder, breast, esophagus, pancreas, lung and skin (melanoma)
Body of Evidence: Moderate
Cost: Low
Recommendation: Treatment – Medium; Prevention – High

Garlic has documented medicinal uses dating back 3,500 years, and a written history of its use as a food going back over 9,000 years (though it probably goes back much further than that). The Bible makes mention of garlic in reference to the Jews' flight from Egypt. Garlic bulbs were found in ancient pharaohs' tombs. Hippocrates considered garlic an essential part of his medicinal supplies, and early Olympiads in Greece used garlic to improve endurance. Ancient Chinese and Indian medicine recommended garlic for everything from digestive health to leprosy. It was commonly used to treat parasite infections and is still used for that today. Garlic also has antibacterial properties, and thus has been used to treat various infections and in the preservation of food. Garlic contains 33 sulfuric compounds, most of which provide benefits of one kind or another.

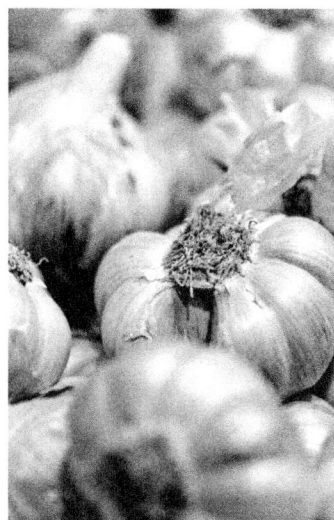

Today, garlic is commonly sold in supplements to improve cardiovascular health, maintain circulatory function, improve the immune system, help the body detoxify, treat high blood pressure, lower cholesterol and for general health purposes.

Of course, garlic is widely used in recipes of all kinds and can be found in foods from many different cultures. With its strong flavor, a little goes a long way.

Now science is finding that garlic has some cancer-preventive and anti-tumor effects as well.

> "In 1990, the U.S. National Cancer Institute initiated the Designer Food Program to determine which foods played an important role in cancer prevention (Dahanukar and Thatte, 1997). They concluded that garlic may be the most potent food having cancer preventive properties. Garlic has a variety of anti-tumor effects, including tumor cell growth inhibition and chemopreventive effects." – PubMed ID#PMC4103721 (2014) [671]

Garlic has been shown to help prevent tumors of the liver, stomach, colon, prostate, bladder, breast, esophagus, lung and even skin cancer (including melanoma).

"Chemoprevention of skin cancer by garlic organosulfur has recently received increased attention… Evidence suggests that the suppression of cancer cell growth by garlic oil and allyl sulfides correlates with apoptosis induction… Taylor et al. were the first to report the antimetastatic effect of garlic sulfur compounds. The result has shown that ajoene inhibits tumor cell growth in vitro, and strongly suppresses metastasis to lung in the B16/BL6 melanoma cell model in C57BL/6 mice. Our studies are in progress to demonstrate that DATS inhibits cell migration, adhesion, and invasion of A375 cells under noncytotoxic concentration… garlic-derived allyl sulfides possess an anticancer effect in several organs, including the skin." – PubMed ID#PMC3499657 (2012) (Open Access license attribution available at the link) [672]

The following is from the National Cancer Institute (an agency under the National Institutes of Health, part of the US Department of Health and Human Services) outlining a few of the many studies that show garlic consumption leading to reduced risk for several types of cancer. Remember that when it comes to natural substances, what can prevent cancer can often help treat it.

"Several population studies show an association between increased intake of garlic and reduced risk of certain cancers, including cancers of the stomach, colon, esophagus, pancreas, and breast. Population studies are multidisciplinary studies of population groups that investigate the cause, incidence, or spread of a disease or examine the effect of health-related interventions, dietary and nutritional intakes, or environmental exposures. An analysis of data from seven population studies showed that the higher the amount of raw and cooked garlic consumed, the lower the risk of stomach and colorectal cancer." – Cancer.gov – "Garlic and Cancer Prevention" [673]

The following paper outlines the research that has been done on garlic and onions, especially in regards to stomach cancer, colorectal cancer, esophageal cancer and prostate cancer, as well as oral cavity/pharynx, larynx, renal cells, breast, ovary and endometrium cancers.

"Allium vegetables and their components have effects at each stage of carcinogenesis and affect many biological processes that modify cancer risk… Approximately 30–40% of cancers are preventable by appropriate food and nutrition, physical activity, and maintenance of healthy body weight… A recent meta-analysis of 19 case-control and 2 cohort studies showed that consumption of large amounts of total Allium vegetables reduced risk of gastric cancer when comparing the highest and lowest consumption groups (odds ratio (OR): 0.54; 95% CI 0.43–0.65)… the fifth quintile of garlic/onion intake was associated with an OR of colorectal adenoma of 0.87 (95% CI 0.77–0.99) compared to the lowest quintile… In addition to the above in colorectal, esophageal, and prostate cancer, the investigators of the Italian and Swiss case-control studies investigated other possible associations between onions or garlic and cancers of the oral cavity/pharynx, larynx, renal cells, breast, ovary, and endometrium" – PubMed ID#PMC4366009 (2015) [674]

In this research out of the National Taiwan University in Taipei, Taiwan, the researchers found that garlic can induce both apoptosis and autophagy in cancer cells.

"Garlic (Dà Suàn; Allium sativum), is one of most powerful food used in many of the civilizations for both culinary and medicinal purpose. In general, these foods induce cancer cell death by apoptosis, autophagy, or necrosis. Studies have discussed how natural food factors regulate cell survival or death by autophagy in cancer cells. From many literature reviews, garlic could not only induce apoptosis but also autophagy in cancer cells… Garlic, which is considered the most powerful anticarcinogenic agent by the Designer Food Program, NCI, 2005, not only induces apoptosis but also autophagy in cancer cells." – PubMed ID#PMC3924985 (2013) (Open Access Attribution available at the link) [675]

Garlic also acts as an immunomodulator that helps the immune system target emerging tumors, while reducing overall inflammation.

"garlic acts as an immune modulator that can shift the balance from a pro-inflammatory and immunosuppressive environment to an enhanced anti-tumor response leading to suppression of an emerging tumor… We propose that long-term supplementation with dietary garlic organosulfur compounds contributes in shifting the balance from a pro-inflammatory to an anti-tumor response by dampening the pro-inflammatory response and/or strengthening the anti-tumor immunity towards tumor eradication." – PubMed ID#PMC3915757 (2014) [676]

Raw garlic consumption (eating it two or more times per week) was shown to lower the risk of developing lung cancer.

"Compared to no intake, raw garlic intake was associated with lower risk of development of lung cancer with a dose-response pattern (aOR for <2 times per week = 0.56, 95% CI: 0.39–0.81 and aOR for ≥2 times per week = 0.50, 95% CI: 0.34 – 0.74; Ptrend = 0.0002). Exploratory analysis showed an additive interaction of raw garlic consumption with indoor air pollution and with any

> supplement use in association with lung cancer… In-vitro and in-vivo experimental studies provided evidence for the anti-cancer properties of garlic against stomach, liver, colon, prostate, skin, bladder, breast and lung cancer… Conclusions: The results of the current study suggest that raw garlic consumption is associated with reduced risk of lung cancer in a Chinese population… the current study reiterated the findings of the previous two studies that raw garlic consumption of 2 or more times per week may be protective against lung cancer." – PubMed ID#PMC4873399 (2016) [677]

Raw garlic was shown to be much better at arresting breast cancer cell growth than boiled garlic. Boiled (or otherwise cooked) garlic may have other benefits not examined in this study.

> "We report here that fresh extracts of garlic (not boiled) arrested the growth and altered the morphology of MCF7 breast cancer cells. Deregulated levels of E-cadherin, cytokeratin, and β-catenin correlated with the altered phenotype… When MCF7 cells were exposed to fresh garlic extract (GE), within 1 hour, the cells began to alter their morphology. After 2-4 hours, GE-treated MCF7 cells became morphologically distinct, attained mesenchyme like phenotype, and lost cell-to-cell contact. In contrast, boiled garlic extract (BGE) failed to alter their morphology… Our results demonstrate that a short exposure to fresh but not boiled garlic extract is sufficient to permanently alter the morphology and trigger the growth arrest of MCF7 cells." – PubMed ID#PMC3463925 (2012) [678]

> "The action of AGE (aged garlic extract) appears to be dependent on the type of cancer cell. On the other hand, AGE enhanced the adhesion of endothelial cells to collagen and fibronectin and suppressed cell motility and invasion. AGE also inhibited the proliferation and tube formation of endothelial cells potently. These results suggest that AGE could prevent tumor formation by inhibiting angiogenesis through the suppression of endothelial cell motility, proliferation, and tube formation. AGE would be a good chemopreventive agent for colorectal cancer because of its antiproliferative action on colorectal carcinoma cells and inhibitory activity on angiogenesis." – PubMed ID#16484577 (2006) [679]

Drugs used to treat childhood precursor-B acute lymphoblastic leukemia (ALL) have been shown to be nonselective against cancer cells (meaning that they can also harm normal cells). The following research shows that garlic is selective and causes apoptosis (programmed cell death) only in malignant cells.

"In conclusion, we show selective apoptosis of malignant cells by garlic compounds that do not alter T-cell immune function and indicate the potential therapeutic benefit of garlic compounds in the treatment of childhood ALL." – PubMed ID#PMC2727784 (2008) [680]

The following paper discusses several studies of garlic's anticancer properties. It is important to point out that allicin, a common supplement, is not the only substance in garlic with anticancer benefits. It is best to consume raw and cooked garlic on a regular basis. Garlic can lead to cancer cell apoptosis, suppresses proliferation and metastasis, inhibits cancer cell migration and suppresses VEGF (a signaling protein that cancer cells use to stimulate the formation of blood vessels to feed the tumor).

"Epidemiologic evidence suggested that high consumption of garlic protected against various cancers... Organo-sulphur compounds (OSC), such as alliin, allicin, diallyl disulfide, diallyl sulfide, allyl mercaptan, and S-allylcysteine, were reported to be major ingredients with anti-tumor properties in garlic... In Hep3B HCC cells, hexane extracts of garlic promoted ROS production and subsequent dysregulation of mitochondrial membrane potential, leading to enhanced apoptotic cell death. Similarly, allicin was also able to induce apoptotic cell death through overproduction of ROS in Hep3B human HCC cell line. The propensity to metastasis of HCC leads to recurrence and poor prognosis... S-allylcysteine was observed to suppress proliferation and metastasis of HCC in a metastatic HCC cell line MHCC97L and in vivo xenograft liver cancer model. The potential mechanisms included to inhibit cancer cell migration and invasion by suppressing VEGF and increasing E-cadherin; to promote cell apoptotic death via downregulating Bcl-2,-xl and upregulating caspase-3, -9 activities; and to induce S cell cycle arrest" – PubMed ID#PMC4808884 (2016, Creative Commons attribution at the link) [681]

This study out of China looked at whether the consumption of raw garlic was associated with a lower risk of developing lung cancer. They found that up to a point, the more garlic one consumed, the lower their risk was of developing lung cancer. Garlic contains 9 major organo-sulfur compounds that are responsible for its cancer fighting properties. Thus, whole garlic may be a better option than supplements.

"Compared with no intake, raw garlic intake was associated with lower risk of development of lung cancer with a dose–response pattern (aOR for <2 times/week = 0.56; 95% CI, 0.39–0.81 and aOR for ≥2 times/week = 0.50; 95% CI, 0.34–0.74; Ptrend = 0.0002). Exploratory analysis showed an additive interaction of raw garlic consumption with indoor air pollution and with any supplement use in association with lung cancer. Conclusions: The results of the current study suggest that raw garlic consumption is associated with reduced risk of lung cancer in a Chinese population." -- DOI: 10.1158/1055-9965.EPI-15-0760 (2016) [682]

S-allylcysteine (SAC) is a water-soluble component of garlic. Water soluble means that no special extraction methods are necessary; when you consume garlic, you can utilize the SAC.

> "SAC (1-100 mmol/L) inhibited the proliferation of A2780 cells in dose- and time-dependent manners (the IC50 value was approximately 25 mmol/L at 48 h, and less than 6.25 mmol/L at 96 h). Furthermore, SAC dose-dependently inhibited the colony formation of A2780 cells... SAC suppresses proliferation and induces apoptosis in A2780 ovarian cancer cells in vitro." – PubMed ID#24362328 (2014) [683]

It is important to use freshly crushed garlic, as this is what produces the beneficial allicin. As explained elsewhere in this section, the important garlic components can quickly break down (oxidize) after they've been crushed.

> "Crushed cloves are rich in sulfur containing compounds collectively termed garlic organosulfur compounds (OSCs) which are the active principles responsible for the biological activity of garlic... In cancer treatment, garlic organosulfur compounds have been shown to inhibit proliferation and induce apoptosis of cancer cells both in culture as well as in mouse xenograft models. Central to this effect are G2/M cell cycle arrest and activation of the mitochondrial-dependent caspase cascade. In cancer prevention, numerous epidemiological studies have demonstrated a link between garlic consumption and decreased risk of cancer... OSCs are reported to exert an immunological effect by eliciting diverse immune responses depending on the particular experimental setting. We propose that garlic OSCs obtained through the diet, may aid in cancer prevention by shifting the overall balance from a tumor-mediated pro-inflammatory to a host-mediated anti-tumor response which may stimulate the immune system towards eradication of an emerging tumor... garlic acts as an immune modulator that can shift the balance from a pro-inflammatory and immunosuppressive environment to an enhanced anti-tumor response leading to suppression of an emerging tumor... the organosulfur compounds of garlic contribute to the prevention or reduction of the immuno-suppressive environment during chronic inflammation with the downstream consequence of assisting the host to escape tumor-mediated immune suppression and to elicit an

---

anti-tumor immune response." – PubMed ID#PMC3915757 (2014) (Creative Common attribution available at the link) [684]

Breast Cancer

An oil-based compound in garlic called diallyl disulfide (DADS) can suppress breast cancer and help reduce side effects from anti-cancer medications used to treat breast cancer.

"Garlic and garlic-derived compounds reduce the development of mammary cancer in animals and suppress the growth of human breast cancer cells in culture. Oil-soluble compounds derived from garlic, such as diallyl disulfide (DADS), are more effective than water-soluble compounds in suppressing breast cancer... DADS synergizes the effect of eicosapentaenoic acid, a breast cancer suppressor, and antagonizes the effect of linoleic acid, a breast cancer enhancer. Moreover, garlic extract reduces the side effects caused by anti-cancer agents. Thus, garlic and garlic-derived compounds are promising candidates for breast cancer control." – PubMed ID#21269259 (2011) [685]

This study only found anticancer benefits in cooked garlic, not boiled. However, they only looked at one very specific type of breast cancer cells, and they were using a garlic extract (not whole cloves). Yet, this shows again how garlic can be beneficial in preventing and treating breast cancer.

"we investigated the effect of various dietary products on morphological differentiation of the breast cancer cell line MCF7 and found that 2-3 hours of exposure to garlic extract (fresh but not boiled) was sufficient to arrest the growth and alter the morphology of MCF7 cells... When MCF7 cells were exposed to fresh garlic extract (GE), within 1 hour, the cells began to alter their morphology. After 2-4 hours, GE-treated MCF7 cells became morphologically distinct, attained mesenchyme like phenotype, and lost cell-to-cell contact... Our results demonstrate that a short exposure to fresh but not boiled garlic extract is sufficient to permanently alter the morphology and trigger the growth arrest of MCF7 cells." – PubMed ID#PMC3463925 (2012) [686]

"Studies have shown that the number of suppressor T cells is increased by garlic and converts the lymphocytes in that form which is cytotoxic to cancerous cells. Metastases are prevented by altering the adhesion and attachment of cancerous cells, circulating in the blood vessels. Harmful effects of carcinogens to DNA are prevented by ripened garlic extract; it improves the immune system of the body, increases the removal of carcinogens from the body, and enhances the detoxifying enzyme's activity... the ripened extract of garlic is also helpful to shield the propagation of several types of cancers such as colon, stomach, breast, lungs and bladder. Complications of chemotherapy and radiotherapy could be lessen with garlic extract." – PubMed ID#PMC4881189 (2016) [687]

"Sulfur containing ingredients are of outmost importance. There is, throughout the literature, a tremendous body of evidence indicating a wide range of different properties for organosulfur compounds of garlic. For instance, it has been shown that diallyltrisulfide (DATS), a sulfur containing ingredient of garlic, induces apoptosis in human breast cancer cells (MCF-7) via ROS-mediated activation of JNK and AP-1. Moreover, when orally administered at a concentration of 1–2 mg/day, thrice/week for 13 weeks, by DASTS markedly suppressed prostate carcinoma and pulmonary metastasis in mouse animal model without any side effects." – PubMed ID#PMC4753037 (2015) [688]

Here an extract of garlic, DATS, inhibited breast cancer cells through apoptosis. Cancer usually disables this; garlic essentially reenabled it.

"Diallyl trisulfide (DATS) is a structurally simple but biologically active constituent of processed garlic with in vivo activity against chemically-induced as well as oncogene-driven cancer in experimental rodents. The present study offers novel insights into the mechanisms underlying anticancer effects of DATS using human breast cancer cells as a model. Exposure of human breast cancer cells (MCF-7 and MDA-MB-231, respectively) and a cell line derived from spontaneously developing mammary tumor of a transgenic mouse (BRI-JM04) to DATS resulted in a dose-dependent inhibition of cell viability that was accompanied by apoptosis induction." – PubMed ID#PMC3594460 (2014) [689]

The following research study looks at numerous cancer cell lines exposed to a "homemade" garlic extract. They also point out that the beneficial ingredients of garlic are very volatile, and garlic should be consumed fresh (once crushed). There is also some research showing that fermented garlic is also beneficial (fermentation is a preservation technique).

"We show that GE inhibits growth of several different cancer cells in vitro, as well as cancer growth in vivo in a syngeneic orthotopic breast cancer model. Multiple myeloma cells were found to be especially sensitive to GE... These activities were lost during freeze or vacuum drying, suggesting that the main anti-cancer compounds in GE are volatile. The anti-cancer activity was stable for

> more than six months in −20 °C. We found that GE enhanced the activities of
> chemotherapeutics, as well as MAPK and PI3K inhibitors. Furthermore, GE
> affected hundreds of proteins involved in cellular signalling, including changes in
> vital cell signalling cascades regulating proliferation, apoptosis, and the cellular
> redox balance." – PubMed ID#PMC5946235 (2018) (Creative Commons
> Attribute at the link) [690]

Strategy

The research is clear that garlic can *Improve Your Odds* in the fight against cancer. This section contains only a small sampling of the many studies available on the subject. However, like anything having to do with cancer, it may not be as simple as popping a garlic supplement.

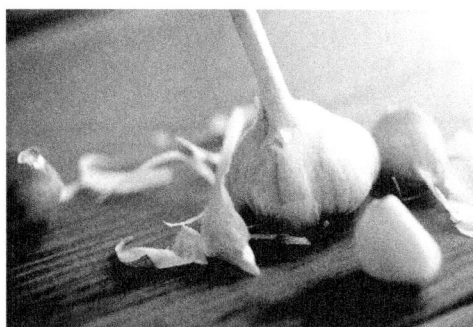

Garlic should be consumed fresh. Research shows that garlic supplements lose many of their beneficial anticancer properties within hours to days of being produced. Garlic maintains its properties until crushed, so the bulbs you purchase at the grocery store will still be viable anticancer agents. Once crushed, the garlic can lose potency within hours if exposed to the air.

Why You Should Consume Freshly Crushed Garlic

Allicin (the main beneficial active ingredient) is made when alliinase (an enzyme) comes into contact with alliin. Both alliinase and alliin are found in whole garlic cloves (allicin is not), but they don't come into contact with each other until the cloves are crushed. Allicin is highly volatile and breaks down within hours of being formed if exposed to air. This is why you can't actually purchase allicin supplements (even those labeled as "allicin" are simply garlic bulb with the *potential* to produce allicin. Or, if it is allicin, it is ineffective by the time it reaches you).

Alliinase (the enzyme) is very sensitive to heat; allicin is not. So, when cooking with garlic it is best to crush the garlic and let it sit for 10 minutes or so before cooking (do not use pre-crushed garlic). This gives allicin time to form. You can then mix the crushed garlic into the food; the dish can then be cooked, and the allicin benefits are preserved! What about leftovers? Allicin loses its potency from oxidation, but the leftover food and refrigeration will help slow this process. If you aren't going to consume the leftovers within 2 days, you should freeze them to get the maximum benefits (PubMed ID#11238815 [691]). Once again, cooking the garlic after the allicin has been released is fine; allicin is heat-tolerant.

> *Baked garlic bulbs, as delicious as they are (I can eat them in about a 50/50 mix of baked garlic and butter! Yummm), will contain little to no allicin. That is because the garlic isn't crushed before cooking, so no allicin will be formed. The heat of the oven will destroy the alliinase enzyme; this means no allicin will be formed as you eat it. Thus, you will not get the most important benefit of garlic when consuming the baked garlic. Workaround? Eat both, baked and raw!*

Garlic supplements that are enteric coated are better than those that are not. The coating allows the capsule to make it through the stomach acid and into the small intestine before opening. However, bile acid (etc.) is also harsh to alliinase, and this inhibits allicin production by about 40% (pubs.acs.org [692]). However, if you do not want to consume fresh raw garlic, an enteric-coated garlic supplement is an option.

So, to summarize, raw garlic (or freshly crushed and then cooked) is best, but enteric-coated garlic bulb will do in a pinch.

I recommend consuming fresh garlic at least twice per week for prevention, and 5 to 7 times per week if fighting cancer (one clove per day or more). You can crush a clove over a salad, on top of many savory dishes, or just chew it and eat it raw. You can also use a garlic crusher, or press, to mix the garlic with butter or olive oil. It can then be used as a spread or topping over a savory food. Baked garlic has other benefits as well, so you can always add this to what you're eating after you've consumed the minimum amount of raw garlic.

GINGER

AKA: *Zingiber officinale*

Ginger has been used to treat disease and inflammation for thousands of years in China and India, probably first originating in China. It made its way to ancient Rome from India and then to the rest of the known world. In ancient times ginger was used to treat the cold, flu, dyspepsia, gastroparesis, headaches, nausea, constipation, slow motility, colic and probably many other ailments. Ginger was often thought of as a cure-all.

Today, in many parts of the world, ginger is still commonly used to treat these conditions. Ginger remains a very popular spice that is used globally, but it is especially popular in Asia (where some of the lowest age-adjusted cancer rates are seen [693]). India, Nepal, Nigeria and Indonesia have the highest ginger consumption per person.

Researchers have found a dose-dependent inhibition of ovarian cancer cells using ginger, reducing in vitro cell viability by over 80% in 72 hours. Though human in vivo studies still need to be done, this is very promising research.

> "The ginger extract significantly inhibited cancer growth in ovarian cancer cell line. The most important attribute was 60 µg/ml concentration which received weights higher than 0.50, 0.75 and 0.95 by 90%, 80% and 50% of feature selection models… High co-expression between P53 and the other apoptosis-inducing proteins such as CASP2 and DEDD was noticeable, suggesting the molecular mechanism underpinning of ginger action… We found that the ginger extract has anticancer properties through p53 pathway to induce apoptosis… ginger extract displayed strong cytotoxicity effects on ovarian cancer cell line" – PubMed ID#PMC5527238 (2017) (Open Access license, attribute at the link) [694]

Creative Common attribution - Pashaei-Asl R, Pashaei-Asl F, Mostafa Gharabaghi P, et al. The Inhibitory Effect of Ginger Extract on Ovarian Cancer Cell Line; Application of Systems Biology. Adv Pharm Bull. 2017;7(2):241–249. doi:10.15171/apb.2017.029

The following graph, from the study above, shows the proliferation of ovarian cancer cells (in vitro) receiving ginger as compared to those in a control group that did not. Ginger extract clearly reduced cancer cell viability in a dose-dependent manner. The control group (far left bar) received no ginger, and the cancer cells remained 100% viable (alive and kicking). The other bars showed various concentrations of ginger and their effects on cell viability.

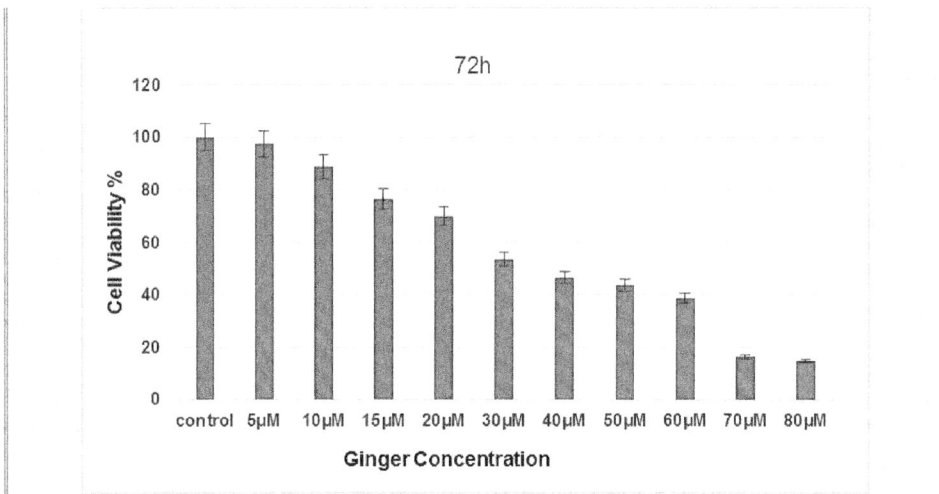

Ginger extract "significantly" reduced key inflammatory markers linked to various types of cancer. In this study, they used rats with liver cancer.

> "ginger extract significantly reduced the elevated expression of NFkappaB and TNF-alpha in rats with liver cancer. Ginger may act as an anti-cancer and anti-inflammatory agent by inactivating NFkappaB through the suppression of the pro-inflammatory TNF-alpha." – PubMed ID#PMC2664283 (2008) [695]

Ginger extract was shown to have antiproliferation effects against pancreatic cancer cells. This study goes on to mention similar benefits obtained against several forms of cancer, including: colon cancer, gastric cancer, lung cancer, breast cancer, leukemia, osteosarcoma, hepatoma, cervical cancer and fibrosarcoma.

> "The extract of ginger (Zingiber officinale Roscoe) and its major pungent components, [6]-shogaol and [6]-gingerol, have been shown to have an anti-proliferative effect on several tumor cell lines… The present study demonstrated that the extract of Syussai ginger (SSHE) had potent growth-inhibitory and cell death-inducing activity against pancreatic cancer cells including Panc-1 cells… the present study demonstrated that ginger extract inhibited cell proliferation and subsequently induced the autotic death of pancreatic cancer Panc-1 cells. The extract suppressed tumor growth without serious adverse effects in a Panc02 peritoneal dissemination mouse model and Panc-1 xenografted mice when administered intraperitoneally." – PubMed ID#PMC4427290 (2015) [696]

Ginger has in vivo (in the body) anticancer benefits against liver, pancreatic, colon, gastric and cholangiocarcinoma cancers. It has shown in vitro benefits against several other forms of cancer.

> "studies showed that ginger and its active components including 6-gingerol and 6-shogaol exert anticancer activities against GI cancer. The anticancer activity of ginger is attributed to its ability to modulate several signaling molecules like NF-κB, STAT3, MAPK, PI3K, ERK1/2, Akt, TNF-α, COX-2, cyclin D1, cdk, MMP-9, survivin, cIAP-1, XIAP, Bcl-2, caspases, and other cell growth regulatory proteins... Although the medicinal properties of ginger have been known for thousands of years, a significant number of in vitro, in vivo, and epidemiological studies further provide substantial evidence that ginger and its active compounds are effective against wide variety of human diseases including GI cancer. Ginger has been found to be effective against various GI cancers such as gastric cancer, pancreatic cancer, liver cancer, colorectal cancer, and cholangiocarcinoma." – PubMed ID#PMC4369959 (2015) (Open Access license, attribute at the link) [697]

The following study looked at using a ginger extract (GE) to treat prostate tumors. The study used prostate xenografts, which involves grafting human prostate cancers into mice, where they then grow and behave very much like prostate cancer in humans. The amount of ginger extract used when scaled to humans would be about 576 to 1,000 mg (depending on the weight of the person), requiring approximately 100 to 200 grams of fresh ginger (about 3.5 to 7 ounces). This is a lot of ginger (however, some other studies have used less). Thus, using a ginger extract (commonly available at health food stores) might be a more practical method of obtaining effective amounts of ginger.

> "Comprehensive studies have confirmed that GE perturbed cell-cycle progression, impaired reproductive capacity, modulated cell-cycle and apoptosis regulatory molecules and induced a caspase-driven, mitochondrially mediated apoptosis in human prostate cancer cells. Remarkably, daily oral feeding of 100 mg/kg body weight of GE inhibited growth and progression of PC-3 xenografts by approximately 56 % in nude mice, as shown by measurements of tumour volume... GE-treated mice showed reduced proliferation index and widespread apoptosis compared with controls... whole GE has been shown to inhibit proliferation of breast and colon cancer cells... Given our anticancer therapeutic doses of GE in reducing tumour burden in mice bearing human prostate xenografts, we performed allometric scaling calculations to extrapolate the mice data to humans, and the human equivalent dose of the GE was found to be approximately 567 mg for a 70 kg adult, which perhaps can be obtained from about 100 g of fresh ginger." – PubMed ID#PMC3426621 (2012) [698]

Ginger extract inhibited inflammation and promoted apoptosis in liver cancer. It also exhibited anti-metastasis benefits. The amount of ginger used in this study, if scaled up for a 70 kg (154 lb) human, would be about 7 grams (1/4 ounce) of ginger per day.

> "The inhibition of inflammation and promotion of apoptosis were implicated in the protection of ginger against liver cancer. For instance, the suppression of inflammatory responses as evidenced by decreased NF-κB and TNF-α was found in ginger (100 mg/kg) treated rat hepatoma model… studies suggested that 6-shogaol and 6-gingerol, two compounds isolated from ginger, exhibited anti-metastasis effects against liver cancer cells.. Moreover, 6-shogaol could also effectively induce ROS-mediated caspase-dependent apoptosis in a multidrug resistance hepatoma cell line" – PubMed ID#PMC4808884 (2016, Open Access attribution at the link) [699]

Ginger was shown here to have chemopreventative and chemotherapeutic benefits. Population studies have shown that people who regularly consume ginger have a lower risk of breast, prostate, gastrointestinal and colon cancers.

> "Population-based studies suggest that Southeast Asians, who regularly consume ginger have a decreased risk for breast, prostate, gastrointestinal, and colon cancers when compared to Americans and Europeans, thus strengthening the notion that ginger phytochemicals work together through common and complementary mechanisms to produce chemopreventive benefits… human clinical trials have indicated the safety profile of GE, suggesting that a daily dose of ginger extract as high as 5 g in its dry form does not cause any toxicity with the exception of mild stomach upset in individuals who infrequently consume spicy foods" – PubMed ID#PMC3925258 (2013) [700]

VEGF stands for vascular endothelial growth factor. Cancer cells upregulate VEGF to produce new blood vessels from preexisting vasculature. These new blood vessels are needed by tumors to sustain their growth. VEGF inhibitors are one of the areas drug companies are investigating for new anticancer drugs. Activation of CD8+ T cells is also a very important anticancer property; see Chapter 2 on Immunotherapy.

> "Ginger and its constituents show a vital effect in the control of tumour development through up regulation of tumour suppressor gene, induction of apoptosis and inactivation of VEGF pathways… Inhibition of VEGF is an important step in the prevention of tumour development/management. Earlier investigation has shown that, 6-gingerol has role in the suppression of the

transformation, hyperproliferation, and inflammatory processes that involve in various steps of carcinogenesis, angiogenesis and metastasis… 6-shogaol has shown to induce apoptosis in human colorectal carcinoma cells… 6-gingerol inhibited pulmonary metastasis in mice bearing B16F10 melanoma cells through the activation of CD8+ T cells. Earlier finding has reported that 6-gingerol showed its anti-tumoral activity through induction of ROS which is also known to trigger activation of p53 and the cell cycle arrest and apoptosis" – PubMed ID#PMC4106649 (2014) [701]

In this study from the *International Journal of Cancer*, it was shown that **6-gingerol (a component of ginger) greatly increased tumor-infiltrating lymphocytes (TILs)**; see Chapter 2 for more information on the importance of TILs. This inhibited tumor growth in several types of cancers. This alone makes ginger an important part of anyone's protocol.

"Tumor-infiltrating lymphocytes (TILs) play critical roles in host antitumor immune responses. It is known that cancer patients with tumor-reactive lymphocyte infiltration in their tumors have better prognoses… administration of 6-gingerol, which is a component of ginger, inhibited tumor growth in several types of murine tumors, such as B16F1 melanomas, Renca renal cell carcinomas and CT26 colon carcinomas… We found that CD8 T cells isolated from 6-gingerol pretreated OT-1 mice, but not from control OT-1 mice, massively infiltrated tumors and tumor draining lymph nodes and divided several times. Our results strongly suggest that 6-gingerol can be used in tumor immunotherapy to increase the number of TILs." – PubMed ID#21792901 (2012) [702]

Recommendation

Ginger should be included in any protocol to treat or prevent cancer, as well as in adjuvant treatments with your oncologist's concurrence. Ginger can be used in cooking, especially in Asian and Indian dishes. It works with garlic and turmeric, which are also very beneficial anticancer herbs. You can also make ginger tea. Simply take about a 2" piece of peeled ginger, slice it to approximately 1/8", boil in water for 10 to 15 minutes, sweeten with stevia and add lemon or lime if you wish. Enjoy. The 2" piece of ginger is approximately equal to ½ ounce, or 14,000 mg, of ginger.

In addition to cooking with ginger, I recommend supplementing a minimum of 1,500 mg per day of ginger root. This can usually be obtained by taking 3 ginger capsules per day. There are also liquid ginger extracts available; the bottle should show how many mg of ginger it is equivalent to. If you drink a cup of ginger tea, you can skip your ginger supplements that day.

❖ GRAPE SEED EXTRACT

Grape seed extract (not to be confused with grapefruit seed extract) is made from the grape waste products of wine production—that is, the grapes' seeds and skins. It has been studied for many years and is prescribed medically in some countries. Health benefits include: reducing high blood pressure, improving blood flow/reducing edema, lower oxidative damage, possibly improving collagen synthesis and bone formation, possibly helping reduce inflammation of the brain, helping to prevent and treat certain intestinal infections, etc. These claims are backed up by multiple research studies, but many of the benefits have only been found in vitro or in animal studies (due to research funding limitations, there have been no human studies that I've seen).

In the below research, grape seed extract (GSE) was studied for its efficacy against colorectal cancer (CRC). They found it to be a "safe, effective, multi-targeted anticancer and chemopreventive agent for CRC." The study also found that GSE interferes with a tumor's ability to convert glucose to energy and with mitochondrial metabolism in cancer cells. Cancer cells have a ferocious need for glucose.

> "GSE, has shown considerable efficacy against CRC… these results indicated the initial mechanism of action of GSE, which was responsible for its anti-cancer efficacy; specifically how GSE targets ER stress response proteins, resulting in an overall down regulation of proteins involved in translation. Specifically, we observed oxidative protein modification, specifically on methionine amino acids residues, and an altered ER (endoplasmic reticulum) stress response protein expression, in human CRC cells, as a result of GSE treatment… this information, combined with the vast pre-clinical GSE efficacy studies, would further solidify GSE as a safe, effective, multi-targeted anti-cancer and chemopreventive agent for CRC." – PubMed ID#PMC4217504 (2014) [703]

GSE exhibits both preventative and treatment potential against hormone-dependent breast cancers.

> "Grape seed extract (GSE) is an aromatase inhibitor and a suppressor of aromatase expression… We believe that these results are exciting in that they show GSE to be potentially useful in the prevention/treatment of hormone-dependent breast cancer through the inhibition of aromatase activity as well as its expression." – PubMed ID#16740737 (2006) [704]

Jurkat cells are human T lymphocyte cells that are used to study acute T cell leukemia.

> "Exposure of Jurkat cells to GSE resulted in dose- and time-dependent increase in apoptosis and caspase activation… Furthermore, treatment of Jurkat cells with GSE resulted in marked increase in levels of phospho-JNK… The result of the present study showed that GSE induces apoptosis in Jurkat cells through a process that involves sustained JNK activation and Cip1/p21 up-regulation, culminating in caspase activation." – PubMed ID#PMC2760842 (2009) [705]

The following journal article reviewed various research studies on grape seed extract (GSE) and found that it helps to prevent and treat various forms of cancer. GSE has the ability to induce apoptosis, inhibit metastasis and inhibit angiogenic capacity in various tumor lines. If you only read one paper on GSE, this would be a good one.

> "dietary feeding of GSP was effective in preventing photocarcinogenesis at both initiation and promotion stages and malignant transformation of skin papillomas to carcinomas… Together, the studies summarized above provide clear evidence for the potential chemopreventive efficacy of GSE/proanthocyanidins against skin cancer with some mechanistic insights… Apart from the anticancer and chemopreventive efficacy of GSE against skin, colorectal, prostate, and breast cancers discussed above in detail, anticancer efficacy of this extract has also been observed against human lung cancer A427, A549, and H1299 cells, human gastric adenocarcinoma CRL-1739 cells, oral squamous cell carcinoma CAL27 and SCC25 cells, Jurkat, U937, and HL-60" – PubMed ID#PMC2728696 (© 2009 – The Journal of Nutrition) [706]

The following study looked at colorectal cancer (CRC) and found that GSE "causes strong growth inhibitory and cell death" in vitro.

> "Grape Seed Extract Induces Cell Cycle Arrest and Apoptosis in Human Colon Carcinoma Cells - GSE produces strong biological effects in different human CRC cell lines, which include growth inhibition, cell cycle arrest, induction of negative regulators of cell cycle progression namely Cip1/p21 and Kip1/p27, and apoptotic cell death. In addition to an aberrant cell cycle progression, loss of apoptotic function is a major contributor towards the resistance of cancer cells to cytotoxic chemotherapeutic agents, and accordingly, an induction of apoptosis under such circumstances is also highly desirable for preventive intervention of various malignancies including CRC." – PubMed ID#PMC2597484 (© 2008 Journal Nutrition and Cancer) [707]

The following research study found that GSE had a strong anticancer effect against liver cancer. GSE achieves these effects through apoptosis, reducing cell proliferation, reducing oxidative stress and downregulating many of the processes cancer needs in order to proliferate. This research looked at both in vitro and in vivo actions of GSE.

"The purpose of this study was to investigate the anti-cancer property of grape seed extract (GSE) during early stages of developing liver cancer… GSE's effects were associated with induced apoptosis, reduced cell proliferation, decreased oxidative stress and down regulation of histone deacetylase activity and inflammation makers, such as cyclooxygenase, inducible nitric oxide synthase, nuclear factor-kappa B-p65 and p- phosphorylated tumor necrosis factor receptor expressions in liver. GSE treatment also decreased the viability of HepG2 cells and induced early and late apoptosis… the present study provides evidence that the GSE's anticancer effect is mediated through the inhibition of cell proliferation, induction of apoptosis, modulating oxidative damage and suppressing inflammatory response… plant extracts have been of a particular interest mainly because of the synergistic effects of the cocktail of plant metabolites and their multiple points of intervention during chemoprevention" – PubMed ID#PMC5775207 (2018 – Creative Commons attribution available at the link) [708]

GSE has been shown to fight various cancers, causing apoptosis, oxidative stress, and DNA damage in cancer cell lines.

"Differential concentrations of GSE may have a differentially antiproliferative function against oral cancer cells via differential apoptosis, oxidative stress and DNA damage… Accumulating evidence of the antiproliferative effect of GSE had been reported in several oral cancer cell lines… We demonstrated that GSE shows differential concentration effects in the antiproliferation of oral cancer cells through differential expressions of apoptosis, oxidative stress, and DNA damage. We showed that the antiproliferative effect of high GSE concentrations is associated with an overproduction of ROS causing DNA damage and apoptosis of cancer cells." – PubMed ID#PMC4393634 (2015) (Creative Commons attribution available at the link) [709]

Recommendations

Grape seed extract shows a lot of promise in fighting cancer. There is not a lot of in vivo evidence (due to funding), so the evidence here is not as strong as with some other botanicals.

If you don't feel like you're taking too many supplements already, this may be another good one to add. Though this will most likely help you to *Improve Your Odds* with cancer, a person can only take so many supplements.

Note: If someone has a COMT enzyme deficiency (see the end of the Green Tea/EGCG section), they may want to avoid GSE as well.

❖ Green Tea/EGCG

AKA: Green tea extract, epigallocatechin-3-gallate, *Camellia sinensis* extract

What most people simply call "tea" is derived from the *Camellia sinensis* evergreen shrub. Whether it is green tea, white tea, oolong tea or black tea, it all comes from the same shrub leaves. The difference depends on the preparation of the leaves and how they were fermented before drying. Tea from this plant has been used in China for at least 3,000 years (probably much longer). It has also been used medicinally for much of that time. Today it is consumed by hundreds of millions of people every day.

Tea has been shown to be beneficial for many conditions and has been shown to help prevent and treat various cancers.

EGCG from green tea inhibited the growth of HCT-116 and SW-480 human colorectal cancer cells by up to 98%, with similar results seen for SW-480 cells. EGCG also increased cancer cell apoptosis by up to 25% (in vitro).

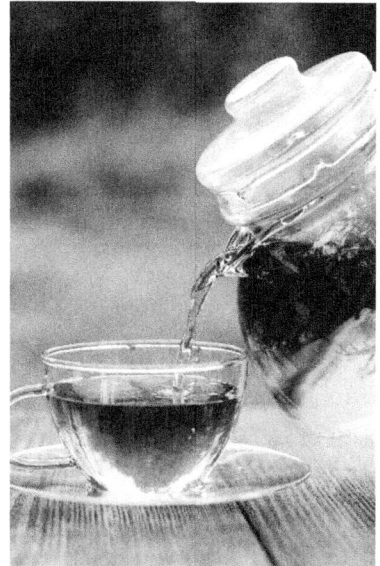

> "Of all the antioxidant compounds found in green tea, the major constituents are polyphenols, including phenolic acids and catechins (Figure 1). Catechins from green tea belong to the family of flavonoids that are powerful antioxidants and free iron scavengers… EGCG is the most abundant and powerful antioxidant in green tea for cancer chemoprevention… green tea could be an effective synergist with anticancer drugs for cancer chemoprevention… 100 µM of CG, ECG, GCG and EGCG inhibited HCT-116 cell growth by 20.2% ± 1.4%, 20.3% ± 1.2%, 79.2% ± 3.4% and 98.4%… The results demonstrate that EGCG significantly induces cell apoptosis." – PubMed ID#PMC3509513 (2012) [710]

Taking the supplement quercetin (discussed later in this chapter) can significantly increase the anticancer (antiproliferation) benefits of green tea.

> "Quercetin increased bioavailability and decreased methylation of green tea polyphenols in vitro and in vivo… The combination of quercetin with EGCG demonstrated the strongest increase in antiproliferation in A549 cells. Cell proliferation was inhibited by 17%, 9% and 42% with the treatment of 40μM of EGCG, 20μM of quercetin and their combination, respectively, at 24h, while by 20%, 32% and 69% at 48h… Our results demonstrated that combined treatment with EGCG and quercetin enhanced the chemopreventive activity of EGCG in different cancer cell lines" – PubMed ID#PMC3590855 (2013) [711]

EGCG from green tea resulted in longer survival times for estrogen receptor-negative breast cancer patients. In addition, EGCG both inhibited proliferation and induced apoptosis of lung cancer stem cells (CSC).

> "EGCG inhibits the growth of ER-negative (estrogen receptor negative) human breast CSCs through down-regulation of ER-α36 expression, indicating that EGCG treatment will result in longer survival of patients with mammary cancers (Pan et al., 2016). The longer survival of patients who drink green tea was reported by Nakachi's group… These results show that EGCG inhibits proliferation and induces apoptosis of lung CSCs (Zhu et al., 2017)" – PubMed ID#PMC5824026 (2018) [712]

COMT Deficiency

Green tea extracts are very safe and lack side effects for most people. However, a small percentage of people have a genetic condition where they do not make enough of the COMT enzyme that breaks down "catechins" in green tea (as well as black teas); this is not an issue with many herbal teas. EGCG is one of those catechins; green tea has 9 of them in total. Without this enzyme, the catechins can build up. For someone with a COMT deficiency, EGCG can be dangerous. It can lead to a wide array of symptoms, including psychological ones such as anxiety, depression and panic attacks, as well as body aches and liver issues (sometimes severe; see the BBC link below). Too much green tea, along with certain other foods (red/purple berries, chocolate, raw red onions) can cause problems for someone with COMT deficiency issues.

Again, this condition is not very common, but it is not "rare," either. Your doctor has most likely never heard of it, so the best way to see if this affects you is genetic testing. I happen to have this condition; through genetic testing, I verified that was the cause of some of my symptoms. I already knew I had an issue with tea and coffee (yes, to a lesser degree coffee is also an issue, even decaffeinated). I used the 23andMe Health + Ancestry test and uploaded the raw data to one of the many free sites to analyze it. I'm "homozygous" on the two main COMT SNPs (areas of DNA), meaning that I produce far less of the COMT enzyme than most people. Most of my immediate family also has obvious symptoms. Easy to manage once you know about it.

COMT is a complicated topic and beyond the scope of this book. However, it is important to avoid EGCG and quercetin supplements if you have a COMT deficiency. For more information on the dangers of EGCG in people with a COMT deficiency, please see the following BBC news article. [713]

Recommendations

Anytime someone can get an anticancer benefit from the food or drink they consume, I'm in favor! The last thing most of us want to do is to consume fistfuls of capsules. For most people, drinking green tea is a great way to *Improve Your Odds* in preventing cancer. However, to get the maximum benefit, you may want to consider adding an EGCG supplement as well. Studies have not shown the most effective long-term dosing for EGCG, so I recommend sticking with the directions on the bottle. Some studies show that taking a quercetin supplement and fish oil can maximize benefits.

Treating Cancer - Because of the possibility of blocking ROS oxidation of tumors (which is beneficial in killing cancer cells), it is recommended that you consult your oncologist before consuming EGCG supplements or drinking more than 2 cups of green tea per day.

Note: Just watch out for new symptoms if you start taking an EGCG supplement. If you are COMT deficient, you will not be able to drink much green tea and should completely avoid taking EGCG or quercetin supplements (quercetin is a COMT inhibitor). See the COMT Deficiency section above.

HONEY

The history of honey is a rich one and goes back thousands of years. A rock painting in Spain from 8,000 years ago shows a honey harvester taking honey from a hive. Other paintings and historic records show people going to great lengths to obtain honey, often at significant risk to life and limb. There are references to honey in the Christian Bible, Jewish Talmud, the Koran and throughout ancient writings. Medicinal uses of honey go back at least 5,000 years. It was used by the Roman armies to dress wounds, ancient Egyptians to dress wounds and in embalming, and it was also frequently used in ancient Ayurvedic and traditional Chinese medicine. Because of the difficulty in obtaining honey, and its expense, it was not consumed daily (or even monthly) by most people until recently.

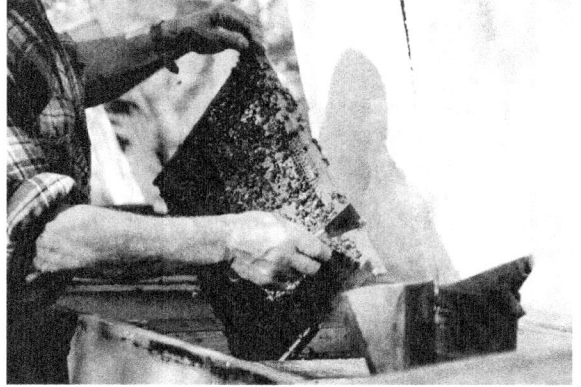

> "And thy Lord taught the bee to build its cells in hills, on trees, and in (men's) habitations; Then to eat of all the produce (of the earth), and find with skill the spacious paths of its Lord: there issues from within their bodies a drink of varying colors, wherein is healing for men: verily in this is a sign for those who give thought" – Quran (609-632 AD)

Honey contains several phenolic acids that are thought to be responsible for its anticancer properties. These phenolic acids include: caffeic acid, ellagic acid, gallic acid, syringic acid, chlorogenic acid, p-coumaric acid, ferulic acid and the flavonoids chrysin, kaempferol, catechin, quercetin, galangin, luteolin, pinocembrin, pinobanksin and myricetin. The primary active ingredients in honey are chrysin and quercetin, both of which are covered elsewhere in this chapter.

This study looked at using honey in vivo (in mice) against human bladder cancer.

> "In vitro studies revealed significant inhibition of the proliferation of T24 and MBT-2 cell lines by 1-25% honey and of RT4 and 253J cell lines by 6-25% honey… In the in vivo studies, intralesional injection of 6 and 12% honey as well as oral ingestion of honey significantly inhibited tumor growth." – PubMed ID#12657101 (2003) [714]

Tualang honey (TH) significantly reduced the size of breast cancer tumors in rats. The honey was diluted in water and given orally to the rats. The study used a rat cancer that was chemically induced.

> "Results showed that breast cancers in the TH-treated groups had slower size increment and smaller mean tumor size (≤ 2 cm3) compared to Controls (≤ 8 cm3). The number of cancers developing in TH-treated groups was also significantly fewer (P<0.05). Histological grading showed majority of TH-treated group cancers to be of grade 1 and 2 compared to grade 3 in controls." – PubMed ID#23725121 (2013) [715]

The following looked at an extract of honey called "chrysin." This compound is also discussed separately earlier in this chapter.

> "In this study, we investigated the antiproliferative role of honey or chrysin on human (A375) and murine (B16-F1) melanoma cell lines… Our results suggest that the anti-proliferative effects of honey are due mainly to the presence of chrysin. Chrysin may therefore be considered a potential candidate for both cancer prevention and treatment." – PubMed ID#20811719 (2010) [716]

There are a few in vitro (in the test tube) studies of the effect of honey on human cancer cells; these studies show significant inhibition of cell growth. However, benefits were found in just some types of cancer, and for other cancer lines it showed no effect. In vivo (in the body) studies have not done as well, with honey often making some cancers worse. Many of the in vivo studies used xenografts, where human tumors were grafted into an animal (usually mice or rats). They often also used special preparations of honey as injections into the test animal. Oral consumption of honey may not work the same way due to digestion, absorption issues and the effects of its high sugar content. The following study was done on mice and rats and used an oral dose of honey.

> "The mice received an oral dose of 2 g/kg, while the dose for the rats was 1 g/kg of wildflower honey from Croatia, for 10 days before and after treatment. Interestingly, when honey was administered two days after tumour cell inoculation, there was no effect on the formation of tumour nodules in mice, while in rats an even more enhanced tumour growth was observed… it remains to be seen whether the concentration achieved in blood is sufficient to intercept the cancer processes in vivo… cancer-associated fibroblasts play an important role in tumour progression; honey has been shown to increase their proliferation" – PubMed ID#PMC5456322 (2016) (Open Access license attribution available at the link) [717]

I was unable to locate any human in vivo cancer studies using honey.

Recommendation

Research studies show mixed results using honey to treat or prevent cancer, with some research showing benefits, and other (in vivo animal) research showing it made cancers worse. Because there are no human in vivo randomized control trials using honey, which might clarify these conflicting results, my recommendation is not to use honey to treat or prevent cancer.

If you are on a low-carb, low-sugar or ketogenic diet to treat cancer, you should avoid honey altogether. Honey is mostly sugar. An extensive body of research shows that all sugar should be avoided when trying to treat or prevent cancer (see Chapter 4 – Diet). Whether it is "natural" or "processed" makes no difference; all sugar gets converted to blood glucose in the body and will feed cancer.

For example, a Snickers candy bar (at 113 grams) has a GI (glycemic index) of 55, but just ONE Tbsp of honey also has a GI of 55! That same Snickers bar (again, 113 grams) has a glycemic load of 35. 113 grams of honey has a glycemic load of 48.4!!!! Almost 50% higher than the Snickers bar!

Honey is 79% sugar and 20% water, with trace amounts of nutrients (less than 1% by weight). Though it has some antimicrobial properties, even these are often offset by the high amounts of sugar it contains. However, honey tastes very good, and for this reason you get a lot of people doing their best to defend it.

My recommendation is to avoid honey due to the high amounts of sugar it contains and its negative effect on blood glucose levels. See Chapter 4 for healthier alternatives. Taking concentrated honey extracts such as chrysin and quercetin would be a much better way of obtaining the cancer fighting properties of honey without the added sugar consumption.

❖ INDIAN GOOSEBERRY

AKA: *Phyllanthus emblica*, emblic, emblic myrobalan, myrobalan, Indian gooseberry, Malacca tree, *Emblica officinalis*, Amla

Indian gooseberry has been shown to have many health benefits and has often been classified as a "superfood." It is indigenous to Southeast Asia. Though classified as a fruit, it is not palatable, and its taste has a strong bitter and sour flavor. It is usually only used in spicy dishes where the bitter flavor is masked.

Like many healthy vegetables and fruit, Indian gooseberry is high in phytochemicals and nutrients (such as ascorbic acid, tannins, phenols, gallic acid and quercetin). Some of these have medicinal properties. Some of the health benefits include: antioxidant properties, liver health, blood sugar control, helping control inflammation, cholesterol lowering properties and, possibly, some anticancer properties.

In this in vivo (mouse xenograft) study, they showed that Indian gooseberry (*Emblica officinalis*, or EO) inhibited skin tumors. This is one of the few in vivo studies on Indian gooseberry.

> "The tumor incidence, tumor yield, tumor burdon and cumulative number of papillomas were found to be higher in the control (without EO treatment) as compared to experimental animals (EO treated). The differences in the values of the results of experimental groups were statistically analysed and found to be significant in comparison to the control group ($p < 0.05$). The present study demonstrates the chemopreventive potential of Emblica officinalis fruit extract on DMBA induced skin tumorigenesis"

Here Indian gooseberry (*P. emblica*) was effective in inhibiting activity against two in vitro cancer cell lines. They also found synergistic effects using it along with the two chemotherapy drugs used in the study.

> "the growth inhibitory activity of the P. emblica and T. bellerica extracts and the chemotherapeutic drugs doxorubicin and cisplatin were investigated in A549, and HepG2 cells. Our results indicate that both plant extracts and chemotherapeutic drugs mediated significant growth inhibitory effects on both cell lines tested in a dose-dependent manner… Our study provides corroborative evidence as it showed that P. emblica and T. bellerica extracts were selectively toxic against two cancer cell lines and that, in combination with doxorubicin and cisplatin, produced an increased growth inhibitory effect in both A549 and HepG2 cells." – PubMed ID#PMC2693740 (2008) [718]

Indian gooseberry was shown to be effective against ovarian cancer in a xenograft mouse model. This might be one of the better studies showing its effectiveness in vivo, as it was also given orally.

> "In contrast to the in vitro studies, there is sparse evidence regarding the tumor repressive activity of Phyllanthus emblica using in vivo models of cancer… However, a striking study has been carried out employing aqueous extracts of the Indian Gooseberry administered orally against an ovarian cancer xenograft model. In this report, the extracts were able to completely ablate the growth of ovarian xenografts, with little or no residual tumor being observed after treatment." – PubMed ID#PMC4477227 (2015) [719]

Gooseberry showed significant inhibition of melanoma cells (in vitro) as well as suppression of pro-inflammatory genes in murine (mouse) macrophage cells.

> "EPE (emblica extract) significantly inhibited the mRNA expressions of tyrosinase, and tyrosinase related proteins (TRP-1 and TRP-2) in B16 murine melanoma cells and suppressed the expression of LPS-induced pro-inflammatory genes (COX-2, iNOS, TNF-α, IL-16 and IL-6) in… murine macrophage cells in a dose-dependent manner." – PubMed ID#24557876 (2014) [720]

Recommendation

Indian gooseberry has some promising in vitro research against various cancer cell lines, along with a small handful of in vivo (mouse model) studies. However, from what I have found, there has been very little research, or discussion, on human dosing. There have also been no in vivo studies on humans. Many of its benefits are probably due to the phytochemicals it contains (see above), and these are also found in many other botanicals that are recommended in this section. For these reasons I am not adding Indian gooseberry to the basic protocol in Chapter 9 (again, a person can only take so many supplements).

There are Indian gooseberry supplements available; it is often called "Amla." Because it is considered to be very safe, it doesn't hurt to take it. I would not exceed the amount directed on the bottle.

❖ I P 6

AKA: Inositol hexaphosphate, myo-inositol hexaphosphate, phytic acid

Inositol hexaphosphate (IP6) is a carbohydrate found in substantial amounts in many plants and mammalian cells. It is very safe to consume and is easily absorbed in the intestinal tract. Foods high in IP6 include: meat, eggs, whole grains, legumes, sprouts, green leafy vegetables, nuts and seeds. Most healthy foods seem to have it.

IP6 seems to enhance the cancer fighting abilities of the immune system, as well as possessing abilities to both directly fight cancers (selectively cytotoxic) and help restore pre-cancerous cells to normal cells. IP6 can reduce cancer cell proliferation, increase differentiation of malignant cells and interfere with angiogenesis (the ability of tumors to create new blood supplies). IP6 is normally found in a healthy human diet, and the body can also make IP6 from inositol (also found in food sources such as nuts, grains and fruit). However, supplementation seems to be needed for optimal benefit in treating cancers.

Phytochemicals are simply plant chemicals (phyto- means "plant" in Greek). Many of these phytochemicals have strong benefits for humans. Though not considered "essential" for life, like vitamins are, they are very important to good health (call me crazy, but I consider anything that might save my life "essential"). Many of the antioxidants fall into this category. Phytochemicals are also known to stimulate the immune system, prevent and repair cellular DNA damage, and provide many anticancer properties. IP6 is one of these phytochemicals.

IP6 was found to have "broad-spectrum" anticancer properties, as well as action against a number of different cancers.

> "IP6 is one of the prime and potential dietary phytochemicals exhibiting broad-spectrum anticancer activities, and its use has been widely described in different tumor types, including breast, pancreas, prostate, lung, liver and colon… studies have shown that IP6 inhibits cell proliferation, cell-cycle progression, metastasis, invasion and angiogenesis. Further studies of prostate carcinoma have shown that IP6 suppresses cell survival, proliferation and angiogenesis… the anticancer effect of IP6 was further confirmed in this in vitro study of colorectal cancer." – PubMed ID#PMC4396237 (2015) [721]

Inositol is known to benefit the actions of IP6, especially when it comes to its anticancer abilities. The IP6 + inositol combination was also shown to enhance conventional chemotherapy and improve the quality of life of people undergoing cancer treatment. This is in addition to its own anticancer benefits.

> Preliminary studies in humans show that IP(6) and inositol, the precursor molecule of IP(6), appear to enhance the anticancer effect of conventional chemotherapy, control cancer metastases, and improve quality of life. Because it is abundantly present in regular diet, efficiently absorbed from the gastrointestinal tract, and safe, IP(6) + inositol holds great promise in our strategies for cancer prevention and therapy. There is clearly enough evidence to justify the initiation of full-scale clinical trials in humans. – PubMed ID#17044765 (2006) [722]

In short, "differentiation" describes how much a cancer cell looks like a normal cell, with well differentiated cancer cells looking more like normal cells. Well differentiated cells tend to be less aggressive than poorly differentiated ones. The following shows that IP6 can cause malignant cells to improve and become better differentiated (and thus less aggressive).

> "Besides decreasing cellular proliferation, IP6 also causes differentiation of malignant cells often resulting in a reversion to normal phenotype. These data strongly point towards the involvement of signal transduction pathways, cell cycle regulatory genes, differentiation genes, oncogenes and perhaps, tumor suppressor genes in bringing about the observed anti-neoplastic action of IP6." – PubMed ID#9244360 (1997) [723]

> "The most consistent and best anticancer results were obtained from the combination of IP6 plus inositol. In addition to reducing cell proliferation, IP6 increases differentiation of malignant cells, often resulting in a reversion to normal phenotype. The data strongly argue for the use of IP6 plus inositol in our strategies for cancer prevention and treatment." – PubMed ID#14608114 (2003 – The Journal of Nutrition) [724]

The following studies showed that IP6 treatment caused a 37% to 65% reduction in breast cancer cells' adhesion ability. This inhibits the cancer cells' ability to metastasize and establish in a new location.

> "IP6 treatment caused a 65% reduction of cell adhesion to fibronection (p = 0.002) and a 37% reduction to collage… The results of this study show that IP6 inhibits the metastasis of human breast cancer cells in vitro through effects on cancer cell adhesion, migration and invasion." – PubMed ID#14666663 (2003) [725]

> "The results of this study indicate that IP6-induced inhibition of cancer cell adhesion, migration and invasion may be mediated through the modulation of integrin dimerization, cell surface expression and integrin-associated signaling pathway." – PubMed ID#14666664 (2003) [726]

Recommendations

The combination of IP6 and inositol seems to have a synergistic effect against many types of cancer. The effect of the two together has been described as exceeding the sum of the two used separately.

Prevention – IP6 is found in many foods, such as grains, legumes and meat. Digestive issues and poor diet can prevent some people from getting adequate levels. One study showed that a good prophylactic (preventative) dose for humans would be 1 to 2 grams per day (combined IP6 + inositol). Eating a healthy diet of fresh vegetables and meat will probably provide all the IP6 most people will need, but a supplement will not hurt.

Treatment – The problem with recommending IP6 is a lack of human in vivo studies to determine cancer treatment dosing. Though very safe, even at high doses, it can be impractical and expensive to take high doses, especially if it isn't necessary. What few studies there are with mice have an extrapolated dosing of 8 to 18 grams per day, suggesting tablespoon amounts. However, some researchers have hypothesized that humans may not need this much, with a human therapeutic dosage of as little as 1 to 2 grams per day (the same as the preventative dose).

Studies indicate that even these very high oral doses are well within the margin of safety, with mouse studies showing 10 g/kg (oral dosing) being safe.

With my "kitchen sink" approach, I have decided on supplementing 1 gram per day. This would be in addition to whatever I am getting from my diet, which is high in vegetables, soluble fiber and high-quality meats.

Note: IP6 has a mild antiplatelet effect, so taking it with antiplatelet or anticoagulant drugs may increase the risk of bleeding. If you take these drugs, you will need to consult your doctor before taking.

IP6 binds to minerals in the stomach and can affect mineral absorption by the small intestine. This is especially true for magnesium, zinc, calcium and iron. This may vary from person to person based on gut health. Long-term use should be monitored for mineral deficiencies. Studies also show that this is rarely a problem unless a person is consuming a minerally deficient diet (PubMed ID#17044765 [727], from the full study). Be sure to consume a healthy, mineral-rich diet if taking high doses of IP6; taking a mineral supplement may also be a good idea. Again, I take this supplement and haven't noticed any problems, but I also make sure I get enough minerals in my diet.

❖ MILK THISTLE

AKA: Silymarin

Milk thistle has been used for centuries to treat liver, spleen and gallbladder disorders. It has also been used as a general detoxifier for snake/bug bites, mushroom poisoning and alcohol poisoning. The silymarin plant can be found growing in northern India, America, Canada and Mexico. It has large leaves with reddish-purple, thorny flowers; the medicinal part of the plant is normally the seeds or fruit. Milk thistle can commonly be found in capsule form as a supplement. It can also be found sold as a tea.

Though there have been many studies of milk thistle, the studies of its uses for treating cancer are somewhat limited. Studies have shown that silymarin is non-toxic, even at large doses, with no LD50 (median lethal dose) defined (though large, chronic dosing has not been studied in humans. So, stick to defined therapeutic doses).

In addition to its anticancer effects, silymarin is able to modulate the immune system. It is also able to enhance the IFN-γ, IL-4 and IL-10 secretions (cytokines important in regulating inflammation and the immune response to cancer) in cultures containing lymphocytes. Lymphocytes are a type of white blood cells that are very important in fighting cancer. As such, milk thistle can be a very important supplement in supporting the immune system's fight against cancer.

Silymarin was shown here to be highly effective against leukemia cells in an in vivo mouse model.

"Silymarin, a flavonoid antioxidant, has high human acceptance being used clinically for the treatment of liver diseases. In this study, Akt activity was inhibited by silymarin without changes in total Akt level associated with a prominent caspases-9 and -3 activation as well as PARP cleavage, accompanied by a strong apoptotic death and growth inhibition of K562 cells… these results clearly indicate that the silymarin concentrations used in the present study showing strong efficacy in K562 leukemia cells are pharmacologically achievable at least in the rodent studies completed. " – PubMed ID#16949716 (2006) [728]

In this study, appearing in the journal *Cell Proliferation*, silymarin blocked proliferation of primary liver cancer (hepatocellular) and induced cancer cell death (through apoptosis—again, this is where cancer cells destroy themselves as damaged cells are supposed to do).

"Our results demonstrate that silymarin treatment inhibited proliferation and induced apoptosis in the human hepatocellular carcinoma cell line HepG2." – PubMed ID#19317806 (2009) [729]

Cell cycle arrest is where cells self-monitor their health and growth status. If they fail these self-checks, the cells will initiate either repairs or apoptosis. In the following study, it was shown that silymarin will induce apoptosis in damaged (cancerous) cells.

"Silymarin induces cell cycle arrest and apoptosis in ovarian cancer cells… The polyphenolic flavonoid silymarin that is the milk thistle extract has been found to possess an anti-cancer effect against various human epithelial cancers… silymarin effectively suppressed cell growth in a dose- and time-dependent manner, and arrested cell cycle progression at G1/S phase… and significantly induced apoptosis in A2780s and PA-1 cells" – PubMed ID#25242120 (2014) [730]

This research paper discusses numerous studies on various forms of cancer. It provides a very good overview of the medicinal uses of silymarin, especially with cancers.

"Effects of silymarin or silybinin on breast cancer, ovarian cancer, lung cancer, skin cancer, prostate cancer, cervical cancer, bladder cancer, liver carcinoma, and colon cancer, have been reported… Silybinin growth inhibitory effects and apoptotic efficacy have been also illustrated in prostate carcinoma cell culture and rat prostate cancer cells… silymarin has the growth inhibitory effect by cell proliferation suppression and apoptosis induction" – PubMed ID#PMC3586829 (2011) [731]

In one of the few in vivo studies, silymarin was found to induce apoptosis in xenografted human melanoma cells in a mouse model. However, the doses used in this study seem to be very high (equating to 35 grams for a 70 kg/150 lb person).

> "The silymarin-induced apoptosis of human melanoma cells was associated with a reduction in the levels of anti-apoptotic proteins (Bcl-2 and Bcl-xl), an increase in the levels of pro-apoptotic protein (Bax), and activation of caspases. Further, oral administration of silymarin (500 mg/kg body weight/2× a week) significantly inhibited (60%, P < 0.01) the growth of BRAF-mutated A375 melanoma tumor xenografts, and this was associated with: (i) inhibition of cell proliferation; (ii) induction of apoptosis of tumor cells; (iii) alterations in cell cycle regulatory proteins; and (iv) reduced expression of tumor angiogenic biomarkers in tumor xenograft tissues. These results indicate that silymarin may have a chemo-therapeutic effect on human melanoma cell growth" – PubMed ID#25174976 (2015) [732]

> "the cancer chemopreventive role of silymarin (Silybum marianum) has been extensively studied and has shown anticancer efficacy against various cancer sites, especially skin and prostate. In skin cancer, silymarin treatment inhibits ultraviolet B radiation or chemically initiated or promoted carcinogenesis. These effects of silymarin against skin carcinogenesis have been attributed to its strong antioxidant and anti-inflammatory action as well as its inhibitory effect on mitogenic signaling. Similarly, silymarin treatment inhibits 3, 2-dimethyl-4-aminobiphenyl-induced prostate carcinogenesis and retards the growth of advanced prostate tumor xenograft in athymic nude mice. In prostate cancer, silymarin treatment down-regulates androgen receptor-, epidermal growth factor receptor-, and nuclear factor-kappaB- mediated signaling and induces cell cycle arrest." – PubMed ID#17548792 (2007) [733]

The following paper outlines a therapeutic dose for cancer treatment.

> "Adult dosage in terms of hepatoprotection is 420 mg/day of extract (standardized to 70-80% silymarin) three times a day for 6-8 weeks. Maintenance dose is 280 mg/day. Intravenous solution is used for cyclopeptid mushroom poison in dose of 33 mg/kg/day for approximately 81.67 hr… Silymarin possess wide range of in vitro and in vivo mechanisms, such as antioxidant, anti-inflammatory, dose dependent anti-apoptotic and modifying cell transporters." – PubMed ID#PMC3586829 (2011) [734]

Strategy

Based on the studies that mentioned human dose levels and common recommendations, I would suggest 400 to 500 mg, taken 2 to 3 times per day. This can be continued throughout the cancer treatment unless advised otherwise by your doctor. I personally take 500 mg of milk thistle per day.

❖ NAC

AKA: N-acetylcysteine

Though there is some evidence of a chemoprotective role for NAC, there is some pretty strong evidence that it should not be used to treat existing cancers—more on this later. Because we can develop cancers without even knowing it (which can often be destroyed by our immune system before we are made aware of their existence), NAC (and some other strong antioxidants) may actually increase the risk of diagnosable cancers.

Beneficial Findings

NAC was administered orally just prior to UV skin exposure. The research subjects had precancerous nevi (moles) that were then removed and studied. The people receiving NAC had less UV-induced damage to the moles and less glutathione (GSH) depletion. Though these are signs of possible cancer prevention, this study didn't look at long-term exposure (with and without NAC supplementation).

> "We found in approximately 50% of patients that nevi removed 3 h following a single 1200 mg dose of NAC, compared to matched nevi removed just prior to drug ingestion, were less susceptible to UV-induced GSH depletion… potential utility of NAC in protecting against pro-carcinogenic oxidative stress induced by UV exposure, and further suggest and support a novel paradigm for melanoma chemoprevention" – PubMed ID#PMC2787788 (2009) [735]

> "NAC as a single agent reduces MCT4 stromal expression, which is a marker of glycolysis in breast cancer with reduced carcinoma cell proliferation… modulating metabolism in the tumor microenvironment has the potential to impact breast cancer proliferation." – PubMed ID#29248134 (2017) [736]

"NAC could inhibit the growth of DU145 and PC3 cells. Suppression of migration and invasion of both human prostrate cancer cells were observed… NAC could have a high potential in attenuating the migration of the human prostate cancer cells from their primary site and their adhesion and invasion to the remote locations." – PubMed ID#23513466 (2012) [737]

Harmful Findings

Much like high doses of vitamin E, NAC has been shown to protect the tumor by reducing ROS (reactive oxygen species) as well as increasing migration and metastasis of tumor cells. Though there may be some benefit to NAC in cancer prevention, this is treading on dangerous territory. As mentioned earlier, we all get microscopic cancer tumors from time to time, which our immune system usually takes care of. Adding NAC may actually protect these tumors and allow them to progress. A lot more research would be needed before I would consider NAC as a preventative treatment.

"administration of N-acetylcysteine (NAC) increases lymph node metastases in an endogenous mouse model of malignant melanoma but has no impact on the number and size of primary tumors. Similarly, NAC and the soluble vitamin E analog Trolox markedly increased the migration and invasive properties of human malignant melanoma cells" – PubMed ID#26446958 (2015) [738]

In this study out of the Department of Molecular and Clinical Medicine at the University of Gothenburg in Sweden, they showed that both NAC and vitamin E increased tumor progression and reduced survival in mouse models of human lung cancer.

"The concept that antioxidants can help fight cancer is deeply rooted in the general population, promoted by the food supplement industry, and supported by some scientific studies. However, clinical trials have reported inconsistent results… supplementing the diet with the antioxidants N-acetylcysteine (NAC) and vitamin E markedly increases tumor progression and reduces survival in mouse models of B-RAF- and K-RAS-induced lung cancer… NAC and vitamin E increase tumor cell proliferation by reducing ROS, DNA damage, and p53 expression in mouse and human lung tumor cells." – PubMed ID#24477002 (2014) [739]

The University of Granada in Spain found that high doses of vitamin C, vitamin E and beta-carotene all decreased the effectiveness of cancer treatments. NAC has the same issues as those described in these studies.

"Increased ROS during cancer development makes tumor cells become highly dependent on antioxidant agents. For this reason, low concentrations of free radicals due to an excessive administration of antioxidants may promote the proliferation of harmful cells in the neoplastic state, promoting the development of cancer rather than interrupting it… In the trial conducted by Bairati et al. with head and neck cancer patients, who were treated with radiotherapy and supplemented with high doses of vitamin C and E, they seemed to improve the adverse effects, but also a loss of effectiveness of the treatment was observed, even an increased mortality in patients who received the treatment with antioxidants " – PubMed ID#PMC4670692 (2016) [740]

"On the basis of our review of the published randomized clinical trials, we conclude that the use of supplemental antioxidants during chemotherapy and radiation therapy should be discouraged because of the possibility of tumor protection and reduced survival." – PubMed ID#18505970 (2008) [741]

See Vitamin E, Melanoma earlier in this chapter for more information and studies on the possible harmful effects of NAC, especially for existing cancers.

Adjuvant Therapy

There is some evidence that NAC (and high-dose vitamin E) can help prevent oxidative stress (and damage to non-cancerous cells) from chemotherapy and radiation treatments. Because of the risks of making the cancer metastasis worse, I recommend that you not make the decision to use NAC (or vitamin E) yourself. Your oncologist will have access to far more information about your health status, your type of cancer and current research than what you'll find in this book; your oncologist should be consulted before starting, or continuing, any of these.

The following study looked at 40 children receiving chemotherapy and NAC. This study is just one of many showing the antioxidant potential of NAC, and oxidation is a known side effect of chemotherapy and radiation therapy.

"Thus we may conclude that vitamin E and NAC supplementation had significantly decreased the level of free radicals resulting from oxidation as evidenced by increasing the level of GLu.Px and lowering level of MAD in ALL patients who took the supplementation… With the combined use of NAC and vitamin E, some improvement in oxidative status had occurred; this could be considered as an encouraging result which paves the way for early combined use of these antioxidants as an adjuvant therapy for cancer chemotherapy." – PubMed ID#PMC2778172 (2009) [742]

Strategy

NAC supplements are found in doses much higher than what one would find in food. Due to the several recent research studies showing that NAC actually protects cancer tumors (from both treatment and the immune system), it is not something I would recommend using. Taking it for prevention also has unacceptable risks. If you have cancer, or have had a metastasizing cancer in the past, you should check with your oncologist before taking NAC. If your oncologist seems unsure, then do not take it.

❖ NEEM LEAF

AKA: *Azadirachta indica, Antelaea azadirachta,* **Arishta, Arishtha, Indian lilac**

Azadirachta indica (neem) is a fast-growing tree native to India but now also found in other parts of the world. In fact, it is considered an invasive species in some parts of Africa and Australia. The bark, seeds and leaves have all been used medicinally. Some of the traditional uses have been to treat: intestinal parasites, loss of appetite, skin ulcers, gum disease, malaria, diabetes and stomach upset.

Neem is thought to have several bioactive substances; however, only azadirachtin and nimbolide have been studied to any degree useful for discussion. Recent research has found that neem and its bioactive compounds have several anticancer properties.

Neem exerts several effects on cancer, including improving apoptosis in cancer cells, suppression of angiogenesis (the formation of new blood supplies to tumors), cell proliferation, etc. It also helps to improve the immune response against cancer cells.

"The key anticancer effects of neem components on malignant cells include inhibition of cell proliferation, induction of cell death, suppression of cancer angiogenesis, restoration of cellular reduction/oxidation (redox) balance, and enhancement of the host immune responses against tumor cells… the anti-proliferative and apoptosis-inducing effects of neem components are tumor selective as the effects on normal cells are significantly weaker. In addition, neem extracts sensitize cancer cells to immunotherapy and radiotherapy, and enhance the efficacy of certain cancer chemotherapeutic agents" – PubMed ID#PMC4734358 (2014) [743]

This excerpt is a bit complicated, but in short, it means that neem improves the immune response to cancer by improving the response of lymphocytes called NK cells (natural killer cells, a type of white blood cell). NK cells are vital in the fight against cancer cells.

> "Neem leaf preparation (NLP) was found to activate natural killer (NK) cells (CD56(+)CD3(-)) to enhance their cytotoxic ability to tumor cells and stimulate the release of interleukin-12 (IL-12) from macrophages from healthy individuals and head-and-neck squamous cell carcinoma patients. NLP upregulated cytotoxic (CD16(+) and CD56(dim)) NK cells, and the cytotoxicity of NK-sensitive K562 cells" – PubMed ID#17961770 (2007) [744]

> "The suppression of tumor growth is associated with the formation of hyalinized fibrous tumor tissue and the induction of cell death by apoptosis. These results suggest that EENL (ethanol extract of neem leaves) containing natural bioactive compounds could have potent anticancer property and the regulation of multiple cellular pathways could exert pleiotrophic effects in prevention and treatment of prostate cancer." – PubMed ID#21560017 (2011) [745]

VEGF is short for vascular endothelial growth factor; this is a signaling protein released by tumors that cause the body to produce new blood supplies to the tumor (angiogenesis). Being able to control VEGF can significantly slow the growth of cancer tumors (and is being studied by pharmaceutical companies). It also shows a range of other anticancer properties that suppress cancer growth and induce apoptosis.

> "Neem modulates the activity of various tumour suppressor genes (e.g., p53, pTEN), angiogenesis (VEGF), transcription factors (e.g., NF-ϰB), and apoptosis (e.g., bcl2, bax)… Neem also plays role as anti-inflammatory via regulation of proinflammatory enzyme activities including cyclooxygenase (COX), and lipoxygenase (LOX) enzyme… neem show(s) a range of activities affecting multiple targets and also play role in the induction of apoptotic cell death in cancer" – PubMed ID#PMC4791507 (2016) [746]

In a 2018 meta-study published by the *International Journal of Molecular Sciences*, they reviewed the current evidence showing chemoprotective and immunomodulatory properties of neem. They reviewed dozens of studies showing that neem has clear cancer prevention properties as well as immune-enhancing/modulating properties when used as adjuvant cancer treatment.

> "neem tree extracts and compounds have great potential for the prevention of cancer. The molecular mechanism of action involves the modulation of cellular

proliferation, differentiation, apoptosis, angiogenesis, and metastasis processes… several in vitro studies have been conducted on cancer cell lines… Chemosensitization of tumor cells by using both neem extracts… This combined approach is able to improve the efficiency of standard cancer therapies by allowing for decreased chemotherapy doses, and neem extracts have also proved to be useful in reducing the toxicity of chemotherapy drugs." – PubMed ID#PMC6321405 (2018) [747]

Neem also exerts immune function benefits. It is our immune system that fights cancer. It is especially important to improve the immune system (but not artificially rev it up) if on any type of immunotherapy.

"Neem (Azadirachta indica) leaf mediated immune activation causes prophylactic growth inhibition of murine Ehrlich carcinoma and B16 melanoma… Flow cytometric evidence suggested that increase in CD4+ and CD8+ T cells accounted for lymphocytosis. The conditional tumor growth retardation, observed in mice treated with NLP before tumor inoculation, may be regulated by NLP mediated immune activation, having prominent role in the cellular immune function of the tumor host." – PubMed ID#15037213 (2004) [748]

"Enhancement of immune responses to neem leaf extract (Azadirachta indica) correlates with antineoplastic activity in BALB/c-mice… In these model systems the number of experimental lung and liver metastases decreased relevantly, however, biometrically non-significantly in neem extract-treated animals, as compared to the control mice which received injections of saline solutions. Neem extract can be regarded as an immunomodulating and antimetastatic substance" – PubMed ID#16634526 (2006) [749]

"Neem leaf preparation enhances Th1 type immune response and anti-tumor immunity against breast tumor associated antigen… NLP is completely safe with no adverse effects on liver and kidney functions (13). Moreover, NLP has been shown to stimulate hematopoiesis. Our earlier reports (13-17) and the experimental data obtained from this study suggest that NLP is a safe, effective and economical adjuvant and can be used in tumor vaccine formulations" – PubMed ID#PMC2935742 (2007) [750]

Recommendations

Neem does have some impressive in vivo studies (mouse xenograft models) showing effectiveness. For this reason, I think it can be worth adding to your regimen, especially if your cancer is one of those mentioned above. Dosing isn't something that has been determined for cancer treatment. Therefore, I would recommend going by the directions on the bottle. Benefits at this dose may (or may not) be minimal, but neem should be beneficial as an adjuvant treatment along with everything else you're doing.

❖ OLIVE LEAF EXTRACT

Olive fruit, seeds and leaves have been used medicinally for hundreds, if not thousands, of years. Olive leaves contain various compounds that have medicinal value, such as oleuropein, tyrosol and hydroxytyrosol, and flavonoids; they are also high in oleic acid. Oleuropein is the most studied component of olive leaf; it has been shown to have antioxidant, antibacterial, anti-inflammatory and immune-stimulating properties. Because of these properties, it has been used to treat colds, influenza, candidiasis, diarrhea and a number of other conditions. It has also been shown in research to benefit diabetes, lower blood sugar levels and lower high blood pressure. Some research has also shown benefits in using olive leaf extract to treat herpes and rotavirus viral infections.

Olive leaf is even thought to be the "tree of life" in the Bible and in this quote: "The fruit thereof shall be for meat, and the leaf thereof for medicine" (Ezekiel 47:12).

Olive leaf extracts (OLE) have been shown to have anticancer properties in several different research studies. It has the ability to increase differentiation in several types of cancer; this helps the immune system to identify cancer cells. It can also help induce apoptosis in cancer cells; this is where defective (or cancerous) cells are programmed to destroy themselves without the aid of the immune system. OLE also exhibits antiproliferative and anti-metastasis properties. Most studies to date have been either in vitro or xenograft in vivo (where human cancer cells are grafted to mice, where they behave very much like they do in humans), rather than human in vivo.

> "Olive leaves contain many potentially bioactive compounds that may have antioxidant, antimicrobial, antihypertensive, antiviral, anti-inflammatory, hypoglycemic, neuroprotective, and anticancer properties… In the prior studies, olive leaf extract has been shown to exhibit an antitumor activity and to induce apoptosis pathways in cancer cells… olive leaf has been reported to exhibit an antileukemia effect by inducing apoptosis in the acute myeloid leukemia HL-60 cells… In this study we give evidence that COLE exhibits its antileukemia effect by both inducing apoptosis and promoting differentiation of the multipotent human leukemia K562 cells." – PubMed ID#PMC3997986 (2014) [751]

Olive leaf is high in a flavonoid called luteolin. The following study looked at both olive leaf extract and luteolin in breast cancer lines (in vitro).

> Incubation with only luteolin showed a significant effect in cell survival. Luteolin induced apoptosis, whereas the whole olive leaf extract incubation led to a significant cell cycle arrest at the G1 phase. The antiproliferative activity of both pure luteolin and olive leaf extract was mediated by the inactivation of the MAPK-proliferation pathway at the extracellular signal-related kinase (ERK1/2). – PubMed ID#25560707 (2015) [752]

Olive leaf and its extracts were studied for their effects on human breast cancers. Human breast cancer cells were xenografted into the mammaries of mice; prostate cells were grafted in the second part of this research. This method allows for in vivo research on mice rather than humans, as the research results would be very similar. They found that olive leaf reduced the volume and weight of tumors, reduced angiogenesis (via VEGF downregulation) and reduced inflammatory markers (which can worsen some cancers).

> "In vivo studies looking at olive leaf polyphenols also appear to support an anti-cancer effect. Oleuropein (125 mg/kg of diet) slowed tumor growth and inhibited cancer metastasis after MCF-7 cell xenograft establishment in mice [110]. OLE dissolved in water (150 and 225 mg/kg/day) reduced tumour volume and weight in mice after breast cancer xenograft… In vivo, luteolin (10 mg/kg/day) reduced both volume and weight of tumors in a prostate xenograft mouse model and in vitro, using the prostate cancer cells PC-3, it down-regulated VEGF phosphorylation of VEGF2 receptor and its downstream inflammatory markers IL-8 and IL-6… There is strong evidence from cell models which demonstrates that olive polyphenols, and specifically the combination found in olive leaf, are able to modulate and interact with molecular pathways and in doing so may inhibit the progression and development of cancer." – PubMed ID#PMC4997426 (2016) [753]

Oleuropein is the major phenolic compound in olive leaf. Besides its anticancer properties, OLE is also known for its antioxidant and anti-inflammatory effects (which can also benefit cancer treatment).

> "Hamdi and Castellon showed that oleuropein inhibits growth of LN-18 cells, a poorly differentiated glioblastoma cell line; TF-1a, a erythroleukemia; and tumor cell lines derived from advanced-grade human tumors (786-O, renal cell adenocarcinoma; T-47D, infiltrating ductal carcinoma of the breast pleural effusion; RPMI-7951, malignant melanoma of the skin-lymph node metastasis; and LoVo, colorectal adenocarcinoma cells) in Swiss albino mice with soft tissue sarcoma… oleuropein aglycone is the most potent phenolic compound in

> decreasing breast cancer cell viability. HER2 oncogene-amplified SKBR3 cells were ~5-times more sensitive to oleuropein aglycone than HER2-negative MCF-7 cells." – PubMed ID#PMC3002804 (2010) [754]

Olive leaf extract has been shown to possess strong anti-melanoma properties in several research studies. It also works well as an adjuvant treatment with chemotherapy and immunotherapy (but always consult your oncologist).

> "The anticancer potential of dry olive leaf extract (DOLE) represents the net effect of multilevel interactions… the results of this study indicate that DOLE possesses strong antimelanoma potential. When DOLE was applied in combination with different chemotherapeutics, various outcomes, including synergy and antagonism, were observed." – PubMed ID#20568104 (2011) [755]

Recommendations

Olive leaf extract exhibits antimicrobial properties. This means that it can reduce the strength, diversity and overall health of the microbiome (as it kills both good and bad bacteria and viruses). Because the microbiome is highly beneficial to immune system health, this can be a problem. The evidence I've seen tends to indicate some selectivity—in other words, OLE seems to kill bad bacteria at a higher rate than most beneficial bacteria.

For this reason, I do not recommend olive leaf extracts for cancer prevention.

For cancer treatment/adjuvant treatment, you can take up to 2,000 mg daily in divided doses (e.g., take two 500 mg capsules, twice per day). While taking olive leaf supplements, be sure to follow the advice in Chapter 2 and Chapter 3 to maintain and improve gut health. A strong microbiome is important, and olive leaf can weaken it.

❖ RESVERATROL

Resveratrol is a natural phenol (a phytochemical) produced by grapes, mulberries, blueberries, raspberries and peanuts. These plants use it as a defense against pathogens such as fungi and bacteria. Red wine and red grape juice have some of the highest concentrations of resveratrol.

The following meta research does an excellent job of outlining the various research on resveratrol's benefits in fighting and preventing cancer. Table 1 in the study outlines 39 in vivo research studies showing its anti-cancer benefits. Most of these studies used xenograft mouse models; this is where human cancers are grafted into the organs of mice, where they grow very much like they would in a human. These types of studies carry far more scientific weight than in vitro studies (which can still be very useful).

> "Resveratrol effectively hindered the development of DMBA/TPA-induced mouse-skin tumors by inducing apoptosis… Resveratrol has exhibited anti-cancer and chemopreventive properties in various animal breast cancer models… Resveratrol, in a xenograft animal model, inhibited the development of ER-β–positive MDA-MB-231 and estrogen receptor (ER)-α–negative tumor explants, raised apoptosis, and lowered angiogenesis… In another study, oral resveratrol at 100 or 200 mg/kg inhibited the development of 4T1 cells and metastasis in mouse lungs… With the use of AR-negative PC-3 human prostate cancer–cell xenografts in the flank regions of mice, post-treatment with oral resveratrol (30 mg/kg/day) decreased the volume of tumors, with lowered tumor-cell proliferation and neovascularization, and induced apoptosis… Resveratrol inhibited hepatic lipogenesis and intracellular ROS, and the results from liver cancer models have been consistently positive, indicating the potential benefit of resveratrol in hepatocellular carcinoma prevention and/or therapy… However, dietary resveratrol had no anti-carcinogenic effect on BOP (N-nitrosobis(2-oxopropyl)amine)-induced pancreatic carcinogenesis in hamsters" – PubMed ID#PMC5751192 (2017) (Open Access attribution available at the link) [756]

Though resveratrol shows some promise, it has been shown in a number of research studies that oral administration may not help very much. In most of these studies, resveratrol was administered intravenously or intraperitoneally (into the abdomen). Resveratrol is not nearly as bioavailable or beneficial when taken orally. Some studies did show benefits to oral dosing, but only at a relatively high dose of 30 mg/kg (so 2 grams/day for a 160 lb person), with one study using 625 mg/kg!

There is also a growing recognition that high doses of certain antioxidants can impede our immune system from fighting existing tumors. As shown with high levels of vitamin E, vitamin C and NAC, high doses of certain antioxidants can interfere with the body's ability to fight cancer. The following study found that low doses of resveratrol may be able to help fight certain types of cancer, especially when combined with a high-fat diet (HFD), but higher amounts can protect cancer cells.

> "With recent results from trials such as SELECT, involving selenium and the antioxidant vitamin E, it is gradually being recognised that complex dose-response relationships exist for dietary-derived agents. Furthermore, the lack of effect or even harm seen in trials with high-dose antioxidant supplements is consistent with the idea that low levels of ROS can trigger cellular defence mechanisms and are actually protective, which is suggestive of a non-linear dose-response, or hormesis… our observations in multiple models of murine and human colorectal cancer provide the first direct evidence that low intakes of

> resveratrol have greater anticancer efficacy than high doses… In summary, we provide compelling evidence of a **bell-shaped dose response** for resveratrol, with low doses having greater efficacy than high doses." – PubMed ID#PMC4827609 (2016) [757]

Recommendation

Taking high-dose resveratrol carries unacceptable risks and would require supplements. Wine is one of the highest food sources of resveratrol, with red wine containing about 1 mg per glass. This means that a 160 lb person would need to drink 2,000 glasses of wine to obtain what was once thought of as an effective therapeutic dose (2 grams). As fun as that sounds, I don't think that it is possible.

Recent research points to a "bell-shaped dose response" where less is better than more. For this reason, I would recommend not taking more than 10 mg per day. This dose may be hard to achieve as food sources do not provide enough, and most supplements will provide far too much. For example, you would need 10 glasses of red wine per day to reach 10 mg. Though this sounds more reasonable than 2,000 glasses, it is still far too much alcohol to drink each day.

Due to the limited research, I decided not to add this supplement to my personal protocol. Proper low doses were difficult to obtain, and high doses carried too much risk (and due to my COMT deficiency, weren't an option).

Note: Resveratrol is a strong antioxidant, so if you are taking high doses of it and you have an existing cancer tumor, you should discuss this with your oncologist. In nearly every situation, if you have an existing cancer, high doses of resveratrol are not recommended and can be dangerous.

Note: Do not take high doses of resveratrol if you have a genetic COMT deficiency (see the COMT discussion under Green Tea/EGCG earlier in this section).

❖ S T E V I A

Most people know of stevia as the sugar substitute. It works very well for this as it is approximately 150 to 300 times as sweet as sugar, while having no effect on blood glucose levels. I often recommend stevia in this book and in my previous book, *The Gut Health Protocol*. [758] Some people find it bitter, but this is usually related to the purity of the product; products with a higher percentage of rebaudioside A (a steviol glycoside) do not have this bitter flavor. Steviol glycosides are the chemical compounds responsible for the sweet taste found in stevia. Stevia is extracted from the leaves of the South American plant *Stevia rebaudiana* (Asteraceae). The leaves of the *S. rebaudiana* plant have been used for more than 1,500 years in South America by the Guaraní native populations.

Now it turns out that stevia also has anticancerous effects against a variety of cancers. The research into this is just beginning, and there aren't a lot of studies yet, but the studies so far are promising.

Stevia should not be relied upon as a cancer treatment, but if you are choosing a sweetener, it is much better to pick one that has research showing anticancerous effects, than to pick one that has been shown to either cause cancer or worsen it (such as sugar—any sugar, including honey). Stevia has only been tested in a few cancers, so it is unknown whether it will have broad-spectrum anticancerous benefits in other cancers or not.

In this study appearing in the *Pharmacognosy Magazine*, steviol glycoside was studied on human breast cancer cells (MCF-7). Steviol showed clear suppression of cancer cell viability, cell cycle arrest (where cell growth is inhibited if the cell is not growing normally) and induction of apoptosis.

> "the present investigation was carried out to study the role of Steviol on human breast cancer cell line (MCF-7). Our results showed that Steviol dose dependently inhibits MCF-7 cell growth and arrests cell cycle arrest at G2/M phase. This study indicates the antineoplastic action of Steviol in breast cancer… The outcome of this study illustrates the cytotoxic or anticancerous effects of Steviol from the plant S. rebaudiana against cultured human breast cancer MCF-7 cells, and its probable mechanisms of action include suppression of cell viability, cell cycle arrest, and induction of apoptosis in cancer cells. Steviol inhibits the proliferation of MCF-7 cells in a dose-dependent manner. Till now, no study has reported on the effect of Steviol on human breast cancer (in vitro or in vivo)" – PubMed ID#PMC5551348 (2017) (Open Access attribution available at the link) 759

In this study out of China (appearing in the *Oncotarget* journal), stevia was shown to "possess intensive anticancer activity on the human gastrointestinal cancer cells." This activity included selectively activating apoptosis in the cancer cells, initiating cell cycle arrest (stopping the growth of cancer cells) and inhibiting tumor angiogenesis in vitro and in vivo.

> "stevia rebaudiana bertoni, was found to possess intensive anticancer activity on the human gastrointestinal cancer cells. Steviol inhibited six human gastrointestinal cancer cells intensively as 5-fluorouracil did at 100 µg/mL. The inhibition mechanism follows mitochondrial apoptotic pathway… Steviol causes phase arrest and apoptosis of the gastrointestinal cancer cells… Taking together, steviol has a wide-spectrum inhibitory activity on the human gastrointestinal cancer cells through leading a mitochondrial apoptotic pathway as evidenced by

> increase of the Bax/Bcl-2 ratio, activation of p21, p53; whereas Caspase 3-independent mechanism was involved." – PubMed ID#PMC5995179 (2018)

Again, stevia was found both to directly cause cancer cell death and to induce apoptosis (cancer cell suicide, a natural process the body uses where deformed cells are culled) while doing no harm to normal cells.

> "Cytotoxic and apoptosis-inducing activities of steviol and isosteviol derivatives against human cancer cell lines." – PubMed ID#23418165 (2013)

Osteosarcoma is cancer that starts in bone; it is most common in teenagers and young adults.

> "The present study demonstrated that steviol inhibits the proliferation of the human osteosarcoma U2OS cell line in a dose- and time-dependent manner, and that the inhibition rate is comparative with that of doxorubicin and 5-fluorouracil." – PubMed ID#29552164 (2018)

Recommendations

There is not strong enough evidence to recommend using stevia supplements to treat or prevent cancer. However, stevia is a very safe food substance and has shown some benefit in treating various cancers. Because most other sweetener choices have been associated with cancer and other health conditions (such as metabolic syndrome, which can interfere with the immune system), stevia should be your sweetener of choice.

I do not recommend supplementing high doses of stevia simply for treating cancer. However, it is my sweetener of choice.

❖ TURMERIC AND CURCUMIN

Turmeric is a spice that has a mild flavor and imparts a bright yellow color to foods. It is the spice that is used to give yellow mustard that bright yellow color. As a major component of curry, it is found in many Indian and Asian dishes. Turmeric is derived from the roots of the *Curcuma longa* plant, which is indigenous to Southeast Asia. Curcumin is a constituent of turmeric and its primary active ingredient. It contains various curcuminoids, which is where most of the benefits are found. Because curcumin is where most of the turmeric's health benefits originate, that is primarily what will be discussed in this section.

However, if you have the opportunity to utilize turmeric in your food, you should. Though curcumin only makes up about 2% to 5% of turmeric per weight, turmeric imparts very mild savory flavors to savory dishes, and every bit of curcumin you can get helps. Turmeric also contains related beneficial turmeric extracts and fractions that may have additional health benefits. The spice curry contains a lot of turmeric, but it gets its heat from other spices in the curry blend. About 90% of the world's turmeric is grown in India, where it is frequently consumed in various dishes, with and without curry.

Research on the health benefits of curcumin has been increasing rapidly. The number of peer-reviewed publications about curcumin was approximately 108 in the year 2000; this increased to about 1,232 in 2015. Extensive research over the last 50 years indicates that curcumin can be used to both treat and prevent various cancers. Some of those studies will be summarized below.

> "In an in vivo study, curcumin demonstrated anticancer activity against chemical induced hepatocarcinogenesis (liver cancer). The administration of curcumin reduced hyper plastic nodule, liver damage markers, body weight loss and hypoproteinemia in the liver... The protective effects of curcumin against liver cancer also involved the enhanced degradation of hypoxia-inducible factor, and curcumin could promote apoptosis" – PubMed ID#PMC4808884 (2016) [760]

This paper out of Switzerland summarizes dozens of recent research studies on curcumin.

> **Nasopharyngeal Cancer (Head and Neck)** - Curcumin induced G2/M phase arrest and apoptosis in human nasopharyngeal carcinoma cells (NPC), which have been associated with mitochondria, apoptosis inducing factor and caspase-3-dependent pathways
>
> **Lung Cancer** - Bax expression was increased while the expression of B-cell lymphoma-2 (Bcl-2) and B-cell lymphoma-xL (Bcl-xL) was decreased by curcumin in small cell lung cancer, thus inducing apoptosis accompanied by increasing intracellular reactive oxygen species (ROS) levels. Mitochondrial membrane potential was decreased, the release of cytochrome c into the cytosol was induced, and then caspase-9 and caspase-3 were activated... it was validated that curcumin treatment to human lung cancer cells could induce DNA damage and inhibit expression of DNA-repair-associated proteins, such as breast cancer susceptibility gene 1 (BRCA1), 14-3-3 protein σ, O6-methylguanine-DNA methyltransferase (MGMT), and mediator of DNA damage checkpoint 1 (MDC1)... studies on animals also confirmed the anti-tumor effects of curcumin in lung cancer... curcumin remarkably inhibited tumor growth of orthotopic human NSCLC xenografts and increased survival of treated athymic mice.

Hepatobiliary Cancer (liver, gall bladder and bile duct cancers) - Curcumin induced antiproliferation and apoptosis in cholangiocarcinoma cells. The apoptosis was significantly related to production of superoxide anion, while the up-regulation of tumor protein 53 (P53) and Bcl-2 associated X protein (Bax) were associated with oxidative stress and apoptosis

Breast Cancers - Curcumin was able to inhibit the proliferation of triple negative breast cancer cells, probably through inhibiting the EGFR signaling pathway… HIF-1α and HIF-2α protein levels in hypoxia were lowered by curcumin. Curcumin also reduced ARNT protein levels and HIF transcriptional activity both in normoxia and hypoxia in MCF-7 breast carcinoma cells… curcumin could be used as an in vivo inhibitor of breast cancer resistance protein [59]. In addition, the recommended dose of curcumin is 6000 mg/day for seven consecutive days every 3 weeks in combination with a standard dose of docetaxel for the combination therapy in advanced and metastatic breast cancer patients.

Gastric Cancers - curcumin inhibited the growth of human colon adeno-carcinoma cell lines and induced apoptosis as evidenced by nuclear fragmentation as well as condensation and DNA fragmentation… induced-dissociation of hexokinase II from the mitochondria led to mitochondrial-mediated apoptosis… curcumin was well tolerated at both 2 g and 4 g in patients, and could decrease ACF number. In addition, curcumin treatment improved the general health of patients with colorectal cancer

Cancer in Uterus - After treatment with curcumin-based cervical cream, HPV+ cervical cancer cells were selectively eliminated, antigen E6 transformation and EGFR expressions were inhibited, and concomitantly p53 was induced.

Hematopoietic Tumor (blood cells) - curcumin could inhibit the growth and promote apoptosis of leukemic cells which were derived from acute promyelocytic leukemia.

Curcumin plays an important role in treatment of many other cancers, such as, peripheral nerve sheath tumors, and oral squamous cell carcinoma"

Zheng J, Zhou Y, Li Y, Xu DP, Li S, Li HB. Spices for Prevention and Treatment of Cancers. Nutrients. 2016 Aug 12;8(8):495. doi: 10.3390/nu8080495. PubMed PMID: 27529277; PubMed Central PMCID: PMC4997408. [761]

Breast Cancer

"We confirmed that curcumin inhibits NF-kB in triple negative breast cancer cells using the HCC1806 line as a model. Curcumin inhibited NF-kB transcription factor function (Fig. 3A) and phosphorylation of p65 NF-kB… The current study demonstrates that curcumin induces DNA damage and apoptosis in triple negative breast cancer cells in association with increased expression, phosphorylation, and cytoplasmic retention of the BRCA1 protein… These results suggest that curcumin may target cancer cells, with limited non-specific toxicity toward non-cancerous cells… Our findings also showed a trend of triple negative breast cancer cells being more sensitive to curcumin than non-TNBCs, suggesting a potential new line of therapy for this subset of breast cancers" – PubMed ID#PMC2756684 (2009) [763]

"More recently, a study showed that treatment of colorectal cancer cells with curcumin and exisulind resulted in a synergistic inhibitory effect of 50-90% on cell growth associated with G2/M arrest and induction of apoptosis… curcumin present in food might act to prevent cancer occurrence and participate in epigenetic control of gene expression." – PubMed ID#22045655 (quote from full study 10.1002/mnfr.201100307) [764]

"Treatment of retinoic acid resistant triple negative breast cancer cells with curcumin sensitized these cells to retinoic acid mediated growth suppression, as well as suppressed incorporation of BrdU. Further studies demonstrated that curcumin showed a marked reduction in the expression level of FABP5 and PPARβ/δ… The combination of curcumin with retinoic acid suppressed PPARβ/δ target genes, VEGF-A and PDK1" – PubMed ID#25260874 (2014) [765]

In the full study discussed in the abstract below, the research concludes that curcumin inhibits NF-κB expression, thus inhibiting cancer cell proliferation. It also induces cancer cell apoptosis through downregulation of various cancer cell genes, cell phase arrest, and modulation of microRNA (miR), DNA, histone and mitochondria. In short, curcumin is multifaceted in how it inhibits cancer.

"Breast cancer is among the most common malignant tumors. It is the second leading cause of cancer mortality among women in the United States. Curcumin, an active derivative from turmeric, has been reported to have anticancer and chemoprevention effects on breast cancer. Curcumin exerts its anticancer effect through a complicated molecular signaling network, involving proliferation, estrogen receptor (ER), and human epidermal growth factor receptor 2 (HER2) pathways. Experimental evidence has shown that curcumin also regulates apoptosis and cell phase–related genes and microRNA in breast cancer cells. Herein, we review the recent research efforts in understanding the molecular targets and anticancer mechanisms of curcumin in breast cancer." – PubMed ID#27325106 [766] Full Study at DOI: 10.1177/2211068216655524 [767] (2016)

Curcumin, like many other natural treatments, has been shown to be a very beneficial adjunct treatment. It not only improves the effectiveness of traditional treatments, but in some cases, the results are better than the sum of those produced by the two treatment types being used individually. Lots of acronyms below; just skip past those you don't recognize. In short, curcumin improved many markers associated with cancer.

"(Curcuma longa) has been proven for its better anticancer potential. In this review different molecular mechanisms including cell cycle arrest; G0/G1 and/or G2/M phase cell cycle arrest by up-regulating Cdk inhibitor, p21/WAF/CIPI and p53, inhibition of transcriptional factors; NFκB, AP-1, TNFα, IL, STAT-3, and PPAR-γ, downstream gene regulation; c-myc, Bcl-2, COX-2, NOS, Cyclin D1, TNFα, interleukins and MMP-9, growth factors; bFGF, EGF, GCSF, IL-8, PDGF, TGFα, TNF, VEGF and cell adhesion molecules; fibronectin, vitronectin, and collagen which are involved in angiogenesis and metastasis, also the effectiveness of curcumin, when given in combination with chemo-therapeutics like cyclophosphamide, doxorubicin, mitomycin etc. in treating breast cancer have been reviewed." – PubMed ID#25553436 (2015) [768]

"A multi-database electronic search was performed to provide an overview of curcumin as an adjunct therapy and miRNA modulator in breast cancer and highlight the significance of observations for the treatment of cancer therapies... The putative anti-tumor properties of curcumin are mediated by diverse mechanisms including inhibition of cell proliferation, metastasis, migration, invasion and angiogenesis, and induction of G2/M cell cycle arrest, apoptosis and paraptosis. Recent evidence implies that curcumin can interact with several oncogenic and tumor suppressive miRNAs involved in different stages of breast cancer. In this context, up-regulation of miR181b, miR-34a, miR-16, miR-15a and miR-146b-5p, and down-regulation of miR-19a and miR-19b have been shown following the treatment of several breast cancer cell lines with curcumin. These effects lead to the suppression of tumorigenesis and metastasis, and induction of apoptosis." – PubMed ID#29189128 (2018) [769]

Melanoma

"Curcumin is a natural polyphenol that shows a variety of pharmacological activities including anti-cancer effects… The anti-cancer effects of curcumin are the result of its anti-angiogenic, pro-apoptotic and immunomodulatory properties… curcumin can blunt epithelial-to-mesenchymal transition and affect many targets that are involved in melanoma initiation and progression (e.g., BCl2, MAPKS, p21 and some microRNAs). However, curcumin has a low oral bioavailability that may limit its maximal benefits. The emergence of tailored formulations of curcumin and new delivery systems such as nanoparticles, liposomes, micelles and phospholipid complexes has led to the enhancement of curcumin bioavailability." – PubMed ID#27280688 (2016) [770]

The following research paper goes on to describe the various mechanisms by which curcumin induces apoptosis in cancer cells, nature's built-in self-destruction mechanism for cells that are damaged or go cancerous. Apoptosis is often dysfunctional in established cancer tumors, and reactivating it is critical to stopping tumor growth and preventing metastasis. To enhance the apoptosis mechanism, curcumin activates caspases 3 and 8, as well as downregulates the JAK-2/STAT3 signaling pathway. In vitro, curcumin has also been found to inhibit melanoma cell migration and invasion.

"Anti-cancer activity of curcumin is mediated by its capacity to modulate several pathways and target multiple genes, transcription factors, inflammatory cytokines, enzymes, growth factors, receptors, adhesion molecules, anti-apoptotic proteins and cell cycle proteins, leading to apoptosis and inhibition of cell proliferation and migration" – PubMed ID#28167449 [771] DOI: 10.1016/j.biopha.2017.01.078 [772] (2017)

Strategy/Usage

Curcumin, the most active ingredient in turmeric, can be a very beneficial supplement. It can improve the immune system and directly fight cancer, all the while supporting general health.

However, curcumin is not very bioavailable in its raw form, meaning it is hard to get it to the cells where it is needed. Supplements that simply include raw extracted curcumin are probably not doing you much good. Luckily, there are now some very good supplements on the market that have proven ways of greatly enhancing bioavailability.

Turmeric contains various active components, but most of the research has been with curcumin. I recommend that you cook with turmeric, but you should also supplement with a good bioavailable form of curcumin. When cooking with turmeric, try to include it in a dish that has some fat and black pepper; this increases the absorption of curcumin. Turmeric is the main ingredient in curry powders, and curry dishes are a good way to get more bioavailable curcumin (as these dishes usually include some fat and pepper). I sometimes sprinkle turmeric on scrambled eggs and other savory dishes.

To achieve the most beneficial effects of curcumin, I recommend that you supplement a highly bioavailable form. I use two different ones; one is called "Theracurmin™." It is a micronized form of curcumin that has been shown in research to be highly bioavailable. This supplement is highly regarded and is mentioned in over 160 research studies and papers. Research shows that this form of curcumin is 27 times more bioavailable than regular curcumin.

> "The area under the blood concentration-time curve of Theracurmin in humans was 27-fold higher than that of curcumin powder." – PubMed ID#25308211 (2014) [773]

The other form of curcumin that I use is an oil-based capsule that contains 95% tetra-hydro-curcuminoids, along with certain herbs that increase bioavailability. Curcumin is fat soluble, so this form also improves effectiveness.

Cancer Prevention – Take one 30 mg capsule of Theracurmin once per day for prevention. You can *Improve Your Odds* even more by adding 1 oil-based curcumin supplement.

Cancer Adjuvant Treatment – Take 1 Theracumin capsule 2 to 3 times per day, as well as 2 oil-based capsules per day. If this gives you gas or gut distress, you may have to start with 1 and 1 and work up to this amount.

Note: Curcumin is a mild natural blood thinner that helps to deliver nutrients to various parts of the body. If you are already taking a blood-thinning medication, please consult with your doctor prior to consuming.

OTHER SUPPLEMENTS

This section will discuss several natural supplements that do not fit other categories but either have anticancer properties or are commonly mentioned in alternative medicine circles as cancer treatments.

If you are on any medications, or have other health issues, be sure to look up any herbal/botanical that you plan to take for contraindications. One of the best ways to do this is on the Memorial Sloan Kettering Herbs and Dietary Supplements website. It is not uncommon for dietary supplements to interfere with certain medications. Your doctor, and especially your oncologist, should also be told of any supplements you plan to take.

❖ pH BUFFERING POTENTIAL

If you have read that "alkalizing" is beneficial for cancer treatment, I highly recommend that you read this entire section. What you see online, and even from many health practitioners, about how to accomplish this is generally incorrect. Simply consuming fruits and vegetables will not "alkalize the body," nor will it alkalize or inhibit cancer tumors. I believe the current alkalizing fad got its start from a misunderstanding of biology and a desire to get people to consume less meat. What you want to do is to increase your pH buffering potential; this will be discussed shortly.

Most "alkaline diets" are not unhealthy. Quite the contrary; they have a lot going for them, but not for reasons having anything to do with the pH of the food. Modern "alkalizing" diets include a lot of healthy vegetables, and they restrict processed foods. I've thought for some time that the healthiest diet is a vegan diet with the addition of some organic meat, fish and eggs! This is how you should think about your diet. The meal's focus shouldn't be the protein; it should be the vegetables. I call this "vegan plus meat." But I digress.

It has been known for some time that cancer tumors, and the microenvironment around them, are acidic. This is due to the tumor's increased metabolism of glucose (cancer cells primarily depend on sugar as an energy source), fast metabolism and poor circulation of their waste products. The cause of this acidity has nothing to do with the food you eat (but food might be part of the solution). Tumor acidity has been shown to be important to a tumor's growth and metastasis. An acidic environment around the tumor suppresses the immune system's ability to destroy cancer cells by affecting T cells and impacting the immune system's ability to detect cancer (this is called "immune escape").

For years it has been theorized that raising the pH (making it more alkaline/base) around tumors may impact them, or perhaps even destroy them. To this end, non-FDA approved oral bicarbonate therapies (and other alkalizing schemes) have been around for some time. Scientists and doctors have always told people to avoid these alternative treatments, as there was no evidence of efficacy and it was feared that people would avoid other treatments.

Research is now finding some validity to the theories of using sodium bicarbonate, or other <u>selective</u> alkalizing methods, in the treatment of some cancers—but not in ways that validate the alternative "alkalizing" treatments you'll find online. When you approach things through scientific methods, you can fine-tune these protocols, so they may actually work in vivo (in the body), not just in a theorist's mind or a grad student's test tube (where many great ideas get started, and many others die a horrible death).

First, a little background. The normal blood pH is tightly regulated in the body to stay between 7.35 and 7.45. Anything even slightly outside this range causes illness and can easily lead to death. The body works very hard at maintaining this pH. Messing with the body's pH is very tricky, and as you can tell, dangerous. Changing the pH by just 10% outside of these norms can be fatal! Lowering the acidity of the tumor's local environment without also lowering the pH of the blood and organs can be difficult. But that is what is necessary to successfully use this type of therapy to prevent or treat cancer (eating lemons and wheatgrass isn't going to do it).

You cannot "alkalize the body," a term I see all too frequently. When you eat food, it first travels through the stomach, which has a pH of around 1.5 (or less—it is very acidic). The pH of the small intestine varies from about 4.0 at the top (the duodenum) to 7.4 at the terminal ileum, while the pH of the large intestine varies from about 5.5 to 7.0, depending on what part of the colon you are measuring. The human vagina maintains an acidic pH of around 4.5; this is due to the large amount of lactic acid-producing bacteria found there (and needed for proper health). As you can see, "alkalizing the body" is not going to happen, and trying to force it will only result in poor health and a disrupted microbiome. What you want to do is to provide the body what it needs to "<u>buffer</u>" acidity as needed (on demand in a regulated manner). Rather than trying to override the body's fine-tuned pH regulatory system, what you want to do is to provide it what it needs to do its job.

When you consume food, the pH of that food is going to be significantly lowered (made to be more acidic) when it passes through the stomach. This is because the stomach bathes the foods in HCl (hydrochloric acid), which lowers the pH of the food chyme to about 1.5 (this is very acidic). So, in this regard, it doesn't make much difference what the original pH is; all food ends up being acidic as it leaves the stomach. Even that giant pile of vegetables you consume would test at about a 2.0 (or less) as it leaves the stomach (assuming a healthy gut). So, it should be clear that the original pH of the food is not significant. One would think that this would doom our chances of alkalizing the tumor micro-environment. However, what is important is how much ability the food has to "buffer" acidity after it leaves the stomach. This may sound confusing at this point, but please read on.

First, let's cover a little of the evidence that changing the pH around the tumor is beneficial (that is what is important; otherwise, we wouldn't need to cover this topic). The following study was undertaken by the Arizona Cancer Center at the University of Arizona and the H. Lee Moffitt Cancer Center and Research Institute in Tampa, Florida. They tested sodium bicarbonate's ability to change the pH of the tumor's micro-environment. The sodium bicarbonate oral dose used was equivalent to 12.5 grams per day for a 70 kg (154 lb) person, which works out to about 3 tsp per day. They found that the sodium bicarbonate had little effect on the blood pH and no effect on the primary tumor (this doesn't sound promising). But they did find that this sodium bicarbonate protocol significantly slowed metastasis for some cancers (that sounds more like what we want).

> "Acid pH has been shown to stimulate tumor cell invasion and metastasis in vitro and in cells before tail vein injection in vivo (in mice)… **oral NaHCO3 (Sodium bicarbonate) selectively increased the pH of tumors and reduced the formation of spontaneous metastases** in mouse models of metastatic breast cancer… In tail vein injections of alternative cancer models, bicarbonate had mixed results, inhibiting the formation of metastases from PC3M prostate cancer cells, but not those of B16 melanoma… Despite a lack of an effect on primary tumor growth, bicarbonate therapy led to significant reductions in the number and size of metastases to lung, intestine, and diaphragm… oral bicarbonate therapy significantly reduced the incidence of metastases in experimental models of breast and prostate cancer" – PubMed ID#PMC2834485 (2009) [774]

It usually isn't the original tumor that kills people; it is the metastasis (spreading) to vital organs. Any improved ability to prevent this is welcome.

To briefly review Chapter 2, one of the limitations of immunotherapy is what happens after tumor cells have been exposed to the immune system (by the therapy). Many of the immunotherapies work by basically uncloaking tumor cells, making them visible to the immune system. The immunotherapy drugs do not actually kill tumor cells; that will be the job of your immune system. But once the tumor cells are visible, the immune system still needs to be able to mount an effective offense against the tumor cells. One of the findings in the following research is that the acidic pH environment around a tumor blocks T cell activation. Thus, the acidity also plays a part in immune suppression. According to this research and others, sodium bicarbonate taken orally does not raise systemic pH, while it does buffer (help raise) the pH just around tumors. Blocking T cells would be a big problem whether a person was using immunotherapy or not, as T cells are an important part of our immune system's ability to fight cancer. So, even if you are not on immunotherapy, this is very important. In this study, bicarbonate treatment was used as adjuvant therapy to CTLA4 and PD1 inhibitors. They found bicarbonate beneficial even for melanomas that were resistant to bicarbonate alone (the bicarbonate still improved the immunotherapy).

> "Neutralization of tumor acidity improves anti-tumor responses to immunotherapies… An acidic pH environment blocked T cell activation and limited glycolysis… neutralizing tumor acidity with bicarbonate monotherapy impaired the growth of some cancer types in mice where it was associated with increased T cell infiltration… our findings show how **raising intratumoral pH through oral buffers therapy can improve responses to immunotherapy**… These results were consistent with prior work in animal models where oral buffers that raise tumor pH were shown to inhibit spontaneous and experimental

metastases… **We observed that combinations of bicarb therapy with anti-CTLA4 or anti-PD1 antibodies significantly improved the anti-tumor effects of these therapies in the B16 melanoma model that was resistant to bicarb alone**… Low pH in the tumor microenvironment works as a "global protection shield" for tumor cells." – PubMed ID#PMC4829106 (2015) [775]

The following research out of Italy looked at cancer cells' ability to avoid the immune system through what are known as "escape pathways." Though several of these pathways exist, they're finding that many are linked to an acidic tumor microenvironment (TME). When the environment around the tumor becomes acidic (as explained above), this negatively impacts various aspects of the immune response. The tumor can then take advantage of these weaknesses to hide from the immune system, or avoid, the immune response. The acidity may also harm the immune cells responding to the cancer, such as T cells, NK (natural killer) cells and antigen-presenting cells. Without a strong immune response, and having the ability to hide from the immune system, cancer cells are much more likely to proliferate. Being able to selectively control, or normalize, the acidity of the TME is thus very beneficial.

"microenvironmental acidity may differentially impact on diverse components of tumor immune surveillance, eventually contributing to immune escape and cancer progression… antitumor effectors such as T and NK cells tend to lose their function and undergo a state of mostly reversible anergy followed by apoptosis, when exposed to low pH environment… Local acidity could also profoundly influence bioactivity and distribution of antibodies, thus potentially interfering with the clinical efficacy of therapeutic antibodies including immune checkpoint inhibitors… tumor acidity acts as a broad immune escape mechanism by which cancer cells, simultaneously wipe out the activity of all antitumor immune effectors (including T cells, NK cells and crucial antigen-presenting cells such as dendritic cells), at the same time favoring the accrual and conversion of regulatory T cells and myeloid cells into immunosuppressive and protumor cells." – ScienceDirect DOI:10.1016/j.semcancer.2017.03.001 (2017) [776]

The following study on mice found that oral dosing of sodium bicarbonate could reduce circulating tumor cells (and thus metastasis).

"Sodium Bicarbonate-Treated Mice Exhibit Lower Circulating Tumor Cells (CTCs)… The frequency of CTC in blood of mice treated with sodium bicarbonate drinking water was significantly less than half of that of untreated mice… Overall, the findings suggest that alkalinization may inhibit tumor invasion from the primary site in part by suppressing the activity of invasion enzymes" – PubMed ID#PMC3722989 (2013) [777]

In vivo testing with mice (using human breast cancers) showed that the pH around breast cancer tumors could be raised by drinking sodium bicarbonate in water. They showed that this could improve the effectiveness of chemotherapy treatment.

> "Furthermore 31P-magnetic resonance spectroscopy (MRS) has shown that the pHe of MCF-7 human breast cancer xenografts can be effectively and significantly raised with sodium bicarbonate in drinking water. The bicarbonate-induced extracellular alkalinization leads to significant improvements in the therapeutic effectiveness of doxorubicin against MCF-7 xenografts in vivo." – PubMed ID#10362108 (1999) [778]

Not all cancers are sensitive to pH manipulation of the tumor microenvironment. Melanoma, lung and colon cancers do not seem to be sensitive to raising the pH levels around the tumor, whereas breast and prostate cancers are (however, other studies showed that these cancers are sensitive to pH increases when combined with immunotherapy drugs; see above).

> "metastasis is not inhibited by buffers in some tumor models, regardless of buffer used. B16-F10 (murine melanoma), LL/2 (murine lung) and HCT116 (human colon) tumors are resistant to treatment with lysine buffer therapy, whereas metastasis is potently inhibited by lysine buffers in MDA-MB-231 (human breast) and PC3M (human prostate) tumors." – PubMed ID#PMC4094835 (2014) [779]

Here they found that perhaps up to 90% of cancer tumors may benefit from buffer therapy. Again, the primary benefit is that of inhibiting metastasis and halting tumor progression.

> "we demonstrated that an acidic microenvironment is critical for carcinogenesis and tumor invasion... systemic buffers reduce intra- and peri-tumoral acidity, inhibit carcinogenesis in transgenic mice, and inhibit metastatic growth in a wide range of cell lines in-vivo... Our data shows that buffer therapy is an effective method of halting tumor progression and metastasis formation... FDG-PET imaging is used to diagnose up to 90% of primary tumors, indicating that the vast majority of patients have glycolytic tumors that may benefit from treatment with buffer therapy" – PubMed ID#PMC4094835 (2014) [780]

There is increasing evidence that raising the pH of the tumor's microenvironment can improve the response rate to modern immunotherapy, such as anti-PD-1 drugs (including Keytruda and Opdivo).

> "The role of the acidic environment in cancer is a serious drawback for natural and induced immunotherapy, and neutralizing this acidity improved immunological defenses in an experimental in vivo setting… the combination of bicarbonate with anti-PD-1 drugs or anti-CTLA-4 drugs improved antitumor responses." – PubMed ID#PMC5074768 (2016) [781]

Obviously, it is important that the body has proper supplies of buffering minerals. This will be discussed below. The acidic environment around a tumor can also be harmful to normal cells, and buffering that acidity may still be beneficial.

Buffer Therapy

Now that we see how important it is to buffer the acidity around tumors, we need to figure out what can be done about it. This mostly involves food and natural substances (which are non-patentable), so there isn't a lot of research in this regard. But there is some, and we're going to go over it here. In keeping with the whole *"Improving Your Odds"* concept, I don't think it is necessary to outline an exact meal-by-meal protocol. Once you read this, you should be able to make tweaks to your normal diet to greatly improve your body's ability to buffer (or alkalize) the acidity around tumors. Again, buffer therapy is not the same thing as the common "alkalizing" protocols that you see on the internet (and those will not work for this).

The following study first looks at what research is available for "Buffer Therapy" and "Dietary Buffer Capacity" (DBC). DBC, in this context, is the property that allows a food or nutrient to acidify or alkalize after it has been digested. The ability to buffer acids in the body is far more important than the original pH of the food, as pH can change considerably during digestion.

> "The most important factor when considering food as adjuvant to pH buffering therapy is not only the initial pH of the foods, but their buffering capacities, i.e. the amount of hydrogen ions consumed to reduce the pH to physiological levels in the GI tract. In addition, subjects on buffer therapy should not consume foods that would counteract the buffer and inhibit therapy." (see attribution below)

The evidence shows that oral administration of alkalizing pH buffers (such as sodium bicarbonate, magnesium, calcium and potassium) can significantly reduce metastases in animal models (in vivo). They believe that this is due to interfering with acidification of the "extracellular matrix and the stromal cell population" (the extracellular matrix helps cancer cells bind together and regulates a number of cellular functions, such as adhesion, migration, proliferation and differentiation). This benefit did not extend to retarding, or reducing, the growth of the primary tumor—it only helped with metastatic cells. But as we know, it is often metastasis that kills people, not the primary tumor. The study goes on to determine that this buffering effect can, at least partially, be achieved through diet alone. This is fortunate as the amount of sodium bicarbonate that must be consumed, and its unpleasant taste, make treatment compliance difficult (people quit taking it). It is also believed that consuming large amounts of sodium bicarbonate can lower the pH of the stomach, which can have a negative impact on digestion and mineral absorption (some minerals in and of themselves are alkalizing buffers, so we don't really want to block their absorption by negatively affecting stomach acid). The good news is that therapeutic levels of sodium bicarbonate have very little negative effect on blood (or systemic) pH (we do not want to mess with that). If changes in the diet can reduce the amount of sodium bicarbonate needed for a therapeutic effect, this might make buffering therapy a viable adjuvant treatment option.

> "Prior to further absorption in the GI tract, the pH of food is restored to ~4.0 at the distal part of the duodenum by secretion of bicarbonate, and the difference between the initial food pH and 4.0 would thus result in a surplus or deficit of bicarbonate anions from the body due to food digestion. The second mechanism consists in the production of acidic or alkaline byproducts from the metabolism of nutrients… **The most important factor when considering food as adjuvant to pH buffering therapy is not only the initial pH of the foods, but their buffering capacities**, i.e. the amount of hydrogen ions consumed to reduce the pH to physiological levels in the GI tract… subjects on buffer therapy should not consume foods that would counteract the buffer and inhibit therapy… while the blood pH in the subjects is unaffected, the bicarbonate concentration in blood and urine pH were significantly lowered… We have evaluated the pH buffering score of various foods to estimate their effect in the whole-body pH buffering system… Our results show that the order of magnitude of **the pH buffering score of a diet containing protein-rich foodstuff such as meats and dairy products is the same as that of the amount of sodium bicarbonate given to cancer patients** in the two clinical trials… For instance, the replacement of 3 servings of carbonated cola by 3 glasses of milk, and an additional 3 servings of meat would increase a person's pH buffering score by $3\times(20 + 3) + 3\times(50 - 5) = 204$ mEq of H+, which is equivalent to approximately 20g of sodium bicarb." – PubMed ID#PMC3872072 (2012) [782]

The following citation applies to the above study and the table below.

Citation: Ribeiro MdLC, Silva AS, Bailey KM, Kumar NB, Sellers TA, et al. (2012) Buffer Therapy for Cancer. Journal of Nutrition and Food Sciences S2:006. DOI: 10.4172/2155-9600.S2-006 [783]

In this study, researchers developed a system for measuring the "buffering capacity" of various foods. This "buffer score" is based on both in vitro and in vivo (in the body) testing. This score is a much more important number than the basic pH of the food. The buffer score indicates how well the food (after digestion and buffering by the small intestine) will be able to buffer acidity in the body (including, and especially, the environment around tumors). This buffering system is based on in vivo (in the body) measurements and shows just how much alkalizing potential a serving of food really has. What they found was very surprising and should change the way we think about using food to "alkalize." On their scale, the higher the (positive) number, the more alkalizing/buffering potential it has, and thus the more ability it has to prevent cancer metastasis. Subsequent research showed that therapeutic benefits of buffer therapy begin at about 50 points. The following is a partial list of foods and their buffering potential. See the full study (link in the citation) for a longer list of foods and their buffering capacities.

- Orange/apple/peach, 1 whole fruit, +0
- Grapes, 1 ounce serving +0
- Tomatoes, 1 Italian, +1.5
- Green beans, ½ cup, +2.0
- Regular coffee, 8 fl oz, +2.4
- Kidney beans, ½ cup, +3.0
- Brussels sprouts, ½ cup, +3.0
- White rice, ½ cup, +4.0
- Cantaloupe, 1 cup cubed, +5.0
- Oatmeal, 1 cup, +5.5
- Eggs, 1 whole, +6.0
- Chicken breast, 5 oz, +15.0
- Low-fat milk, 8 oz, +19
- Hamburger patty (fatty, probably 80/20), 1 patty, +52
- 1 gram of sodium bicarbonate, +11 (1 tsp = 4 grams = +44 points)

Some foods can subtract from the buffering potential (reducing the body's ability to buffer acids); you will want to avoid these when possible.

- White wine, 5 fl oz, -4.5
- Caffeine-free cola, 12 fl oz, -3.0
- Apple juice, 1 cup, -2.5
- Red wine, 5 fl oz, -1.5
- Caffeine-free and sugar-free cola, 12 fl oz, -1.5 (this probably applies to any sugar-free carbonated beverage)

As you can see above, when it comes to preventing metastasis (one of the most dangerous aspects of cancer), meat—and especially fatty meat—has more alkalizing (or buffering) potential than any fruit or vegetable (per serving). One hamburger patty (+52) is equal to nearly 5 grams of sodium bicarbonate! I know which one I would rather consume!

> "The fruits and vegetables group showed the lowest pH buffering score, while the meats group showed the highest buffering score." -- PubMed ID#PMC3872072 (citation above)

This does not mean that hamburger is overall better for you than vegetables. But if your goal is to alkalize the environment around tumors and help prevent metastasis, research shows that fatty meat is a better option that either fruit or vegetables. I would certainly want to consume high-quality meat (grass-fed, organic) as well as continue to consume lots of vegetables (for the other benefits found throughout this book). None of the vegetables had negative buffering numbers, so they will not make the pH around the tumor worse. You certainly want to avoid carbonated drinks, fruit juices, sugar (of any kind, including "natural") and alcohol (as all of these have negative buffering numbers, meaning that they acidify even after digestion). At a very minimum, make sure you consume these in moderation and offset their negative buffering score with something with a much higher value. You should not use this as an excuse to eat an unhealthy diet, especially if you continue to consume any foods with a negative buffering score. As the following quote indicates, a ketogenic diet (high fat, moderate protein) works well in this regard, as most of the foods will have a high buffering potential. Chargrilling food, especially to the point of any black sear, causes the meat to lose buffering potential, and it also creates carcinogens.

> "These results suggest that a highly buffered, high-protein diet prepared at a high pH can increase the systemic buffering system and potentially delay metastases." -- PubMed ID#PMC3872072 (citation and endnote link above)

The study below builds on the one discussed above and gives the buffering potential of more foods. Their point system differs from that above, with 1 gram of sodium bicarbonate equaling 1 point (rather than 11 points in the study above). They too found buffer therapy significantly inhibited metastasis and improved patients' response to checkpoint immunotherapy.

> "Thus, in a therapeutic setting, 11 g of bicarbonate can be eliminated for every 100 g of protein ingested… Tumor acidity can be neutralized with oral buffers, reversing some of the sequelae of acidity, including local invasion, metastasis, and immune inhibition. For example, 200 mM ad lib sodium bicarbonate has been shown to neutralize tumor acidity, and inhibit in vivo invasion as well as spontaneous and experimental metastasis in a variety of systems and to improve response to checkpoint blockade immune therapy… if buffer therapy was initiated after the emergence of spontaneous cancers in this system, metastasis was significantly inhibited… treatment of cancers with buffers, such as sodium bicarbonate (bicarb) is strong evidence in favor of clinical translation. Based on data from mice, and inter-species PK conversion, the target dose in humans would be 0.7 g/kg/d, or about 50 g/d for a 70 kg human. In prior therapeutic trials, 21 grams per day (0.4 g/kg) were administered orally to children with Sickle Cell Anemia for one year without complication. Complications from sodium bicarbonate administration are rare in the dose ranges proposed."

Citation: Pilot C, Mahipal A, Gillies RJ (2018) Buffer Therapy → Buffer Diet. J Nutr Food Sci 8: 685. DOI: 10.4172/2155-9600.1000685 [784]

Though not discussed at length in the studies above, the dietary minerals magnesium, potassium and calcium have very high buffering potential.

> "The current investigation demonstrated a significant increase in RAST performance of elite soccer players supplemented with sodium and potassium bicarbonate along with calcium phosphate, potassium citrate, and magnesium citrate ingested twice a day over a nine-day training period. The improvements in anaerobic performance were caused by increased resting blood pH and bicarbonate levels." – PubMed ID#PMC6266022 (2018) [785]

So, be sure to eat foods high in these minerals and take a mineral supplement. If you enjoy organ meats, they will be much higher in minerals than ground beef. Something we do from time to time is mix about 20% ground beef liver in with our ground meat. It is barely noticeable and gives it those added minerals. The amino acid l-lysine has been shown to decrease metastasis; this is thought to be due to its strong buffering ability.

Recommendations

It is important to reiterate that eating a diet high in foods with excess buffering capacity is not the same thing as the popular "alkalizing diet," where the goal is simply to eat foods with a high pH. Foods with a high pH but low buffering potential, or the disproven "ash" theory (where acidic foods, like lemons, are said to become an alkaline ash), will not increase the pH around a cancer tumor. However, foods with a high buffering potential will—and this is what we want; we want the environment around the tumor to be made selectively less acidic, and this is done through buffering.

I recommend not getting too wrapped up in all the numbers above. There are a lot of factors that go into this, and there has not been as much research as would be needed for a true point system protocol. I think the best strategy is simply to try to consume foods with a high buffering capacity and avoid those with negative numbers (as discussed above). Foods high in the minerals calcium, magnesium and potassium provide even more acid buffering.

Protein, including animal protein, is not the problem certain vegan websites would have you believe. As discussed in Chapter 4, the main problem with a high-protein diet is that it can leave no room for vegetables, which have plenty of health benefits not related to alkalizing or buffering. So, eat your low-sugar fruit and your healthy vegetables, but do not avoid proteins. If you ate animal protein before you got cancer, you can continue to do so. Dairy also has a very high buffering capacity, but care should be taken if you are the least bit lactose intolerant. Cheeses are a good choice here, especially hard cheeses, as they have a high buffering capacity (+18 to +25) while having very little lactose. Also see the Dairy section at the end of Chapter 4. Organic is always best, especially when it comes to dairy.

Though this is separate from the pH/buffering discussion, when consuming cooked animal protein, it should not be charred on the outside. In fact, grilling meat has been found to contribute to cancer risk. This method of cooking does decrease its buffering capacity and may even push it into negative numbers. Meats should be baked, pressure cooked, sous-vide cooked, or cooked in liquid (e.g., soups and stews). Charring vegetables is also not a good idea. Personally, I still grill meat from time to time, but I try to avoid over-charring and trim off any burnt pieces.

Sodium Bicarbonate – Before adding sodium bicarbonate to your regimen, you should consult your oncologist. This is relatively new research, and because there is very little funding for dietary cancer interventions, there just aren't a lot of practical implementation strategies. The tips above are a good start. But if you feel that you need additional buffering, taking a teaspoon of sodium bicarbonate (baking soda) mixed in a glass of water (or low-sugar smoothie) can give that to you. Always take sodium bicarbonate at least an hour away from meals. Sodium bicarbonate can neutralize stomach acid (HCl), and you do want this acid when digesting a meal; you want your food, especially proteins, to be fully digested. One teaspoon of sodium bicarbonate equals 4 grams, or +44 points of buffering capacity. This can be taken up to 3 times per day—again, away from meals. If you plan to do this, please read these online precautions. [786]

Sodium bicarbonate does contain sodium, but you may not be able to take it if you are on a salt-restricted diet. One tsp of sodium bicarbonate (baking soda) contains 1.2 grams of sodium. Many health guidelines tell people with hypertension to consume no more than 5 grams of sodium per day from all sources. Recent research shows that people with normal blood pressure do not need to restrict dietary sodium (though sodium poisoning is possible at higher levels, e.g., >50 grams per day).

For the first week or two, you'll find the taste of sodium bicarbonate is not very pleasant; this gets better with time, but it is still not great. I suggest that you simply chug it; sipping will just extend the agony. Drinking more water afterwards does help get rid of the taste.

> *Taking sodium bicarbonate is something that I started doing late in my treatment protocol but stopped once I was declared cancer-free. I will still take ½ to 1 tsp if I've been consuming foods (drinks) with a negative buffering potential (which I still try to avoid).*

❖ COLOSTRUM/LACTOFERRIN

Colostrum is the first milk a new mammal mother makes for her offspring. It is full of health benefits for the newborn. Some of these benefits include immune factors, growth and tissue repair factors, antibody factors, lactoferrin (antimicrobial and immune system benefits), leukocytes, nutrients, etc. Bovine colostrum and lactoferrin are also sold as supplements and tout immune system and disease prevention benefits.

Improving the immune system, without forcing it into overdrive, is almost always beneficial. Strengthening the functionality and potential of the immune system is especially beneficial during immunotherapy.

The following study compares colostrum to the flu vaccination and found that colostrum can be more effective in fighting the flu (this does not mean you should avoid the flu shot; that is a totally different subject). The two together are even more potent. This goes to show how much colostrum can help the immune system do its job.

> "Vaccinations have generally produced a striking improvement in public health, reducing mortality and morbidity through an improvement in specific immunity… The efficacy of flu vaccination and its cost effectiveness is probably questionable… In many instances, flu starts from the intestinal tract, and protection in situ may be one of the advantages given by colostrum… We conclude from our observations that colostrum appears to offer a more effective protection." — PubMed #17456621

Liposomal lactoferrin (from colostrum) is a form that improves the delivery to where it is needed. Here the study showed that liposomal lactoferrin helped to inhibit tumor cells, activate natural killer (NK) cells and improve apoptosis.

> "Liposomalization of lactoferrin enhanced its anti-tumoral effects on melanoma cells… A number of studies have reported the anti-tumoral activity of lactoferrin, a property mediated by a variety of mechanisms such as inhibitory effects on tumor cell growth, NK cell activation, and enhancement of apoptosis." – PubMed ID#20191307 (2010) [787]

Native monomeric bovine lactoferrin (NM-bLf, the most common form of lactoferrin supplements) was shown to increase apoptosis and decrease the proliferation of some breast cancer lines, with similar effects seen in melanoma tumors (in vivo), lymphoma and Lewis lung cancer.

> "it has been shown that NM-bLf decreased the viability of breast cancer cell lines HS578T and T47D by inducing a 2-fold increase in apoptosis, and decreased the proliferation rates as well in both the cell lines. A similar effect of bLf was seen on colon carcinoma and in vivo on tumors of melanoma, EL-4 T-cell thymic lymphoma and Lewis lung cancer cells" – PubMed ID#PMC4164354 (2014) [788]

Recommendation

Improving the immune system is something that can be very beneficial in fighting cancer, especially if you are on immunotherapy. As with everything in this book, it is best to discuss this with your oncologist. If you are taking part in a medical trial (study), they will most likely not allow you to take any supplements, as this will throw off the results.

Colostrum contains some lactoferrin and has additional immuno-benefits not seen in lactoferrin. For this reason, I advise sticking to colostrum supplements. I'm taking 500 mg twice per day (35% immunoglobulins). A liposomal form is best, though it is also more expensive.

❖ D-LIMONENE

D-limonene is a common terpene found in several citrus fruits. As its name implies, it is found in lemons, but also limes, oranges, grapefruit and tangerines. It is commonly used to flavor foods, chewing gum and beverages. It has also been used for symptom relief from acid reflux and GERD. There is some evidence that it has benefits for preventing certain cancers and possibly reducing metastasis. Most studies in this regard have been in vitro or in vivo mouse models, with the most promising benefits seen with lung and melanoma cancers.

> "d-limonene is a plant extract with widespread application, and it has been recently reported to have antiproliferative and proapoptotic effects on cancer cells… d-limonene inhibited the growth of lung cancer cells and suppressed the growth of transplanted tumors in nude mice. Expression of apoptosis and autophagy-related genes were increased in tumors after treatment with d-limonene… Cell growth in A549 and H1299 cells was inhibited in a dose-and time-dependent manner after treatment with d-limonene when compared to the control cells… Moreover, d-limonene inhibits the proliferation and clone formation of the other three lung cancer cell lines H1975, H520, and PC9. Taken together, these data indicate that d-limonene inhibits the proliferation of lung cancer cells." – PubMed ID#PMC5894671 (2018) [789]

> "The effects of naturally occurring monoterpenes on lung metastasis induced by B16F-10 melanoma cells were studied in C57BL/6 mice. Administration of monoterpenes such as limonene (100 micromoles/kg body wt. 10 doses i.p.) and perillic acid (50 micromoles/kg body wt 10 doses i.p.) remarkably reduced the metastatic tumour nodule formation by 65% and 67%, respectively." – PubMed ID#18072821 (2007) [790]

After consumption, D-limonene is found at much higher concentrations in body fat, adipose, than in the blood. Therefore, it is most likely to have cancer-preventative potential in cancers such as breast cancer and melanoma.

"Our data suggests that d-limonene may accumulate in the breast, given the high adiposity of breast tissue. Further research is needed to determine the effects of d-limonene on the expression and secretion of adipose-derived cytokines and hormones and its effects in breast tissue and thus its potential as a cancer preventive agent." – PubMed ID#PMC6262896 (2010) [791]

Any cancer-preventative potential seems likely to be limited to breast cancer and melanoma. However, research is limited. Consuming more lemons and low-sugar lemonade can't hurt.

❖ DMSO

DMSO was researched and not included in this book due to concerns regarding toxicity. Use in animals has been linked to changes in the lens of the eye. The fear is this might happen with humans as well. There is limited research showing the safety and effectiveness of DMSO.

❖ Ginkgo biloba

There are a few studies showing that *Ginkgo biloba* has some chemopreventive and therapeutic effects; they seem to be limited to very specific types of cancer and certain situations. This is not the type of adjuvant treatment I would recommend, in large part due to research that shows that *Ginkgo biloba* can also increase the risks of certain cancers and worsen metastasis. For this reason, I would not recommend *Ginkgo biloba* for cancer unless advised to use it by your oncologist.

"EGb (extract of Ginkgo biloba) significantly increased the rate of metastasis in mouse liver and decreased the number of necrotic and apoptotic cells in the metastatic liver when compared to the control. Meanwhile, EGb **significantly induced proliferation of tumor cells** in the metastatic liver" – PubMed ID#PMC5712166 (2017) [792]

"A total of 3069 GEM (Ginkgo Evaluation of Memory research study) participants 75+ years of age were randomized to twice-daily doses of either 120 mg Ginkgo extract (EGb 761) or placebo and followed for a median 6.1 years. We identified hospitalizations for invasive cancer by reviewing hospital admission and discharge records for all reported hospitalizations over follow-up… Overall, these **results do not support the hypothesis that regular use of Ginkgo biloba reduces the risk of cancer**." – PubMed ID#20582906 (2010) [793]

> "Two companion studies were conducted to explore possible mechanisms of
> carcinogenicity of GBE using mouse liver tissue from these two year studies… In
> the hepatocellular carcinoma study, Hoenerhoff et al., observed dose-related
> mutations in β-catenin (Ctnnb1) genes in GBE-treated carcinomas, while
> mutations occurred predominantly in H-ras genes in the control group
> carcinomas. These mutations are common events in both human and mouse
> hepatocarcinogenesis (Ctnnb1)" – PubMed ID#PMC3929544 (2014) [794]

❖ I N D O L E - 3 - C A R B I N O L

I3C is derived from the breakdown of a compound in cruciferous vegetables called
glucobrassicin. Though there are numerous studies showing an inverse relationship between
cancer and consuming cruciferous vegetables (such as cauliflower, broccoli, Brussels sprouts,
cabbage, kale and bok choy), there are few studies on I3C.

Several studies show benefits of supplemental I3C in the prevention and treatment of various
cancers. However, due to some in vivo animal studies showing that it can worsen some cancers
under certain circumstances, I would not recommend taking this supplement unless advised to
do so by your oncologist.

> "many studies showed that I3C suppresses the proliferation of various cancer cell
> lines, including breast, colon, prostate, and endometrial cancer cells. One example
> of its anti-proliferative properties comes from a study conducted on non-
> tumorigenic and tumorigenic breast epithelial cells… In vivo studies showed that
> I3C inhibits the development of different cancers in several animals when given
> before or in parallel to a carcinogen. However, **when I3C was given to the
> animals after the carcinogen, I3C promoted carcinogenesis**. This concern
> regarding the long-term effects of I3C treatment on cancer risk in humans
> resulted in some caution in the use of I3C as a dietary supplement in cancer
> management protocols" – PubMed ID#PMC5989150 (2018) [795]

Katz, E., Nisani, S., & Chamovitz, D. A. (2018). Indole-3-carbinol: a plant hormone combatting
cancer. F1000Research, 7, F1000 Faculty Rev-689. doi:10.12688/f1000research.14127.1

❖ M A N N O S E

Mannose is a simple sugar similar to glucose. It has been used for years in the treatment of urinary
tract infections (UTIs) and has been found to be safe when used by otherwise healthy people. It
is also showing some benefits in the treatment of cancer. Cancer cells have 10 to 17 times the
intake of glucose compared to normal cells. Mannose is brought into cells in the same way

glucose is utilized. While mannose seems to have no impact on normal cells, it appears to interfere with the cancer cell's ability to utilize glucose.

The full study for the following research showed that mannose appeared to interfere with the way cancer cells break down glucose. This significantly slowed their growth. They tested this with colorectal, skin cancer, lung cancer and pancreatic cancer cells. The supplements were given to mice 3 times per week. They also found that mannose significantly improved the efficacy of chemotherapy treatment. Mice treated with doxorubicin (a chemotherapy drug) plus mannose had a significantly increased life expectancy when compared to untreated mice or those treated with either doxorubicin or mannose alone. Mannose induced growth inhibition in tumor cells but not cell death.

"mannose causes growth retardation in several tumour types in vitro, and enhances cell death in response to major forms of chemotherapy… these effects also occur in vivo in mice following the oral administration of mannose… mannose is taken up by the same transporter(s) as glucose3 but accumulates as mannose-6-phosphate in cells, and this impairs the further metabolism of glucose in glycolysis… We consider that the administration of mannose could be a simple, safe and selective therapy in the treatment of cancer, and could be applicable to multiple tumour types." – PubMed ID#30464341 (2018) [796]

Recommendation

This is very new research, and mannose hasn't been tested with all cancers. From the research, it is clear that mannose may have some benefits against skin, lung and pancreatic cancers (in vitro and in vivo mouse experiments). However, it seems to have little or no benefit against ovarian cancer and leukemia. Because research is limited, this is something I would not give a strong recommendation to. Mannose supplementation doesn't seem to hurt anything; therefore, it is something you can add if you are following the other recommendations in the book and find yourself not taking enough supplements.

It appears that when translating the doses given to mice, it works out to about 8 grams, 3 times per week for humans. This dose may be too high to take long term until further testing is done on humans.

❖ MELATONIN

Melatonin is a hormone created by the pineal gland in humans; it is best known for regulating sleep and wakefulness. This hormone is found in many animals, not just humans, and serves some of the same purposes. In animals it is also used for a variety of other timing functions, such as seasonal reproduction and hibernation. Although melatonin is primarily produced by the pineal gland, it is also produced by the gut, retina, skin and leukocytes. Lucky for us, melatonin is also found in many foods, such as cherries, corn, broccoli, rice and barley. Melatonin is also available as a nutritional supplement.

There are many high-quality studies on melatonin. Not only can it be used as adjuvant treatment, but it has shown benefits of its own in treating cancer (e.g., apoptosis, slowing metastasis, etc.) The following paper takes an in-depth look at the dozens of research studies of melatonin and its effect on cancer. These studies have shown that melatonin can help fight cancer by several different mechanisms, including: stimulation of apoptosis (programmed cell death that triggers cancer cells to kill themselves), inhibits tumor induced angiogenesis (cutting off new blood vessels to cancer cells), helping to prevent metastasis (stopping cancer from spreading), etc.

> "Melatonin could be an excellent candidate for the prevention and treatment of several cancers, such as breast cancer, prostate cancer, gastric cancer and colorectal cancer… melatonin could exert growth inhibition on some human tumor cells in vitro and in animal models. The underlying mechanisms include antioxidant activity, modulation of melatonin receptors MT1 and MT2, stimulation of apoptosis, regulation of pro-survival signaling and tumor metabolism, inhibition on angiogenesis, metastasis, and induction of epigenetic alteration. Melatonin could also be utilized as adjuvant of cancer therapies, through reinforcing the therapeutic effects and reducing the side effects of chemotherapies or radiation." – PubMed ID#PMC5503661 (2017, Creative Commons attribution available at the link) [797]

The Nurses' Health Study is one of the largest prospective studies of risk factors for major disease in women. The original study started in 1976 and continues to this day with over 275,000 women participating. The study below looked at 18,643 cancer-free women from this study and followed them over time. What they found was a strong inverse relationship between melatonin levels and breast cancer; those with the highest levels of melatonin (over time) had the lowest risk of developing breast cancer.

> "We conducted a nested case-control study in the Nurses' Health Study cohort. First spot morning urine was collected from 18,643 cancer-free women… An increased concentration of urinary aMT6s [a melatonin metabolite] was statistically significantly associated with a lower risk of breast cancer… Results from this prospective study add substantially to the growing literature that supports an inverse association between melatonin levels and breast cancer risk."
> – PubMed ID#19124483 (2009) [798]

I think the key here was that a lack of melatonin resulted in increased cancer proliferation, and tumor growth rates were negatively correlated with melatonin levels.

> "studies showcasing absence or lack of melatonin exhibit an increased proliferative cellular state. Conversely, administration of melatonin inhibits tumor growth in melanoma cells. Associations between tumor progression and decreased levels of melatonin have been established… tumor growth rates were negatively correlated with melatonin concentrations in the different exposure groups in a dose-response fashion… The circadian control of melatonin and, in particular, DNA repair mechanisms provides more robust evidence for supporting the link between circadian dysrhythmia and skin cancer development."
> -- Int. J. Mol. Sci. 2016, 17(5), 621; doi:10.3390/ijms17050621 [799]

This paper looked at several research studies and found that melatonin used as adjuvant therapy (i.e., alongside traditional therapies) was very effective. This was especially true in breast cancer and malignant melanoma.

> "in breast cancer melatonin appears to be useful as adjuvant in the therapy of this malignancy. We have also performed initial testing of melatonin in the C1-4 squamous cell carcinoma line of cervical origin and found inhibition of cell viability by increasing concentrations… Several clinical studies have reported positive results with melatonin in patients with metastatic malignant melanoma… an overall response rate of 30%… In a clinical study of 13 patients with metastatic malignant melanoma, melatonin was used in combination with cisplatin and IL-2 as a second-line therapy after failure of the first-line therapy with dacarbazine and interferon alpha. The objective tumor response-rate (CR + PR) was 31% with stable disease occurring in five patients." – PubMed ID#PMC1317110 (2005) [800]

> "melatonin acts as an anti-inflammatory and reactive oxygen species inducer agent which suppresses the growth of tumors. It also has apoptosis induction characteristics… Thus, adding melatonin to chemo- and radiotherapy may have synergistic therapeutic effects and increase the survival time in patients with skin cancer." – PubMed ID#30618091 (2019) [801]

Melatonin has been shown to significantly suppress the toxicity of chemotherapy drugs to normal cells and to increase their anticancer cytotoxicity. This again shows that melatonin may be very beneficial as adjuvant therapy when the patient is also undergoing traditional treatments such as chemotherapy and radiation therapy.

> "melatonin has been shown to reduce the toxicity and increase the efficacy of a large number of drugs whose side effects are well documented. Herein, we summarize the beneficial effects of melatonin when combined with the following drugs: doxorubicin, cisplatin, epirubicin, cytarabine, bleomycin, gentamicin, ciclosporin, indometacin, acetylsalicylic acid, ranitidine, omeprazole, isoniazid, iron and erythropoietin, phenobarbital, carbamazepine, haloperidol, caposide-50, morphine, cyclophosphamide and L-cysteine… Considering the low toxicity of melatonin and its ability to reduce the side effects and increase the efficacy of these drugs, its use as a combination therapy with these agents seems important and worthy of pursuit." – PubMed ID#12396291 (2002) [802]

Melatonin was found to directly inhibit melanoma in vitro.

> "The effects of melatonin on the growth of two highly tumorigenic rodent melanoma cells were studied in vitro. PG19, an amelanotic mouse melanoma cell line, and B16BL6, a melanotic melanoma cell line selected for its invasive potential… These results support the hypothesis that, at physiological concentrations, melatonin exerts a direct inhibitory effect on PG19 and B16BL6 cells proliferation." – PubMed ID#11333131 (2001) [803]

Melatonin has been shown to be "pro-apoptotic," meaning that it triggers defective (cancer) cells to kill themselves (as cells normally do when they become damaged or grow old). Cancer cells usually turn off this process, which is one of the mechanisms that allows them to grow in spite of the immune system.

> "Melatonin plays different physiological functions ranging from the regulation of circadian rhythms to tumor inhibition, owing to its antioxidant, immunomodulatory and anti-aging properties. Due to its pleiotropic functions, melatonin has been shown to elicit cytoprotective processes in normal cells and trigger pro-apoptotic signals in cancer cells." – PubMed ID#28978121 (2017) [804]

> "Melatonin and its metabolites accumulate in the human epidermis in vivo and inhibit proliferation and tyrosinase activity in epidermal melanocytes in vitro… Testing of their phenotypic effects in normal human melanocytes show that melatonin and its metabolites (10(-5) M) inhibit tyrosinase activity and cell growth, and inhibit DNA synthesis in a dose dependent manner… In melanoma cells, they inhibited cell growth" – PubMed ID#25168391 (2015) [805]

"We demonstrated that melatonin treatment significantly inhibits S-91 melanoma cell proliferation in vitro (EC50 = 10-7 m) as well as reduces tumor growth in vivo. We also demonstrated that melatonin directly increases the activity of the antioxidant enzymes catalase and glutathione peroxidase… These results suggest that expression of the MT-1 melatonin receptor in melanoma cells is a potential alternative approach to specifically target cells in cancer therapeutic treatment." – PubMed ID#15009512 (2004) [806]

This review out of Tulane University School of Medicine does a very good job of covering most of the research available on melatonin and cancer. If you are researching this topic, you certainly want to read this paper; it has a wealth of information.

"Numerous studies have documented the oncostatic properties… in human breast tumor cell lines in vitro and in animal models including human breast tumor xenografts in athymic nude mice and nude rats, carcinogen-induced mammary tumors in rats, and genetically engineered models of breast cancer in mice… The broad action of melatonin on breast cancer including its inhibition of tumor metabolism, signaling, and genomic instability, its activity as a scavenger of ROS, synergism with other cancer therapeutic agents, lack of toxicity, and wide availability and minimal cost, should make its movement into clinical trials a high priority." – PubMed ID#PMC4457700 (2015) [807]

The following study from Emory University School of Medicine showed that "melatonin as an adjuvant therapy to (breast) cancer may lead to improvement in tumor remission and survival and may improve the side-effects of chemotherapy or radiotherapy."

"Melatonin counteracts tumor occurrence and tumor cell progression in vivo and in vitro in animal and human breast cancer cell cultures. It acts predominantly through its melatonin MT1 receptor… Melatonin also exerts anti-invasive and anti-metastatic effects through blockade of 38 phosphorylation and matrix metalloprotein expression… There was an enhanced anti-proliferation effect on these cells through a combination of valproic acid and melatonin… Randomized controlled trials of melatonin treatment, including breast cancer, have been evaluated in two meta-analyses of published reports [77, 78]. It was concluded that melatonin as an adjuvant therapy to cancer may lead to improvement in tumor remission and survival and may ameliorate the side-effects of chemotherapy or radiotherapy." – PubMed ID#PMC3552359 (2012) [808]

> "Melatonin (MLT) has been proven to counteract chemotherapy toxicity, by acting as an anti-oxidant agent, and to promote apoptosis of cancer cells, so enhancing chemotherapy cytotoxicity." – <u>PubMed ID#10674014</u> (1999) [809]

Recommendations

If your oncologist approves, I recommend taking 3 to 6 mg at bedtime (3 mg if you are considered underweight or sleep well, or if 3 mg improves your sleep). For me, the effects last about 8 to 8 ½ hours, so I generally take 3 mg about an hour before I go to bed. Do not take melatonin at any other time of the day, as it will throw off your circadian rhythms. Taking more is unlikely to exhibit additional benefits and may hinder cancer treatments due to its strong antioxidant abilities. Melatonin is very safe, especially at this dosage, but proper use is important for maximum benefit.

❖ MSM

AKA: Methylsulfonylmethane, methyl sulfone, methyl sulfonyl methane

Methylsulfonylmethane (MSM, an organosulfur compound) is a popular supplement as it has been shown to help many health conditions, including: inflammation, joint/muscle pain, muscle cramps, headaches, allergies, arthritis, muscle recovery after exercise, hair growth and several other health conditions. These claims all have some level of supporting research.

There is also quite a bit of evidence that MSM can benefit cancer treatment.

In this study, they xenografted human breast cancer cells into mice (where they grow very much like they would in humans). They found that oral MSM significantly inhibited the growth of cancer tumors. MSM not only had an impact on a number of important cancer markers, but also inhibited triple-negative breast cancer gene expression.

> "Breast cancer is the most aggressive form of all cancers, with high incidence and mortality rates… MSM is an organic sulfur-containing natural compound without any toxicity. In this study, we demonstrated that MSM substantially decreased the viability of human breast cancer cells in a dose-dependent manner. MSM also suppressed the phosphorylation of STAT3, STAT5b, expression of IGF-1R, HIF-1α, VEGF, BrK, and p-IGF-1R and inhibited triple-negative receptor expression in receptor-positive cell lines… Concurring to our in vitro analysis, these xenografts showed decreased expression of STAT3, STAT5b, IGF-1R and VEGF. Through in vitro and in vivo analysis, we confirmed that MSM can effectively regulate multiple targets including STAT3/VEGF and STAT5b/IGF-1R. These are the major molecules involved in tumor development, progression,

and metastasis. Thus, **we strongly recommend the use of MSM as a trial drug for treating all types of breast cancers including triple-negative cancers.**" – PubMed ID#PMC3317666 (2012) [810]

MSM was found to inhibit various prostate cancers, even at low doses, by inducing apoptosis and helping halt cancer cell development through a normalization of the cell cycle checkpoints.

"Methylsulfonylmethane (MSM), also known as organic sulfur, is a dietary supplement used for various clinical purposes, mostly known for its anti-inflammatory properties. Therefore, we decided to evaluate the effect of MSM on PC (prostate cancer) cells LNCaP, PC3 and DU-145 which represent different in vitro models of PC. We observed that MSM decreases the viability and invasiveness of PC cells through the induction of apoptosis and cell cycle arrest in the G0/G1 cell cycle phase. Moreover, MSM in a low dose (200 mM) is able to reduce the migration and invasion of PC cells. Considering the low overall body toxicity and insignificant side effects of MSM, its apoptosis-inducing properties might be used in PC treatment" – PubMed ID#30339981 (2018) [811]

MSM was found to induce cell cycle arrest (stop the process of normal cells becoming cancerous) in metastatic melanoma. The same was found with metastatic breast cancer cells. MSM also improved healing of the tumor area.

"In the metastatic Cloudman S-91 (M3) melanoma cell line, methyl sulfone induces cell cycle arrest, proper melanocyte structure including melanosome-filled arborization, cellular senescence, and loss of ability to migrate through an extracellular matrix. We demonstrated anticancer activity with methyl sulfone in the metastatic breast cell line, 66cl-4, as well as in cancerous tissue of 17 breast cancer patients, again with decreasing metastatic phenotypes and increasing normal phenotypes. Normal breast tissue from the 17 patients retained proper healthy breast structure for at least 90 days in culture in the presence of methyl sulfone… we showed that metastatic and normal breast tissue, 66cl-4 breast cancer cells and M3 melanoma cells carry out proper wound healing in the presence of methyl sulfone, but not in the absence of the molecule." – PubMed ID#PMC4633041 (2015) [812]

Open Access license attribution - Caron JM, Caron JM. Methyl Sulfone Blocked Multiple Hypoxia- and Non-Hypoxia-Induced Metastatic Targets in Breast Cancer Cells and Melanoma Cells. PLoS One. 2015;10(11):e0141565. Published 2015 Nov 4. doi:10.1371/journal.pone.0141565

In this study of various liver cancer cell lines, MSM was again found to increase apoptosis of cancer cells. This significantly reduced cancer cell progression.

"MSM decreased the growth of HepG2, Huh7-Mock and Huh7-H-rasG12V cells in a dose-dependent manner. That was correlated with significantly increased apoptosis and reduced cell numbers in MSM treated cells… MSM decreased the growth of HepG2, Huh7-Mock and Huh7-H-rasG12V cells in a dose-dependent manner. That was correlated with significantly increased apoptosis and reduced cell numbers in MSM treated cells." – PubMed ID#PMC3934636 (2014) [813]

Foods High in MSM

- Raw milk
- Tomatoes
- Sprouts
- Green leafy vegetables
- Green tea
- Apples
- Raspberries
- Beer
- Whole grains
- Legumes

Recommendation

It is always best to obtain nutrition from the foods you eat; the foods will contain more bioavailable forms, other nutritional compounds and any cofactors needed for proper utilization. Several of the foods high in MSM are also very healthy and contain other cancer fighting properties.

Taking 3 to 5 grams per day as a supplement is generally regarded as safe for the vast majority of adults and should be enough to provide benefits. In another case of "more is not better," one study looking at allergy relief showed that people taking 12 grams per day reported less benefit than those taking 3 grams per day.

MSM is a low-cost, very safe supplement. When purchased in powder form, it can easily be added to low-sugar smoothies. Because of its well-established benefits in fighting cancer, and the fact that it fights it in ways that are not duplicative of other supplements in this book, I would recommend (in addition to a good diet) trying to supplement 500 mg to 3 grams per day.

❖ QUERCETIN

Quercetin is a plant pigment, polyphenol, antioxidant and flavonoid. It is found in a variety of foods, including: apples, green tea, berries (and concentrated in wine, especially red wine), pomegranates, onions and capers (which have the highest concentration of it). Quercetin has been studied and shows various levels of benefit to several health conditions, including brain health (including possibly helping to prevent Alzheimer's disease), inflammation, anti-aging, leaky gut (where the intestinal barrier allows more through than it should), calming abnormal histamine responses, antibacterial properties, diabetes, arthritis, hypertension and, of course, cancer.

The cancer benefits of quercetin have received quite a bit of research. It lowers TNF-a levels (which can stimulate cancer cell growth, proliferation, invasion and metastasis, and tumor angiogenesis), induces cell-cycle arrest, and/or initiates apoptosis in cancer cells.

> "Quercetin can inhibit the growth of cancer cells with the ability to act as chemopreventers. Its cancer-preventive effect has been attributed to various mechanisms, including the induction of cell-cycle arrest and/or apoptosis as well as the antioxidant functions… Quercetin has received increasing attention as a pro-apoptotic flavonoid with specific and almost exclusive activity on tumor cells rather than normal, nontransformed cells" – PubMed ID#PMC4378141 (2015 – Open Access attribution at the link) [814]

Though this paper primarily focuses on melanoma, it also discusses breast, colon, hepatoma (liver), prostate and esophageal cancers.

> "Quercetin has great potential to be used an antitumor agent in melanoma, and various preventative and therapeutic options can be developed. This review has outlined four specific areas, that with further investigation, could facilitate the development of quercetin into an anticancer compound… with reduced cell viability, increased apoptosis, and enhanced nuclear translocation of NF-$\varkappa$B" – PubMed ID#PMC5086580 (2016) [815]

Quercetin was shown to induce cytotoxicity in leukemia and breast cancer cells. Quercetin led to a 5-fold increase in the lifespans of mice that had (xenografted) human breast cancer tumors.

> "Besides leukemic cells, quercetin also induced cytotoxicity in breast cancer cells, however, its effect on normal cells was limited or none… administration of quercetin lead to ~5 fold increase in the life span in tumor bearing mice compared to that of untreated controls. Further, we found that quercetin interacts

with DNA directly, and could be one of the mechanisms for inducing apoptosis in both, cancer cell lines and tumor tissues by activating the intrinsic pathway… Hence, our results show that quercetin induced significant toxicity in both leukemic and breast cancer cell lines, however, its effect on normal cells was minimal." – PubMed ID#PMC4828642 (2016 – Creative Commons Attribution 4.0, attribution available at the link) [816]

COMT Advisory – People who have a deficiency of the COMT enzyme caused by a genetic variation (single nucleotide polymorphisms, or SNP) on COMT V158M and COMT H62H may need to avoid quercetin supplements. They may even need to cut back on foods containing quercetin. Quercetin is a COMT inhibitor, just what someone with this issue does not need. For more information on COMT, see the Green Tea/EGCG section earlier in this chapter.

Recommendations

If you tolerate quercetin (i.e., you do not have a COMT enzyme deficiency), this may be something you want to include in your regimen. Some medical sources recommend up to 500 mg twice per day. Foods high in quercetin include: capers, kale, yellow/red onions, apples, tomatoes, black/green tea, grapes, red wine, elderberry juice concentrate and cilantro. The following list shows the top 100 quercetin-containing foods: superfoody.com. [817]

❖ Soursop

AKA: *Annona muricata*, graviola, Brazilian paw paw, guanabana, custard apple

The fruit of the graviola tree, commonly known as soursop, is a long, prickly fruit. It has a mild taste similar to a fruity yogurt flavor. It is native to Mexico, Central and South America, and the Caribbean. Most of the research on soursop has been on its fatty acid derivatives called annonaceous aceteogenins. Soursop is getting quite a bit of attention in the alternative medicine arena; however, the limited amount of research and possible harmful side effects should be strongly considered before using.

The ability of soursop to decrease pancreatic tumor growth and retard metastasis was shown in vitro and was confirmed with in vivo xenograft studies on mice (where human pancreatic tumors were transplanted into mice).

"Graviola extract inhibits tumor growth and metastasis of pancreatic cancer (PC) cells… Graviola extract reduces the viability of PC cells and tumors by inducing necrosis and cell cycle arrest, and by inhibiting PC cell motility (i.e. cytoskeleton rearrangement), migration, and metabolism. Overall, in vitro experiments revealed that the compounds present in the natural extract inhibited several pathways involved in PC cell proliferation and metabolism, simultaneously. Such inhibitions ultimately led to a decrease in tumor growth and metastasis in orthotopically transplanted pancreatic tumor-bearing mice." – PubMed ID#PMC3371140 (2012) [818]

"the in vivo anti-cancer study was conducted where mice were fed with extract after inducing the tumor… Annona muricata crude extract samples exhibited different level of cytotoxicity toward breast cancer cell lines. The selected B1 AMCE reduced the tumor's size and weight, showed anti-metastatic features, and induced apoptosis in vitro and in vivo of the 4 T1 cells… while also increased the level of white blood cell, T-cell, and natural killer cell population… The results suggest that, B1 AMCE is a promising candidate for cancer treatment especially in breast cancer" – PubMed ID#PMC4997662 (2016) [819]

"Graviola leaves inhibited the proliferation of A549 cells and human breast cancer cells by arresting the cell cycle and inducing apoptosis… our findings suggest that GE (Graviola leaf extracts) can activate the innate immune system by inducing macrophage activation and production of cytokines… These results indicate that GE has immunostimulatory potential and can be applied to boost the innate immune system in immunocompromised patients." – PubMed ID#PMC5209628 (2016) [820]

This study from 1997 (below) found that compounds from the soursop fruit were up to 250 times more powerful than adriamycin (a chemotherapy) in certain drug-resistant cancer cell lines. This study was done completely in vitro, and the research was done to show if these compounds were safe for normal human tissue. It was also only tested on cell lines that were resistant to adriamycin (so it wouldn't be too difficult for something else to show better effectiveness). Studies like this are designed simply to screen substances for potential and require far more research before a treatment can be recommended. This study is often used in alternative treatment circles to show that soursop is far better than chemotherapy. However, it shows no such thing (it has had no in vivo testing or safety testing and has only been tested against chemo-resistant cell lines). As I've mentioned before, bleach can kill cancer cells, but it will also kill normal cells (and will kill you if consumed at high enough quantities to kill cancer). One needs to be very careful when reading these studies to make sure the research has a practical application and has been sufficiently tested for safety; this study did neither.

"Fourteen structurally diverse Annonaceous acetogenins, representing the three main classes of bis-adjacent, bis-nonadjacent, and single-THF ring(s), were tested for their ability to inhibit the growth of adriamycin resistant human mammary adenocarcinoma (MCF-7/Adr) cells. This cell line is resistant to treatment with adriamycin, vincristine, and vinblastine and is, thus, multidrug resistant (MDR)… those with the stereochemistry of threo-trans-threo-trans-erythro (from C-15 to C-24) were the most potent with as much as 250 times the potency of adriamycin." – PubMed ID#9207950 (1997) [821]

Harmful Findings

Soursop is probably not a good natural supplement to consume at therapeutic doses, at least not in its natural state. It has been found to lead to Parkinson's-like symptoms. In parts of the world where soursop consumption is common, people are often thought to have Parkinson's when in fact their symptoms were brought on by soursop consumption. This is one of those foods that may have the potential to help fight cancer, but it will probably need to wait for drug companies to isolate, or synthesize, safer extracts.

"relation of atypical parkinsonism in the French West Indies with consumption of tropical plants: a case-control study… investigate a postulated link with consumption of herbal tea and fruits from the Annonaceae family (Annona muricata and Annona squamosa), which contain neurotoxic benzyltetrahydroisoquinoline alkaloids… Chronic exposure to neurotoxic alkaloids could be an important aetiological factor because these compounds induce parkinsonism" – PubMed ID#10440304 (1999) [822]

There is also research showing that soursop use can lead to myeloneuropathy (neuropathy that affects the myelin nerve sheath). This might explain the Parkinson's-like symptoms above.

"In the French West Indies there is an abnormally high frequency of levodopa-resistant parkinsonism, suggested to be caused by consumption of fruit and infusions of tropical plants, especially Annona muricata (corossol, soursop). To determine whether toxic substances from this plant can cause the neuronal degeneration or dysfunction underlying the syndrome, we exposed mesencephalic dopaminergic neurons in culture to the total extract (totum) of alkaloids from Annona muricata root bark and to two of the most abundant subfractions, coreximine and reticuline. After 24 hours, 50% of dopaminergic neurons degenerated… consumption could cause the neuronal dysfunction and degeneration underlying the West Indian parkinsonian syndrome." – PubMed ID#11835443 (2002) [823]

Recommendation

I would avoid this one. There is very little evidence of in vivo benefits, and too much evidence of health and safety issues. There are just plenty of better alternatives.

Updates at - https://improvingyourodds.com/

Support at - https://www.facebook.com/groups/cancer.improving.your.odds

◆❖◆

Chapter 7
Detoxification and Our Environment

It's far more important to know what person the disease has,
than what disease the person has. ~ Hippocrates

Detoxification is a very important function in the body and is far more complicated than most people understand. The body has a number of mechanisms in place to handle detoxification, but nature is very efficient and first utilizes what is at hand: gut bacteria, infrared light, exercise and sweat. Then for the toxins that are left, it has developed more complex mechanisms, which involve our liver and kidneys.

Our bodies are constantly detoxifying the byproducts of our metabolism, natural toxins from the food we eat (even organic vegetables), toxins in alcoholic beverages, trace toxins in the air we breathe, cellular byproducts, byproducts from bacterial fermentation in our gut, and even toxins created by cancer tumors we may be unaware of. It is a huge process, but one our bodies are pretty good at. Detoxification helps the body cleanse the internal organs of toxins and waste products; it isn't simply a trendy buzzword, but an important natural process that occurs all the time.

It never ceases to amaze me how complex we are. Even waste elimination is complex! If we lived life like our ancestors, we wouldn't have to learn how to help detoxification, or even what foods are best for us. However, I for one am not willing to live outside, hunt all my food and do without my electronics.

In our modern world we are exposed to far more toxins than our ancestors were, and these toxins are of a variety that our ancestors' bodies probably never had to deal with (e.g., petrochemicals, medications, heavy metals, man-made chemicals of all sorts, etc.). At times our detoxification processes simply cannot keep up. When this happens, the toxins are often stored in the organs and fat, the biologic logic being that detoxification of these toxins would take place the next time we suffer through a fast, or starvation period, and have to burn the polluted fat for energy. This is just one of the reasons why intermittent fasting can be so beneficial (see Chapter 4). When toxins are detoxified, they are mixed with our food waste and eliminated from the body in our stool and urine.

When we can't keep up with detoxification, these toxins can impede the function of our normal cells. Some of these toxins are also carcinogens and thus can promote cancers in the body. If we already have cancer, detoxification can help our general health and enable our immune system to detoxify the waste products created by these cancers. There isn't a lot of evidence that detoxifying actually helps kill cancer cells, but any time you can help your immune system work better, you're "*Improving Your Odds*" of beating cancer!

For millions of years, humans (and all other animals on the planet) took care of detoxification while giving it no thought at all (other than knowing they had to eliminate waste a few times per day). Today we are exposed to a lot more toxins in the environment, but most of the time our bodies can still handle this pretty well. However, this assumes that we are otherwise living like our ancestors—getting enough sleep, exercising, eating right, sweating, intermittently fasting, exposing ourselves to infrared light from the sun, etc., all of the things they would have done daily. Do you remember Ötzi, the Iceman, from Chapter 6? Evidence shows that he would have done all the things to properly detoxify routinely. All of that was a natural part of living for our ancient ancestors, and it was an important part of natural detoxification; if we aren't doing those things (or emulating them), then we are not properly detoxifying.

There are many ways to help our bodies with the detoxification process. There are also probably just as many internet detoxification recommendations that really don't help. I'm going to briefly cover both categories below.

- **Exercise** – Nature's #1 method of detoxification. Exercise ramps up your metabolic rate, burns fat (and the toxins stored there), improves circulation (of both the blood and lymphatic systems), can cause you to sweat, etc. The lymphatic system is very important for the detoxification process (removing cellular debris and other waste), but it requires the movement of the body to function properly (there is no lymphatic "pump" like the heart for blood circulation). Exercise also helps keep the lungs cleaned out; again, there are no housekeeping robots taking care of things. For example, people who are bedridden and cannot properly exercise are far more prone to lung infections. You do not need to become a runner or weightlifter in order to experience significant benefits from exercise, and you don't even need an expensive gym membership. A simple 15-minute brisk walk per day can be beneficial. The topic of exercise is discussed more in Chapter 5; just know that it is also vitally important for detoxification. If you can sweat and get infrared light exposure at the same time, so much the better.

> *Do you or your neighbor have a dog? They would LOVE to go for a walk with you. We have to spell the word "walk" around our little dog, and she's starting to catch on to that! She would rather go for a walk than eat.*

- **Fasting** – Traditionally, this means water only. Fasting is probably the second-best thing a person can do to help remove toxins from the body. It not only gives our organs a rest from detoxifying the chemicals in the food we eat (and there are a lot of them; most are 100% natural), but it also primes our biology to focus on the task of detoxification. If you happen to burn some fat during this process, you will be detoxifying at an even higher rate (and removing possible carcinogens from your fat stores). Though an actual fast is the best method, a ketogenic diet will also engage most of the same processes. Fasting is nature's way of making the best of a bad situation; nobody really wants to starve, but nature uses this time to play catch-up on detoxing and to do some basic housecleaning. Due to the possible intensity of the detoxification process, I recommend starting with intermittent fasting (see below), and working up to fasting for occasional longer periods of time. Personally, I like to take a soluble fiber supplement when fasting; this starves us (as the fiber has no calories that we can utilize) while feeding our microbiota (or beneficial gut bacteria).
  - o **Intermittent fasting** – Again, see Chapter 4 for details. This is very much like fasting above, just for shorter periods of time. It can take advantage of the fact that you are already "fasting" 7 to 8 hours per day while you're sleeping; it just tacks a few more hours onto that. If intermittent fasting is combined with a ketogenic diet, the process will work even better, as you'll be burning fat for energy and that fat has stored toxins that will be removed.
  - o **Juicing** – Though this is very popular, a juice diet is probably not quite as effective as a water fast (especially not how most people do juicing, with sugary fruit). The soluble fiber, vitamins and minerals in the juice will have some health benefits, but they too can trigger metabolic processes within us that have to be detoxified. Fruits and vegetables contain phytonutrients; plants utilize them as insecticides, and although they are mostly healthy for us, they need to be detoxified. Combining a small amount of juicing with a water fast is probably a good compromise; taking 1 shot of vegetable juice, 2 to 3 times per day, will provide our body the nutrients it needs to help the detoxifying process, while at the same time not contributing too much to the toxic load. I would avoid most fruits during this due to the amount of sugar they contain.
- **Sleep** – Sleep is vital for the brain's "glymphatic system" (the brain's waste disposal system). This process is necessary to remove toxins and other waste products, including the toxic protein amyloid-beta, which has been strongly implicated in Alzheimer's disease. Sleep is when the body is at rest and produces the least amount of waste and physiological stress; it is when our bodies best

perform maintenance tasks, such as detoxifying tasks. Do not underestimate the importance of enough sleep.

- **Sweating** – We've known for many, many years that a hot sauna helps to detoxify us and makes us feel good. Sweating has been shown scientifically to remove toxins and heavy metals from the body.

> "No person is without some level of toxic metals in their bodies, circulating and accumulating with acute and chronic lifetime exposures… Sweating was induced by sauna, exercise, or pilocarpine iontophoresis to measure the concentration of the heavy metals in the sweat, while sauna and exercise were used for therapy… On average, arsenic was 1.5-fold (in males) to 3-fold (in females) higher in sweat than in blood plasma… Stauber and Florence concluded that sweat may be an important route for excretion of cadmium… Haber et al. found that prolonged endurance workouts (rowing) ameliorated elevated blood lead levels… Arsenic, cadmium, lead, and mercury may be excreted in appreciable quantities through the skin, and rates of excretion were reported to match or even exceed urinary excretion in a 24-hour period." – PubMed ID#PMC3312275 (2012) [824]

- **Near Infrared (NIR)** – This is covered in much more detail later in this chapter. For now, just know that even though near infrared will cause you to sweat, there is more to it than that. NIR light exposure is what makes you feel good and relaxed after a day on the beach; it has been a natural part of human existence for as long as we've been around. So naturally, our bodies have figured out how to utilize it to our advantage. Even though NIR is a natural part of sunlight, it is not what is responsible for cancer or skin damage; that dubious honor belongs to UV-A and UV-B (though a little of those, especially UV-B, is good for us, too).

- **Gut Health** – See Chapter 3 for more information on this. The bacteria in our gut actually help detoxify heavy metals and can break down other toxins before they are absorbed into the body. Several research studies have shown that the bacteria in our gut are a very important part of detoxification and can break down mercury, lead, cadmium and a wide range of organic and inorganic toxins. In some cases, the liver will first conjugate (bind) these substances for transport to the gut. If the bacteria are not there to break down the toxins (for elimination in the stool), they can get reabsorbed by the body. For many reasons, it is very important to have a healthy microbiome, and detoxifying is one them. – *The Gut Health Protocol* [825]

❖ HYPERBARIC OXYGEN

Many of you may be familiar with the term "hyperbaric oxygen chamber" from movies or the news. They have been used for decades to help prevent, or treat, "the bends" in deep-sea divers. They can look like a room with a safe-like door, or simply a sealed tube that someone lies inside. The chamber's atmospheric pressure (AP) can then be adjusted. A hyperbaric oxygen (HBO) chamber is not inexpensive; a 1.3 atmosphere model can be purchased for $5,000 to $20,000 (and more). However, there are clinics that offer this treatment. But 1.3 AP may not be enough to help much, and higher-pressure units can cost much more. Spoiler alert: After reviewing the evidence, I end up not recommending hyperbaric oxygen treatments (so if you want to skip this section, I'll understand), though they might have some limited benefit used as adjuvant therapy alongside chemotherapy and other medical treatments (but they can make cancer worse when used by themselves).

Hyperbaric oxygen chambers and hyperbaric oxygen therapy (HBOT) have also been used for many years to help speed healing of wounds and burn injuries. HBOT has been moderately effective in this regard. These chambers increase the pressure on a person by a factor of normal atmospheric pressure (AP, with normal pressure being equal to 1 AP). Most hyperbaric oxygen chambers range from 1.3 AP to 3 AP. Most home-style HBOTs are 1.3 AP (or 4.4 PSI). This is a much lower atmospheric pressure than what most of the studies used (1.3 AP is only 30% more than standard atmospheric pressure). The study below used 2.4 atmospheres, which is 140% above standard atmospheric pressure. This does not mean that a home-style HBOT won't help in some situations; it might, but to what degree is unknown.

This study out of Tufts University School of Medicine looked at using hyperbaric oxygen on 4 different cancer lines at 2.4 atmospheres, which is much higher than home hyperbaric chambers can reach.

> "HBO (97.9% O_2, 2.1% CO_2, 2.4 atmospheres absolute) inhibited the proliferation of all 4 cell types as measured by light microscopy... HBO enhanced the anti-proliferative effects of melphalan ($p < 0.05$), gemcitabine ($p < 0.001$) and paclitaxel ($p < 0.001$). The clonogenicity assay demonstrated that the effects of HBO were still evident 2 weeks after the exposure ($p < 0.01$ for all 4 cell types). Experiments using Hoechst-propidium iodide or annexin V-propidium iodide staining showed no HBO-induced increases in necrosis or apoptosis...

The conclusion was that hyperbaric oxygen therapy inhibits proliferation but does not enhance cancer cell death.

> CONCLUSION: HBO inhibits benign and malignant mammary epithelial cell proliferation, but does not enhance cell death." – PubMed ID#16312043 (2005) [826]

This 2010 study out of China found that HBO treatment showed a significant benefit when using HBO along with chemotherapy. They found significant synergism in cancer cell proliferation (nasopharyngeal carcinoma (NPC) cell line CNE2Z). However, they found no benefits when HBO was used by itself.

> "Simple HBO2 treatment after 48 and 72 hours could inhibit the proliferation of nasopharyngeal carcinoma CNE2Z cells. The combination of HBO2 with 5-FU exhibited significant synergism in the suppression of NE2Z cell proliferation only after 48 hours of treatment compared to 5-FU. Simple HBO2 treatment could not reduce the high expressions of MMP-9 and VEGF and inhibit the metastasis of human NPC CNE2Z cells, and no synergistic effect was observed for the combination of HBO2 with 5-FU compared to 5-FU alone."

Artemisinin is an antimalarial drug that has shown some benefits in treating certain cancers. Here they showed that adding HBO treatment increased the effectiveness of artemisinin by 22%.

> "Combined artemisinin and HBO treatment resulted in an additional 22% decrease in growth." – PubMed ID#21115894 (2010) [827]

The following study looked at HBO treatment as adjuvant treatment with chemotherapy in osteosarcoma-bearing mice. Osteosarcoma is one of the most common bone cancers in children and young adults. Note that this study did not look at standalone HBO treatment.

> "hyperbaric oxygen has been shown to enhance the efficacy of radiotherapy and chemotherapy for the treatment of several malignant tumors… In vivo, C3H mice were subcutaneously inoculated with osteosarcoma cells… After 5 weeks, increase in both tumor volume and number of lung metastases was significantly suppressed in the hyperbaric oxygen group. Concomitant hyperbaric oxygen clearly enhanced the chemotherapeutic effects of carboplatin on both tumor growth and lung metastasis" – PubMed ID#19787219 (2009) [828]

I took a look at the full study associated with the above abstract (DOI 10.3892@or 00000534, [829]). HBO alone decreased tumor size as well as carboplatin (CBDCA) chemotherapy. The two combined cut the tumor size at week 6 by 50% that of either CBDCA or HBO used alone, and the two combined cut tumor size by a total of about 600% (compared to the control group). Life expectancy was also greatly enhanced. Only 20% of the HBO mice were still alive at the end of 6 weeks, versus 30% of those that had chemotherapy alone (30% of the controls were still alive as well). Therefore, neither HBO nor CBDCA improved life expectancy when used alone. However, 60% of the mice given both HBO and CBDCA were alive at the end of 6 weeks. The two treatments combined showed a significant synergy. This is more evidence that **HBO, when used alone, can actually make cancer worse**. This should be considered when contemplating HBO treatment; unless HBO is used in combination with another treatment (proven to work synergistically with HBO), it should not be used.

The full study associated with the abstract below suggests that HBO may help carboplatin (chemotherapy) pass through the blood-brain barrier, thus improving the effectiveness of carboplatin.

> "These results suggest that HBO therapy prolongs the biological residence time of carboplatin. MRT for carboplatin may be useful for predicting continuation or modification of chemotherapy and/or clinical antitumor effects in patients with malignant gliomas." – PubMed ID#19465788 (2009) [830]

The following study looked at tumor growth of breast cancer tumors inserted into mice (xenograft) over 12 days. They found the tumor increased to 180% of the original size in the controls and 140% in the 5-FU chemo group, but fell to 80% (of the size of the original tumor) with HBO, and fell to almost 60% of the original size with HBO and 5-FU combined. In the full study, they concluded that HBO alone decreased DMBA-induced tumors by 17% to 24%, and that it reduced the number of blood vessels in the tumor by 72% to 87%.

> "Tumor size fell by 17-24.2% in the HBO groups and by 35.5% when combined with 5-FU (P < 0.05 compared to HBO). HBO treatment reduced the total number of blood vessels in the tumors." – PubMed ID#15172118 (2004) [831]

This was confirmed in the following 2009 study out of Norway. Here HBO treatment was administered to 20 rats, with 20 more rats as controls, all with breast cancer tumors (induced beginning 5 weeks prior). HBO was administered for 11 days. During this time the size of the tumors in the control grew over 90%. In the rats administered HBO, the tumors shrank by nearly 20%. This study was conducted with 2 bars (nearly 2 atmospheres).

> "A total of 20 controls and 20 HBO treated tumors were measured. The measurements of tumor volume started approximately 5 weeks post DMBA induction, when the tumors were approximately 1.0–2.5 cm3. During the observation period of 11 days, tumor volume increased significantly in controls (p<0.0001), whereas a marked reduction in tumor volume (p<0.0001) was found in HBO treated tumors compared to pre-treatment sizes at day 1" – PubMed ID#PMC2712688 (2009) [832]

The following study showed that HBO treatment actually increased gastric cancer cell proliferation (the cell line used in the study; this may very well be the case for other cancers as well).

> "the effect of hyperbaric oxygen treatment alone on tumor treatment remains controversial… The results indicated that, following HBO treatment, the increase in SGC7901 cell proliferation was significant compared with that in the control group, and in addition, there was a significant increase level in autophagosome marker LC3-II, as well as prosurvival molecule BiP level. However, there was a significant decrease in the levels of apoptosis-related molecule, CHOP." – PubMed ID#PMC5374952 (2017) [833]

Combining HBO treatment with a ketogenic diet has also shown significant benefits.

> "The KD alone increased mean survival time by approximately 17 days (56.7%), and when combined with HBO2T, mice exhibited an increase in mean survival time of approximately 24 days (77.9%)… KD+HBO2T mice demonstrated a trend of reduced metastatic tumors in animals compared to the SD group… Our study strongly suggests that combining a KD with HBO2T may be an effective non-toxic therapy for the treatment of metastatic cancer." – PubMed ID#PMC3673985 (2013) [834]

Recommendations

Currently, there just does not seem to be enough evidence to recommend hyperbaric oxygen treatments, especially with home-style (1.3 AP) chambers. Some of the recent evidence indicates that HBO may make some cancers worse. There may be combination treatments in the future that involve hyperbaric oxygen treatment, but standalone HBO treatment most likely provides little or no benefit in treating or preventing cancer. HBO usefulness seems limited to being able to "push" chemotherapy (and perhaps other drugs) into cells or through the blood-brain barrier. The current studies showing benefit are in vitro (where cells react very differently to pressurized oxygen than they do in vivo) or on mice. HBO equipment or treatments can be very expensive and time consuming.

Remember, if there is no reliable independent evidence that something works, you should assume it does not. There is just far too much monetary incentive for some unscrupulous clinics to push unproven and possibly dangerous treatments. There is no vast conspiracy to hide these treatments from you. Remember that countries such as China, Cuba and Iran (etc.,

etc., etc.) would not participate in such a conspiracy, as they have financial incentives to find inexpensive cancer treatments (as they have socialized medical systems).

❖ NEAR INFRARED (NIR)

Near infrared photobiomodulation (PBM) may only have applications for skin cancers, though other cancers have not been studied, especially not in vivo. However, there is the possibility that infrared sauna treatments can enhance other treatments due to their ability to help detoxify toxins from the body. Near infrared (NIR) has an advantage over traditional saunas in that it does not heat the air around you; NIR creates heat in the body. You still sweat, but you are not breathing hot air. As discussed earlier, sweating releases toxins from the body, and this can improve the immune system and remove carcinogens. It is believed that NIR has other direct benefits that extend beyond the heating effect. Some of this has been shown in studies on Alzheimer's.

> *One huge advantage of NIR is that it is a pretty inexpensive treatment to try at home. A simple two-light setup can be purchased for about $130. This is exactly what I did. I've seen some rather elaborate NIR sauna setups (both commercial and DIY), and that is fine, but a simple setup of bulbs and brooder clamps can be just as effective. Infrared saunas can also be found in some massage clinics and chiropractor offices, where you can pay for their use by the half hour.*

The benefits of near infrared have been known for many years, but recent research has provided a good deal of scientific evidence verifying these benefits.

> "It has been known for almost 50 years that low energy exposure to visible and NIR wavelengths is beneficial to humans via the promotion of healing processes. This low level light therapy (so called LLLT or PBM) has been reported in thousands of peer reviewed articles since 1968... It is also used as a photodynamic therapy light source to photoactivate a photosynthetizer (Protoporphyrin IX or PpIX) when treating actinic keratosis, basal cell carcinoma and acne... NIR photobiomodulation of tissue pathologies is associated with increased proliferation of specific cells, gene expression of anti-inflammatory cytokines and suppression of the synthesis of pro-inflammatory mediators" – PubMed ID#PMC4745411 [835] (Creative Common / Open Access License, attribution can be found at https://doi.org/10.1016/j.jphotobiol.2015.12.014 [836])

Here are just a few of the benefits provided by near infrared PBM.

- **Muscle and joint pain relief** – There are several studies showing the efficacy of infrared for muscle and joint pain. In one placebo-controlled study, patients showed relief for chronic lower back pain with one treatment per week for 7 weeks (PubMed ID#PMC2539004 [837]).

- **Skin and breast cancer treatment** – See studies below.

- **Metabolism improvements** – "NASA Light Emitting Diode Medical Applications From Deep Space to Deep Sea" – Marquette University/NASA Marshall Space Flight Center (2001) [838]

- **Improved detoxification** – "Detox" seems to be the darling treatment du jour for most anything. People blame all their troubles on their perceived inability to detoxify. Often, toxins in the body are a symptom, not a cause. The body is constantly detoxifying everything from cellular waste to normal low-level toxins found in almost all the foods we eat. Our bodies are normally very good at detoxifying. However, sometimes parts of this detoxification process don't work as well as they should, and we may even be born with very slight differences in genetics that make it hard for us to detoxify certain things. Or we may have an imbalance of gut bacteria that produce low-level toxins 24/7, which can overwhelm our ability to detoxify them quickly. Cancer tumors can also produce toxins and free radicals that need to be detoxified for us to feel better. Infrared can help with this process and has been a natural part of detoxification for as long as there have been mammals on this planet (and maybe longer).

- **Skin rejuvenation** – Studies have shown that near infrared can improve the look and elasticity of skin. Part of this is the improved detoxification of cellular waste mentioned above, improved blood flow and improved fibroblast activity (which manufactures collagen and other fibers necessary for skin elasticity and fullness), resulting in healthier looking skin.

- **Wound healing** – NIR has been used since the early 1970s by NASA and the military to help facilitate wound healing. Several studies on this have been done over the years.

- The FDA has approved infrared devices for "temporarily relieves minor pain, stiffness, and muscle spasm," as well as "temporarily increases local blood circulation."

> "There is preliminary but high-quality support of FIRS therapy for treatment of NYHA class II and III CHF and systolic hypertension, and there is fair preliminary support for its role in reducing chronic pain. There is weak preliminary support for FIRS therapy in treating chronic fatigue syndrome. There are inconsistent data regarding the effects of FIRS on weight loss, diastolic BP, and fasting blood glucose levels" – PubMed ID# PMC2718593 (2009) [839]

In this small and very short-term (28-day) study of NIR treatment on Alzheimer's patients, some benefits were noted. A larger and longer study is in the works.

"Our study investigated the potential effect of Photobiomodulation on Alzheimer's dementia with results suggestive a trend of improvement in executive functioning; clock drawing, immediate recall, praxis memory, visual attention and task switching (Trails A&B) as well as improved EEG amplitude and connectivity measures." – PubMed ID#PMC5459322 (2017) [840]

Though this study mentions other types of cancer cells that were killed by NIR, it is unlikely that NIR will work in vivo (in the body) for anything other than skin cancer, and perhaps some breast and brain cancers. This is because NIR does not penetrate far enough into the body to make it useful in treating other types of cancer. The useful penetration for NIR energy is approximately 2", perhaps a little more for 250-watt incandescent bulbs. There are some theories that NIR may help kill metastasizing cancer cells that are traveling in the blood and lymphatic system, but this has yet to be shown in vivo (however, it can't hurt to try).

"In in vitro study, five kinds of cultured cancer cell lines (MCF7 breast cancer, HeLa uterine cervical cancer, NUGC-4 gastric cancer, B16F0 melanoma, and MDA-MB435 melanoma) were irradiated using the infrared device, and then the cell proliferation activity was evaluated… we have shown that infrared irradiation significantly inhibited the tumor growth of MCF7 breast cancer transplanted in severe combined immunodeficiency mice and MDA-MB435 melanoma transplanted in nude mice in vivo. Significant differences between control and irradiated groups were observed in tumor volume and frequencies of TUNEL-positive and Ki-67-positive cells. These results indicate that infrared, independent of thermal energy, can induce cell killing of cancer cells… As this infrared irradiation schedule reduces discomfort and side effects, reaches the deep subcutaneous tissues, and facilitates repeated irradiations, it may have potential as an application for treating various forms of cancer." – PubMed ID#20345484 (2010) [841]

In the following study, they show that near infrared (NIR) can directly kill cancer cells, even without heating them; this shows that NIR's benefits extend beyond detoxification. This may be especially useful for malignant melanoma, as it isn't as deep inside us as other cancers (in the beginning stages, especially before we even notice it). You may be able to *Improve Your Odds* of beating melanoma, without even knowing that you have it! NIR from higher wattage sauna-type incandescent bulbs can penetrate tissue and bone up to 2 inches, and therefore, NIR should have applications for treating some breast cancer as well (this would depend on where the tumor is located).

"Both near-infrared and doxorubicin inhibited the tumor growth of MDA-MB435 melanoma cell xenografts in nude mice and increased the phosphorylation of p53 at Ser, Chk1 at Ser, SMC1 at Ser, and H2AX at Ser compared with control mice. These results indicate that near-infrared irradiation can non-thermally induce cytocidal effects in cancer cells as a result of activation of the DNA damage response pathway. The near-infrared irradiation schedule used here reduces discomfort and side effects. Therefore, this strategy may have potential application in the treatment of cancer." – PubMed ID#22515193 (2012) [842] Full Study [843] (Open Access Attribute a the Full Study link. © 2012 Japanese Cancer Association)

Figure 1 from the study above shows cancer cell viability after 1 to 5 rounds of near infrared (NIR) treatment. Cancer cell viability plummeted after only 4 rounds of treatment.

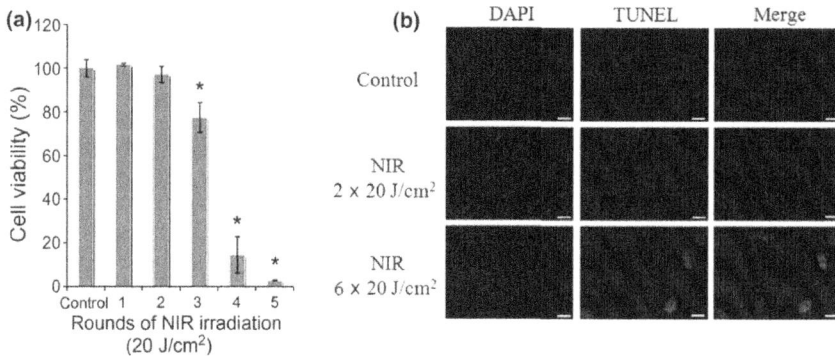

Notice how the melanoma cells went from 100% viability (in the controls) to under 10% after 5 treatments of near infrared. Remember that near infrared can penetrate up to 2", and this is plenty deep to treat melanoma cells (in primary skin tumors) and some breast cancer cells.

Though not included in the following quote, this study examined the use of NIR on pancreatic cancer. This type of cancer is very aggressive and difficult to treat. The study found that "the combination of gemcitabine and irradiation significantly increased the percentage of apoptotic cells compared with either treatment alone." Though the authors acknowledge that it is technically not currently possible to treat pancreatic cancer with NIR in vivo (due to the cancer being located too deep in the body for NIR to penetrate), they noted that the development of such a device could be useful for the treatment of pancreatic cancer in the future.

"Near-infrared radiation (NIR) is a low-energy form of radiation that exerts multiple effects on mammalian cells. Previous studies have reported that NIR induces DNA double-strand breaks and apoptosis of cancer cells... NIR induces the proliferation of keratinocytes, promotes cell attachment, attenuates the infarct size following myocardial infarction in rats and dogs and regenerates and induces the proliferation of skeletal muscle. In addition, NIR has been demonstrated to have an inhibitory effect on advanced neoplasia. Broad-spectrum irradiation ranging between 1,100 and 1,800 nm resulted in apoptosis in multiple cancer cell types in vitro, independent of thermal energy. These previous studies have indicated that NIR may be useful for cancer treatment" – PubMed ID#26622761 (2015) [844]

Even though the following research utilized infrared laser, there is no evidence that other infrared sources would not also work well. The goal is to get infrared light into the tumor without generating too much heat. This study xenografted human melanoma cells into the skin of mice, let those cells grow into tumors, and then used infrared light to destroy them. They found the infrared treatment to be very effective on one type of melanoma and moderately effective on the other. In addition, the infrared treatment improved the immune system's response to melanoma, possibly making this a good adjuvant treatment as well.

"Treatment of cutaneous melanoma (M-3 and B16-F10 implanted in mice) with rapidly-scanned, tightly-focused near infrared light elicits selective destruction of tumor tissue. A single laser treatment yielded complete eradication in >90% of B16-F10 tumors with thicknesses of approximately 3 mm; amelanotic M-3 tumors proved less responsive (ca 25% clearance rate). In addition to local tumor destruction, laser treatment of B16-F10 tumors in immunocompetent mice stimulated enhanced cytokine levels (interleukin-2 and interleukin-10) within treated tumor tissues and rejection of tumor cells upon a subsequent challenge dose. Such an antitumor immune response may lead to improved outcomes at both the treatment site and at sites of distant metastasis." – PubMed ID#11950096 (2002) [845]

Safety

Infrared lamps have been used in saunas for many years, often with no explanation provided for how to use them. Hospitals also use them in postnatal wards on preemies to keep the infants warm. You may have also seen these lamps on timers in hotel bathrooms. Some of these, especially older ones, were far infrared (FIR), which has the same inherent safety as NIR but lacks some of the benefits. Though near infrared is a very safe technology, some precautions should be taken.

- Never look directly at the lights for more than a couple of seconds. Your eye will focus this light into a narrow beam, and this can possibly damage the eye (through heat, much like a magnifying glass on ants). If sitting directly in front of the lamp, you should wear IR shades (or a black sleep mask) when facing it; they are very inexpensive and available on Amazon. Even with your eyelids closed, your eye can focus the infrared that makes it through them.

- Once you start feeling really warm, that is enough. Skin hyperthermia is probably the biggest risk. You do not want your tissue temperature to increase by more than a couple of degrees (Fahrenheit), so 15 to 25 minutes of use (per body area) at a time is plenty, even if you aren't feeling overly warm (more does not equate to better). If you want to do more, wait at least an hour to allow yourself to cool off internally. Again, this is not a regular sauna; the heat is traveling deeper and your surface skin area cools faster than the tissue 2 inches below the skin. Though this sauna heating effect may feel great, too much can be a problem.

- Never touch the incandescent bulb when it is on, and for at least 30 minutes after turning them off. Also, do not allow any water or sweat to come in contact with a hot bulb. They get very hot and will shatter if water touches them.

- Sit or stand about 18" to 36" from the bulbs. You don't want to sit too close as this can cause too much heat internally. Remember, even though it feels good, it is the infrared light that is providing the long-term benefits, not the heat. Do not sit too close to your bulbs; the closer you sit, the more light is concentrated on a small area. This will increase heat without increasing benefit.

- Do not focus a bulb on your head (under 12" distance) for more than 3 to 4 minutes. This is too intense and may generate too much heat for your brain to cool.

- Stay hydrated; infrared may cause you to sweat (even if you still feel cool). The increased detoxification caused by infrared can also use additional fluids.

- Follow all instructions that come with your bulbs and lamps.

The following study shows that near infrared is very safe when the flesh temperature is maintained at 37 °C (98.6 °F). When I use my NIR bulbs, I have a ceiling fan going above me to help cool me. I also do not use NIR for more than 20 to 25 minutes at a time, per body area. If your space is already warm, you may want to turn the A/C down (cooler) while using your NIR lamps. Remember that NIR is good, but overheating is not.

> "IR-A, applied over 30 min to the skin at an irradiance of 190 mW/cm2, with the skin temperature maintained at 37 °C (98.6 °F) by convective cooling from air ventilation, did not significantly affect the cell viability, the inflammatory status, the free radical content, or the antioxidant defense systems of the skin. This is of clinical relevance since the irradiance exceeded the maximum solar IR-A irradiance at the Earth's surface more than 5 times."

This study points out that any deleterious effects are due to thermal (heat) effects, not due to infrared. Again, it is very important not to overheat the tissue. You want the benefits of IR without the possible negative consequences of your cells overheating.

> "the irradiance used in the in vitro experiments showing IR deleterious effects must be considered to be unnaturally high. Actually, the effects observed are most likely thermal effects (due to the increased temperature of the cells),

which are not related to specific properties of IR-A radiation." – PubMed ID#PMC4745411 [846] (Creative Common License, attribution can be found at https://doi.org/10.1016/j.jphotobiol.2015.12.014 [847])

Strategy

This, like many topics discussed in this book, can be somewhat complex. There are different types of bulbs (LED and incandescent), there are different bulb power ratings, there are physical safety issues (incandescent bulbs get very hot and can break), etc. So, let me start by telling you what I'm doing.

I decided to go with two near infrared (NIR) 250-watt incandescent sauna-type bulbs. These bulbs cause warmth within the body (you can sweat, even though your skin may stay cool). Each bulb will cover a skin surface area of about 2 to 3 feet (60 to 90 cm). I say "each" bulb because many people create their own sauna effect by using 2 to 6 bulbs at once. Though not necessary, it may be a practical way to treat the whole body at once (e.g., if worried about skin cancer). For breast cancer, 1 bulb may be all you need to treat one tumor area. The incandescent bulbs produce a lot more infrared, over a larger area of the body, than do LED devices.

My two bulbs are screwed into a clamp-on reflector lamp, called a "brooder" lamp (as heat lamps are often used to keep chickens warm). Each lamp clamps onto furniture 2 to 4 feet from me (like a chair back or table edge); you can also clamp them to a tripod if you have one. I then let the light cover bare skin for 20 minutes (per area). You can use it up to 2 to 3 times per day, giving the skin time to completely cool between uses. I generally use it once per day. That's it.

So why not LED NIR devices? They're OK, but they cover much less surface area, can burn the skin if used improperly (as some LEDs can be hot to the touch, and the LEDs generally come into contact with the skin when using the device), the infrared from LEDs does not travel as deeply, and they cost a lot more. They might be OK to use when traveling, if you only need to treat a small area of the body.

Though the evidence of efficacy for some cancers isn't very strong, I still feel that this is one of those things that might "*Improve Your Odds*" of beating or preventing cancer. It is something that I continue to do. Besides, it feels great.

❖ ELECTROMAGNETIC FIELDS (EMF)

> *"When a distinguished but elderly scientist states that something is possible, he is almost certainly right. When he states that something is impossible, he is very probably wrong." ~ Arthur C. Clarke*

Electromagnetic fields (EMF) have been suspected of causing cancer for decades, especially those from power lines and cell phones. Many studies have looked at this issue and have mostly shown little to no association. An exception to this is childhood leukemia, which I will cover below. EMF are something you should strive to avoid; they are not a treatment.

I would like to start with my opinion from reading the research. My advice is to avoid frequent, or prolonged, close contact with sources of strong EMF. Most research studies have been relatively short term, studying healthy animals or healthy people—or otherwise, they were in vitro (focusing on cells outside the body). Long-term exposure studies (running 10 years or more) have not been done, especially on humans already fighting cancer or other diseases. There are a few studies that show that non-ionizing EMF (e.g., the type given off by power lines and home appliances) can cause cancer, but I think the only questions are how much exposure, at what frequencies, and at what strength are necessary to cause harm.

Just like you can't necessarily trust what industry scientists are telling you, you also can't trust much of what you read on the internet on this topic. There is a <u>lot</u> of fearmongering on this subject, from those looking to get more hits for their website, to people wanting to sell you a fraudulent product to block EMF, as well as from some well-meaning people who obviously know very little about the topic. I happen to have a background on this topic (Google "military TEMPEST"—I worked in that field for 12 years a number of years ago) and certainly know enough about the topic to discuss it.

There is much debate on EMF, and many people in industry, government and the medical profession will tell you that non-ionizing EMF (the type we're discussing here) cannot cause cancer. I don't agree with that assertion; there are research studies that dispute this. There is now little doubt that non-ionizing EMF above a certain level can increase the risk of childhood leukemia. This should tell those experts that non-ionizing radiation <u>can</u> cause cancer; there is clear evidence of it. The laws of physics and basic biology aren't different for children and adults; non-ionizing EMF can cause cancer. However, many questions remain regarding how much exposure is safe; since most of us really cannot escape them, knowing how to live with them becomes important.

Childhood Leukemia

There are studies showing a clear correlation between childhood leukemia and how close the children live to power lines. The following study indicates a 100% increase in risk for children exposed to background levels of EMF (e.g., power lines) equal to or above 0.4 micro-T (μT, micro-tesla, a unit of measure for a magnetic field). In other words, they face double the risk compared to children not living close to power lines.

> "In summary, the 99.2% of children residing in homes with exposure levels < 0.4 microT had estimates compatible with no increased risk, while the 0.8% of children with exposures >/= 0.4 microT had a relative risk estimate of approximately 2, which is unlikely to be due to random variability." – PubMed ID#10944614 (2000) [848]

The following confirms the conclusions of the study above. A meta-analysis of 15 studies observed a 1.7 times increase in childhood leukemia among children with exposures of 0.3 μT or higher. A little more than 3% of children in the studies experienced this level of exposure (on a positive note, both of these studies indicate that children receiving less than 0.4 μT have no added risk of leukemia from power lines).

> "estimates from 12 studies that supplied magnetic field measures exhibited little or no association of magnetic fields with leukemia when comparing 0.1-0.2 and 0.2-0.3 microtesla (microT) categories with the 0-0.1 microT category, but the Mantel-Haenszel summary odds ratio comparing >0.3 microT to 0-0.1 microT was 1.7 (95% confidence limits = 1.2, 2.3)… an estimate of the U.S. population attributable fraction of childhood leukemia associated with residential exposure is 3%" – PubMed ID#11055621 (2000) [849]

A more recent meta-analysis (appearing in the *British Journal of Cancer*) of seven studies with a total of 10,865 childhood leukemia cases and 12,853 controls came up with pretty much the same conclusion.

> "We conclude that recent studies on magnetic fields and childhood leukaemia do not alter the previous assessment that magnetic fields are possibly carcinogenic." – PubMed ID#20877339 (2010) [850]

Most people have little to worry about from standard neighborhood power lines. These usually do not have the current necessary to generate the very powerful EMF levels necessary to travel into homes at levels high enough to cause problems. However, if you happen to live very near high-tension power lines, you may want to have your home's EMF levels tested, especially if you have young children (or are wanting children).

This study by the Division of Cancer Epidemiology and Genetics at the National Cancer Institute evaluated the EMF cancer risk from home appliances (which give off EMF to some degree or another). **Electric blanket use by the mothers during pregnancy increased risk of their children contracting lymphoblastic leukemia by nearly 60%. If a child used an electric blanket or electric mattress pad, the risk was 175% higher than for children who did not use the electric blanket** (see my own measurements of electric blankets below). An increase in risk was also associated with other appliances, such as hair dryers, video games, etc., but the risk was much lower as the devices give off less EMF and are not (generally) used as long per day as an electric blanket. Increased risk was always associated with how much EMF a device gives off, how close it was to the person during use, and how much time it was used. In other words, a TV set across the room has far less risk than one 2 feet away.

> "Mothers were interviewed regarding use of electrical appliances during their pregnancy with the subject and the child's postnatal use. The risk of acute lymphoblastic leukemia was elevated in children whose mothers reported use of an electric blanket or mattress pad during pregnancy [odds ratio (OR) = 1.59… The risk of acute lymphoblastic leukemia was increased with children's use of electric blankets or mattress pads (OR = 2.75; 95% CI = 1.52-4.98) and three other electrical appliances (hair dryers, video machines in arcades, and video games connected to a television)… Risks rose with increasing number of hours per day children spent watching television" – PubMed ID#9583414 (1998) [851]

Adult EMF Exposure

Government and industry have been saying for years that power lines and home appliances only produce non-ionizing radiation and therefore cannot cause cancer. Yet the studies above show that this simply is not true. If exposure to relatively low power line EMF (0.3 to 0.4 µT) can increase the odds of contracting childhood leukemia by 170% (1.7 times), this is strong evidence that non-ionizing, low-frequency EMF can induce cancer. However, unless you live under very high-power power lines, you can control the amount of EMF you receive each day and thus lower your risk to negligible levels. Unless you want to live in the middle of a large forest with no electronics, mitigating EMF risk is the next best thing.

Exposure time and EMF strength are the two most important measures we need to pay attention to. Brief exposures to EMF in the 0.3 µT to 5 µT range are not much of a risk. Living under this level of EMF 24/7 is a much higher risk.

I've come up with this very simple risk formula based on daily exposure time and µT (microtesla units). Simply multiply the µT number times the number of hours of exposure per day, and then add up all of these daily exposures. This leaves you with your Daily EMF Risk number.

Now, assuming that the risk of EMF increasing cancer begins at 0.4 μT for 24-hour-per-day exposure (e.g., living under power lines, such as in the studies above for childhood leukemia risk), then danger begins at a Daily EMF Risk number of 9.6 (0.4 μT times 24). Any Daily EMF Risk number higher than 9.6 should thus be considered problematic, and the higher the number, the more risk.

I purchased an EMF tester (30 to 300 Hz) and measured some common household appliances in my own home. This device does not test for higher-frequency RF noise (RF = radio frequency, such as from a WiFi router), but such equipment is at a much lower wattage and still outside of the ionizing (dangerous) frequencies (the 60 Hz EMF wattage emitted from the power cord would exceed that of the WiFi signals, so the measurements should still be useful to determine risk). Thus, exposure from your WiFi router, smart power meter and Bluetooth devices will not significantly add to your total Daily EMF Risk number unless you put it under your pillow at night, or perhaps on your bedside night table.

All of the EMF sources in your home are <u>non-ionizing</u> radiation, so they do not have the energy to release electrons from orbit (which is a well-known health risk). The exception to that is your microwave oven; however, it is shielded to eliminate the risk from those frequencies (although it is not shielded to eliminate regular 60 Hz power line EMF, which is non-ionizing). Home electronics emitting high-frequency RF EMF (such as from cell phones) are very low wattage. Though testing is still being done, the risks from such low-power devices are very low and really only apply if you are talking on the phone with it up against your ear. Bluetooth, though still an RF frequency technology, has a much lower wattage than even the cell phone. Therefore, Bluetooth earbuds, or even better, headphones, are a good option to greatly reduce risk from a cell phone. Wired headphones almost completely eliminate any risk if the cell phone is placed 2 to 3 feet from you. All in all, I do not worry very much about cell phones, but I do take some precautions. I use Bluetooth headphones or the speakerphone at home, and the Bluetooth-enabled stereo speakers in my vehicle. This greatly reduces my exposure. When I do have to use the phone against my ear, I don't worry about it—again, the risks are already very low, and the less you use it against your ear, the lower the risks are (worry and stress are known contributors to cancer). I'm certain that the cancer risks from using a modern cell phone for an hour or two per day are lower than those of consuming sugary treats every day.

Below is an example of this scoring system for exposure to common household appliances and electronics. If you spend twice the amount of time using one of these devices as you need to, double your score for that device. Readings were taken from various locations at the distance specified (the further you are from an EMF source, the lower the amount of EMF you receive). The reading shown is the highest reading measured at the specified distance. The following may look complicated, but it isn't; just remember that your Daily EMF Risk score should total less than 9.6, and the EMF Risk score is the μT number times the number of hours (or fraction of an hour) you're exposed per day.

- Electric blanket #1 –This is the inexpensive electric blanket (name brand) that we were using before I started writing this book. Assume you will have direct contact with the blanket, 8 hours per night. The risk score below is very high but can be completely mitigated by using your blanket to warm your bed starting an hour before getting in, and then turning it off before getting into bed. This way you still get the benefits of getting into a warm bed, but without the EMF risk!

- This blanket measured 42.1 μT at zero inches, for a Daily EMF Risk score of 336.8! This is 35 times higher than the amount known to cause childhood leukemia! This is obviously too high.
- Electric blanket #2 – After determining the above risk, we originally were turning off the old blanket before getting into bed. We live in Minnesota and decided we needed a low-EMF electric blanket. So, we purchased a new one. It works just as well and we like it better. Here are the results from the new blanket. Needless to say, the blanket now stays on overnight during the winter months! We're <u>very</u> happy with this new blanket.
    - 0.0 μT, or a Daily EMF Risk score of 0 (zero)
- Controller for electric blanket #2 – The controller unit for the low-EMF electric blanket does emit some EMF. However, it dissipates very quickly as you move away from it. Because of this, I'm not at all concerned about EMF from the controller. We're probably about 18" from either controller (there are two of them), and from that distance, the measured EMF is zero, so there is no additional risk from the controller.
    - 0" – 3.1 to 7.2 μT
    - 3" – 0.11 μT
    - 6" – 0.0 μT, no EMF detected, Daily EMF Risk score of 0 (zero)
- 26" LCD computer monitor, measured from the front, used for 8 hours per day. I found I sit 18" to 21" from my monitor, so my Daily EMF Risk score is 0 (zero) for this.
    - 1" – 19.5 μT, or a score of 156
    - 9" – 0.13 μT, or a score of 1.04
    - 12" – 0.08 μT, or a score of 0.64
    - 18" – 0.0 μT, or a score of 0.0
- 1,500 watt space heater, used 2 hours per day during the winter months. I keep the heater about 48" away and try to limit usage.
    - 2" – >200 μT (my meter maxes out at 200 μT!), a Daily EMF Risk score of 400+
    - 6" – 180 μT, a score of 360
    - 12" – 32.1 μT, a score of 64.2
    - 36" – 0.35 μT, a score of 0.7
    - 48" – 0.22 μT, a daily EMF score of 0.44 at 2 hours per day, or 0.88 at 4 hours per day
- Hair blow drier – Because you need to hold the hair drier, I used the reading for the handheld area, since it was the highest reading (other than the back of the unit and the cord). The handheld area's reading was 41 μT for 15 minutes per day, for **a score of 10.25** (41 μT * 0.25 hours). My recommendation would be to towel-dry your hair as much as possible, and perhaps cut your blow-dry time by half (this will cut your score in half as well). Also, do not hold the electric cord, because due to the high current going through the wire, the EMF level of the cord is very high. There is not much you can do about the handheld area; you must hold the hair drier. EMF dissipates very quickly with distance; therefore, the main risk here would be to cancers of the blood, as the EMF will not reach other parts of the body. If you are a hairstylist, you are receiving a very large amount of EMF each day (41 μT * 3 hours of blow drier time = a Daily EMF Risk score of 123),

but there is probably not much you can do about it. Because the EMF number was too high, we purchased a new, lower-EMF blow drier and tested it next (see this book's website for recommendations).

- High heat/high fan – 1.2 µT at 3," 0.35 at 6" (measured from airflow area)
- Warm heat/low fan – 1.1 µT at 3," 0.30 at 6" (measured from airflow area)
- Combination of cord and hot air – 88.8 µT at 3"
- Handheld area – 41 µT
- Back of the blower – 50 µT

- Low-EMF hair drier – While writing this book, I purchased my wife a new, lower-EMF hair drier. This is an inexpensive ($21) hair drier found on Amazon. It uses far infrared rather than heating coils. As you can see, it generated about ½ to ¼ the amount of EMF compared to the old heating-coil model. The handheld area again generates the most EMF that you are likely to be exposed to. Again, for the hairstylist, 17.5 µT * 3 hours of blow drier time = a Daily EMF Risk score of 52.5, less than half that of the traditional heating-coil drier (for someone using it 15 minutes per day, the Daily EMF score is 4.375; cut the usage time in half, and you half this number).

  - High heat/fan – 0.69 µT at 3" (measured from front airflow area)
  - Low heat/fan – 0.65 µT at 3" (measured from front airflow area)
  - Handheld area – 11 µT on low, 17.5 µT on high
  - Back of the blower at 1" – 19.2 µT on low, 19.2 µT on high; at 12", both low and high were 0.25 µT

- Hair straightener – 0 µT at any distance

- Cell phone – Measurements are in direct contact with the phone. The score is 2 hours of use per day. I now use wireless Bluetooth headphones with my cell phone, and the EMF on those are very low. A cell phone will also produce EMF at higher than 300 Hz, and it was not tested at these frequencies; however, the concept of using wireless headphones to reduce EMF exposure still applies.

  - Idle/texting – 0.15 µT, a score of 0.3
  - Voice call – 4.4 µT, a score of 8.8 at 2 hours per day with no headphones

- Ceiling fan – Very little risk due to the distance

  - 4" – 0.4 µT
  - 12" and beyond – 0.00 µT

- Microwave oven – A microwave oven emits a lot of EMF. On our Panasonic microwave, even when not microwaving anything, the display panel emits a considerable amount of EMF, but it dissipates quickly the further away from it you are. I'm giving this a Daily EMF Risk score of 0.9 (using 3" exposure for 30 minutes per day), but this can vary a lot depending on how it is used (such as little noses pressed against the glass). In our house we just try to stand about 5 feet from it when it's in use.

  - Microwaving –75 µT at 0" from the glass (Daily EMF Risk of 37.5 @ 30 minutes/day)
  - Microwaving – 63.2 µT at 2" (Daily EMF Risk of 31.6 @ 30 minutes/day)
  - Microwaving – 54 µT at 5" (Daily EMF Risk of 27 @ 30 minutes/day)
  - Microwaving – 1.8 µT at 3' (Daily EMF Risk of 0.9 @ 30 minutes/day)
  - Microwaving – 0.08 µT at 5' (Daily EMF Risk of 0.04 @ 30 minutes/day)

- Idle - Control panel while the microwave was <u>not</u> in use measured 140.3 μT at zero inches, 0.4 μT at 12", and none at 24"
- Glass door area while the microwave is <u>not</u> in use – 21.5 μT

- Desktop computer – This will vary depending on how close it is to you. At 9" nothing was detectable from my computer, for a score of zero.

  - Front – Nothing detectable at 6"
  - Side – 0.38 μT at 0", 0.18 μT at 6"
  - Top – 0.35 μT at 6" (there is a large computer fan in the top of the case)

- Laptop computer – An average from the keyboard's home keys was 0.15 μT. This gives us an EMF Risk score of 1.2 (0.15 μT at 8 hours/day). Again, less time equals less risk. Using an external keyboard lowers this risk to zero.

  - 0 μT at the wrist rest
  - 0 to 0.3 μT at the home keys (fluctuates based on CPU usage)
  - 0 μT from the screen and laptop at 6"

- Laser mouse – 0.0 μT while moving, with the meter touching the mouse. No risk.

- Wireless keyboard – 0.0 μT at the home keys, 0.15 μT where the USB cord plugs into the keyboard (and while charging). This essentially has no effect on me, as it measures zero where I'm typing. No risk.

- USB charging station – With two USB battery backups charging, 1" = 91.4 μT, 6" = 9.3 μT, and 12" = 3.6 μT. The EMF was very directional, so it was very sensitive to how I held the meter. The charging station was about 12" from my keyboard (and my hands). I'm giving this a **score of 28.8** (3.6 μT * 8 hours per day). I have since moved the charging station about 4" further back, and my keyboard position about 2" over. **My score has now fallen to 1.44** at my left hand and zero at my right. Making some simple adjustments can make a world of difference.

As you can see, the biggest risk in a home comes from a standard electric blanket (unless you are hugging your space heater all night!). When used as directed, a standard electric blanket produced a very large amount of EMF, and it will have direct contact with the body for 6 to 9 hours per day! My advice is to turn the blanket on high an hour before going to bed, and then turn it off before you get in bed. This gives you a nice warm bed to get into and no EMF risk. Or you can do what we did and purchase a low-EMF blanket (see the <u>book's website</u> for recommendations).

The next highest appliance surprised me; it was the microwave oven. Though microwaves are shielded to prevent the microwave radiation from escaping, they are not shielded against lower-frequency EMF (such as household current). Though our daily exposure time in front of the microwave is probably pretty low, this high level of EMF is still concerning. We now stand off to the side of the microwave and a few feet back—never directly in front. Though most people already know this, I wouldn't let children stick their nose against the microwave door and watch it cook the food.

I spend a lot of time beside my desktop computer. It sits under my desk, and my left leg (the one where I had a malignant melanoma) sits right beside it. I have now moved the computer further back and to the outside of my desk, significantly reducing my EMF exposure. Most of the EMF was coming from the side fan (fans generate a lot of EMF, and this is where there are holes in the case for airflow. The solid metal case is grounded and provides very good shielding from EMF). This has reduced my exposure from 0.38 µT to 0.18 µT, going from a Daily EMF Risk score of 3.04 down to 1.44.

In the winter months, the room that I use as my office gets cooler than the rest of the house. Therefore, I use a space heater in there. As you can see, it produces a considerable amount of EMF. But moving it back 4 to 5 feet from me helps tremendously. I used to have it about 3 feet from me for up to 4 hours per day, for a score of 2.8; now that I've moved it back to 5 feet, that score has dropped to zero.

The hair drier is my wife's. She uses it for about 5 minutes per day and has no plans of giving it up. This added about 3.41 to her Daily EMF Risk score, but the new hair drier cut this by more than half to 1.46 µT.

Scams

Do not purchase devices claiming to reduce EMF in your home; they do not work. The military has been studying EMF for decades, not so much for health reasons but because EMF can give away vital secrets. Any electronic device, including your monitor, keyboard and even your printer, gives off EMF. But this signal isn't static; it changes based on usage. For example, every key on your keyboard gives off a slightly different electronic signature. An adversary with the right equipment can pick up these unique signals, run them through a computer to analyze the signals, and determine exactly what you are typing. However, there is no need for most people to worry about eavesdropping; the equipment to pick up EMF and translate the signal into readable text is very expensive and not commonly available. The signals also don't travel very far, and the more walls the signals must go through, the less distance it can travel. But if a simple, inexpensive plugin device was available to stop all EMF, the military wouldn't have to spend billions of dollars hardening their equipment (they would find something else to spend that money on, probably things that go boom). Besides, others have opened those EMF blockers and examined them; they contain about 10 cents worth of very inexpensive components that could not possibly block EMF. They're total scams.

EMF (electromagnetic fields) are simply radio waves, usually with no intelligible information. Your local AM or FM radio station broadcasts radio waves with audio superimposed on the wave, as does your cell phone. EMF signals from electronics (such as from a space heater) have no such intelligence on the wave. If these EMF blocking devices worked, they would stop not only AM/FM radio signals, but all cell phone signals as well. If it cannot block these signals, it is not going to block other electromagnetic fields either.

To stop EMF once it is generated, you need grounded shielding—something metal between you and the source of the EMF, connected to ground. One of the best such shields is what is called a Faraday cage; this is a grounded metal mesh (much like a screen door) made out of a highly conductive metal (such as copper or silver). For lower frequencies such as household currents, a shield made from high-magnetic-permeability metal alloys must be used. These solutions are bulky (e.g., they would need to cover your entire home to protect it from powerline EMF), expensive and impractical as a means of blocking EMF from outside your home.

I've seen fraudulent whole-house EMF devices selling for hundreds and even thousands of dollars! I even came across a $130 pendant said to neutralize EMF for 6 feet around the wearer. None of these devices work, not even in the slightest. There are dozens of vendors on Amazon selling them, and apparently people are buying them. There are plenty of obviously fake reviews, but there are also some placebo effect reviews (the sugar pill effect where people convince themselves that something they are taking or doing is working). There are also photos from people who took their device apart and found very simple electronics; inside were only the electronics that are necessary to light the LEDs on the device itself. Simple tests quickly show that the devices block no EMF, and in fact, sometimes they emit small amounts of their own EMF.

Save your money—they don't work.

Strategy

Most people do not have much to worry about from EMF in their homes, especially if you make some simple adjustments to how you use these EMF-producing devices. If you don't use an electric blanket, don't sit 2 to 3 feet from a space heater, don't press your nose up against the microwave oven glass and don't talk on your cell phone for hours per day, you're probably OK.

However, avoidance is still a good idea where practical. I recommend looking at the wattage rating on appliances; anything using 250 watts or more of electricity has the <u>potential</u> for generating significant amounts of EMF when in use. Try to rearrange your environment to keep high-current/high-wattage electronics away from you. If you need reading glasses, use them; this will allow you to sit further back from your monitor. Often for low-wattage electronics, just moving back 3" to 4" can help significantly.

- If you normally use a standard electric blanket or heating pad on your bed in the winter months, turn it on an hour before bed, and then turn it off before getting into bed.

- Avoid sitting or sleeping near space heaters. Try to stay at least 3 feet from them.

- Try to sit at least 18" back from your computer monitor. If you need to use computer glasses to see it from that distance, then it is best to use them.

- Rearrange your office, or home office, to keep charging stations and charging devices as far from you as possible.

- When using the microwave oven, try to stay at least 3 feet from it while it is in use. Never allow children to watch the food cook or press their noses against the glass (even when not microwaving food).

- Keep your WiFi router and cable box 3 to 4 feet or more from where you spend time.

- Do not worry about any low-power (e.g., battery operated) or low-wattage device that you don't spend an hour or more using per day. The Daily EMF Risk score should be negligible. Much like natural toxins in the environment, the body is used to dealing with such insults, and devices with a very low score should probably count as zero towards a daily total.

- Relax about brief exposures to EMF, and focus on devices with the highest Daily EMF Risk. Remember that stress and worry are very bad for the immune system, much worse for you than low levels of EMF.

- Most of all, do not treat EMF like a poison. People think that the more electronic devices they have in their house, the more these devices are poisoning their bodies. Not necessarily. EMF dissipates, and it usually dissipates quickly. Once it is gone, it's gone. When it drops below certain levels, it is truly harmless. Education about the science involved will help you learn what to avoid; again, it mostly means putting a few feet between you and EMF emitting appliances, or limiting exposure time.

Humans are living longer and longer lives, and yet we're exposed to much more EMF than ever before. Though some cancer rates are going up, there are plenty of other reasons for that (e.g., high-sugar diets, insecticides, stress, using blue light electronics at night, lack of sleep, etc., etc.), and those are the areas you should be focusing on the most. However, limiting overall daily EMF exposure is not a bad idea. Focus on those areas that have the highest Daily EMF Risk. It often isn't difficult to make some small changes to greatly reduce your total Daily EMF Risk.

Updates at - https://improvingyourodds.com/

Support at - https://www.facebook.com/groups/cancer.improving.your.odds

◆❖◆

--- This Page Intentionally Left Blank ---

Chapter 8
Natural Treatment Hoaxes

"I know that most men, including those at ease with problems of the greatest complexity, can seldom accept even the simplest and most obvious truth if it be such as would oblige them to admit the falsity of conclusions which they have delighted in explaining to colleagues, which they have proudly taught to others, and which they have woven, thread by thread, into the fabric of their lives." ~ Tolstoy

The problem with most medical hoaxes is that people <u>want</u> to believe in them, so they really don't have to be convinced. It is ever so inviting to think that a simple machine, drug or treatment, free of side effects, will cure us. We won't have to lose our hair, file for bankruptcy or even change our eating habits (much less die!). This desire to believe in a magic cure has been around for literally thousands of years. We want it to be true so badly that we are willing to believe that there is a massive conspiracy to keep this magical cure from us.

Today, the huckster has teamed up with the conspiracy nut. Now you get not only a great sales pitch, but a contagious dose of paranoia as well. According to them, the reason why the medical establishment and the government are railing against their magic is that these actors are in bed with "big pharma." If only the world listened to these hucksters, they would put big pharma out of business. If every doctor started using (for example) a Rife machine to cure cancer (and every other medical condition, including the common cold), that would put the drug companies out of business overnight. According to the conspiracy theories, even scientific researchers (including those in universities and countries with socialized medicine) are in on the scam to deprive these magic treatments of their day in the sun. Apparently, big pharma is meeting scientists, doctors and government regulators in Walmart parking lots with wheelbarrows full of cash.

It is quite easy to dispute the hucksters' claims scientifically and logically. There are thousands of research studies on natural treatments; there are nearly a thousand of them summarized in this book alone (and I read at least two thousand more). Some of these studies have even shown that some natural treatments are more effective than medical chemotherapies or can enhance the benefits of medical therapies and reduce their side effects. There is no vast conspiracy to block research on natural treatments.

Today's world is <u>very</u> competitive. If Western countries aren't keeping up with research on natural therapies, I can assure you that other countries will pick up the slack. Countries such as China, Iran, Cuba, etc. are doing a lot of research into natural therapies, as they stand to save a lot of money on their socialized medicine programs if they can find inexpensive natural therapies that work. Effective natural treatments would also help support their political systems with their populace. Non-Western capitalist countries are also providing a lot of research on natural botanicals; Japan, Taiwan and South Korea are examples of this (they also have government-run medical systems). "One-upping" the larger Western countries is also a huge incentive to continue this research.

The theory that Western countries suppress natural cancer research simply doesn't hold up to scrutiny. Natural treatments certainly don't receive as much funding as drugs do, but there is still a lot of research being done. We can wish there was more such research, but to say there is a massive conspiracy to suppress it doesn't seem to be supported by evidence.

However, as previously discussed, there are a number of reasons why the research being done on natural treatments never makes it into your oncologist's medical bag of treatment options.

1. The primary one being (what I call) liability diversion; if something goes wrong with an approved drug treatment, the drug company gets sued, and usually not the doctor. If something goes wrong with a natural treatment, the doctor gets sued. Whether anything will go wrong with a natural treatment is beside the point; doctors are constantly worried about liability.
2. There is also big money in standard medical treatments; oncologists get paid big bucks and have a lot of bills to pay (including student loans). Telling people to go home and take curcumin won't pay those bills. Besides, these drugs and the oncologists are very valuable to cancer treatment.
3. Doctors simply are not educated in natural treatments. They already spend a lot of time and money getting educated on established medical treatments. I wouldn't call it *brainwashing*, but if all you ever learn about is one way of doing things, that is what you're going to believe works, often to the exclusion of everything else.

No conspiracy is necessary for all the oncologists to figure out what is safer from a liability perspective and what has a higher profit margin. Rather than blame doctors for not knowing something, we should try to educate them. Just don't forget that doctors are people of science, and most will only respect a scientific point of view. Thus, this book.

Because our doctors are not educating us on natural treatments, this leaves the internet and books. We all should know the internet is a perfect vehicle for scammers and hucksters from around the world to reach us. This all makes it difficult to tell the difference between a snake oil hoax treatment and something that may have significant benefits. That is what this book is

---

about: separating the beneficial natural treatments from the hoaxes. This works a lot like drug approval; if there are several well run, peer-reviewed research studies showing safety and efficacy, then perhaps a treatment is worth trying. If there are no scientific, peer-reviewed, double-blind studies showing efficacy, then chances are it is a hoax and you should avoid it. And remember, all things being equal, in vivo research always trumps in vitro.

I can certainly understand why some people don't trust government, don't trust doctors and can't trust the food they eat. All of these have let us down at one time or another. However, that does not mean you should trust a huckster or some random person on the internet. I also wouldn't blindly trust testimonials; methamphetamines can really help people have more energy, and many people have fallen for their appeal, but the long-term consequences are terrible—and yet many people swear by them (at least at first). There is also the placebo effect; people want to believe something is helping them, and they can end up thinking the sugar pill cured them (and don't forget, our bodies are capable of curing cancer, and some people will get well with, or without, the sugar pill). For decades snake oil salesmen have been able to get thousands of people to believe in their products and give testimonials. Faith healers have been "laying hands" to cure people for thousands of years.

> *As a child growing up in a small town in northern Louisiana, I remember watching these flamboyant faith healers when they came through with their circus tents. Even at 13 years old, I found it sad that people would fall for this, and many did.*

Therefore, we need scientifically controlled studies and peer review of those studies; though it may not always be perfect, it is the best method we have of researching treatment and prevention options.

There are several Facebook groups that tout natural cures for cancer. In researching this book, I joined several of these groups. Today one of them had posted about 10 different foods and botanicals that could "cure" lung cancer. The title was "Scientifically Proven Natural Lung Cancer Cures," and below each food picture it would say something like, "Celery Compound is an 86% Cure For Lung Cancer," and then list a PubMed webpage. Well, when you go to the PubMed webpage, it would say nothing about "curing," nor would it mention a "percentage," or even an adjective suggesting how well it worked. The study would be about a compound in that food, involved **in vitro** testing, and included no hint as to how this translated to in vivo human dosing (or even if it might work in humans). The research was taken very much out of context (to the extent of making stuff up), and yet, who wouldn't simply want to eat 10 different foods and have a minimum of a 97% chance of curing their lung cancer (this was said to be the cure rate of just one of those foods)? Combining 10 foods that listed 80% or higher cure rates must no doubt equal at least a 99% cure rate! All from just making minor adjustments to one's diet (who needs doctors with results like this?). Of course, none of these rates were for humans; it was all in the test tube (most poisons kill cancer in the test tube, but that doesn't mean we should take them to cure our cancer). Also, none of the studies used the whole food; instead, they used highly refined extracts in doses that would not be possible to obtain from eating the whole food. At the concentrations listed for the extract, if a person consumed enough of it to obtain those blood concentrations they would die. These studies are used to identify chemicals for further research and possible patentable derivatives (I exclude them from this book).

> *So, what did that Facebook group admin say when someone told him that these memes weren't a fair reading of the research? "This has nothing to do with fair or unfair. These aren't my opinions or suggestions. These are scientifically proven studies that are true, you'll never hear about them in the mainstream media. There it is. Take it for what's it's worth or ignore it."*

"Scientifically proven" my big fat chair warmer! Often, these memes are posted by "health coaches" who profit from advising people about how to cure their cancer naturally (with no regards to objective science). Or sometimes it is just someone with a big ego who loves followers (but apparently hates science). So, you should be very careful about what you read on the internet; if it sounds too good to be true, it probably is. Always insist on seeing the science, and always try to verify that what is being claimed is what the research actually shows.

In short, if there isn't good scientific evidence of safety and efficacy, don't waste your time and money on it.

What follows are a few of the better-known cancer cure hoaxes (there are at least hundreds, if not thousands, more). I know I'm going to get hate mail, bad reviews, and maybe even a threat or two for disparaging these sacred cows. But I go where the science takes me; I'm not in this for popularity.

❖ ALKALIZING

"Alkalizing" is the misguided attempt to change the pH of the body (blood and organs) through dietary means. This is not the same thing as improving the "buffering potential" that is discussed in Chapter 6.

Whenever I've discussed the alkalizing myth in my book, *The Gut Health Protocol*, and in its Facebook group, you would think I was insulting someone's religion. Yes, not only does "alkalizing" not help, but it's impossible to actually alkalize the body without getting very ill or dying. It is especially difficult to change the pH of the body simply by changing your diet. In fact, some of the techniques used in alkalizing can reduce the body's buffering potential and are counterproductive to treating cancer (because they protect the tumor).

The pH of the blood and organs in the human body is tightly regulated to stay within the narrow range of pH 7.35 to 7.45. Deviating from this even a little can be very unhealthy and possibly deadly. You can consume all the alkalizing foods you want; it won't change the pH of the body, but only that of your urine, and to some degree, your gut. So, throw away those pH

---

test sticks; the pH of your urine is meaningless in this regard as it has no relation to the pH of the body as a whole.

There may be some benefit to increasing the urine pH for bladder cancer, but apparently only in smokers (no reduction in bladder cancer risk was found in non-smokers who increased their urine pH).

> "Urine pH is determined primarily by a combination of body surface and dietary intake, where fruits and vegetables contribute to alkalinizing urine pH, whereas meat, fish and dairy products contribute to lowering urine pH. We observed a dose–response relationship in bladder cancer risk with increasing urinary acidity, with no association among non-smokers, a weak association among former smokers, a strong association among current smokers and with evidence of interaction between having consistently acidic urinary pH and heavy smoking." – PubMed ID#PMC3106435 (2011) [852]

If you go too far in your alkalizing efforts in an attempt to change your systemic pH, you may end up overwhelming your gut's ability to compensate. This will raise the pH (alkaline) of your intestines. This is a very bad idea. The body (and the microbiota of the gut) normally keep the pH of the intestine below 7.0 (7 is neutral)—so, slightly acidic. The pH of the small intestine ranges from about 4.0 to about 6.3 (relatively acidic); the pH of the colon slowly increases to about 6.7 at the rectum. This acidic pH is necessary to deter both bad bacteria and intestinal yeast. This may be the opposite of what you've heard on the internet, but there is plenty of actual scientific research behind this (and it can be easily verified by using a smart pill that you swallow to measure the pH). This study is concerning *Candida albicans*, a very problematic yeast that can colonize the colon and small intestine when the conditions are favorable.

> "It is well established that a pH around neutrality favours hyphal development of *C. albicans* in vitro, while a low pH (pH < 6.5) blocks hyphal formation" — ojmm.2013.33028 [853]

Your body has very good systems in place to maintain proper pH throughout the body; the main things it needs to do this are proper mineral levels. To achieve proper mineral levels, your gut needs to be functioning properly, especially in digestion and the small intestine for mineral absorption. The body uses minerals to reduce acidity; it is part of its overall buffering system. So, as part of a healthy diet, consume lots of vegetables and don't worry about the pH of your urine (and if you smoke, quit). Vegetables have many different health benefits, and most of those have some positive influence on the immune system and fighting cancer.

❖ RIFE MACHINE

The Rife machine was invented in 1920 by Royal Raymond Rife. The inventor proposed that the Rife machine could kill any pathogen or parasite, as well as cure cancer and most disease, simply by tuning it to the correct frequency—all the while not harming a single normal human cell. His claims have never been proven by any scientific study, and many researchers (around the world) have tried. Rife claimed that the American Medical Association (AMA) and other establishment medical organizations were conspiring to discredit his work.

The Rife machine is a favorite topic among conspiracy-minded people in the alternative medicine world. To this day, many believe that the Rife machine is a miracle device that not only cures cancer, but also thousands of other diseases. It is these people's belief that the Rife machine is being held back by the medical establishment as it would put thousands of doctors and pharmaceutical companies out of business.

The Rife machine, and the underlying theory behind it, has been studied dozens of times, all over the world. Each time the results have been the same: no evidence of efficacy for treating any disease. The machine is banned in several countries as people have died from forgoing other treatment, believing the hype that their new $1,000 (US dollars) Rife machine would cure their cancer or AIDS. In the US several people have gone to jail for selling the device while making false claims about curing cancer. Today the Rife machine is still sold in many countries. Website claims artfully mention that Royal Raymond Rife cured the cancers of thousands of people, while making no definitive claims about the machine that they are selling today (and yet they list the frequency settings for cancer, AIDS and hundreds of other diseases in their instruction manuals).

A Rife machine is a simple signal generator, not unlike those that have been used since the early 1900s in electronic repair. It simply generates a specific radio frequency (or frequencies) at a specified voltage. They are pretty simple devices. Yet to the average person not trained in electronics, they probably seem just as sophisticated as the medical equipment in an ICU; however, they don't even come close. Anyone with a simple oscilloscope (a device to visually show radio frequency signals, often shown in the background of pictures of Mr. Rife) can see exactly what the Rife machine is doing and easily emulate it with their own signal generator (nice ones can be purchased for $50 to $100—much nicer than what Mr. Rife had available in the early 1900s).

Mr. Rife, if alive today, would argue that it is the precise frequencies he determined that kill disease, and this is the genius behind the invention/discovery. A point worth discussing. So, exactly how did he determine these precise frequencies for thousands of organisms and diseases? He wasn't a doctor; he didn't have the resources for huge scientific studies, and he had no government approvals for doing studies on humans. He also didn't have access to all the bacteria, yeasts, viruses, parasites and cancer cells to test these frequencies. Again, we're talking about thousands of different diseases, and presumably tests would have to be done on multiple subjects for each disease. In short, there is no evidence that these studies were ever conducted. The frequencies were just made up.

When these devices are dissected, electronic engineers have often simply found a battery, wiring, a switch or two, a very simple electronic timer and two lengths of copper tubing. This copper tubing is used to deliver an "almost undetectable" current that is so minute that it may not even penetrate the skin (source: Electronics Australia, via Wikipedia). There is nothing special about the device, and again, the technology is very common in electronics and has been used for decades.

The frequencies that Mr. Rife came up with seem to have been made up at random, and there is no evidence that these specific frequencies kill pathogens or cancer cells, especially at the voltages used in a Rife machine (voltages low enough not to cause any shock—I'm sure the marketing genius didn't want to dissuade customers from purchasing the device).

The question remains today as to exactly how Rife came up with these frequencies. In the 1920s to 1950s, the ability to visualize viruses via a standard microscope was very crude, and most could not be seen at all. So how did Mr. Rife overcome this problem? He invented his own microscope, one that he claimed was 15 times more powerful than the other microscopes of the time, matching the power of electron microscopes produced decades later. The problem is that only 5 of these microscopes were ever produced, and none were ever tested to verify his claims; of course, none of these exist today. It too was a hoax. Even though Rife told the world that he could cure cancer with his machine, he never was able to examine cancer cells under a microscope and believed that cancer was an ultra-small bacillus bacteria, rather than human cells that have run amok (as we know today).

The actual Rife machine, plans and theories have been examined many times. It is a very simple device by today's standards. Researchers around the world have tried to verify whether it can kill bacteria, viruses and cancer cells, and every study has shown that it cannot. Today, unlike in Mr. Rife's time, it is very easy to verify if such a simple device works or not. It does not. Please do not waste your money on such a device, nor risk your life by using one rather than other treatments.

Note: The Rife machine should not be confused with an investigative treatment called pulsed electromagnetic field (PEMF) therapy. PEMF sounds similar in concept, but it is being scientifically validated. Currently there have been a few small in vivo PEMF clinical trials involving humans, and the results of these studies have shown some promise. However, much more research needs to be done before it can be recommended.

❖ OZONE THERAPY

Though not a complete hoax, ozone therapy is way overhyped. It isn't hyped so much by medical doctors, but by alternative doctors, practitioners and (so-called) internet "experts." Ozone treatments can have some uses in disease and skin infection, but their use in cancer treatment shows very little (in vivo) evidence of efficacy.

This isn't to say that ozone can't kill cancer cells; it can. But it also kills normal cells. This puts it in a category similar to chemotherapy, with the goal being to kill more cancer cells than normal ones while trying not to kill the patient in so doing. However, getting ozone to where it needs to go is tricky. Ozone is very volatile; you can't simply drink some ozonated water and hope the ozone gets to the cancer cells. Much like drinking a carbonated beverage, where the

CO_2 leaves the beverage about the same second it hits your stomach (sometimes causing you to belch), so too with ozonated water (the ozone will escape the water, become gas again and be expelled).

The studies on ozone to date have been in vitro, on cancer cells examined by microscope (etc.), or in vivo on research animals (mostly mice). In the in vivo studies, the ozonated water is injected directly into the tumor, which isn't always possible.

In the following study, researchers injected ozonated water directly into the tumors of research mice. They found that this reduced tumor size and decreased metastasis.

> "Necrosis of the tumor cells was observed following local injection of ozonated water directly into the tumor tissues. Moreover, the tumor growth rate was significantly decreased and there was a significant increase in the tumor necrotic area." – PubMed ID#PMC4632793 (2015) [854]

However, this does not kill the cancer cells outside of the tumor area (metastasis cells that cause cancer to spread), and doesn't seem to be able to kill the tumor on its own. The ozonated water must be injected into the tumor; simply drinking it will not work (ozone is very volatile, and the ozonated water will not make it to the site of the tumor after oral consumption). This makes ozone a possible adjunct treatment, to be used alongside traditional treatments, and it must be administered by a doctor. Since surgery would achieve the same goal, this would primarily be used in sensitive areas where surgery wasn't possible. This type of treatment will not work at all for blood cancers or cancers that have already metastasized to other locations.

> "An array of ill-effects are observed owing to the reactivity of O_3 viz oxidation, peroxidation or generation of free radicals and giving rise to cascade of reactions like peroxidation of lipids leading to changes in membrane permeability, lipid ozonation products (LOP) act as signal transducer molecules… which activates the lipases triggering the release of endogenous mediators of inflammation. The loss of functional groups in enzymes leading to enzyme inactivation. These reactions further results in cell injury or eventual cell death. Combinations of O3 and NO2 occur in photochemical smog, have hazardous effects on lung alveoli and act additively or synergistically." – PubMed ID#PMC3312702 (2011) [855]

Much like chemotherapy, ozone is a poison; it does not nourish the body, nor improve the immune system. Though not completely a hoax, it is something I do not recommend.

> *"The dose makes the poison"* ~ Paracelsus (1493-1541)

❖ VITAMIN B17 (LAETRILE)

AKA: Laetrile, amygdalin, madelonitrile, amygdaloside

This is another subject that will cause me to get hate mail. However, once again we must go with the evidence. Western countries do not have a monopoly on apricots or scientific research, and there is no vast conspiracy to keep this treatment from you (as evidenced by the hundreds of research studies in this book on some near-miraculous natural treatments!). I'm afraid Laetrile (amygdalin or vitamin B17) simply is not a miracle cure, and it may even be dangerous.

First let's start with the most basic science: "Vitamin B17" is not a vitamin. It first got this nomenclature in the 1950s from a charlatan trying to avoid the FDA. "B17" is not required by the body, and it isn't recognized by any medical body in any country as a "vitamin." There is no physiological "deficiency" state for amygdalin (B17). However, this isn't the primary issue; most of the nutrients in this book are not "vitamins." The biggest reasons to avoid it are that it doesn't work, and it can be dangerous. There have been many studies on amygdalin, and none have found it to be effective in treating cancer; all have pointed to safety concerns. FDA regulations require significant evidence of safety and efficacy before a new drug is approved for medical use (or sold making medical claims); amygdalin was not able to meet these standards, so the hucksters tried to market it as a vitamin.

Amygdalin (AKA: B17) is a chemical found in the kernels of some stone fruit, such as apricots, peaches and plums. It has been promoted as a cancer cure since the early 1950s. It was first tried as a cancer treatment in Germany in 1892, but it was abandoned due to it being shown to be ineffective and toxic (yes, even way back then, they knew it was toxic). Since the 1950s, amygdalin/Laetrile/vitamin B17 has been tested for cancer treatment efficacy in more than 20 studies; no studies to date have shown that it has any benefit in the treatment of cancer in vivo, and its anticancer abilities in vitro are very limited.

Laetrile is a patented semisynthetic derivative of amygdalin; Laetrile and amygdalin are not the same thing. The "Laetrile" found in Mexican clinics is usually not true Laetrile; it is amygdalin and often is a crude mixture made from crushed apricot pits. However, both Laetrile and amygdalin contain cyanide (or it can be converted to cyanide in the body), and both are dangerous. Oral forms (usually ground-up apricot pits) are much more dangerous than purified injectable forms. This is because the oral form gets broken down by gut bacteria; some bacteria in the gut contain an enzyme called beta-glucosidases, and this enzyme activates the release of hydrogen cyanide (a potent poison) from amygdalin. Though this does not occur with the injected forms, some cyanide is still released. Never consume oral forms of amygdalin or ground apricot pits.

You'll often hear claims that apricot kernels contain no cyanide. Technically this is true; however, the bacteria in our guts convert amygdalin into cyanide.

> "When conventional rats were given single oral doses of amygdalin (600 mg/kg), they sometimes experienced lethargy and convulsions, and usually died within 2 to 5 hr. Rats affected in this way had high concentrations of cyanide in

their blood (2.6–4.5 µg/ml). Germfree rats receiving the same dose of amygdalin did not exhibit these symptoms and had blood cyanide concentrations indistinguishable from those of conventional rats which did not receive amygdalin." – DOI:10.1016/0006-2952(80)90504-3 (1980) [856]

Also see PubMed ID#3089225. [857]

Because there is no reliable research showing that Laetrile can safely treat cancer, it is banned by the US FDA as unsafe, ineffective and often marketed with unproven health claims (FDA.GOV [858]).

There have been many studies looking at amygdalin/Laetrile, and no reputable (reproducible) in vivo study has ever found any benefit in the treatment (or prevention) of any cancer. One study has shown very limited benefit in vitro (in the test tube), but over 20 other studies have shown no benefits. The studies also confirmed that oral administration of amygdalin is associated with far more toxicity than intravenous, intraperitoneal or intramuscular injections, making this very unsafe for DIY applications.

If you research amygdalin online, you will undoubtably find many websites, and even a few books, promoting its miracle healing properties. What you won't find is much, if any, scientific research to back up any of their claims. Without peer-reviewed research to back up these claims, they should be considered worthless (and dangerous). Anyone can make assertions; many (seemingly) commonsense theories have later been proven incorrect when put to the test. Even something that shows promise in one study must be reproducible in scientific peer review. If a medical claim cannot pass this rigor, it should be avoided. I find it ironic that today "B17" is mostly promoted by people very much opposed to chemotherapy; however, this is exactly how Laetrile was originally promoted: as a chemotherapy (at least until those pushing it failed to prove that it actually worked). I've even seen advice on some of these online sites to take amygdalin along with vitamin C; however, research shows that this can make the risks of amygdalin even worse!

"Cancer patients should be informed about the high risk of developing serious adverse effects due to cyanide poisoning after laetrile or amygdalin, especially after oral ingestion. This risk could increase with concomitant intake of vitamin C and in vegetarians with vitamin B12 deficiency." – doi:10.1002/14651858.CD005476.pub3 (2011) [859]

Also see "Cyanide Production From Laetrile in the Presence of Mega-doses of Ascorbic Acid" JAMA (1979). [860]

In 1982 there was a relatively large (178 patients) phase II medical study of Laetrile (*New England Journal of Medicine*, Jan 28th, 1982), where they found that Laetrile had no effect on cancer (in vivo). All of the patients in this study had normal progression of their cancer within a few months. Toxicity was reported in some of them, and blood cyanide levels increased dramatically (doi:10.1056/nejm198201283060403). [861] Remember that the alternative medicine crowd would have you believe that cyanide is only created when amygdalin contacts cancer cells, and thus it does not damage normal cells. If that were the case, whole blood cyanide levels should not increase; however, that was not the case, and blood cyanide levels increased dramatically.

> "The primary objective of this study was to detect evidence that amygdalin... was capable of producing a favorable effect on patients with malignant disease... We purposely chose patients who were in good general condition in order to maximize the possibility of observing benefit. Our data indicated that no therapeutic benefit was produced. Only one questionable, partial, and transient objective response was observed among 171 completely evaluable patients. Even if this response rate was real, a response rate less than 1 per cent certainly can not be regarded as salutary" --
> doi:10.1056/nejm198201283060403 (1982) [862]

I would like to especially advise people to avoid homemade oral apricot kernel treatments, as these can be very dangerous. The whole (unproven) concept of amygdalin is that cancer cells contain an enzyme that creates hydrogen cyanide from amygdalin and kills the cancer cell, whereas normal cells do not contain this enzyme and thus are not harmed (again, this has not been shown by science). However, if you take an oral formulation, your gut bacteria will break down the amygdalin and release the hydrogen cyanide into your gut, where it is then absorbed through the intestine. From there it gets into the bloodstream where it does damage systemically (e.g., all over the body). By taking oral formulas you are simply harming yourself and not even getting the theoretical benefits of amygdalin. If you are bound and determined to take this treatment and ignore all of the research studies/warnings, you will need to shell out the tens of thousands of dollars for intravenous treatments in Mexico or another country that doesn't regulate such substances (though "unregulated" also sounds dangerous to me). Again, even for the intravenous treatments, there is very little evidence that amygdalin helps, and considerable credible evidence that it is ineffective against cancer.

> "In both studies, the animals were treated with intraperitoneal injections of amygdalin, with or without the enzyme beta-glucosidase. None of the solid tumors or leukemias that were investigated responded to amygdalin at any dose that was tested. No statistically significant increase in animal survival was observed in any of the treatment groups. Similar results were obtained in another study using human breast cancer and colon cancer cells implanted into mice (xenograft models). Amygdalin at every dose level tested produced no response either as a single agent or in combination with beta-glucosidase." –
> PubMed ID#NBK65988 (2017) [863]

The following meta-study looked at over 200 research studies of Laetrile or amygdalin. It was undertaken by the Division of Oncology and Hematology at Paracelsus Medical University in Nuremberg, Germany. Out of these 200 studies, they evaluated the 63 that met the criteria of being "randomized control trials" (where those receiving the treatment are compared to a control group not receiving the treatment). Here is what they found.

> "The claims that laetrile or amygdalin have beneficial effects for cancer patients are not currently supported by sound clinical data. There is a considerable risk of serious adverse effects from cyanide poisoning after laetrile or amygdalin, especially after oral ingestion. The risk-benefit balance of laetrile or amygdalin as a treatment for cancer is therefore unambiguously negative." – PubMed ID#25918920 (2015) [864]

There are a small number of in vitro studies showing limited results against a few cancer cell lines (bladder, prostate, cervical and promyelocytic leukemia (HL-60) cells). However, the amygdalin concentrations used in vitro were at high concentrations, and these studies have not worked out how this could be achieved in vivo (in the body) without running into significant issues of cyanide poisoning to non-cancerous cells.

> "In the present study, assessment of cell viability using MTT assay confirmed that amygdalin at high concentrations exhibits a dose-dependent cytotoxicity on the DU145 and LNCaP prostate cancer cells... treatment with high concentrations of amygdalin on the human DU145 and LNCaP prostate cancer cells induced apoptotic cell death" – DOI #10.1248/bpb.29.1597 (2005 – Kyung Hee University)

> "The aim of this review is to summarize all types of clinical data related to the effectiveness or safety of laetrile interventions as a treatment of any type of cancer... Thirty six reports met our inclusion criteria. No controlled clinical trials were found... None of these publications proved the effectiveness of laetrile... the claim that laetrile has beneficial effects for cancer patients is not supported by sound clinical data." – PubMed ID#17106659 (2007) [865]

I took a look at the website of one of the best-known Laetrile clinics in Mexico. One of the first things I saw was a graph showing cancer survival rates for various forms of cancer; they list a 100% 1-year survival rate for breast cancer patients. Further down the page, they have some patient testimonials. Being the researcher that I am, I couldn't help but see if I could find information about these patients (their full names are listed on the website, but I won't use them here). The first one I looked up was a Catherine S.; I was able to find her obituary, and she died in August 2017 of metastatic breast cancer. I was able to find a few more of the patients'

---

obituaries as well. Now to be fair, this outcome is probably possible for people seeing oncologists as well, and these people may have lived for more than a year after receiving treatment. My point is: don't believe the hype, because that is not a valid way to judge the success of cancer treatments. Stick to independent scientific research.

Recommendation

My recommendation is to avoid Laetrile/B17/amygdalin treatments. I would especially avoid homemade oral apricot kernel treatments; these can be very dangerous, especially over time. Where these treatments are allowed by local governments, they are poorly regulated, and preparations are not reliably or independently tested. However, if you insist on seeking out these treatments, I again highly recommend avoiding any oral-based treatments. I would also avoid taking any vitamin C while taking Laetrile, and make sure you get enough vitamin B12.

❖ CARRAGEENAN

AKA: Carrahan, caragahen, pearl moss, Irish moss

One of the hardest things about writing this book is debunking some of the myths. I've found people feel much more strongly about the myths they believe in than they do about those things supported by valid science. I'll leave it to the experts to figure out that mystery.

Carrageenan has been used for centuries for food and medicinal purposes. During the 19th century famine in Ireland, it was consumed by many to supplement their diet. In recent times it has been used in the food industry as a thickener in foods such as ice cream, beer, toothpaste, alternative milks (such as almond and soy milk) and even in diet soda to enhance the flavor. It can often be found in vegan foods as a thickening agent. This hoax claims carrageenan is a carcinogen; it is not.

In 2001 a little-known researcher named Joanne Tobacman released a paper blaming carrageenan for inflammation. Since inflammation has been linked to cancer, Alzheimer's disease, Parkinson's disease and heart diseases, that is not a small matter. However, Tobacman's research has never been replicated, and several studies have shown that food-grade carrageenan does not present an inflammation risk. Researchers now believe that what she used was "poligeenan," a degraded form of carrageenan that behaves very differently from natural food-grade carrageenan in the body. It is like making bioplastic from vegetable matter and then feeding the plastic to people (and saying that vegetables are poison); the vegetables have been denatured and are no longer edible. Poligeenan is used in medical imaging and is not a food; it is a denatured form of carrageenan. Carrageenan has a very high molecular weight; this prevents it from being absorbed through the intestinal wall. Poligeenan has gone through a complicated chemical, heat and mechanical process to turn carrageenan into something that has a very low molecular weight. Because of its low molecular weight, poligeenan can enter the systemic environment and lead to inflammation and possibly other nasty conditions. In fact, researchers use poligeenan to induce inflammation in research animals and in vitro cells so they can test anti-inflammation drugs. Poligeenan should never be consumed by humans.

However, the myth that carrageenan is dangerous has been maintained on the internet. The FDA doesn't consider carrageenan the least bit dangerous, hundreds of scientific researchers do not believe carrageenan is dangerous, and the medical community doesn't consider carrageenan dangerous, but one researcher thought so almost 20 years ago, and thus the myth continues.

> "Food additive carrageenan: Part I: A critical review of carrageenan in vitro studies, potential pitfalls, and implications for human health and safety… Carrageenan (CGN) has been used as a safe food additive for several decades. Confusion over nomenclature, basic CGN chemistry, type of CGN tested, interspecies biology, and misinterpretation of both in vivo and in vitro data has resulted in the dissemination of incorrect information regarding the human safety of CGN." – PubMed ID#24456237 (2014) [866]

> Review of several studies from numerous species indicates that food grade CGN does not produce intestinal ulceration at doses up to 5% in the diet… Based on the many animal subchronic and chronic toxicity studies, CGN has not been found to affect the immune system, as judged by lack of effects on organ histopathology, clinical chemistry, hematology, normal health, and the lack of target organ toxicities. In these studies, animals consumed CGN at orders of magnitude above levels of CGN in the human diet… Dietary CGN has been shown to lack carcinogenic, tumor promoter, genotoxic, developmental, and reproductive effects in animal studies. CGN in infant formula has been shown to be safe in infant baboons and in an epidemiology study on human infants at current use levels." – PubMed ID#24467586 (2014) [867]

If you want to avoid carrageenan, it shouldn't be too difficult, especially if you avoid processed foods. However, there is little scientific evidence that shows food-grade carrageenan causes any human disease.

◆❖◆

Chapter 9
Natural Treatment Protocols

"New opinions are always suspected, and usually opposed, without any other reason but because they are not already common." ~ John Locke

If you've made it this far through the book, you've learned that there is a lot of scientific research that should leave no doubt that you can "*Improve Your Odds*" of preventing—and helping to beat—cancer using nothing but natural foods, supplements and other healthy interventions. Much of the information in this book you've probably never heard before, and some of it your oncologist has never heard before. As I've said many times, none of this information means you should give up on your oncologist! Traditional medical treatments also *Improve Your Odds*, and nearly everything discussed in this book can work synergistically with those treatments—1+1=3 or more! Our medical system is set up to follow one particular path, but there are several paths that can be beneficial. This book also only covers one path, a natural one that can be used as an "adjuvant" (alongside) medical treatments.

What follows is a basic protocol that you can either use as is or adapt to your specific cancer and lifestyle. It serves more as a review of what you've already read than a step-by-step protocol. Remember that the goal of this book is to "*Improve Your Odds*"; I think I've laid out enough evidence to convince you (and probably your oncologist) that this is truly possible. What you want to do is to attack the cancer from as many different directions as you can.

Many of the recommendations in this book involve food that you can add to your diet. You don't have to consume every food, every day; alternate and eat a variety of foods, and don't freak out if you must skip a day. You can also add small amounts of these foods to other dishes: medicinal mushrooms in a casserole, broccoli and flaxseed in a smoothie, larch tree fiber in iced tea, turmeric in scrambled eggs, etc. But if you are serious and want to "*Improve Your Odds*" as much as possible, you'll step outside of your normal comfort foods and try to consume as many of these foods as possible, as frequently as you can.

BASELINE PROTOCOL

> *"Ill-health, of body or of mind, is defeat.*
> *Health alone is victory. Let all men, if they can manage it,*
> *contrive to be healthy!"* ~ *Thomas Carlyle*

The baseline is what everyone should be doing, whether you are treating cancer or trying to prevent it. Remember, this book focuses on the immune system (such as natural immunomodulators) and not on toxins that happen to kill certain cancers (at perhaps a somewhat higher rate than normal cells). Here, what treats cancer can also prevent cancer (unless noted). The immune system is <u>highly</u> selective in what it kills, whereas most drugs are not (with the exception being newer immunotherapy drugs that work with the immune system, rather than against it). As such, the following have been shown in research studies to benefit a wide range of cancers (most likely many more cancers than have been studied to date). All show benefits to general health and the immune system. Therefore, they meet the criterion of "*Improving your Odds*."

What follows is a summary of what has been discussed earlier. Please read the full section for each of these, as dosing, preparation, cautions, etc., may not be fully represented below. Reading the evidence for the efficacy of each of these is very eye-opening and inspiring.

In addition to what follows, you should use the index to search for references to your particular type of cancer; hopefully, you have also been highlighting for your particular cancer. There will likely be other supplements or foods you'll want to add to this protocol for maximum benefit.

Remember, this should not replace your medical treatment.

Supplements

The following is a baseline supplement list. This is where most people start unless there are reasons not to (genetic issues, allergies, etc.) Recommendations of brands/forms can be found on the book's website (address listed at the bottom of every other page).

1. **Mushrooms** – Consume a variety of medicinal mushrooms each and every day. The importance here is hard to overstate. See the full recommendations in Chapter 6. In addition to regularly consuming mushrooms, I recommend taking a powdered supplement with a mix of medicinal mushrooms. We need a variety of good mushrooms, not a large amount of any one type. The supplements and powder mix I currently take, and recommend, are listed on the website at https://www.improvingyourodds.com/wp/supplements/ I also recommend

consuming chaga tea daily. See the following link at *The Gut Health Protocol* for <u>how to make it</u>. Because it is concentrated, I can make a week's worth at a time. [868] Highest recommendation.

2. **Beta-Glucans** - Consume a wide variety of beta-glucans from foods. In addition to those in the mushroom powder, you can also take a beta-glucan supplement. This is explained in much more detail in Chapter 6. Food sources are what will provide diversity.

3. **Bifidobacteria** – Take a good probiotic that contains Bifidobacterium probiotics (see Chapter 2); these are very important for tuning the immune system to fight cancer. Our understanding of this topic is just now starting to show how truly important this is. I recommend one that contains a "phage complex." Normally when you take a probiotic, the beneficial bacteria die in the first few feet of the colon and are not measurable in the stool. The phage complex kills some of the bad competition, and these dead bacteria feed the Bifidobacterium throughout the gut (the cells are in part made of beta-glucans). Studies have shown this can amplify the amount of Bifidobacteria by 10 to 100 times (from what you take as a capsule, to what is measured in the stool). As you can tell from Chapter 2, having good Bifidobacteria levels is very important for the immune system to fight and prevent cancer. See the book's website for a recommendation. Highly recommended.

4. **Larch Tree Arabinogalactan** – 1.5 grams/twice daily. With the brand that I use, this is one scoop of powder, twice per day. It can be mixed into any liquid and wet foods (e.g., in a casserole recipe). Everyone should be taking this. Great for the immune system (as well as gut health) and has good evidence of efficacy. Highly recommended.

5. **Cinnamon Oil** – 1 to 2 drops per day. Be sure to read the section in Chapter 6 for more details, because it is important to take the correct type in the right way. This is for treatment, though for prevention, you can take one drop 2 to 3 times per week to spice a smoothie, tea, coffee, etc. I recommend taking the probiotic supplement at least 2 hours away from cinnamon oil.

6. **Turmeric and Curcumin** – Absorption is key with curcumin. If you cook with turmeric, always include some fat and black pepper, as both help with absorption. I recommend one of the highly assimilated supplements that have evidence of efficacy (see Chapter 6). Because of its improved absorption, not a lot is needed. For prevention, I recommend 30 mg (1 small capsule per day) of Theracumin; for treatment I recommend 2 to 6 capsules per day (60 to 180 mg). You will need to start slowly and increase the dose by 1 capsule every week. Try not to take more than 2 capsules every 3 hours (e.g., if you decide to take 6 capsules, take 2 in the morning, 2 at noon and 2 at dinner). There is an oil-based form with a highly absorbable form of curcumin called tetra-hydro-curcuminoids; I take this one as well.

7. **Modified Citrus Pectin (MCP)** – If you are eating the "vegan + meat" diet and taking other prebiotic supplements, you probably don't need this one for prevention. For treatment you can take 5 to 10 grams per day. Mix with chaga tea, smoothies, etc.

8. **Fucoidan** – Great for strengthening the immune system, and it can also fight cancer through various mechanisms. Risk of side effects is very low. I recommend 500 mg once per day for prevention and twice per day for treatment. Fucoidan supplements will contain varying amounts of iodine. If you have Hashimoto's disease, see the cautions in the Iodine section of this book and discuss supplementing with your doctor.

9. **Omega-3** – 2 to 5 grams per day. See the "Strategy" section under Omega-3 in Chapter 6. Take a dosage on the low end for prevention and on the high end for treatment.

10. **Melatonin** – 3 mg before bed is all you need; more is not better. Also see the section on melatonin for more information and why it is so important. If you are following the circadian rhythm recommendations and sleep well, you only need 3 mg on cloudy days.

11. **Minerals** – We should all try to eat a healthy diet, full of organic vegetables and tubers high in minerals. But taking a good mineral supplement can be helpful as well. Just make sure it is a "supplement" to what you are doing through diet, and not a replacement. I take added magnesium due to a history of deficiency. Prevention and treatment are the same: Try to get enough, but don't overdo it; more is not better.

12. **Vitamin D** –5,000 IU per day. Unless you work outside or sunbathe, it is hard to get enough vitamin D. Nearly everyone needs this. More than 5,000 IU is needed if you have confirmed low vitamin D levels and you need to catch up. Work with your healthcare provider for a catchup protocol. It is best to get some from the sun; see the section in Chapter 6 for more information. Be sure to also take a magnesium and K2 supplement (as discussed in Chapter 6).

13. **Vitamin K2** – 75 to 150 mcg. I take this in a supplement combined with vitamin D3. You can take up to 300 mcg per day (though no toxicity level has been defined), but more may not provide additional benefits. Everyone can take this.

14. **Vitamin A** – Few of us get enough retinol, so a supplement is useful here. On days you consume liver, skip your vitamin A supplement. See Chapter 6 for more information.

15. **Vitamin C** – I do not supplement additional vitamin C; can you believe it!? Chaga is supposed to be high in vitamin C, but I haven't seen reliable information on how much it contains. The vegetables and low-sugar fruit I consume are also high in vitamin C. Obtain it from food when possible. See Chapter 6 as to why I don't take added vitamin C.

16. **Vitamin E** – I take 170 mg of mixed natural tocopherols and tocotrienols (it contains only 19 mg of d-alpha-Tocopherol). The goal here is to obtain high-quality mixed tocopherols and tocotrienols. Taking too much synthetic vitamin E can interfere with the immune system's ability to kill tumors, so mega-dose amounts are not recommended (and that is what most vitamin E supplements contain). If you eat plenty of nuts, green leafy vegetables, avocado and ocean fish, you are probably getting enough vitamin E, especially for prevention.

17. **Folate** – Eating a diet with lots of healthy green vegetables will provide for most of your folate needs. For treatment, you may also want to take a supplement; see Chapter 6 for details. Try to avoid "folic acid" as many people have trouble converting this synthetic version to the natural version the body can use, and that can prevent absorption of natural folate.

18. **Bilberry/Blueberry** – 1 tsp per day of a concentrated bilberry or blueberry powder supplement. I take ½ tsp, twice per day.

---

19. **Green Tea** – 2 to 3 cups per day. See cautions under Green Tea/EGCG in Chapter 6. Some people should avoid or limit consumption.

20. **Black Seed Extract (*Nigella sativa*)** – 1,500 to 2,000 mg per day (usually 4 capsules), divided doses (e.g., 500 mg, 3 times per day), take with a meal or food. Start with 1 capsule per day and work up slowly; watch for gut irritation.

21. ***Boswellia serrata*** – Also known as frankincense. Take 500 mg twice per day.

22. **Chrysin** – 500 mg, twice per day. This is especially important for melanoma and colon cancer adjuvant treatment and prevention.

23. **Ginger** – Consume fresh ginger in food when possible and drink ginger tea. In addition, supplement a minimum of 1,500 mg (1.5 grams) of ginger per day for best results.

Foods to Consume

- **Mushrooms** – Try to include various types of mushrooms in cooking; they go well with most savory dishes. This is in addition to a medicinal mushroom powder. You can also add mushroom powders to various foods prior to cooking (such as a casserole, soups and stews). It adds that "umami" flavor to savory dishes.

- **Sweet Potato** – Try to consume at least a little, 3 to 4 times per week. No need to purchase supplements. Sweet potato is easy to sneak into casseroles, soups, stews, hash or by itself. Purple sweet potatoes are best if you can find them.

- **Garlic** – Fresh is best, and this means eating raw garlic whenever possible. Consume within two hours of crushing. Try to consume at least 3 cloves of raw garlic per week. See its section in Chapter 6 for more details on how to consume it (how it's prepared is important).

- **Ginger** – Great in stir-fries or as a tea.

- **Fish** – High in omega-3s. See the list of low-mercury options in Chapter 6, Foods and Food Fractions, Omega-3 Fatty Acids.

- Lots of **cruciferous vegetables**, especially their sprouts. These should be consumed raw or fermented when possible. Great for making slaws or mixed into any salad.

- Lots of **vegetables**. Remember, the best diet is "vegan + meat." Be adventurous and try new things as often as possible. Consume about 70% cooked vegetables and 30% raw. The nutrition in cooked vegetables is more bioavailable, and the soluble fiber is more available to our microbiome. Make those raw vegetables cruciferous ones when possible.

- Use **stevia** to sweeten; it is the only natural sweetener with evidence of fighting cancer (rather than causing it). Monk fruit is OK but doesn't have the benefits. Avoid all artificial sweeteners!

See Chapter 4 for more diet recommendations.

Other

Sleep and Exercise – Are very important and should not be ignored. See Chapter 5 for much more on these topics. More sleep can be an easy one; for many people it is simply allocating less time to TV or the computer and going to bed earlier. Of course, for those with insomnia or other sleeping problems, it may not be so easy. Exercise is no less important; it has been shown to be highly beneficial to our immune system and healing. Even though not a lot of time has been spent on these two subjects, it doesn't mean they aren't important.

Diet – Ketogenic and/or intermittent fasting. Low-sugar/low-glycemic index foods are very important. See Chapter 4 for more information. Way too much to cover here.

Positive Thinking – It is more important than we even know at this point. Many people who show improvements from the placebo effect are actually getting better due to positive thinking. Skip the placebo and just enjoy every minute of every day! Focus on spiritually uplifting, fun and funny movies, shows and events. Avoid anything dark, upsetting, horror, frightening, etc.

Detoxification – Most of what you hear about "detox" in the public media is probably garbage. We do need to detoxify, and there are things we can do to improve detoxifying, but some of the popular internet media ideas (e.g., green coffee bean enemas, high-dose vitamin C, ozone treatments, etc., etc.) not only have no scientific basis, but may be dangerous. Stick to the science on this one.

Near Infrared – I have a very inexpensive setup (as described in Chapter 7) and enjoy it. When I turn it on, I can instantly feel a soothing effect even before feeling the heat. My whole mood changes within seconds.

EMF – I advise everyone to try to reduce their EMF exposure and to be aware of what the major sources of EMF are in their home. I do <u>not</u> think people need to remove all sources of EMF from their home! We have whole-house WiFi coverage, and I plan to keep it! There simply is not good science showing that these very low-power, high-frequency devices are a problem, especially if kept a few feet away from where we spend time.

Avoid – I can't summarize this one. Please read the end of Chapter 4 for what you should avoid in your diet, Chapter 7, and Chapter 8 for the short list of hoaxes. Just keep in mind that there is a LOT of false information on the internet. If there isn't good science behind it, it's probably just made up. Apparently, there are a lot of lonely people in their parents' basements with nothing better to do than make things up.

Alcohol – I would avoid alcohol while treating cancer and always consume in moderation if you care about preventing cancer. There are a lot of reasons for this. Alcohol has a direct correlation with several cancers, including: stomach, colon, esophagus, rectum, liver, breast and ovarian. But one of the most important reasons to avoid alcohol is that has a seriously negative effect on the immune system, as well as the all-important gut microbiome.

Updates at - https://improvingyourodds.com

Support at - https://www.facebook.com/groups/cancer.improving.your.odds

"Clinicians have long observed an association between excessive alcohol consumption and adverse immune-related health effects such as susceptibility to pneumonia… This issue of Alcohol Research: Current Reviews (ARCR) summarizes the evidence that alcohol disrupts immune pathways in complex and seemingly paradoxical ways. These disruptions can impair the body's ability to defend against infection, contribute to organ damage associated with alcohol consumption, and impede recovery from tissue injury… Alcohol consumption also **damages** epithelial cells, **T cells, and neutrophils** in the GI system, disrupting gut barrier function and facilitating leakage of microbes into the circulation" – NIH.GOV [869]

Gut Health – A very important topic. Again, this is hard to summarize, and you will at least need to read Chapter 3. But don't forget to take care of your gut; it is extremely important for a well-functioning immune system, especially those Bifidobacteria. It would be difficult for me to overemphasize this. Oncologists are now starting to stress the importance of gut health when discussing immunotherapy (mine did. We really geeked out on it).

In addition to the above, you should **use the index to search for your particular cancer**. There may be other supplements or foods you'll want to add to this protocol for maximum benefit.

If you would like more information on gut health, I would like to highly recommend my book, The Gut Health Protocol, available on Amazon. [870] I also have a specially formulated probiotic/prebiotic called "Phage Complete"; I formulated this myself and both my wife and I take it twice daily! [871] In accordance with FDA regulations, I make no cancer claims for this product. This product is not intended to diagnose, treat, cure, or prevent any disease.

Updates at - https://improvingyourodds.com/

Support at - https://www.facebook.com/groups/cancer.improving.your.odds

◆❖◆

--- This Page Intentionally Left Blank --

Appendix Y
Glossary/List of Abbreviations

In this glossary, I've included some of the more common medical words I thought people might want to look up. However, the research studies include many complex words that the average person may never have heard before. As I mentioned at the beginning of this book, it is not always necessary to understand every word of the abstract in order to understand the point being made. However, if you wish to look up these words, you can use one of the following online medical dictionaries: The Free Dictionary (medical), [872] Merriam-Webster – Medical Dictionary, [873] Medical-Dictionary, and [874] MediLexicon. [875]

Adjuvant	A treatment given in conjunction with another, primary, treatment to either improve its effectiveness, decrease recurrence or reduce side effects.
Angiogenesis	The process by which new blood vessels are formed. Cancer tumors can release angiogenesis-signaling chemicals to cause the body to provide them with more blood vessels.
Antiproliferation	To inhibit or prevent the growth of cancer tumors or the development of malignant cells.
Apoptosis	This is a function of normal cells often referred to as "preprogrammed cell death." When a cell becomes cancerous, damaged or even just too old, it is supposed to automatically kill itself. This function is often defective in cancer cells, allowing them to grow uncontrolled. Returning the apoptosis function to normal in cancer cells has the potential to rid the body of that cancer or at least prevent metastasis. You can read more about this here. [876]

Ayurvedic medicine	One of the world's oldest medical systems, it got its start over 3,000 years ago in India. It is based on natural and holistic approaches.
Cancer	A term used to describe nearly 100 different diseases. What each of these have in common is uncontrolled growth of cells. Cancer also has the ability to migrate from the original location and spread to distant sites within the body.
CBD	Cannabidiol – A naturally occurring constituent of cannabis. Cannabis, or marijuana, contains at least 113 different cannabinoids. THC is the psychoactive cannabinoid found in marijuana.
CD8+ T cell	A cytotoxic T cell / T lymphocyte (a type of white blood cell and vital part of the immune system) that can kill cancer cells, cells that are infected (particularly by viruses), or cells that are damaged in some other way.
Cemiplimab	Libtayo – An immunotherapy drug, PD-1 inhibitor
CFU	The abbreviation for colony-forming units. For example, it is often used to describe how many bacteria are found in a probiotic.
Contraindicated	Something that one would be ill advised to take with another supplement or medicine. For example, it may be contraindicated to take aspirin along with a blood thinning agent.
Cytotoxic	Something that is toxic or damaging to cells. Often used to describe a substance that can kill cancer cells (though it may also kill non-cancer cells).
Dendritic cells	The main function of these cells is to process antigen material and present it on the cell surface for T cells. They are known as antigen-presenting cells (APC). Once activated, dendritic cells interact with T cells and B cells and help shape the adaptive immune response.

Differentiation	Differentiated cancer cells look more like normal cancer cells (under a microscope) and are less dangerous than undifferentiated cells. Poorly differentiated cells tend to grow and spread more quickly.
Disaccharide	A sugar (or carbohydrate) made up of two monosaccharides. They are held together by a glycosidic bond. Disaccharides are water soluble molecules.
Endocannabinoids	Cannabinoids that are native to the human body. They activate the same receptors in the body as the drug THC (found in marijuana) does. They are one of the brain's natural messengers, perhaps used in stress-related situations with possible applications in eating, disease treatment and social behavior. Their exact uses in the brain are not well understood at this time.
Exocannabinoids	Cannabinoids originating outside the body. This would include the 113 different cannabinoids found in cannabis, including THC.
FDA	Abbreviation for the Food and Drug Administration. Regulates some food products, drugs, vaccines and medical devices within the USA.
FMT	Abbreviation for "Fecal Matter Transplant." A procedure for transferring fecal matter from one person's colon to another's. This is used to transfer beneficial bacteria (and other organisms) from one person to another with the goal of improving the health of the recipient.
Glioblastoma	A very aggressive brain cancer. You can find out more about it on the Mayo Clinic's website. [877]
Glioma	A type of tumor that starts in the glial cells of the brain or the spine. Glioblastoma is one type of glioma.
Immunomodulator	Something that modulates, or changes, the immune response. Usually used when discussing something beneficial. Such as foods that can feed beneficial bacteria that help train T cells. The food has no direct relation with the T cells (a component of the immune system), but it has an indirect benefit by causing a change to the T cells.

Immunosurveillance	The ability of the immune system to detect and respond to threats or aberrant cells. This would include the ability to detect cancer cells (this is where immunotherapy can help; see Chapter 2).
Immunotherapy	Any therapy that improves the immune system or the immune response. Cancer immunotherapy uses the body's own immune system to fight cancer. The therapy may stimulate the immune system to work harder or help the immune system "see" cancer cells better.
Intraperitoneal	Usually refers to an injection method where the substance is injected into the peritoneum (body cavity), rather than a blood vessel. In cancer therapy this often is done through a previously installed "port."
In vitro	In the test tube. For example, experiments done outside the living body and in an artificial environment.
In vivo	In the body. For example, experiments done inside the body of either animals or humans.
Ketogenic	Something that produces the state of ketosis, a biochemical process by which ketone bodies are created by the breakdown of fatty acids. This is usually done by the body rather than burning glucose for energy.
Ketones	Your body produces ketones when it doesn't have enough insulin to turn sugar (or glucose) into energy <u>or</u> when it doesn't have enough carbohydrates to convert to glucose (and therefore it burns fat for energy). The first example occurs in diabetics and can be dangerous. The second example occurs in people who are on a ketogenic (low carbohydrate/high fat) diet, and this second form of ketosis is not dangerous (see Chapter 4).
Lymphocytes	A type of white blood cell that can fight bacteria, viruses, cancer cells, etc. One of the more important types of lymphocytes for cancer treatment are "T cells." Also see "TIL" below.

Updates at - https://improvingyourodds.com

Support at - https://www.facebook.com/groups/cancer.improving.your.odds

Melanoma	A very aggressive and dangerous form of skin cancer.
Metastasis	The ability of cancer cells to move from the primary tumor site to a different, or secondary, site. When this occurs in the body, the cancer is said to have "metastasized."
Metastatic	A type of cancer that has spread from one location to another.
Microbiome	A community of microorganisms that inhabit a specific environment. Often this refers to the microorganisms living within the human (or animal) gut.
Microbiota	The actual microorganisms living in the microbiome. See "microbiome" above.
Microenvironment	In the context of this book, this refers to the environment surrounding the tumor (known as the "tumor microenvironment" or TME). This includes the surrounding blood vessels, immune cells, fibroblasts, signaling molecules and the extracellular matrix.
Microvilli	Microscopic projections of absorptive cells that line the small intestine. The villi and microvilli absorb the vitamins, minerals, sugars, etc., into the bloodstream.
Monosaccharide	A simple sugar that is the most basic form of carbohydrate. Glucose and fructose are examples of monosaccharides.
Nivolumab	Opdivo – An immunotherapy drug and PD-1 inhibitor.
Oncologist	A type of medical doctor who specializes in the prevention, diagnosis and treatment of cancer.
OR	Odds ratio. A statistic that defines the odds associated between two variables. See the Wikipedia article for a more lengthy explanation. [878]

Paywall	A method of restricting access to academic papers and research studies by charging a fee for access.
PD-1/PD-L1	Types of proteins found on the surfaces of cells (PD-1 is found on T cells; PD-L1 is found on normal human cells and cancer cells). The interaction between PD-1 and PD-L1 instructs immune system T cells not to attack the cell. Some cancer cells produce large amounts of PD-L1 in order to hide from the immune system.
Peer review	A process where research is independently reviewed by someone (or some organization) competent to judge the research presented to them. This is often done by subject matter journals (such as the *Journal of Clinical Oncology*).
Pembrolizumab	Keytruda – An immunotherapy drug and PD-1 inhibitor.
PubMed	PubMed is a free search engine run by the US government's National Institutes of Health. PubMed comprises more than 30 million citations for biomedical literature from MEDLINE, life science journals, and online books. Citations may include links to full-text content from PubMed Central and publisher web sites.
NED	No Evidence of Disease. This means that the cancer appears to be in full remission and the doctors can find no evidence of any viable cancer.
Neoplasm	A type of abnormal growth of tissue caused by the rapid division of cells that have undergone some form of mutation. A neoplasm can either be benign or pre-cancerous.
NK cells	Natural killer cells. A type of lymphocyte (white blood cell) that plays a major role in fighting both tumors and virally infected cells.
Phages	AKA: Bacteriophages. A type of virus that infects and replicates within bacteria. They cannot infect human or animal cells and thus

	are not harmful to humans. Some types of phages kill bacteria cells very quickly after infecting them.
Polysaccharide	A large, complex molecule made of many smaller monosaccharides. Polysaccharides are complex sugars or carbohydrates and can have many functions within the body, some of which are medicinal in nature.
Prebiotic	Generally, prebiotics are carbohydrates that are not digestible by humans and go on to feed beneficial bacteria.
Probiotic	Probiotics are live microorganisms intended to provide health benefits to the host when consumed, generally by improving or restoring the microbiome (gut flora).
RCC	Renal cell carcinoma. A type of kidney cancer.
ROS	Reactive oxygen species. Chemically active prooxidant molecules that are generated by incomplete reduction of oxygen. ROS are involved in a variety of physiological and pathological processes in the cell. ROS can either be beneficial or detrimental to tumors depending on the level of ROS activity.
SCFA	Short-chain fatty acid. Fatty acids produced in the gut by beneficial bacteria. May be cancer-preventative for colon cancer. They also help to maintain a healthy balance of gut bacteria, which are important for the immune system.
SLNB	The abbreviation for sentinel lymph node biopsy. This is where the lymph nodes that the area of the tumor drains into are removed and examined for cancer. If the nodes are found to be cancerous, the cancer is then usually staged at stage III or higher.
Stage	As in cancer stage. A process for determining how widespread cancer is in the body and how severe it is. How cancer is staged varies from cancer to cancer. The stages range from stage 0, the least dangerous, to stage IV, meaning that cancer has metastasized to organs or spread throughout the body. See the following Wikipedia article for more information. [879]

T cells	A type of immune system lymphocyte (or white blood cell). Responsible for killing targeted invaders, such as cancer cells, bacteria and viruses. A major component of our immune response.
TCM	Traditional Chinese medicine
THC	Tetrahydrocannabinol, one of 113 cannabinoids found in cannabis. THC is the active component in marijuana that is responsible for its mind-altering effects.
TIL	Tumor-infiltrating lymphocytes. An important measure of how well the immune system is attacking tumors. It shows how well lymphocytes (white blood cells such as T cells) are leaving the bloodstream and reaching the tumor. They are commonly seen on tumor biopsies rated as "absent," "non-brisk," and "brisk," with "brisk" being the best rating.
Tumor	A tumor is an abnormal mass of tissue that may be solid or fluid-filled. Some tumors are benign (not cancerous and cannot spread, although they may still cause harm), while others may be malignant (cancerous).
WLE	Wide local excision. A surgical procedure that removes a small area of disease or cancer, along with a margin of tissue around the tumor area. Often used with melanoma and other skin cancers.
Xenograft	When tissue or an organ is transplanted from one species (e.g., a human) to another (e.g., a mouse). Commonly used to test new cancer treatments, as effectiveness against human cancers can be tested in mice.

◆ ❖ ◆

Appendix Z
Disclaimer and Usage Permissions

Neither the author of this book, nor the contributors, are doctors or medical professionals. This book is not intended as medical advice, nor is it meant to treat, cure, or prevent any medical condition. The nutritional information presented here is for educational use only. The author will not be held liable for any issues that arise if someone applies the information here to their medical condition.

It is my hope that everyone is receiving proper medical treatment and/or monitoring of their condition. This protocol should not be used as a substitute for the services of a licensed practitioner. Feel free to share this information with your healthcare professional to get their opinion and advice. The information provided here may not even apply to your condition or situation, which is why you should be treated by a doctor. Because children and people with other medical conditions are normally excluded from the research studies quoted in this book, people in those groups should always be seen by a medical professional before changing their diet, taking any supplements or trying to self-treat their condition.

The research information included in this book has been specially formatted so that your doctor can look up the research studies from the PubMed or DOI document IDs. This makes it easy for you to highlight the information and share it with your doctor. There should be no excuse for not doing so.

❖ Usage Permissions

For further information, email <herronj@improvingyourodds.com>

You may share snippets of information in this book with your medical practitioner in order to seek medical advice. Like any other book, you are welcome to loan it to friends and family.

❖ UPDATES AND DISCUSSION

You can find me at https://improvingyourodds.com, where I will be posting updates, relevant stories and new research studies.

For support and discussion on the topic of *Improving Your Odds* of treating or preventing cancer, join us on Facebook at:

https://www.facebook.com/groups/cancer.improving.your.odds

Here there are plenty of people with health issues very similar to your own and plenty of people, including myself, ready to lend advice.

> *If you would like more information on gut health, I would like to highly recommend my book, The Gut Health Protocol, available on Amazon. [880] I also have a specially formulated probiotic/prebiotic called "Phage Complete"; I formulated this myself, and both my wife and I take it twice daily! [881] In accordance with FDA regulations, I make no cancer claims for this product. This product is not intended to diagnose, treat, cure, or prevent any disease.*

❖ NOTE REGARDING STUDIES IN THIS BOOK

Due to the complexities around copyrighted research studies, most of the study excerpts in this book were taken from the abstracts appearing on nih.gov's PubMed site and other repositories of research document abstracts. In many cases the full studies were reviewed for the author's educational purposes and comment. In some situations, very small sections of these full studies are quoted here under the copyright "Fair Use Doctrine" where discussion and commentary were necessary. Larger portions of studies were used from those that are licensed under an appropriate "Creative Commons" license agreement. Every effort was made to give proper citation to these studies and authors, and I appreciate them making this research available to the public.

All excerpts from cited material are used for criticism and review. Appropriate attribution is determined by the authors and may be found at the cited location.

If you believe a study or paper in this publication was used improperly, please contact me at herronj@improvingyourodds.com

❖ REVISIONS

12/2019 - 1st Revision

Updates at - https://improvingyourodds.com/

Support at - https://www.facebook.com/groups/cancer.improving.your.odds

◆ ❖ ◆

--- This Page Intentionally Left Blank ---

Index/Endnotes

◆❖◆

Notes

[1] https://www.mskcc.org/cancer-care/diagnosis-treatment/symptom-management/integrative-medicine/herbs

[2] https://www.ncbi.nlm.nih.gov/pmc/articles/PMC5679595/

[3] https://www.washingtonpost.com/news/wonk/wp/2014/11/18/does-it-really-cost-2-6-billion-to-develop-a-new-drug/

[4] https://www.ncbi.nlm.nih.gov/pmc/articles/PMC5067200/

[5] https://www.ncbi.nlm.nih.gov/pmc/articles/PMC1994798/

[6] https://www.ncbi.nlm.nih.gov/pmc/articles/PMC4369959/

[7] https://ourworldindata.org/cancer

[8] http://bit.ly/2XpJETz

[9] https://www.webmd.com/cancer/immunotherapy-treatment-types

[10] https://www.ncbi.nlm.nih.gov/pubmed/29097493

[11] https://www.ncbi.nlm.nih.gov/pmc/articles/PMC5845387/

[12] https://www.ncbi.nlm.nih.gov/pmc/articles/PMC6423251/

[13] https://ascopubs.org/doi/10.1200/JCO.2017.35.15_suppl.3008

[14] https://www.ncbi.nlm.nih.gov/pmc/articles/PMC4873287/

[15] https://www.imperial.ac.uk/news/192887/antibiotics-reduce-survival-rates-cancer-patients/

[16] https://www.ncbi.nlm.nih.gov/pubmed/31513236

[17] https://www.ncbi.nlm.nih.gov/pmc/articles/PMC3339609/

[18] https://www.ncbi.nlm.nih.gov/pmc/articles/PMC5937616/

[19] https://www.ncbi.nlm.nih.gov/pmc/articles/PMC5592279/

[20] https://www.ncbi.nlm.nih.gov/pubmed/12211223/

[21] https://www.ncbi.nlm.nih.gov/pmc/articles/PMC6044372/

---

[22] https://www.ncbi.nlm.nih.gov/pmc/articles/PMC5834761/

[23] https://www.ncbi.nlm.nih.gov/pmc/articles/PMC5973856/

[24] https://www.ncbi.nlm.nih.gov/pmc/articles/PMC5069311/

[25] https://www.ncbi.nlm.nih.gov/pubmed/27057439/

[26] https://www.ncbi.nlm.nih.gov/pmc/articles/PMC4597191/

[27] https://www.ncbi.nlm.nih.gov/pmc/articles/PMC5130043/

[28] http://amzn.to/2f5RRec

[29] https://ubiome.com/blog/post/can-microbiome-affect-effectiveness-cancer-treatment/

[30] https://www.ncbi.nlm.nih.gov/pmc/articles/PMC2515351/

[31] https://www.ncbi.nlm.nih.gov/pubmed/29061314

[32] https://www.ncbi.nlm.nih.gov/pmc/articles/PMC6267863/

[33] https://www.ncbi.nlm.nih.gov/pmc/articles/PMC4873287/

[34] https://www.ncbi.nlm.nih.gov/pubmed/29097494

[35] https://science.sciencemag.org/content/364/6446/1179.full

[36] https://www.ncbi.nlm.nih.gov/pmc/articles/PMC3145055/

[37] http://amzn.to/2f5RRec

[38] http://amzn.to/2f5RRec

[39] https://www.ncbi.nlm.nih.gov/pubmed/22575588

[40] https://www.ncbi.nlm.nih.gov/pmc/articles/PMC5408367/

[41] http://bit.ly/2NW19en (New York University)

[42] https://www.ncbi.nlm.nih.gov/pmc/articles/PMC4690201/

[43] https://www.ncbi.nlm.nih.gov/pmc/articles/PMC5856380/

[44] https://www.ncbi.nlm.nih.gov/pubmed/15806096/

[45] https://www.ncbi.nlm.nih.gov/pmc/articles/PMC3511874/

[46] http://bit.ly/2ECIuzE (Targeted Oncology)

[47] https://www.ncbi.nlm.nih.gov/pubmed/24382758/

[48] https://www.ncbi.nlm.nih.gov/pubmed/24333719

[49] https://www.ncbi.nlm.nih.gov/pubmed/25625500

[50] https://www.ncbi.nlm.nih.gov/pubmed/19722233

[51] https://www.ncbi.nlm.nih.gov/pubmed/12216068

[52] http://amzn.to/2f5RRec

[53] http://bit.ly/phagecomplete

[54] https://www.ncbi.nlm.nih.gov/pmc/articles/PMC4780226/

[55] https://www.ncbi.nlm.nih.gov/pmc/articles/PMC2687095/

[56] https://www.ncbi.nlm.nih.gov/pubmed/18469262

[57] https://www.ncbi.nlm.nih.gov/pmc/articles/PMC2849637/

[58] https://www.cell.com/current-biology/fulltext/S0960-9822(18)30703-6

[59] https://charliefoundation.org/

[60] https://knowthecause.com/ketogenic-diet-confusion/

[61] https://www.ncbi.nlm.nih.gov/pmc/articles/PMC4215472/

[62] https://www.ncbi.nlm.nih.gov/pmc/articles/PMC5450454/

[63] https://www.ncbi.nlm.nih.gov/pubmed/23755243/

[64] https://www.ncbi.nlm.nih.gov/pubmed/23743570/

[65] https://www.ncbi.nlm.nih.gov/pmc/articles/PMC5110522/

[66] https://www.ncbi.nlm.nih.gov/pubmed/26053068/

[67] https://www.ncbi.nlm.nih.gov/pubmed/25773851/

[68] https://www.ncbi.nlm.nih.gov/pubmed/25228990/

[69] https://www.cell.com/cell/fulltext/S0092-8674(11)00127-9

[70] https://www.ncbi.nlm.nih.gov/pmc/articles/PMC2408928/

[71] https://www.ncbi.nlm.nih.gov/pmc/articles/PMC5624453/

[72] https://www.ncbi.nlm.nih.gov/pubmed/28653283

[73] https://www.ncbi.nlm.nih.gov/pmc/articles/PMC3826507/

[74] https://www.ncbi.nlm.nih.gov/pmc/articles/PMC3654894/

[75] https://clinicaltrials.gov/ct2/show/NCT01535911

[76] https://www.ncbi.nlm.nih.gov/pmc/articles/PMC4371612/

[77] https://www.ncbi.nlm.nih.gov/pmc/articles/PMC4235292/

[78] https://www.ncbi.nlm.nih.gov/pubmed/19049606

[79] https://www.ncbi.nlm.nih.gov/pmc/articles/PMC4235292/

[80] https://www.ncbi.nlm.nih.gov/pmc/articles/PMC3267662/

[81] https://www.ncbi.nlm.nih.gov/pmc/articles/PMC2716748/

[82] https://www.ncbi.nlm.nih.gov/pmc/articles/PMC5608861/

[83] https://www.ncbi.nlm.nih.gov/pubmed/21794124

[84] https://amzn.to/2YJs9hj

[85] https://amzn.to/33fcqtJ

[86] https://amzn.to/2T9Swf3

[87] https://amzn.to/31GcBg8

[88] https://www.webmd.com/vitamins/ai/ingredientmono-915/medium-chain-triglycerides-mcts

[89] http://journal.waocp.org/?sid=Entrez:PubMed&id=pmid:25773851&key=2015.16.5.2061

[90] https://www.ncbi.nlm.nih.gov/pmc/articles/PMC5630289/

[91] https://www.ncbi.nlm.nih.gov/pubmed/18447912

[92] https://www.ncbi.nlm.nih.gov/pmc/articles/PMC4669977/

[93] https://www.ncbi.nlm.nih.gov/pubmed/3219268

[94] https://www.ncbi.nlm.nih.gov/pmc/articles/PMC5622605/

[95] https://www.ncbi.nlm.nih.gov/pubmed/15298947/

[96] https://www.ncbi.nlm.nih.gov/pubmed/22323820/

[97] https://en.wikipedia.org/wiki/Intermittent_fasting

[98] https://www.healthline.com/nutrition/intermittent-fasting-guide

[99] https://www.ncbi.nlm.nih.gov/pmc/articles/PMC4875377/

[100] https://www.ncbi.nlm.nih.gov/pmc/articles/PMC6035072/

[101] https://www.ncbi.nlm.nih.gov/pmc/articles/PMC3766524/

[102] https://www.ncbi.nlm.nih.gov/pmc/articles/PMC3959866/

[103] https://www.ncbi.nlm.nih.gov/pmc/articles/PMC3199852/

[104] https://www.ncbi.nlm.nih.gov/pmc/articles/PMC4124826/

[105] https://www.ncbi.nlm.nih.gov/pubmed/26740253

[106] http://dx.doi.org/10.1016/j.nut.2015.10.008

[107] https://phys.org/news/2016-06-unraveling-food-web-gut.html

[108] http://dx.doi.org/10.1038/nmicrobiol.2016.88

[109] https://www.ncbi.nlm.nih.gov/pmc/articles/PMC4829739/

[110] https://www.ncbi.nlm.nih.gov/pmc/articles/PMC2360254/

[111] https://chriskresser.com/rest-in-peace-china-study/

[112] https://deniseminger.com/2010/07/07/the-china-study-fact-or-fallac/

[113] http://freetheanimal.com/2010/07/t-colin-campbells-the-china-study-finally-exhaustively-discredited.html

[114] http://perfecthealthdiet.com/2010/07/the-china-study-evidence-for-the-perfect-health-diet/

[115] https://www.ncbi.nlm.nih.gov/pmc/articles/PMC1905232/

[116] https://www.ncbi.nlm.nih.gov/pmc/articles/PMC4728637/

[117] https://www.ncbi.nlm.nih.gov/pubmed/25412153

[118] https://www.ncbi.nlm.nih.gov/pubmed/22765297/

[119] http://www.dietandfitnesstoday.com/fruits-high-in-vitamin-b12.php

[120] https://goaskalice.columbia.edu/answered-questions/fruitarian-teens-are-they-stunting-their-growth

[121] https://www.ncbi.nlm.nih.gov/pmc/articles/PMC5657107/

122 https://www.ncbi.nlm.nih.gov/pmc/articles/PMC4829739/

123 https://www.ncbi.nlm.nih.gov/pmc/articles/PMC4829739/

124 https://www.cancer.net/blog/2014-04/foods-avoid-during-cancer-treatment

125 https://www.ncbi.nlm.nih.gov/pmc/articles/PMC4690201/

126 https://www.ncbi.nlm.nih.gov/pubmed/15531672/

127 https://www.ncbi.nlm.nih.gov/pmc/articles/PMC5093066/

128 https://www.ncbi.nlm.nih.gov/pmc/articles/PMC1118103/

129 https://www.ncbi.nlm.nih.gov/pmc/articles/PMC5655300/

130 https://www.ncbi.nlm.nih.gov/pubmed/22449736

131 https://www.ncbi.nlm.nih.gov/pmc/articles/PMC4937962/

132 https://www.ncbi.nlm.nih.gov/pmc/articles/PMC3933667/

133 https://www.ncbi.nlm.nih.gov/pmc/articles/PMC2715202/

134 https://nutritionfacts.org/2016/01/07/the-dietary-link-between-acne-and-cancer/

135 https://www.ncbi.nlm.nih.gov/pubmed/23975508

136 https://www.ncbi.nlm.nih.gov/pubmed/28956261

137 https://www.ncbi.nlm.nih.gov/pmc/articles/PMC3021092/

138 https://www.ncbi.nlm.nih.gov/pmc/articles/PMC3409927/

139 https://www.ncbi.nlm.nih.gov/pubmed/17975006

140 https://www.ncbi.nlm.nih.gov/pubmed/28366336

141 https://www.ncbi.nlm.nih.gov/pubmed/27611440

142 https://www.ncbi.nlm.nih.gov/pubmed/28417334

143 https://www.ncbi.nlm.nih.gov/pmc/articles/PMC4346497/

144 https://www.ncbi.nlm.nih.gov/pubmed/23395427

145 https://www.ncbi.nlm.nih.gov/pmc/articles/PMC1557490/

146 https://www.ncbi.nlm.nih.gov/pubmed/23007867/

147 https://www.ncbi.nlm.nih.gov/pmc/articles/PMC5924733/

148 https://www.ncbi.nlm.nih.gov/pubmed/15520194/

149 http://cancerres.aacrjournals.org/content/64/21/7879.long

150 https://www.ncbi.nlm.nih.gov/pmc/articles/PMC2831986/

151 https://www.ncbi.nlm.nih.gov/pmc/articles/PMC4449937/

152 https://www.ncbi.nlm.nih.gov/pmc/articles/PMC4681241/

153 https://justgetflux.com/

154 https://www.ncbi.nlm.nih.gov/pubmed/11560181

155 https://www.ncbi.nlm.nih.gov/pmc/articles/PMC3317043/

156 https://www.ncbi.nlm.nih.gov/pmc/articles/PMC4326238/

157 https://www.ncbi.nlm.nih.gov/pmc/articles/PMC3037818/

158 https://www.ncbi.nlm.nih.gov/pubmed/9741836/

159 https://www.ncbi.nlm.nih.gov/pubmed/1654166/

160 https://www.ncbi.nlm.nih.gov/pmc/articles/PMC4432778/

161 https://www.ncbi.nlm.nih.gov/pmc/articles/PMC4972115/

162 https://www.ncbi.nlm.nih.gov/pubmed/15914748/

163 https://www.ncbi.nlm.nih.gov/pubmed/18711185/

164 https://www.ncbi.nlm.nih.gov/pmc/articles/PMC5406418/

165 http://bit.ly/physicalactivityandcancer

166 https://www.mskcc.org/cancer-care/diagnosis-treatment/symptom-management/integrative-medicine/herbs

167 https://www.ncbi.nlm.nih.gov/pmc/articles/PMC4012169/

168 https://en.wikipedia.org/wiki/Beta-glucan

169 https://www.ncbi.nlm.nih.gov/pmc/articles/PMC3977804/

170 https://www.ncbi.nlm.nih.gov/pubmed/10477568/

171 https://www.ncbi.nlm.nih.gov/pmc/articles/PMC2685877/

[172] https://www.ncbi.nlm.nih.gov/pubmed/15240666/

[173] https://www.ncbi.nlm.nih.gov/pubmed/17895634

[174] https://www.ncbi.nlm.nih.gov/pmc/articles/PMC3202617/

[175] https://www.ncbi.nlm.nih.gov/pubmed/23140352

[176] https://nutritionj.biomedcentral.com/articles/10.1186/1475-2891-13-38

[177] https://www.ncbi.nlm.nih.gov/pubmed/16849475

[178] https://www.ncbi.nlm.nih.gov/pubmed/26092171

[179] https://www.ncbi.nlm.nih.gov/pmc/articles/PMC4231372/

[180] https://www.ncbi.nlm.nih.gov/pmc/articles/PMC5118454/

[181] https://www.EpiCorimmune.com/what-is-EpiCor/

[182] https://www.ncbi.nlm.nih.gov/pmc/articles/PMC4350453/

[183] https://www.ncbi.nlm.nih.gov/pmc/articles/PMC4209333/

[184] https://www.ncbi.nlm.nih.gov/pmc/articles/PMC3880197/

[185] https://www.ncbi.nlm.nih.gov/pmc/articles/PMC3157306/

[186] https://www.ncbi.nlm.nih.gov/pmc/articles/PMC5618583/

[187] https://www.ncbi.nlm.nih.gov/pmc/articles/PMC5118454/

[188] https://www.ncbi.nlm.nih.gov/pmc/articles/PMC3226611/

[189] https://www.ncbi.nlm.nih.gov/pubmed/28605319

[190] https://www.ncbi.nlm.nih.gov/pubmed/26559858

[191] https://www.ncbi.nlm.nih.gov/pmc/articles/PMC5973856/

[192] https://www.ncbi.nlm.nih.gov/pubmed/19048616

[193] https://www.ncbi.nlm.nih.gov/pmc/articles/PMC4491205/

[194] https://www.ncbi.nlm.nih.gov/pmc/articles/PMC4878560/

[195] https://www.nature.com/articles/nature21674.epdf

[196] https://www.ncbi.nlm.nih.gov/pubmed/19020714/

[197] By Nathan Wilson at Mushroom Observer, a source for mycological images, via Wikimedia Commons.

[198] https://www.ncbi.nlm.nih.gov/pmc/articles/PMC3730566/

[199] https://www.ncbi.nlm.nih.gov/pubmed/20130735

[200] https://www.ncbi.nlm.nih.gov/pubmed/19243740

[201] https://www.ncbi.nlm.nih.gov/pmc/articles/PMC3168293/

[202] https://www.ncbi.nlm.nih.gov/pmc/articles/PMC4946216/

[203] https://www.ncbi.nlm.nih.gov/pubmed/22135889

[204] https://www.ncbi.nlm.nih.gov/pmc/articles/PMC2895696/

[205] https://www.ncbi.nlm.nih.gov/pubmed/26210065

[206] https://www.ncbi.nlm.nih.gov/pubmed/18992843

[207] https://www.ncbi.nlm.nih.gov/pubmed/22135889

[208] https://www.ncbi.nlm.nih.gov/pubmed/25861415

[209] https://www.ncbi.nlm.nih.gov/pmc/articles/PMC4388940/

[210] https://www.ncbi.nlm.nih.gov/pubmed/19367670

[211] https://www.ncbi.nlm.nih.gov/pmc/articles/PMC2681140/

[212] https://www.ncbi.nlm.nih.gov/pubmed/23561137

[213] http://bit.ly/2zBPHxp

[214] http://koreascience.or.kr/article/ArticleFullRecord.jsp?cn=POCPA9_2013_v14n3_1571

[215] https://www.ncbi.nlm.nih.gov/pubmed/15630179

[216] https://www.ncbi.nlm.nih.gov/pmc/articles/PMC3430291/

[217] https://www.ncbi.nlm.nih.gov/pubmed/19041933

[218] https://www.ncbi.nlm.nih.gov/pubmed/23149251

[219] By natureluvr01 (Chaga) [CC BY 2.0 (https://creativecommons.org/licenses/by/2.0)], via Wikimedia Commons

[220] https://www.theguthealthprotocol.com/wp/chaga-tea-recipe/

[221] https://www.ncbi.nlm.nih.gov/pmc/articles/PMC4491205/

[222] https://www.ncbi.nlm.nih.gov/pmc/articles/PMC4878560/

[223] https://www.ncbi.nlm.nih.gov/pubmed/29253616

[224] https://www.ncbi.nlm.nih.gov/pubmed/24789042

[225] https://www.spandidos-publications.com/ijo/45/1/209

[226] https://www.ncbi.nlm.nih.gov/pubmed/20944118

[227] https://www.ncbi.nlm.nih.gov/pubmed/1597083

[228] https://www.ncbi.nlm.nih.gov/pubmed/10230862

[229] https://www.ncbi.nlm.nih.gov/pubmed/24762485

[230] https://www.ncbi.nlm.nih.gov/pmc/articles/PMC3909570/

[231] https://www.ncbi.nlm.nih.gov/pmc/articles/PMC4509066/

[232] https://www.ncbi.nlm.nih.gov/pubmed/19909827/

[233] https://www.ncbi.nlm.nih.gov/pubmed/16894961/

[234] https://www.ncbi.nlm.nih.gov/pubmed/16391863/

[235] https://www.ncbi.nlm.nih.gov/pmc/articles/PMC5141589/

[236] https://www.ncbi.nlm.nih.gov/pubmed/24274472

[237] https://www.ncbi.nlm.nih.gov/pubmed/19645242

[238] https://www.ncbi.nlm.nih.gov/pmc/articles/PMC4808884/

[239] By Henk Monster, CC BY 3.0, https://commons.wikimedia.org/w/index.php?curid=58676751

[240] http://bit.ly/2GVdHxT

[241] https://www.ncbi.nlm.nih.gov/pubmed/23668749

[242] https://www.ncbi.nlm.nih.gov/pubmed/21846141

[243] https://www.ncbi.nlm.nih.gov/pubmed/22624604

[244] https://www.ncbi.nlm.nih.gov/pubmed/24631140

[245] https://www.ncbi.nlm.nih.gov/pmc/articles/PMC4707368/

[246] https://www.ncbi.nlm.nih.gov/pubmed/20554107

[247] https://www.ncbi.nlm.nih.gov/pubmed/26547693

[248] https://www.ncbi.nlm.nih.gov/pubmed/29168863

[249] https://www.ncbi.nlm.nih.gov/pubmed/28266682

[250] https://www.ncbi.nlm.nih.gov/pubmed/14977447

[251] https://www.ncbi.nlm.nih.gov/pubmed/12126464

[252] https://www.ncbi.nlm.nih.gov/pubmed/9616756

[253] http://www.jhoonline.org/content/1/1/25

[254] http://www.jhoonline.org/content/1/1/25

[255] https://www.ncbi.nlm.nih.gov/pubmed/12499658

[256] http://bit.ly/2kNHTld

[257] https://www.ncbi.nlm.nih.gov/pubmed/19253021

[258] https://www.ncbi.nlm.nih.gov/pubmed/19477214

[259] https://www.ncbi.nlm.nih.gov/pubmed/28618133

[260] https://www.cancer.gov/types/brain/research/immunotherapy-glioblastoma

[261] https://www.ncbi.nlm.nih.gov/pubmed/25268766

[262] https://www.ncbi.nlm.nih.gov/pubmed/24228611

[263] https://www.ncbi.nlm.nih.gov/pubmed/21630638

[264] https://www.ncbi.nlm.nih.gov/pubmed/28981104

[265] https://www.ncbi.nlm.nih.gov/pubmed/15635158

[266] https://www.ncbi.nlm.nih.gov/pubmed/24001891

[267] https://www.ncbi.nlm.nih.gov/pubmed/15533593

[268] https://www.ncbi.nlm.nih.gov/pmc/articles/PMC3154178/

[269] https://www.ncbi.nlm.nih.gov/pmc/articles/PMC3907864/

[270] https://www.ncbi.nlm.nih.gov/pubmed/12117774/

[271] https://www.ncbi.nlm.nih.gov/pubmed/25827476

Updates at - https://improvingyourodds.com

Support at - https://www.facebook.com/groups/cancer.improving.your.odds

[272] https://www.ncbi.nlm.nih.gov/m/pubmed/28008810/

[273] https://www.ncbi.nlm.nih.gov/pubmed/24189312/

[274] https://www.ncbi.nlm.nih.gov/pubmed/19020765

[275] https://www.ncbi.nlm.nih.gov/pubmed/16822205

[276] https://www.ncbi.nlm.nih.gov/pubmed/9538185

[277] https://www.ncbi.nlm.nih.gov/pubmed/16413114

[278] https://www.ncbi.nlm.nih.gov/pubmed/17961926

[279] https://www.ncbi.nlm.nih.gov/pubmed/9130004

[280] https://www.ncbi.nlm.nih.gov/pubmed/22324408

[281] https://www.ncbi.nlm.nih.gov/pubmed/16782541

[282] https://www.ncbi.nlm.nih.gov/pubmed/25892617

[283] https://www.ncbi.nlm.nih.gov/pubmed/22234986

[284] http://www.breastcancer.org/tips/immune/cancer/chemo

[285] https://www.ncbi.nlm.nih.gov/pubmed/14713328

[286] https://www.ncbi.nlm.nih.gov/pmc/articles/PMC3585368/

[287] https://www.ncbi.nlm.nih.gov/pubmed/21888505/

[288] https://www.ncbi.nlm.nih.gov/pmc/articles/PMC3201987/

[289] https://www.ncbi.nlm.nih.gov/pmc/articles/PMC4735696/

[290] https://www.ncbi.nlm.nih.gov/pubmed/15525457

[291] https://www.ncbi.nlm.nih.gov/pubmed/12408995/

[292] https://www.ncbi.nlm.nih.gov/pubmed/28264501

[293] https://www.ncbi.nlm.nih.gov/pubmed/28427938

[294] https://www.ncbi.nlm.nih.gov/pmc/articles/PMC4206800/

[295] https://www.ncbi.nlm.nih.gov/pubmed/16566671

[296] https://www.ncbi.nlm.nih.gov/pmc/articles/PMC3664515/

[297] https://www.ncbi.nlm.nih.gov/pubmed/12470439

[298] https://www.ncbi.nlm.nih.gov/pmc/articles/PMC3339609/

[299] https://www.ncbi.nlm.nih.gov/pubmed/10190187

[300] https://www.ncbi.nlm.nih.gov/pubmed/25866155

[301] https://www.ncbi.nlm.nih.gov/pubmed/28845769

[302] https://www.ncbi.nlm.nih.gov/pubmed/18670743

[303] https://www.ncbi.nlm.nih.gov/pmc/articles/PMC2845472/

[304] https://www.ncbi.nlm.nih.gov/pmc/articles/PMC3369477/

[305] http://bit.ly/2udtO1Z

[306] https://www.ncbi.nlm.nih.gov/pubmed/18313195

[307] https://www.ncbi.nlm.nih.gov/pubmed/21603625/

[308] http://bit.ly/2JeYPr4

[309] https://www.ncbi.nlm.nih.gov/pubmed/21603625/

[310] https://www.ncbi.nlm.nih.gov/pmc/articles/PMC5592279/

[311] https://www.ncbi.nlm.nih.gov/pubmed/8008044

[312] https://www.ncbi.nlm.nih.gov/pubmed/7737599

[313] https://www.ncbi.nlm.nih.gov/pubmed/19005974

[314] https://www.ncbi.nlm.nih.gov/pubmed/17178902

[315] https://www.ncbi.nlm.nih.gov/pubmed/22217303

[316] https://www.ncbi.nlm.nih.gov/pubmed/11739882

[317] https://www.ncbi.nlm.nih.gov/pmc/articles/PMC2649035/

[318] https://academic.oup.com/jn/article/131/12/3288/4686305

[319] https://www.ncbi.nlm.nih.gov/pmc/articles/PMC3976240/

[320] https://mayocl.in/2B4FLe1

[321] https://www.ncbi.nlm.nih.gov/pmc/articles/PMC5327366/

---

[322] https://www.ncbi.nlm.nih.gov/pmc/articles/PMC3204293/

[323] https://www.ncbi.nlm.nih.gov/pubmed/10395237

[324] https://www.ncbi.nlm.nih.gov/pmc/articles/PMC3976240/

[325] https://www.ncbi.nlm.nih.gov/pmc/articles/PMC5464505/

[326] https://www.ncbi.nlm.nih.gov/pmc/articles/PMC3883964/

[327] https://www.ncbi.nlm.nih.gov/pmc/articles/PMC3204293/

[328] http://ourradioactiveocean.com/results.html

[329] https://www.ncbi.nlm.nih.gov/pmc/articles/PMC5637834/

[330] https://www.ncbi.nlm.nih.gov/pmc/articles/PMC4759402/

[331] https://www.ncbi.nlm.nih.gov/pmc/articles/PMC2902380/

[332] https://www.ncbi.nlm.nih.gov/pmc/articles/PMC4705892/

[333] https://www.ncbi.nlm.nih.gov/pmc/articles/PMC4443096/

[334] https://www.ncbi.nlm.nih.gov/pubmed/17114811/

[335] https://www.ncbi.nlm.nih.gov/pubmed/15621924/

[336] https://www.ncbi.nlm.nih.gov/pubmed/11819232

[337] https://www.ncbi.nlm.nih.gov/pmc/articles/PMC4767765/

[338] https://www.ncbi.nlm.nih.gov/pubmed/22980353

[339] https://www.ncbi.nlm.nih.gov/pmc/articles/PMC3705316/

[340] https://www.ncbi.nlm.nih.gov/pubmed/24683040

[341] https://www.ncbi.nlm.nih.gov/pubmed/19352569

[342] https://www.ncbi.nlm.nih.gov/pmc/articles/PMC3705340/

[343] https://www.ncbi.nlm.nih.gov/pmc/articles/PMC3705340/

[344] https://www.ncbi.nlm.nih.gov/pubmed/9634050/

[345] https://www.ncbi.nlm.nih.gov/pubmed/9315315

[346] http://bit.ly/2ueCvJr

[347] https://www.ncbi.nlm.nih.gov/pmc/articles/PMC4441528/

348 https://www.ncbi.nlm.nih.gov/pubmed/8971064

349 https://www.ncbi.nlm.nih.gov/pmc/articles/PMC4387950/

350 https://www.ncbi.nlm.nih.gov/pubmed/15476854/

351 https://www.ncbi.nlm.nih.gov/pubmed/21079797/

352 https://www.ncbi.nlm.nih.gov/pmc/articles/PMC4265016/

353 https://www.ncbi.nlm.nih.gov/pubmed/24239628

354 https://www.ncbi.nlm.nih.gov/pubmed/12757023

355 https://www.ncbi.nlm.nih.gov/pubmed/15134535

356 https://www.ncbi.nlm.nih.gov/pmc/articles/PMC4053099/

357 https://www.ncbi.nlm.nih.gov/pubmed/12452454

358 https://www.ncbi.nlm.nih.gov/pubmed/19124479

359 https://www.ncbi.nlm.nih.gov/pmc/articles/PMC4265016/

360 https://www.ncbi.nlm.nih.gov/pmc/articles/PMC3352977/

361 https://www.ncbi.nlm.nih.gov/pmc/articles/PMC4105469/

362 https://www.ncbi.nlm.nih.gov/pmc/articles/PMC4586774/

363 https://www.ncbi.nlm.nih.gov/pubmed/22377763/

364 https://www.ncbi.nlm.nih.gov/pmc/articles/PMC4265016/

365 https://www.ncbi.nlm.nih.gov/pubmed/12787812

366 https://www.ncbi.nlm.nih.gov/pubmedhealth/PMH0030452/

367 https://www.ncbi.nlm.nih.gov/pubmedhealth/PMH0030452/

368 https://onlinelibrary.wiley.com/doi/full/10.1002/ijc.25008

369 https://www.ncbi.nlm.nih.gov/pmc/articles/PMC3991754/

370 https://www.ncbi.nlm.nih.gov/pmc/articles/PMC4570783/

371 https://www.ncbi.nlm.nih.gov/pubmed/7647689

---

[372] https://www.ncbi.nlm.nih.gov/pmc/articles/PMC4570783/

[373] https://www.ncbi.nlm.nih.gov/pmc/articles/PMC3757421/

[374] https://www.ncbi.nlm.nih.gov/pmc/articles/PMC3757421/

[375] https://www.ncbi.nlm.nih.gov/pmc/articles/PMC5489781/

[376] https://www.ncbi.nlm.nih.gov/pmc/articles/PMC3742263/

[377] https://www.ncbi.nlm.nih.gov/pubmed/18302908

[378] https://www.ncbi.nlm.nih.gov/pmc/articles/PMC3850026/

[379] https://www.ncbi.nlm.nih.gov/pmc/articles/PMC4515619/

[380] https://www.ncbi.nlm.nih.gov/pubmed/28829668

[381] https://healthsupplementsnutritionalguide.com/recommended-daily-allowances/

[382] https://www.ncbi.nlm.nih.gov/pmc/articles/PMC3795437/

[383] https://www.ncbi.nlm.nih.gov/pubmed/20544289

[384] https://www.ncbi.nlm.nih.gov/pmc/articles/PMC3795437/

[385] https://www.ncbi.nlm.nih.gov/pubmed/20544289

[386] https://www.ncbi.nlm.nih.gov/pubmed/10746348

[387] https://www.ncbi.nlm.nih.gov/pubmed/10575908

[388] https://www.ncbi.nlm.nih.gov/pmc/articles/PMC2790187/

[389] https://www.ncbi.nlm.nih.gov/pubmed/20085565

[390] https://www.ncbi.nlm.nih.gov/pubmed/17063929

[391] https://www.ncbi.nlm.nih.gov/pmc/articles/PMC4059748/

[392] https://www.ncbi.nlm.nih.gov/pmc/articles/PMC2790187/

[393] https://www.ncbi.nlm.nih.gov/pmc/articles/PMC3082037/

[394] https://www.ncbi.nlm.nih.gov/pmc/articles/PMC3695824/

[395] https://www.ncbi.nlm.nih.gov/pubmed/25601965

[396] https://www.ncbi.nlm.nih.gov/pmc/articles/PMC4103214/

[397] https://www.ncbi.nlm.nih.gov/pubmed/18348443

[398] https://www.ncbi.nlm.nih.gov/pubmed/19269856/

[399] https://www.ncbi.nlm.nih.gov/pubmed/25882019

[400] https://www.ncbi.nlm.nih.gov/pubmed/16886659

[401] https://www.ncbi.nlm.nih.gov/pmc/articles/PMC4571149/

[402] https://www.ncbi.nlm.nih.gov/pmc/articles/PMC4572477/

[403] https://www.ncbi.nlm.nih.gov/pmc/articles/PMC3899831/

[404] https://www.ncbi.nlm.nih.gov/pmc/articles/PMC4572477/

[405] https://www.ncbi.nlm.nih.gov/pubmed/24402695

[406] https://www.ncbi.nlm.nih.gov/pubmed/25856702

[407] http://bit.ly/2mgeXzL

[408] https://www.ncbi.nlm.nih.gov/pmc/articles/PMC3897598/

[409] https://www.ncbi.nlm.nih.gov/pmc/articles/PMC5802611/

[410] https://www.ncbi.nlm.nih.gov/pmc/articles/PMC5713297/

[411] https://www.ncbi.nlm.nih.gov/pubmed/29374749

[412] https://www.ncbi.nlm.nih.gov/pmc/articles/PMC5938036/

[413] https://www.ncbi.nlm.nih.gov/pmc/articles/PMC4586774/

[414] https://www.ncbi.nlm.nih.gov/pmc/articles/PMC5351676/

[415] https://www.ncbi.nlm.nih.gov/pubmed/25437008/

[416] https://www.ncbi.nlm.nih.gov/pubmed/6257495/

[417] https://www.ncbi.nlm.nih.gov/pubmed/25813525/

[418] http://cancerpreventionresearch.aacrjournals.org/content/8/8/675.long

[419] https://www.ncbi.nlm.nih.gov/pubmed/21309673

[420] https://www.ncbi.nlm.nih.gov/pmc/articles/PMC4890569/

[421] https://www.ncbi.nlm.nih.gov/pubmed/23700865

[422] https://www.ncbi.nlm.nih.gov/pmc/articles/PMC5664083/

[423] https://www.ncbi.nlm.nih.gov/pmc/articles/PMC5802611/

[424] https://www.ncbi.nlm.nih.gov/pmc/articles/PMC5100621/

[425] https://www.ncbi.nlm.nih.gov/pmc/articles/PMC5713297/

[426] https://www.ncbi.nlm.nih.gov/pubmed/27632371

[427] http://bit.ly/2xngDg4

[428] https://www.vitamindcouncil.org/how-much-vitamin-d-is-needed-to-achieve-optimal-levels/

[429] https://www.ncbi.nlm.nih.gov/pubmed/18722618/

[430] https://www.ncbi.nlm.nih.gov/pmc/articles/PMC5683003/

[431] https://www.ncbi.nlm.nih.gov/pmc/articles/PMC3502042/

[432] https://www.ncbi.nlm.nih.gov/pmc/articles/PMC4365088/

[433] https://www.ncbi.nlm.nih.gov/pubmed/15769967

[434] https://www.ncbi.nlm.nih.gov/pubmed/27383327

[435] http://bit.ly/2KNYlxH

[436] https://www.ncbi.nlm.nih.gov/pmc/articles/PMC4586774/

[437] https://www.ncbi.nlm.nih.gov/pubmed/25316441

[438] https://www.ncbi.nlm.nih.gov/pubmed/11812968/

[439] https://gupea.ub.gu.se/handle/2077/55966

[440] https://www.nature.com/news/antioxidants-speed-cancer-in-mice-1.14606

[441] https://doi.org/10.1016/j.redox.2014.12.017

[442] https://doi.org/10.1016/S1382-6689(02)00003-0

[443] https://www.ncbi.nlm.nih.gov/pmc/articles/PMC2566998/

[444] https://www.ncbi.nlm.nih.gov/pubmed/24647393

[445] https://www.ncbi.nlm.nih.gov/pubmed/20335553

[446] https://www.ncbi.nlm.nih.gov/pmc/articles/PMC5958717/

[447] https://www.ncbi.nlm.nih.gov/pmc/articles/PMC3767046/

[448] https://www.ncbi.nlm.nih.gov/pubmed/26082424

[449] https://www.ncbi.nlm.nih.gov/pmc/articles/PMC4600246/

[450] https://www.ncbi.nlm.nih.gov/pubmed/11455981

[451] https://www.ncbi.nlm.nih.gov/pubmed/10482991

[452] https://www.ncbi.nlm.nih.gov/pmc/articles/PMC5593683/

[453] https://www.ncbi.nlm.nih.gov/pubmed/15586222

[454] https://www.ncbi.nlm.nih.gov/pmc/articles/PMC4600246/

[455] https://www.ncbi.nlm.nih.gov/pubmed/24089220

[456] https://www.ncbi.nlm.nih.gov/pubmed/29196151

[457] https://www.ncbi.nlm.nih.gov/pubmed/29429532

[458] https://www.ncbi.nlm.nih.gov/pmc/articles/PMC4808884/

[459] https://www.ncbi.nlm.nih.gov/pubmed/30156381

[460] https://www.ncbi.nlm.nih.gov/pubmed/24310501

[461] https://www.ncbi.nlm.nih.gov/pmc/articles/PMC5492086/

[462] https://www.ncbi.nlm.nih.gov/pubmed/12502387/

[463] https://www.ncbi.nlm.nih.gov/pubmed/20564502/

[464] https://www.ncbi.nlm.nih.gov/pmc/articles/PMC3641647/

[465] https://www.ncbi.nlm.nih.gov/pubmed/23890760

[466] https://www.ncbi.nlm.nih.gov/pubmed/28680383

[467] https://www.ncbi.nlm.nih.gov/pmc/articles/PMC6007476/

[468] https://www.ncbi.nlm.nih.gov/pubmed/24160296

[469] https://www.ncbi.nlm.nih.gov/pubmed/26224132

[470] https://www.ncbi.nlm.nih.gov/pmc/articles/PMC5669027/

[471] https://www.ncbi.nlm.nih.gov/pubmed/16109447/

Updates at - https://improvingyourodds.com

Support at - https://www.facebook.com/groups/cancer.improving.your.odds

472 https://www.ncbi.nlm.nih.gov/pmc/articles/PMC4443161/

473 https://www.ncbi.nlm.nih.gov/pmc/articles/PMC1379496/

474 https://www.ncbi.nlm.nih.gov/pubmed/18327874/

475 https://www.ncbi.nlm.nih.gov/pmc/articles/PMC5460521/

476 https://www.ncbi.nlm.nih.gov/pubmed/8877066/

477 https://www.ncbi.nlm.nih.gov/pmc/articles/PMC2874783/

478 https://www.ncbi.nlm.nih.gov/pubmed/23679237

479 http://cancerpreventionresearch.aacrjournals.org/content/11/8/451.long

480 https://www.ncbi.nlm.nih.gov/pubmed/21649489

481 https://www.ncbi.nlm.nih.gov/pubmed/24289589

482 https://www.ncbi.nlm.nih.gov/pmc/articles/PMC4354933/

483 https://www.ncbi.nlm.nih.gov/pubmed/28735362

484 https://www.ncbi.nlm.nih.gov/pmc/articles/PMC5099878/

485 https://www.ncbi.nlm.nih.gov/pubmed/23411305

486 https://www.ncbi.nlm.nih.gov/pmc/articles/PMC5808339/

487 https://www.ncbi.nlm.nih.gov/pubmed/12588699/

488 https://www.ncbi.nlm.nih.gov/pmc/articles/PMC4375225/

489 https://www.ncbi.nlm.nih.gov/pubmed/9500208

490 https://www.ncbi.nlm.nih.gov/pmc/articles/PMC4517353/

491 http://www.ams.ac.ir/AIM/NEWPUB/15/18/12/0011.pdf

492 https://www.ncbi.nlm.nih.gov/pubmed/17369232/

493 https://www.ncbi.nlm.nih.gov/pmc/articles/PMC5739168/

494 https://www.ncbi.nlm.nih.gov/pmc/articles/PMC3064404/

495 https://www.ncbi.nlm.nih.gov/pubmed/28956261

496 https://www.ncbi.nlm.nih.gov/pmc/articles/PMC5739168/

497 https://www.theguthealthprotocol.com/wp/kefir-instructions/

[498] https://www.ncbi.nlm.nih.gov/pmc/articles/PMC5669027/

[499] http://bit.ly/2zBqot5

[500] https://www.ncbi.nlm.nih.gov/pmc/articles/PMC5585139/

[501] https://www.ncbi.nlm.nih.gov/pubmed/28152473

[502] https://www.ncbi.nlm.nih.gov/pubmed/10231609

[503] https://www.ncbi.nlm.nih.gov/pubmed/2785214

[504] https://www.ncbi.nlm.nih.gov/pubmed/30471400

[505] https://www.ncbi.nlm.nih.gov/pubmed/8439987

[506] https://www.ncbi.nlm.nih.gov/pubmed/10231609

[507] https://www.ncbi.nlm.nih.gov/pmc/articles/PMC4888479/

[508] https://www.ncbi.nlm.nih.gov/pubmed/8310409/

[509] https://www.ncbi.nlm.nih.gov/pubmed/8076711/

[510] https://www.ncbi.nlm.nih.gov/pubmed/1315652

[511] https://www.ncbi.nlm.nih.gov/pmc/articles/PMC3534294/

[512] http://polarispharma.com/adi-peg-20/

[513] https://www.ncbi.nlm.nih.gov/pmc/articles/PMC4368604/

[514] https://www.ncbi.nlm.nih.gov/pmc/articles/PMC2782490/

[515] https://www.ncbi.nlm.nih.gov/pubmed/29769742

[516] https://www.ncbi.nlm.nih.gov/pubmed/30043669

[517] https://www.ncbi.nlm.nih.gov/pmc/articles/PMC2778124/

[518] https://www.ncbi.nlm.nih.gov/pmc/articles/PMC4662425/

[519] https://www.ncbi.nlm.nih.gov/pmc/articles/PMC3500452/

[520] https://www.ncbi.nlm.nih.gov/pmc/articles/PMC4870717/

[521] https://www.ncbi.nlm.nih.gov/pmc/articles/PMC4808858/

[522] https://www.ncbi.nlm.nih.gov/pmc/articles/PMC5776638/

[523] https://www.ncbi.nlm.nih.gov/pubmed/12442909

[524] https://www.ncbi.nlm.nih.gov/pmc/articles/PMC4773771/

[525] http://seafood.edf.org/

[526] https://www.ncbi.nlm.nih.gov/pmc/articles/PMC4418048/

[527] https://www.theguthealthprotocol.com/wp/5-minute-homemade-mayonnaise/

[528] http://www.lifeextension.com/Protocols/Cancer/Alternative-Cancer-Therapies/Page-07

[529] https://www.ncbi.nlm.nih.gov/pubmed/23919747

[530] https://www.ncbi.nlm.nih.gov/pubmed/27161216

[531] https://www.ncbi.nlm.nih.gov/pubmed/14628433

[532] https://www.ncbi.nlm.nih.gov/pmc/articles/PMC3671082/

[533] https://www.ncbi.nlm.nih.gov/pubmed/28714369

[534] https://www.ncbi.nlm.nih.gov/pubmed/20408878

[535] https://www.ncbi.nlm.nih.gov/pubmed/29039512

[536] https://www.ncbi.nlm.nih.gov/pubmed/26509161

[537] https://www.ncbi.nlm.nih.gov/pubmed/24921903

[538] https://www.ncbi.nlm.nih.gov/pmc/articles/PMC3671082/

[539] https://www.ncbi.nlm.nih.gov/pmc/articles/PMC5429338/

[540] https://link.springer.com/chapter/10.1007/978-3-319-15126-7_15

[541] https://www.ncbi.nlm.nih.gov/pmc/articles/PMC5840730/

[542] https://www.ncbi.nlm.nih.gov/pubmed/25395275

[543] https://www.ncbi.nlm.nih.gov/pmc/articles/PMC4486811/

[544] https://www.ncbi.nlm.nih.gov/pubmed/18296370

[545] https://www.ncbi.nlm.nih.gov/pmc/articles/PMC4560032/

[546] https://www.ncbi.nlm.nih.gov/pmc/articles/PMC5137221/

[547] https://www.ncbi.nlm.nih.gov/pubmed/9786231?dopt=Abstract

[548] https://www.ncbi.nlm.nih.gov/pmc/articles/PMC4121755/

[549] https://www.ncbi.nlm.nih.gov/pubmed/30979659

[550] https://www.ncbi.nlm.nih.gov/pmc/articles/PMC3738245/

[551] https://www.ncbi.nlm.nih.gov/pubmed/24847854

[552] https://www.ncbi.nlm.nih.gov/pubmed/11122711

[553] https://www.ncbi.nlm.nih.gov/pubmed/17125538/

[554] https://www.mskcc.org/cancer-care/diagnosis-treatment/symptom-management/integrative-medicine/herbs

[555] https://www.ncbi.nlm.nih.gov/pubmed/30027204

[556] https://www.ncbi.nlm.nih.gov/pubmed/25854386

[557] http://journal.waocp.org/journal/about

[558] https://www.ncbi.nlm.nih.gov/pubmed/20839215

[559] https://www.ncbi.nlm.nih.gov/pubmed/22343391/

[560] https://www.ncbi.nlm.nih.gov/pubmed/20932247/

[561] https://www.ncbi.nlm.nih.gov/pubmed/19941474/

[562] https://www.ncbi.nlm.nih.gov/pmc/articles/PMC5494088/

[563] http://dergipark.gov.tr/download/article-file/454178

[564] https://www.ncbi.nlm.nih.gov/pmc/articles/PMC3728063/

[565] https://www.wikihow.com/Extract-Aloe-Vera

[566] https://www.ncbi.nlm.nih.gov/pmc/articles/PMC5872176/

[567] https://www.ncbi.nlm.nih.gov/pubmed/18956140

[568] https://www.ncbi.nlm.nih.gov/pubmed/15330172

[569] https://www.ncbi.nlm.nih.gov/pubmed/16185154

[570] https://www.ncbi.nlm.nih.gov/pubmed/25579554

[571] https://www.ncbi.nlm.nih.gov/pubmed/26230090

[572] https://www.ncbi.nlm.nih.gov/pubmed/20840055

[573] https://www.ncbi.nlm.nih.gov/pubmed/17003952

[574] https://www.ncbi.nlm.nih.gov/pubmed/25368231

[575] https://www.ncbi.nlm.nih.gov/pubmed/23821767/

[576] https://www.ncbi.nlm.nih.gov/pmc/articles/PMC4867258/

[577] https://www.ncbi.nlm.nih.gov/pubmed/30685490

[578] https://www.ncbi.nlm.nih.gov/pmc/articles/PMC3214041/

[579] https://www.ncbi.nlm.nih.gov/pubmed/22182427

[580] https://www.ncbi.nlm.nih.gov/pmc/articles/PMC3573577/

[581] https://www.ncbi.nlm.nih.gov/pmc/articles/PMC4270108/

[582] https://www.ncbi.nlm.nih.gov/pmc/articles/PMC4689484/

[583] https://www.ncbi.nlm.nih.gov/pubmed/27731799

[584] https://www.ncbi.nlm.nih.gov/pmc/articles/PMC6426520/

[585] https://www.ncbi.nlm.nih.gov/pubmed/25544381

[586] https://www.ncbi.nlm.nih.gov/pmc/articles/PMC5535724/

[587] http://dx.doi.org/10.1038/aps.2016.125

[588] https://www.ncbi.nlm.nih.gov/pubmed/25212656

[589] https://www.ncbi.nlm.nih.gov/pubmed/21953764

[590] https://www.ncbi.nlm.nih.gov/pmc/articles/PMC5309756/

[591] https://www.ncbi.nlm.nih.gov/pmc/articles/PMC5839379/

[592] https://www.ncbi.nlm.nih.gov/pubmed/20843118

[593] https://www.ncbi.nlm.nih.gov/pubmed/12230008

[594] https://www.ncbi.nlm.nih.gov/pmc/articles/PMC5751158/

[595] https://www.ncbi.nlm.nih.gov/pmc/articles/PMC5067200/

[596] https://www.ncbi.nlm.nih.gov/pmc/articles/PMC5052360/

[597] https://www.ncbi.nlm.nih.gov/pmc/articles/PMC3252704

[598] https://www.ncbi.nlm.nih.gov/pmc/articles/PMC5466966/

[599] https://www.ncbi.nlm.nih.gov/pubmed/23583630

[600] https://www.ncbi.nlm.nih.gov/pmc/articles/PMC3258268/

[601] https://www.ncbi.nlm.nih.gov/pubmed/23237355

[602] https://www.ncbi.nlm.nih.gov/pubmed/17001517

[603] https://www.ncbi.nlm.nih.gov/pubmed/19737966

[604] https://www.ncbi.nlm.nih.gov/pmc/articles/PMC4142179/

[605] http://bit.ly/2P027BW

[606] https://www.ncbi.nlm.nih.gov/pmc/articles/PMC5739138/

[607] https://www.ncbi.nlm.nih.gov/pubmed/28549801

[608] https://www.ncbi.nlm.nih.gov/pubmed/29109091

[609] https://www.ncbi.nlm.nih.gov/pmc/articles/PMC2664784/

[610] https://www.ncbi.nlm.nih.gov/pmc/articles/PMC3246525/

[611] https://www.ncbi.nlm.nih.gov/pmc/articles/PMC4791148/

[612] https://www.ncbi.nlm.nih.gov/pubmed/12514108

[613] https://www.ncbi.nlm.nih.gov/pubmed/15313899

[614] https://www.ncbi.nlm.nih.gov/pubmed/20053780

[615] https://www.ncbi.nlm.nih.gov/pmc/articles/PMC5928848/

[616] https://www.ncbi.nlm.nih.gov/pmc/articles/PMC5852356/

[617] https://www.ncbi.nlm.nih.gov/pubmed/18199524

[618] https://www.ncbi.nlm.nih.gov/pubmed/19589225

[619] https://www.ncbi.nlm.nih.gov/pubmed/12182964

[620] https://www.ncbi.nlm.nih.gov/pmc/articles/PMC1576089/

[621] https://www.ncbi.nlm.nih.gov/pubmed/9771884

[622] https://www.ncbi.nlm.nih.gov/pmc/articles/PMC2673842/

[623] https://www.ncbi.nlm.nih.gov/pubmed/19480992

[624] https://www.ncbi.nlm.nih.gov/pubmed/14640910

[625] https://www.ncbi.nlm.nih.gov/pubmed/12958205

[626] http://cancerres.aacrjournals.org/content/67/9_Supplement/4749

[627] https://www.ncbi.nlm.nih.gov/pubmed/15026328/

[628] https://www.ncbi.nlm.nih.gov/pubmed/15749859/

[629] https://www.ncbi.nlm.nih.gov/pubmed/10861074/

[630] http://www.jimmunol.org/content/165/1/373.long

[631] https://www.ncbi.nlm.nih.gov/pmc/articles/PMC4791144/

[632] https://www.ncbi.nlm.nih.gov/pubmed/18199524

[633] https://www.ncbi.nlm.nih.gov/pubmed/29482741

[634] https://www.ncbi.nlm.nih.gov/pmc/articles/PMC5961457/

[635] https://www.ncbi.nlm.nih.gov/pmc/articles/PMC5879974/

[636] https://www.wthr.com/article/dea-feds-wont-arrest-cbd-oil-users-neither-should-indiana

[637] https://www.ncbi.nlm.nih.gov/pmc/articles/PMC5176373/

[638] https://www.ncbi.nlm.nih.gov/pubmed/29352974

[639] https://www.ncbi.nlm.nih.gov/pubmed/20811719

[640] https://www.ncbi.nlm.nih.gov/pmc/articles/PMC5228444/

[641] https://www.ncbi.nlm.nih.gov/pmc/articles/PMC5492241/

[642] https://www.ncbi.nlm.nih.gov/pmc/articles/PMC4488098/

[643] https://www.ncbi.nlm.nih.gov/pubmed/19203831

[644] https://www.ncbi.nlm.nih.gov/pmc/articles/PMC2920880/

[645] https://www.ncbi.nlm.nih.gov/pubmed/27253180

[646] https://www.ncbi.nlm.nih.gov/pmc/articles/PMC2901047/

[647] https://www.ncbi.nlm.nih.gov/pmc/articles/PMC3105590/

[648] http://bit.ly/2JfAXDN

[649] https://www.ncbi.nlm.nih.gov/pubmed/19203831

[650] https://www.ncbi.nlm.nih.gov/pmc/articles/PMC2893107/

[651] https://www.ncbi.nlm.nih.gov/pubmed/12860272

[652] https://www.ncbi.nlm.nih.gov/pubmed/26677144

[653] https://www.ncbi.nlm.nih.gov/pubmed/26677144

[654] https://www.ncbi.nlm.nih.gov/pubmed/20653974

[655] https://www.ncbi.nlm.nih.gov/pmc/articles/PMC4466762/

[656] https://www.ncbi.nlm.nih.gov/pubmed/15353028

[657] https://www.ncbi.nlm.nih.gov/pubmed/17640165

[658] https://www.ncbi.nlm.nih.gov/pmc/articles/PMC4413214/

[659] https://www.ncbi.nlm.nih.gov/pubmed/12929574

[660] https://www.ncbi.nlm.nih.gov/pubmed/19754176/

[661] https://www.ncbi.nlm.nih.gov/pubmed/16201850

[662] https://www.ncbi.nlm.nih.gov/pubmed/12504793

[663] https://www.ncbi.nlm.nih.gov/pubmed/18239813

[664] https://journals.plos.org/plosone/article?id=10.1371/journal.pone.0027441

[665] https://onlinelibrary.wiley.com/doi/full/10.1111/j.1750-3841.2011.02099.x

[666] https://www.ncbi.nlm.nih.gov/pmc/articles/PMC6266495/

[667] https://www.ncbi.nlm.nih.gov/pubmed/22866084

[668] https://www.ncbi.nlm.nih.gov/pmc/articles/PMC4061164/

[669] https://www.ncbi.nlm.nih.gov/pubmed/28627320

[670] https://www.ncbi.nlm.nih.gov/pmc/articles/PMC5408268/

[671] https://www.ncbi.nlm.nih.gov/pmc/articles/PMC4103721/

---

672 https://www.ncbi.nlm.nih.gov/pmc/articles/PMC3499657/

673 https://www.cancer.gov/about-cancer/causes-prevention/risk/diet/garlic-fact-sheet

674 https://www.ncbi.nlm.nih.gov/pmc/articles/PMC4366009/

675 https://www.ncbi.nlm.nih.gov/pmc/articles/PMC3924985/

676 https://www.ncbi.nlm.nih.gov/pmc/articles/PMC3915757/

677 https://www.ncbi.nlm.nih.gov/pmc/articles/PMC4873399/

678 https://www.ncbi.nlm.nih.gov/pmc/articles/PMC3463925/

679 https://www.ncbi.nlm.nih.gov/pubmed/16484577

680 https://www.ncbi.nlm.nih.gov/pmc/articles/PMC2727784/

681 https://www.ncbi.nlm.nih.gov/pmc/articles/PMC4808884/

682 http://cebp.aacrjournals.org/content/25/4/624.long

683 https://www.ncbi.nlm.nih.gov/pubmed/24362328/

684 https://www.ncbi.nlm.nih.gov/pmc/articles/PMC3915757/

685 https://www.ncbi.nlm.nih.gov/pubmed/21269259

686 https://www.ncbi.nlm.nih.gov/pmc/articles/PMC3463925/

687 https://www.ncbi.nlm.nih.gov/pmc/articles/PMC4881189/

688 https://www.ncbi.nlm.nih.gov/pmc/articles/PMC4753037/

689 https://www.ncbi.nlm.nih.gov/pmc/articles/PMC3594460/

690 https://www.ncbi.nlm.nih.gov/pmc/articles/PMC5946235/

691 https://www.ncbi.nlm.nih.gov/pubmed/11238815

692 https://pubs.acs.org/doi/abs/10.1021/jf00057a004

693 http://bit.ly/2Ajb7O0

694 https://www.ncbi.nlm.nih.gov/pmc/articles/PMC5527238/

695 https://www.ncbi.nlm.nih.gov/pmc/articles/PMC2664283/

696 https://www.ncbi.nlm.nih.gov/pmc/articles/PMC4427290/

697 https://www.ncbi.nlm.nih.gov/pmc/articles/PMC4369959/

[698] https://www.ncbi.nlm.nih.gov/pmc/articles/PMC3426621/

[699] https://www.ncbi.nlm.nih.gov/pmc/articles/PMC4808884/

[700] https://www.ncbi.nlm.nih.gov/pmc/articles/PMC3925258/

[701] https://www.ncbi.nlm.nih.gov/pmc/articles/PMC4106649/

[702] https://www.ncbi.nlm.nih.gov/pubmed/21792901

[703] https://www.ncbi.nlm.nih.gov/pmc/articles/PMC4217504/

[704] https://www.ncbi.nlm.nih.gov/pubmed/16740737

[705] https://www.ncbi.nlm.nih.gov/pmc/articles/PMC2760842/

[706] https://www.ncbi.nlm.nih.gov/pmc/articles/PMC2728696/

[707] https://www.ncbi.nlm.nih.gov/pmc/articles/PMC2597484/

[708] https://www.ncbi.nlm.nih.gov/pmc/articles/PMC5775207/

[709] https://www.ncbi.nlm.nih.gov/pmc/articles/PMC4393634/

[710] https://www.ncbi.nlm.nih.gov/pmc/articles/PMC3509513/

[711] https://www.ncbi.nlm.nih.gov/pmc/articles/PMC3590855/

[712] https://www.ncbi.nlm.nih.gov/pmc/articles/PMC5824026/

[713] https://www.bbc.com/news/stories-45971416

[714] https://www.ncbi.nlm.nih.gov/pubmed/12657101/

[715] https://www.ncbi.nlm.nih.gov/pubmed/23725121/

[716] https://www.ncbi.nlm.nih.gov/pubmed/20811719

[717] https://www.ncbi.nlm.nih.gov/pmc/articles/PMC5456322/

[718] https://www.ncbi.nlm.nih.gov/pmc/articles/PMC2693740/

[719] https://www.ncbi.nlm.nih.gov/pmc/articles/PMC4477227/

[720] https://www.ncbi.nlm.nih.gov/pubmed/24557876

[721] https://www.ncbi.nlm.nih.gov/pmc/articles/PMC4396237/

[722] https://www.ncbi.nlm.nih.gov/pubmed/17044765

[723] https://www.ncbi.nlm.nih.gov/pubmed/9244360

[724] https://www.ncbi.nlm.nih.gov/pubmed/14608114

[725] https://www.ncbi.nlm.nih.gov/pubmed/14666663

[726] https://www.ncbi.nlm.nih.gov/pubmed/14666664

[727] https://www.ncbi.nlm.nih.gov/pubmed/17044765

[728] https://www.ncbi.nlm.nih.gov/pubmed/16949716

[729] https://www.ncbi.nlm.nih.gov/pubmed/19317806

[730] https://www.ncbi.nlm.nih.gov/pubmed/25242120

[731] https://www.ncbi.nlm.nih.gov/pmc/articles/PMC3586829/

[732] https://www.ncbi.nlm.nih.gov/pubmed/25174976

[733] https://www.ncbi.nlm.nih.gov/pubmed/17548792

[734] https://www.ncbi.nlm.nih.gov/pmc/articles/PMC3586829/

[735] https://www.ncbi.nlm.nih.gov/pmc/articles/PMC2787788/

[736] https://www.ncbi.nlm.nih.gov/pubmed/29248134

[737] https://www.ncbi.nlm.nih.gov/pubmed/23513466

[738] https://www.ncbi.nlm.nih.gov/pubmed/26446958

[739] https://www.ncbi.nlm.nih.gov/pubmed/24477002

[740] https://www.ncbi.nlm.nih.gov/pmc/articles/PMC4670692/

[741] https://www.ncbi.nlm.nih.gov/pubmed/18505970/

[742] https://www.ncbi.nlm.nih.gov/pmc/articles/PMC2778172/

[743] https://www.ncbi.nlm.nih.gov/pmc/articles/PMC4734358/

[744] https://www.ncbi.nlm.nih.gov/pubmed/17961770

[745] https://www.ncbi.nlm.nih.gov/pubmed/21560017

[746] https://www.ncbi.nlm.nih.gov/pmc/articles/PMC4791507/

[747] https://www.ncbi.nlm.nih.gov/pmc/articles/PMC6321405/

[748] https://www.ncbi.nlm.nih.gov/pubmed/15037213

[749] https://www.ncbi.nlm.nih.gov/pubmed/16634526

[750] https://www.ncbi.nlm.nih.gov/pmc/articles/PMC2935742/

[751] https://www.ncbi.nlm.nih.gov/pmc/articles/PMC3997986/

[752] https://www.ncbi.nlm.nih.gov/pubmed/25560707/

[753] https://www.ncbi.nlm.nih.gov/pmc/articles/PMC4997426/

[754] https://www.ncbi.nlm.nih.gov/pmc/articles/PMC3002804/

[755] https://www.ncbi.nlm.nih.gov/pubmed/20568104

[756] https://www.ncbi.nlm.nih.gov/pmc/articles/PMC5751192/

[757] https://www.ncbi.nlm.nih.gov/pmc/articles/PMC4827609/

[758] https://amzn.to/2kYN7uL

[759] https://www.ncbi.nlm.nih.gov/pmc/articles/PMC5551348/

[760] https://www.ncbi.nlm.nih.gov/pmc/articles/PMC4808884/

[761] https://www.ncbi.nlm.nih.gov/pmc/articles/PMC4997408/

[762] https://creativecommons.org/licenses/by/4.0/

[763] https://www.ncbi.nlm.nih.gov/pmc/articles/PMC2756684/

[764] https://www.ncbi.nlm.nih.gov/pubmed/22045655

[765] https://www.ncbi.nlm.nih.gov/pubmed/25260874/

[766] https://www.ncbi.nlm.nih.gov/pubmed/27325106

[767] http://journals.sagepub.com/doi/pdf/10.1177/2211068216655524

[768] https://www.ncbi.nlm.nih.gov/pubmed/25553436

[769] https://www.ncbi.nlm.nih.gov/pubmed/29189128

[770] https://www.ncbi.nlm.nih.gov/pubmed/27280688

[771] https://www.ncbi.nlm.nih.gov/pubmed/28167449

[772] http://bit.ly/2KQg5c0

[773] https://www.ncbi.nlm.nih.gov/pubmed/25308211/

[774] https://www.ncbi.nlm.nih.gov/pmc/articles/PMC2834485/

[775] https://www.ncbi.nlm.nih.gov/pmc/articles/PMC4829106/

[776] https://www.sciencedirect.com/science/article/pii/S1044579X17300366

[777] https://www.ncbi.nlm.nih.gov/pmc/articles/PMC3722989/

[778] https://www.ncbi.nlm.nih.gov/pubmed/10362108/

[779] https://www.ncbi.nlm.nih.gov/pmc/articles/PMC4094835/

[780] https://www.ncbi.nlm.nih.gov/pmc/articles/PMC4094835/

[781] https://www.ncbi.nlm.nih.gov/pmc/articles/PMC5074768/

[782] https://www.ncbi.nlm.nih.gov/pmc/articles/PMC3872072/

[783] https://www.longdom.org/open-access/buffer-therapy-for-cancer-2155-9600.S2-006.pdf

[784] https://doi.org/10.4172/2155-9600.1000685

[785] https://www.ncbi.nlm.nih.gov/pmc/articles/PMC6266022/

[786] https://www.webmd.com/drugs/2/drug-11325/sodium-bicarbonate-oral/details

[787] https://www.ncbi.nlm.nih.gov/pubmed/20191307

[788] https://www.ncbi.nlm.nih.gov/pmc/articles/PMC4164354/

[789] https://www.ncbi.nlm.nih.gov/pmc/articles/PMC5894671/

[790] https://www.ncbi.nlm.nih.gov/pubmed/18072821

[791] https://www.ncbi.nlm.nih.gov/pmc/articles/PMC6262896/

[792] https://www.ncbi.nlm.nih.gov/pmc/articles/PMC5712166/

[793] https://www.ncbi.nlm.nih.gov/pubmed/20582906

[794] https://www.ncbi.nlm.nih.gov/pmc/articles/PMC3929544/

[795] https://www.ncbi.nlm.nih.gov/pmc/articles/PMC5989150/

[796] https://www.ncbi.nlm.nih.gov/pubmed/30464341

[797] https://www.ncbi.nlm.nih.gov/pmc/articles/PMC5503661/

[798] https://www.ncbi.nlm.nih.gov/pubmed/19124483/

[799] http://www.mdpi.com/1422-0067/17/5/621/htm

[800] https://www.ncbi.nlm.nih.gov/pmc/articles/PMC1317110/

[801] https://www.ncbi.nlm.nih.gov/pubmed/30618091

[802] https://www.ncbi.nlm.nih.gov/pubmed/12396291/

[803] https://www.ncbi.nlm.nih.gov/pubmed/11333131

[804] https://www.ncbi.nlm.nih.gov/pubmed/28978121

[805] https://www.ncbi.nlm.nih.gov/pubmed/25168391

[806] https://www.ncbi.nlm.nih.gov/pubmed/15009512

[807] https://www.ncbi.nlm.nih.gov/pmc/articles/PMC4457700/

[808] https://www.ncbi.nlm.nih.gov/pmc/articles/PMC3552359/

[809] https://www.ncbi.nlm.nih.gov/pubmed/10674014

[810] https://www.ncbi.nlm.nih.gov/pmc/articles/PMC3317666/

[811] https://www.ncbi.nlm.nih.gov/pubmed/30339981

[812] https://www.ncbi.nlm.nih.gov/pmc/articles/PMC4633041/

[813] https://www.ncbi.nlm.nih.gov/pmc/articles/PMC3934636/

[814] https://www.ncbi.nlm.nih.gov/pmc/articles/PMC4378141/

[815] https://www.ncbi.nlm.nih.gov/pmc/articles/PMC5086580/

[816] https://www.ncbi.nlm.nih.gov/pmc/articles/PMC4828642/

[817] https://www.superfoodly.com/quercetin-foods/

[818] https://www.ncbi.nlm.nih.gov/pmc/articles/PMC3371140/

[819] https://www.ncbi.nlm.nih.gov/pmc/articles/PMC4997662/

[820] https://www.ncbi.nlm.nih.gov/pmc/articles/PMC5209628/

[821] https://www.ncbi.nlm.nih.gov/pubmed/9207950

822 https://www.ncbi.nlm.nih.gov/pubmed/10440304

823 https://www.ncbi.nlm.nih.gov/pubmed/11835443

824 https://www.ncbi.nlm.nih.gov/pmc/articles/PMC3312275/

825 https://www.theguthealthprotocol.com/wp/nature-detoxifies-mercury-gut/

826 https://www.ncbi.nlm.nih.gov/pubmed/16312043/

827 https://www.ncbi.nlm.nih.gov/pubmed/21115894/

828 https://www.ncbi.nlm.nih.gov/pubmed/19787219/

829 https://doi.org/10.3892/or_00000534

830 https://www.ncbi.nlm.nih.gov/pubmed/19465788/

831 https://www.ncbi.nlm.nih.gov/pubmed/15172118/

832 https://www.ncbi.nlm.nih.gov/pmc/articles/PMC2712688/

833 https://www.ncbi.nlm.nih.gov/pmc/articles/PMC5374952/

834 https://www.ncbi.nlm.nih.gov/pmc/articles/PMC3673985/

835 https://www.ncbi.nlm.nih.gov/pmc/articles/PMC4745411/

836 https://doi.org/10.1016/j.jphotobiol.2015.12.014

837 https://www.ncbi.nlm.nih.gov/pmc/articles/PMC2539004/

838 http://bit.ly/2L6tpsa

839 https://www.ncbi.nlm.nih.gov/pmc/articles/PMC2718593/

840 https://www.ncbi.nlm.nih.gov/pmc/articles/PMC5459322/

841 https://www.ncbi.nlm.nih.gov/pubmed/20345484

842 https://www.ncbi.nlm.nih.gov/pubmed/22515193

843 http://bit.ly/2NK8CZz

844 https://www.ncbi.nlm.nih.gov/pubmed/26622761

845 https://www.ncbi.nlm.nih.gov/pubmed/11950096

846 https://www.ncbi.nlm.nih.gov/pmc/articles/PMC4745411/

847 https://doi.org/10.1016/j.jphotobiol.2015.12.014

[848] https://www.ncbi.nlm.nih.gov/pubmed/10944614

[849] https://www.ncbi.nlm.nih.gov/pubmed/11055621

[850] https://www.ncbi.nlm.nih.gov/pubmed/20877339

[851] https://www.ncbi.nlm.nih.gov/pubmed/9583414

[852] https://www.ncbi.nlm.nih.gov/pmc/articles/PMC3106435/

[853] http://www.scirp.org/journal/PaperDownload.aspx?paperID=37056

[854] https://www.ncbi.nlm.nih.gov/pmc/articles/PMC4632793/

[855] https://www.ncbi.nlm.nih.gov/pmc/articles/PMC3312702/

[856] https://www.sciencedirect.com/science/article/abs/pii/0006295280905043

[857] https://www.ncbi.nlm.nih.gov/pubmed/3089225/

[858] https://www.accessdata.fda.gov/scripts/plantox/detail.cfm?id=5342

[859] https://www.cochranelibrary.com/cdsr/doi/10.1002/14651858.CD005476.pub3/full

[860] https://jamanetwork.com/journals/jama/article-abstract/1722420

[861] https://www.nejm.org/doi/10.1056/NEJM198201283060403

[862] https://www.nejm.org/doi/10.1056/NEJM198201283060403

[863] https://www.ncbi.nlm.nih.gov/books/NBK65988/

[864] https://www.ncbi.nlm.nih.gov/pubmed/25918920/

[865] https://www.ncbi.nlm.nih.gov/pubmed/17106659/

[866] https://www.ncbi.nlm.nih.gov/pubmed/24456237

[867] https://www.ncbi.nlm.nih.gov/pubmed/24467586

[868] https://www.theguthealthprotocol.com/wp/chaga-tea-recipe/

[869] https://pubs.niaaa.nih.gov/publications/arh25-4/263-270.htm

[870] http://amzn.to/2f5RRec

[871] http://bit.ly/phagecomplete

Updates at - https://improvingyourodds.com

Support at - https://www.facebook.com/groups/cancer.improving.your.odds

[872] https://medical-dictionary.thefreedictionary.com/

[873] https://www.merriam-webster.com/medical

[874] https://medical-dictionary.com/

[875] https://www.medilexicon.com/dictionary

[876] https://academic.oup.com/carcin/article/28/2/233/2476711

[877] https://www.mayoclinic.org/diseases-conditions/glioblastoma/cdc-20350148

[879] https://en.wikipedia.org/wiki/Cancer_staging

[880] http://amzn.to/2f5RRec

[881] http://bit.ly/phagecomplete

Printed in Great Britain
by Amazon

24415209R00302